Psychiatric
Words and Phrases

Second Edition

by

Mary Ann D'Onofrio, CMT, AMLS

and

Elizabeth D'Onofrio, BFA

Health Professions Institute • Modesto, California • 1998

Psychiatric Words and Phrases
Second Edition

by Mary Ann D'Onofrio, CMT, AMLS
and Elizabeth D'Onofrio, BFA

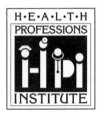

Sally Crenshaw Pitman
Editor & Publisher
Health Professions Institute
P. O. Box 801
Modesto, CA 95353-0801
Phone 209-551-2112
Fax 209-551-0404
E-mail: hpi@ainet.com
Web site: http://www.hpisum.com

Printed by
Parks Printing & Lithography
Modesto, California

ISBN 0-934385-70-X

Last digit is the print number: 9 8 7 6 5 4 3 2

In loving memory of

Dominic,

beloved husband and father

Acknowledgments

We are grateful to Beverly Ormsbee, CMT, Marti Rovan, and Nikki Briere, CMT, for their contributions of psychiatric words and phrases; to Diane Durand for her lists of phobias; and to Carolanne Overshiner for her contribution of words and phrases regarding neurolinguistics. We appreciate the encouragement and patience that Sally C. Pitman, MA, Linda Campbell, CMT, and the staff of Health Professions Institute have shown us as we brought this project to its conclusion. Thank you all.

Mary Ann D'Onofrio, CMT, AMLS
Elizabeth D'Onofrio, BFA

Contents

Preface

For *Psychiatric Words and Phrases*, Second Edition, we have expanded our primary source material. While still garnering words and phrases from actual transcripts of psychiatric admissions and discharges, psychiatric social histories and therapy notes, we have culled many terms from the new DSM-IV, revisions of the ICD-9-CM, as well as dictionaries, and current journals in psychiatry and psychopharmacology.

Continuing to feature and update our lists of street names of drugs, we also include in the body of the text many street terms currently in use. The updated list of drugs by their street name and chemical name is found under the main entry "drugs, street." These street drug terms are also listed under the main entry for each substance, e.g., amobarbital, amphetamine, and cannabis.

The list of phobias has been expanded, although surely not complete to everyone's satisfaction. These are listed under both "phobia" and "fear of" in the main text.

The DSM-IV lists learning disorders and mental retardation as part of the AXIS II criteria. We have, therefore, expanded the terms for the communication disorders (speech, language, and hearing) in this second edition of *Psychiatric Words and Phrases*. Professionals in the area of neurolinguistics who work closely with psychologists and psychiatrists may also find this book useful.

We have included two appendices to make this book more valuable to paraprofessionals in the fields of psychiatry, psychology, and neurolinguistics. Appendix I contains the multiaxial criteria of the DSM-IV as well as sample reports for illustrating the acceptable form for reporting that criteria. Appendix II lists muscles of the larynx, palate, pharynx, respiration and tongue—all involved in the speech process.

How to Use This Book

The words and phrases in this book are alphabetized letter by letter of all words in the entry, ignoring punctuation marks and words or letters in parentheses. The possessive form ('s) is often omitted from eponyms and ignored when present for ease in alphabetizing. Numbers are alphabetized as if written out, with the exception of subscripts and superscripts which are ignored.

Diagnostic tests may be located alphabetically as well as under the main entry *test*. The quick-reference list of over two thousand tests includes various alternative and related terms, such as *analysis, appraisal, assessment, battery, checklist, evaluation, examination, index, indicator, interview, inventory, measurement, profile, scale, score, screen*, and *survey*.

A, a

"A," "A's" (amphetamine sulfate)
AA (Academic Alertness)
AA (achievement age)
AA (Alcoholics Anonymous)
AAA (acute anxiety attack)
AABT (Association for Advancement of Behavior Therapy)
AACAP (American Academy of Child and Adolescent Psychiatry)
AACDP (American Association of Chairmen of Departments of Psychiatry)
AADPRT (American Association of Directors of Psychiatric Residency Training)
AAF (altered auditory feedback)
AAFP (American Academy of Family Physicians)
AAGP (American Association for Geriatric Psychiatry)
AAGT (Association for the Advancement of Gestalt Therapy)
AAMD (American Association on Mental Deficiency) Adaptive Behavior Scale, School Edition
AAMFT (American Association for Marriage and Family Therapy)

AAO (awake, alert, and oriented)
AAP (American Academy of Pediatrics)
AAP (Association of Academic Psychiatry)
AAPA (American Association of Psychiatric Administrators)
AAPAA (American Academy of Psychiatrists in Alcoholism and Addictions)
AAPL (American Academy of Psychiatry and the Law)
AAPS (Arizona Articulation Proficiency Scale)
AAT (Academic Aptitude Test)
abalienate
abalienatio mentis
abalienation
abandoner
abandonment
    fear of
    imagined
    perceived emotional
    real
abandonment concerns
Abbreviated Conners Rating Scale

1

Abbreviated Conners Teacher
Questionnaire
ABC (Aberrant Behavior Checklist)
ABC (Assessment of Basic Com-
petencies)
ABC Inventory—Extended
ABCD (The Arizona Battery for
Communication Disorders of
Dementia)
abdominal-diaphragmatic respiration
abducens (cranial nerve VI)
abducent
abductor paralysis
  bilateral
  unilateral
"Abe" (re: drug value)
"Abe's cabe" (re: currency)
aberrant behavior
Aberrant Behavior Checklist (ABC)
aberrant gene
aberration, mental
ABES (Adaptive Behavior Evaluation Scale)
ABFP (American Board of Family
Practice)
ABIC (Adaptive Behavior Inventory
for Children)
abilities (see *ability)*
abilities test (see *test*)
ability (pl. abilities*)*
  abstracting
  abstractive
  attention shift
  attentional
  auditory
  cognitive
  communication
  conceptual
  concrete
  constructional
  coping
  disturbance in perceptual motor

ability *(cont.)*
  disturbance in word-finding
  drawing
  focal
  general learning (G)
  impaired
  intellectual
  language
  learning
  mathematical
  memory
  mental
  nonverbal abstractive
  nonverbal synthesizing
  oral sensory
  perceptual
  perceptual motor
  positive
  premorbid
  reality testing (Rorschach)
  reduced attention
  spatial
  thinking
  writing
ability battery (see *test*)
ability test (see *test*)
Ability-to-Benefit Admissions Test
ability to take criticism
ABLB (Alternate Binaural Loudness
Balance) test
ABLE (Adult Basic Learning
Examination)
ablutomania
abnormal asymmetry
abnormal development
abnormal EEG tracing
abnormal involuntary movement
disorder (AIMD)
abnormal involuntary movement
scale (AIMS)
abnormalities in sleep-wake timing
mechanisms

abnormalities of affect
abnormality (pl. abnormalities)
  brain
  cranial nerve
  electrolyte
  eye movement
  food intake
  gait
  inherited
  laboratory
  lateralizing
  metabolic
  performance
  polysomnographic
  sleep
  sleep-wake
  structural brain
  vocal pitch
abnormal mood
abnormal movements
abnormal pathologic condition
abnormal perceptions
abnormal positioning of distal limbs
abnormal psychology
abnormal responsiveness
abnormal sleep-wake schedule
abnormal stoppage of sound
abolic (veterinary steroid)
abortion
above-average intelligence
ABPN (American Board of
  Psychiatry and Neurology)
ABR (auditory brainstem response)
ABR audiometry
abreaction, hypnotic
abrupt onset
abrupt topic shift
ABS (Adaptive Behavior Scale)
abscond
absence epilepsy
absence episode
absence of feeling

absence seizure
  atonic
  atypical
absence status
absence syndrome
absenteeism
absentia
absentia epileptica
absent without leave (AWOL)
absinthe addiction or dependence
absolute agraphia
absolute construction of phrases
absolute quantity
absolute scotoma
absolute threshold
absorption of drug
absorption of inhalants
abstinence
  alcohol
  drug
  nicotine
  sexual
abstinence syndrome
  alcohol
  drug
abstractability
abstract attitude
abstract concept
abstracting ability
abstract intelligence
abstract interpretation
abstraction ladder
abstractive ability
  concrete
  nonverbal
abstract reasoning
abstract terms
abstract thinking
absurd
absurdity
abulia, cyclic
abulic

abuse or dependence
  adolescent
  adult
  aerosol spray
  alcohol
  amphetamine
  amyl nitrate
  antidepressant-type
  anxiolytic
  barbiturate
  caffeine
  cannabis
  chemical
  child
  childhood physical
  childhood sexual
  chronic alcohol
  cocaine
  drug
  elder
  emotional
  hallucinogen
  hashish
  hypnotic (drug)
  inhalant
  laxative
  "laxative habit"
  LSD
  marijuana
  mental
  methamphetamine
  mixed drug
  morphine-type
  nonprescription drug
  opioid
  parent
  patent medicinal
  perpetuator of
  phencyclidine (PCP)
  physical
  polydrug
  problems related to

abuse *(cont.)*
  psychoactive substance
  psychological
  ritual
  sadistic
  sedative
  sexual
  spousal
  spouse
  substance
  sympathomimetic
  tobacco
  tranquilizer
  verbal
  victim
  vocal
abuse counseling
abuse criteria
abused child
abused drugs (see *dependence*; *drugs, street*; and *medications*)
abuser
  anxious substance
  child
  drug
  spouse
  substance
abusive vocal behavior
abutting consonants
AC (air conduction)
AC (alternating current)
a.c. (before meals)
ACA (Adult Child[ren] of Alcoholics)
Academic Alertness (AA)
Academic Aptitude Test (AAT)
academic difficulty
academic functioning
  marked decline in
  subaverage
academic inhibition
Academic Instruction Measurement System

academic performance
academic preparation
academic problem
academic psychiatry
academic underachievement disorder
academically understimulating
   environment
Academy of Certified Social
   Workers (ACSW)
Academy of Psychosomatic Medicine
   (APM)
Academy of Religion and Mental
   Health (ARMH)
acalculia
   aphasic
   visual-spatial
"Acapulco gold" (cannabis)
"Acapulco red" (cannabis)
acarophobia
acatalepsy
acatamathesia
acataphasia
acathexis
Acc (accommodation)
accelerated interaction
accelerated speech
accelerometer
accented vowel
accent, word
acceptable behavior
Acceptance of Disability Scale (AD
   Scale)
accessing cues
Access Management Survey (AMS)
accessory nerve, spiral
access to health care services
ACCI (Adult Career Concerns
   Inventory)
accident
   alcohol-related risk for
   cerebrovascular (CVA)
accidental affair

accidental pregnancy
accidental suicide
accident neurosis
accident-prone behavior
accidents as major childhood
   stressors
accommodation (Acc)
according to (per)
acculturation problem with
   expression of customs
   expression of habits
   expression of political values
   expression of religious values
accusative case
accusatory hallucination
ACD (Assessment of Career
   Development)
ACDM (Assessment of Career
   Decision Making)
ACE (American Council on
   Education)
"ace" (cannabis; phencyclidine)
acenesthesia
ACER Advanced Test B90, New
   Zealand Edition
ACER Applied Reading Test
acerbophobia
acerophobia
ACER Test of Basic Skills—
   Blue Series
ACER Test of Basic Skills—
   Green Series
ACER Test of Reasoning Ability
acetylcholine as neurotransmitter
acetylcholine cholinergic receptors
ACG (Assessment of Core Goals)
achievement (see also *test*)
   educational
   exaggerated
   math
   reading
   school
   vocational

achievement age (AA)
achievement behavior
achievement motive
achievement need (n-Ach)
achievement quotient (AQ)
achievement test (see *test*)
achluophobia
acid
  gamma aminobutyric (GABA)
  homovanillic (HVA)
  plasma homovanillic (HVA)
"acid" (lysergic acid diethylamide)
acid-base balance
"acid" flashbacks
"acid head" (re: lysergic acid
  diethylamide user)
Ackerman-Schoendorf Scales for
  Parent Evaluation of Custody
  (ASPECT)
ACL (Achievement Check List)
ACL (Adjective Check List)
ACLC (Assessment of Children's
  Language Comprehension)
ACN (American College of Neuropsychiatrists)
ACO (Assessment of Conceptual
  Organization)
ACO: Improving Writing, Thinking,
  and Reading Skills
ACOA (Adult Child[ren] of
  Alcoholics)
acouesthesia
acoupedic rehabilitation
acoupedics
acousma
acousmatagnosis
acousmatamnesia
acoustic agnosia
acoustic agraphia
acoustical
acoustic-amnestic aphasia
acoustic analysis

acoustic aphasia
acoustic area
acoustic energy
acoustic evoked potential
acoustic feedback
acoustic gain, peak
acoustic immittance measurement
  test
acoustic impedance, static
acoustic input
acoustic interface
acoustic meatus
  external
  internal
acoustic nerve
acoustic neurilemoma
acoustic neuroma
acoustic noise
acousticopalpebral reflex
acousticophobia
acoustic output, maximum
acoustic papilla
acoustic phonetics
acoustic radiation
acoustic ratio, the oral-nasal
  (TONAR)
acoustic reflex
  sensitivity prediction from the
    (SPAR)
  stapedial
acoustic reflex threshold
acoustics
acoustic signal
acoustic spectrum
acoustic stria
acoustic trauma deafness
acoustic tubercle
ACP (American College of
  Physicians)
acquiescence, social (SA)
acquired aphasia
acquired dyslexia

acquired epileptic aphasia (Landau-Kleffner syndrome)
acquired fluent aphasia
acquired sexual dysfunction
acquisition device, language (LAD)
acrolect
acromania
acromegaly
acronym
acrophase
acrophobia
across identity states
ACS (acute confusional state)
ACSW (Academy of Certified Social Workers)
act (pl. acts)
  biological
  frequency of violent
  instrumental avoidance (theory in stuttering)
  rape
  sadistic rape
  serious assaultive
  sensorimotor
  speech
  suicide
  violent
ACT (Anxiety Control Training)
act and volition
ACTeRS (ADD-H: Comprehensive Teacher's Rating Scale, Second Edition)
ACT Evaluation/Survey Service (ESS)
ACTH (adrenocorticotropic hormone)
acting out
  asocial
  passive-aggressive
  sexual
acting-out behavior
acting-out potential

acting-out tendencies
action
  amphetamine-like
  compulsive
  course of
  duration of drug
  effective
  intensified
  legal
  morphine-like
  semiautomatic
  unacceptable
  uncontrollable
action on first messengers, lithium
action on membranes, lithium
action on second messengers, lithium
action potential
action tremor
activated epilepsy
active bilingualism
active desire
active displacement of emotive energy
active filter
active modification
active passivity
active phase of schizophrenia
active-phase symptoms of schizophrenia
active psychoanalysis
active psychotic symptom
active sleep
active therapist
active treatment
active voice
activities (see activity)
activities of daily living (ADLs)
  normal
  simulated (SADL)
activities of daily living skills (ADLS)
Activities Therapist (AT)

Activities Therapist, Registered
(ATR)
activity (pl. activities)
  alpha
  alpha EEG
  antisocial
  autonomic
  background
  beta
  brain wave
  constricted
  cross-gender
  daily
  day-to-day
  decreased
  diminished pleasure in everyday
  EEG alpha
  EEG delta
  EEG theta
  electromyographic
  electro-oculographic
  emotional
  excessive motor
  fast
  focus of
  goal-directed
  gross motor (GMA)
  group
  hedonistic
  high risk
  homosexual
  impulsive
  leisure
  limited
  major life
  masochistic sexual
  masturbatory
  mental
  motor
  neglect of pleasurable
  nighttime
  nonproductive

activity (cont.)
  occupational
  organized
  paroxysmal
  pharyngeal motor
  phasic REM
  pleasurable
  political
  psychomotor
  random
  rapid change in
  reduced physical
  religious
  repetitious
  restricted
  role-play
  self-care
  self-initiated
  sexual
  slow-frequency (delta) EEG
  slowing
  slow-wave
  solitary
  stereotyped
  stream of mental
  sweat gland
  voyeuristic
activity and attention disturbance
  with hyperkinesis
activity and behavior
activity group therapy (AGT)
activity-interview group psychotherapy (A-IGP)
activity level
Activity Losses Assessment (ALA)
activity mapping
Activity Pattern Indicators (APIs)
activity-reactivity, autonomic
activity restriction
acts (see act)
ACT Study Power Assessment and
  Inventory (SPA; SPI)

ACT Study Skills Assessment and
Inventory (SSA; SSI)
actual derailment
actualization
Actualizing Assessment Battery I
and II: The Interpersonal
Inventories
actual neurosis
acuity
auditory
sensory
visual
acuity-level masking technique
aculalia
aculturated into a system (e.g., a
gang)
acusticus externus meatus
acusticus internus meatus
acute anxiety attack (AAA)
acute confusional state (ACS)
acute depression
recurrent episode
single episode
acute discomfort in close relationships
acute drunkenness
acute exacerbation schizophrenia
acute intoxication
acute movement disorder
Acute Panic Inventory
acute stress disorder
acute toxic effects
ad lib (as desired)
"Adam" (analog of amphetamine/
methamphetamine)
ADAMHA (Alcohol, Drug Abuse
and Mental Health
Administration)
Adaptability Test
adaptation reaction
adaptation, social
adaptational approach

adaptational syndrome, general
(GAS)
Adapted Sequenced Inventory of
Communication Development
(A-SICD)
adapting, difficulty in
adaption, auditory
Adaptive Behavior Evaluation Scale
(ABES)
Adaptive Behavior Inventory
Adaptive Behavior Inventory for
Children (ABIC)
Adaptive Behavior Scale (ABS)
adaptive functioning
adaptive level
adaptive response
adaptive scale norms
adaptive skill domains
ADAS (Alzheimer's Disease
Assessment Scale)
ADAS noncognitive subscale
ADC (AIDS dementia complex)
Scale
ADD (attention-deficit disorder)
ADDBRS (Attention Deficit Disorder
Behavior Rating Scales)
added purpose task
ADDES (Attention Deficit Disorders
Evaluation Scale)
ADDH (attention-deficit disorder
with hyperactivity)
ADD-H: Comprehensive Teacher's
Rating Scale, Second Edition
(ACTeRS)
addict, drug (DA)
addiction (adxn)
absinthe
alcohol
biological roots of
cocaine
drug
ethyl alcohol

addiction *(cont.)*
  heroin
  iatrogenic
  Internet
  methyl alcohol
  methylated spirit
  morphine-type
  nicotine
  opium
  polysurgical
  proneness to
  relation
  relationship
  sex
  sympathic mimetic
  sympathomimetic
  tobacco
addiction-prone personality (APP)
addiction psychiatry
Addiction Severity Index (ASI)
addiction syndrome
addiction-type organic psychosis
addictive behavior
Addictive Disease Unit (ADU)
addictive disorders
addictive potential of drug
addictologist
addictology
addition articulation
adductor paralysis
  bilateral
  unilateral
adductor spasmodic dysphonia
A-delta fibers
adenohypophysis
adenosine monophosphate
adenoidectomy, lateral
adenoid, lateral rim of the
adenylate cyclase
adequacy
adequate treatment
ADFM (Association of Departments
  of Family Medicine)

ADH (antidiuretic hormone) for
  bedwetting
ADHD (attention-deficit hyperactivity disorder)
adhesive otitis media
ADI (Adolescent Diagnostic Interview)
ADI (Adolescent Drinking Index)
adiadochokinesia
adiadochokinesis
adjective (parts of speech)
  derived
  predicate
Adjective Check List (ACL)
adjunctive therapy
adjustment
  cultural
  life-cycle
  premorbid
  psychological
  vocational (V Adj)
adjustment disorder
  anxiety
  conduct disturbance
  depressed mood
  depressive
  emotional disturbance
  mixed conduct/emotional
    disturbance
adjustment following migration
adjustment interface disorder
adjustment measure
adjustment reaction
  anxious mood
  conduct disturbance
  depressive
  dysthymic
  elective mutism
  emotional disturbance
  mixed conduct/emotional
    disturbance
  physical symptoms
  withdrawal

adjustment situational reaction
adjustment therapy
adjuvant therapy
ADL or ADLs (activities of daily
    living)
ADL index
ADL scale
ADL test
Adler, Alfred (1870-1937)
adlerian psychoanalysis
adlerian psychology
adlerian psychotherapy
Adler theory
ADLS (activities of daily living
    skills)
adm (admission)
administration
    avenues of
    method of
administrative psychiatry
admiration
    excessive
    need for
admission (adm)
    prior to (PTA)
    voluntary (Vol Adm)
admittance
adol (adolescent)
adolescence
    disorder of
    GID of
    late
    sensitivity reaction of
    withdrawal reaction of
adolescent (pl. adolescents)
    communication with
    evaluation of
    limit-setting for
adolescent abuse
Adolescent Alienation Index
adolescent antisocial behavior
adolescent behavior

adolescent conduct disorder
Adolescent-Coping Orientation for
    Problem Experiences
adolescent crisis
adolescent cross-gender behavior
Adolescent Diagnostic Interview
    (ADI)
Adolescent Drinking Index (ADI)
adolescent dyssocial behavior
Adolescent-Family Inventory of Life
    Events and Changes
adolescent group therapies
adolescent guardedness
adolescent insanity
adolescent language quotient
Adolescent Language Screening Test
Adolescent Life Change Event
    Questionnaire (ALCEQ)
Adolescent Multiphasic Personality
    Inventory
adolescent neurotic delinquency
adolescent onset
adolescent personal identity
adolescent psychiatry
adolescent psychology
adolescent risk-taking behavior
Adolescent Separation Anxiety Test
adolescent sexual identity
adolescent suicide
adolescent voice
adoption
adoptive family
adrenal hyperplasia, congenital
adrenergic
adrenocorticotropic hormone
    (ACTH)
adrenoleukodystrophy
AD Scale (Acceptance of Disability
    Scale)
ADU (Addictive Disease Unit)
adult (pl. adults)
    consenting
    nonconsenting

adult abuse
adult antisocial behavior
Adult Basic Learning Examination
 (ABLE)
Adult Career Concerns Inventory
 (ACCI)
Adult Child(ren) of Alcoholics
 (ACOA)
adult criminal behavior
adult cross-gender behavior
adult dyssocial behavior
adulterer
adulteress
adult group therapies
adult-life psychosexual identity
 disorder
Adult Neuropsychological Questionnaire (ANQ)
adult obstructive sleep apnea
 syndrome
adult-onset-type conduct disorder
Adult Performance Level Survey
 (APLS)
Adult Personal Adjustment and Role
 Skills
adult personal data inventory (APDI)
Adult Personality Inventory (API)
Adult Protective Services (APS)
Adult Suicidal Ideation Questionnaire
 (ASIQ)
adult survivor of child abuse
adult survivor of neglect
adulterous
adultery
adulthood, GID of
adulthood psychiatry
adultomorphic behavior role
adultomorphic stance
adultomorphism
advanced dementia
Advanced Measures of Music
 Audiation

Advanced Placement Program (APP)
Advanced Progressive Matrices
advanced sleep-phase pattern
advanced sleep-phase syndrome
adventitious movement
adverb (parts of speech)
adverse effects of medication
advice (noun); advise (verb)
advice
 against medical (AMA)
 excessive need for
adxn (addiction)
adynamia
adynamic
aego-dystonic
aelurophobia
AEP (auditory evoked potential)
AERA (average evoked response
 audiometry)
aerasthenia
aerodromophobia
aerodynamic analysis
aerodynamics
aerodynamic speech analysis
aeroneurosis
aerophagia
aerophagy
aerophobia
aerosol spray (inhalation) dependence
affair (pl. affairs)
 accidental
 extramarital
 instrumental
 love
 withdrawal from social
affect (noun)
 abnormalities of
 ambivalent
 angry
 apathetic
 appropriate

affect *(cont.)*
  assessment of
  bland
  blunted
  congruent
  constricted
  depressed
  depressive
  diminution of
  dramatic
  dysphoric
  elated
  emptiness of
  euphoric
  flat
  fluctuating
  garrulous
  impaired
  inappropriate
  incongruous
  infantile
  intense
  intense painful
  isolation of
  labile
  labile range of
  modulated
  negative
  normal
  predominant
  preservation of
  removed
  restricted
  restricted range of
  shallow
  short-lived schizophrenic
  silly
  solemn
  superficial
  vacuous
Affect Balance Scale
affect displacement

affected by feelings
affect-fantasy
affection
affectional life change
affective and paranoid state
affective arousal
affective bipolar disorder
affective depressive reaction
affective disease
affective disorder
  atypical
  atypical bipolar
  major
  organic
  primary (PAD)
affective disorder syndrome
affective dyscontrol
affective experience
affective expression
affective flattening
affective function
affective imagery
affective incontinence
affective insanity
affective instability
affective interaction
affective lability
affective melancholia
affective/paranoid organic psychosis
affective personality
affective psychosis
  bipolar
  depressive
  involutional
  major depressive
  manic
  manic-depressive
  melancholia
  mixed-type
  mood swings
  senile
affective reaction

affective reactivity
affective responsiveness
affective/schizophrenia psychosis
affective schizophreniform psychosis
affective set of disturbances
affective syndrome
affectivity, flattened
affectivity ratio
affect-laden delusion
affect memory
affect modulation
affectomotor
affect response
affect state
afferent feedback
afferent motor aphasia
afferent nerve
affiliation
affix
afflict
affliction
affricate consonant formation
affrication
affricative sounds
"Afghanistan black" (cannabis)
African American vernacular English
"African black" (cannabis)
"African bush" (cannabis)
"African woodbine" (cannabis ciga-
    rette)
aftercare
aftereffect, figural
aftereffects of drinking
after-glide
afterimages
aftermath of trauma
after meals (p.c.)
afternoon (P.M., PM, p.m.)
against medical advice (AMA)
age
    achievement (AA)
    basal

age *(cont.)*
    Binet
    biologic
    characteristic
    chronological (CA)
    critical
    developmental
    educational (EA)
    emotional
    functional
    individual's
    mental (MA)
    middle
    relation to
    social (SA)
    typical
age-appropriate societal norms
age at onset
age correction
age features
age group
ageism
age-level behavior
age-matched individual
age mate
agency
    health systems (HSA)
    social service
agenesis
agent (drug)
    antianxiety
    antidipsotropic
    antihypertensive
    antimanic
    antipsychotic
    azaspirodeconedione
    butyrophenone
    causative
    dibenzoxozepine
    etiological
    MAOI-serotonergic
    monoamine oxidase inhibitor

agent *(cont.)*
  monoamine oxidase inhibitor-
    serotonergic
  monoamine oxidase inhibitor-
    tricyclic
  neuroleptic
  offending
  phenothiazine
  possessing
  psychedelic
  psychotomimetic
  sedative-hypnotic
  therapeutic
  transmissible
agent-action
agent-object
agent of change
Agent Orange
age peer
Age Projection Test (APT)
age-related cognitive decline
age-related deterioration
age-related hearing loss
age-related pharmacodynamic
  changes
age-related pharmacokinetic changes
age-specific features
ageusia
ageusic aphasia
aggregation, familial
aggression
  domestic
  husband-to-wife
  passive
  physical
  wife-to-husband
aggression to animals
aggression without provocation
aggressive behavior, de-escalating
aggressive disorder
aggressive drive
aggressive immaturity reaction

aggressive impulses
aggressive instinct
aggressive invasion
aggressiveness, hostile
aggressive outburst
aggressive personality
aggressive-type conduct disorder
aggressive-type personality disorder
aggressive undersocialized reaction
aggressor
aging process, normative
agitans, paralysis
agitata
  amentia
  melancholia
agitate
agitated behavior
agitated depression
agitated melancholia
agitated patient
agitated state
agitation
  emotional
  extreme
  mental
  nighttime
  onset of
  physical
  psychomotor
  purposeless
  unpredictable
  unrelieved
  untriggered
  violent
agitative features
agitographia
agitolalia
agitophasia
aglossia
AGLP (Association of Gay and
  Lesbian Psychiatrists)
agnathia

agnathous
agnosia
  acoustic
  apperceptive visual
  associative visual
  auditory
  autotopagnosia
  color
  corporal
  facial
  finger
  generalized auditory
  object
  selective auditory
  tactile
  topographical
  verbal
  verbal auditory
  visual
agnostic alexia
agnostic behavior
"agonies" (re: drug withdrawal)
agonist medication
agonist, partial
agonist therapy
agoramania
agoraphobia
agoraphobic avoidance
AGP (Archive of General
  Psychiatry)
AGPA (American Group Psychotherapy Association)
agrammalogia
agrammatic speech
agrammatica
agrammatism
agrammatologia
agraphia
  absolute
  acoustic
  amnemonic
  aphasic

agraphia *(cont.)*
  apractic
  apraxic
  atactic
  cerebral
  developmental
  jargon
  lexical
  literal
  mental
  motor
  musical
  optic
  phonological
  pure
  spatial
  verbal
agraphia amnemonica
agraphia atactica
agraphic
agreeableness
agreement
  separation
  subject-verb
agromania
AGS Early Screening Profiles
AGT (activity group therapy)
agyiomania
agyiophobia
AH (ataxic hemiparesis)
AH4 Group Intelligence Test
AH5 Group Test of High Grade
  Intelligence
AH6 Group Test of High Level
  Intelligence
AHIMA (American Health Information Management Association)
AHPAT (Allied Health Professions
  Admission Test)
"ah-pen-yen" (opium)
AI (anxiety index)
aichmophobia

aid
  air-conduction hearing
  binaural hearing
  body hearing
  bone-conduction hearing
  canal hearing
  contralateral routing of signals
    (CROS)
  digital hearing
  external memory
  in-the-ear (ITE) hearing
  monaural hearing
  vibrotactile
  Y-cord hearing
aidoiomania
AIDS dementia complex (ADC)
AIDS encephalopathy
ailuromania
ailurophobia
AIM (Artificial Intelligence in
  Medicine)
AIMD (abnormal involuntary movement disorder)
"aimies" (amphetamine; amyl
  nitrite)
aimless behavior
aimless motor activity
aimless wandering
AIMS (abnormal involuntary movement scale)
Ainsworth Strange Situation Test
"AIP" (heroin from Afghanistan,
  Iran, and Pakistan)
air
  complemental
  tidal
air-blade sound
"air blast" (inhalant)
air-bone gap
air conduction (AC), pure tone
air-conduction hearing aid
air-conduction receiver

air-conduction threshold, pure tone
"airhead" (re: cannabis user)
air hunger, psychogenic
"airplane" (cannabis)
airplane glue (sniffing) dependence
airstream mechanism
air wastage
airway dysfunction, lingual
AKA, a.k.a. (also known as)
akathisia
  neuroleptic dose-dependent
  neuroleptic-induced
akinesia
akinesis
akinesthesia
akinetic apraxia
akinetic autism
akinetic mania
akinetic mutism
akinetic seizure
Al-Anon
ala cerebelli
ala (pl. alae), nasal
ALA (Activity Losses Assessment)
alalia prolongata
alalic
alar flutter
alarm-clock headache
alarm reaction
alaryngeal speech
albuminurophobia
ALC (Alternate Lifestyle Checklist)
Alcadd Test
ALCEQ (Adolescent Life Change
  Event Questionnaire)
alcohol (EtOH, ETOH), toxic effects
  of
alcohol abuse
alcohol addiction
alcohol amnestic disorder
alcohol amnestic syndrome
alcohol as cause of seizure

Alcohol Assessment and Treatment
  Profile
alcohol binge
alcohol consumption
alcohol dependence syndrome
alcohol drinking
Alcohol, Drug Abuse and Mental
  Health Administration (ADAMHA)
alcohol effects, fetal (FAE)
alcohol habits
alcoholic
  Child(ren) of (CoA)
  detoxified
  inactive (IA)
  newly abstinent
alcoholic amentia
alcoholic amnesia
alcoholic ataxia
alcoholic brain syndrome, chronic
  (CABS)
alcoholic coma
alcoholic confusional state
alcoholic delirium
  acute
  chronic
alcoholic delirium tremens
alcoholic delirium withdrawal
alcoholic dementia
alcoholic deterioration
alcoholic drunkenness
alcoholic epilepsy
alcoholic hallucination
alcoholic hallucinosis
alcoholic insanity
alcoholic intoxication with dependence
alcoholic jealousy
alcoholic liver disease-type organic
  psychosis
alcoholic mania
  acute
  chronic
alcoholic paranoia

alcoholic paranoid psychosis
alcoholic psychosis
  abstinence syndrome
  amnestic confabulatory
  amnestic syndrome
  delirium tremens
  hallucinosis
  Korsakoff
  paranoid-type
  pathological intoxication
  polyneuritic
  withdrawal delirium
  withdrawal hallucinosis
  withdrawal syndrome
Alcoholics Anonymous (AA)
alcoholic wet brain syndrome
alcohol idiosyncratic intoxication
alcohol-induced anxiety disorder
alcohol-induced nighttime sleep
alcohol-induced persisting amnestic
  disorder
alcohol-induced persisting dementia
alcohol-induced psychotic disorder
alcohol-induced sexual dysfunction
alcohol-induced paranoid state
alcohol-induced sleep disorder
alcohol intoxication
  acute
  idiosyncratic
  pathological
  signs of
alcohol intoxication delirium
alcohol intoxication organic
  psychosis
alcoholism
  acute
  chronic
  delirium
  mental disorder due to
alcoholism associated with dementia
alcoholism organic psychosis
alcohol level, blood

alcoholomania
alcohol on breath (AOB)
alcoholophilia
alcoholophobia
alcohol poisoning
alcohol-precipitated epilepsy
alcohol problem
alcohol-related disorder
alcohol-related risk for accidents
alcohol-related risk for suicide
alcohol-related risk for violence
alcohol-related seizure
alcohol syndrome, fetal
alcohol use disorder
Alcohol Use Inventory (AUI)
alcohol use questionnaire
alcohol withdrawal delirium
alcohol withdrawal seizure
alcohol withdrawal syndrome
ALD (Appraisal of Language
  Disturbances)
alert and oriented times four (x 4)
  (to person, place, time, and future
  plans or situation) (A+Ox4)
alert and oriented times three (x 3) (to
  person, place, and time) (A+Ox3)
alert awake state
alerting stimulus
alertness
  level of
  state of
Alexander, Franz (1891-1964)
Alexander's deafness
alexia (dyslexia)
  agnostic
  anterior
  auditory
  central
  cortical
  incomplete
  motor
  musical

alexia *(cont.)*
  optical
  posterior
  pure
  sensory
  subcortical
  tactile
  visual
alexia with agraphia
alexia without agraphia
alexic
alexithymia
alexithymic personality
algera, apraxia
algophilia
algophily
algophobia
algopsychalia
ALI (American Law Institute) Test
aliases, use of
"Alice B. Toklas" (cannabis brown-
  ie)
Alice in Wonderland syndrome
alien
alienating
alienation, social
alienism
alienist
alien obsession
alien thoughts
alkalosis, metabolic
"all-American drug" (cocaine)
"all lit up" (re: drug influence)
"all star" (re: drug user)
allenian theory
allenian therapy
allergic disorder, psychogenic
allergic encephalopathy
alleviating aggressive behavior
alleviating violence in aggressive
  behavior

alliance
 therapeutic
 working
Alliance for Mentally Ill Chemical
 Abusers
allied health professional
Allied Health Professions Admission
 Test (AHPAT)
alliteration (figure of speech)
 consonantal
 vocalic
allomorph
allophone tabulation
allotropic personality
Allport group relations theory
allusion (figure of speech)
alogia
alogical thinking
aloneness
aloof
alopecia
 psychogenic
 trichotillomania-induced
alopecia areata
alpha activity
alpha-adrenergic receptor
alphabet
 American Manual
 initial teaching
 International Phonetic (IPA)
 International Standard Manual
 (ISMA)
 manual
 phonetic
alpha EEG activity
alpha-ethyltryptamine (street names)
 alpha-ET
 ET
 love pearls
 love pills
 trip
alpha frequency

alpha index
alpha interferon
alpha-methyldopa-induced mood
 disorder
alpha rhythm
alpha state
alpha wave
alpha wave strains
ALPS (Aphasia Language Performance Scales)
ALS (amyotrophic lateral sclerosis)
 (Lou Gehrig's disease)
ALSD (Alzheimer-like senile
 dementia)
also known as (a.k.a., AKA)
alteration in identity
alteration in rate of speech
alterations in time perception
alterations, NMDA receptor
altered auditory feedback (AAF)
altered level of consciousness
altered life circumstances
altered mental status
altered sensation
altered state
altered vision
altered voice
alterego
alteregoism
Alternate Binaural Loudness Balance
 (ABLB)
alternate forms reliability coefficient
alternate identity
Alternate Lifestyle Checklist (ALC)
Alternate Monaural Loudness
 Balance (AMLB)
alternate motion rate (AMR)
alternating bipolar disorder
alternating current (AC)
alternating insanity
alternating manic-depressive
 psychosis

alternating personality
alternating psychosis
alternating pulse
alternative criterion B for dysthymic
    disorder
alternative dimensional descriptors
    for schizophrenia
altophobia
altruism
altruistic suicide
alveolar angle
alveolar arch
alveolar area
alveolar border of mandible
alveolar canal
alveolar consonant placement
alveolar hypoventilation syndrome
alveolar nerve
alveolar point
alveolar process of maxilla
alveolar ridge
alveolar sac
alveolar septum
alveolar space
alveolar supporting bone
alveolar wall
alveolar yoke
alveolingual
alveolitis
alveolodental canal
alveololabial
alveololingual
alveolopalatal
alveolus (pl. alveoli)
Alzheimer dementia
Alzheimer disease
Alzheimer Disease Assessment Scale
    (ADAS)
Alzheimer-like senile dementia
    (ALSD)
Alzheimer syndrome
Alzheimer tangles

Alzheimer-type, senile dementia
    (SDAT)
AM (amplitude modulation)
AMA (against medical advice)
    sign-out
amathophobia
amaurotic axonal idiocy
amaurotic familial idiocy
amaurotic idiocy
amaxomania
amaxophobia
ambidexterity
ambidextrous
ambient noise
ambiguity
    lexical
    role
    structural
ambiguous genitalia
ambilaterality
ambisyllabic
ambitendency
ambivalence
ambivalent affect
ambivalent feelings
ambivalent quotient
ambiversion
ambivert
amblyopia, toxic
ambulation index
ambulatory schizophrenia
amelioration, tendency toward
a-methyl-paratyrosine (for mania)
amenomania
ament
amentia
    nevoid
    phenylpyruvic
    Stern alcoholic
amentia agitata
amentia attonita
amentia occulta

amentia paranoides
Americamania
American Academy of Child and
Adolescent Psychiatry (AACAP)
American Academy of Family
Physicians (AAFP)
American Academy of Pediatrics
(AAP)
American Academy of Psychiatrists
in Alcoholism and Addictions
(AAPAA)
American Academy of Psychiatry
and the Law (AAPL)
American Association for Geriatric
Psychiatry (AAGP)
American Association for Marriage
and Family Therapy (AAMFT)
American Association of Chairmen
of Departments of Psychiatry
(AACDP)
American Association of Directors
of Psychiatric Residency Training
(AADPRT)
American Association of Psychiatric
Administrators (AAPA)
American Association of Teachers
of Spanish and Portuguese
National Spanish Examinations
American Association on Mental
Deficiency (AAMD)
American Board of Family Practice
(ABFP)
American Board of Psychiatry and
Neurology (ABPN)
American College of Neuropsychia-
trists (ACN)
American College of Physicians
(ACP)
American Council on Education
(ACE)
American Drug and Alcohol Survey
American Group Psychotherapy
Association (AGPA)

American Health Information Man-
agement Association (AHIMA)
American Indian Sign Language
(Amerind)
American Journal of Psychiatry
American Law Institute (ALI)
Formulation
American Law Institute (ALI) Test
American Manual Alphabet
American Medical Society on Alco-
hol and Other Drug Dependencies
(AMSAODD)
American National Standards Institute
(ANSI)
American Nurses Association (ANA)
American Occupational Therapy
Association (AOTA)
American Occupational Therapy
Association, Inc., Fieldwork
Evaluation for the Occupational
Therapist
American Orthopsychiatric Associ-
ation (AOA)
American Psychiatric Association
(APA)
American Psychiatric Press
American Psychoanalytic Association
(APA)
American Psychological Association
(APA)
American Psychological Society
(APS)
American Psychopathological Associ-
ation (APA)
American Psychosomatic Society
(APS)
American Sign Language (ASL)
(Ameslan)
American Sleep Disorders Associ-
ation (ASDA)
American Society for Adolescent
Psychiatry (ASAP)

American Society of Clinical
  Hypnosis (ASCH)
American Speech-Language-Hearing
  Association (ASHA)
Amerind (American Indian Sign
  Language)
"ames" (amyl nitrite)
Ameslan (American Sign Language)
  (ASL)
ametamorphosis
AMHC (Association of Mental Health
  Clergy)
AMI (Athletic Motivation Inventory)
"amidone" (methadone hydrochloride)
amimia
  amnesic
  ataxic
amimic
amine, biogenic
amine hypothesis, biogenic
amino acids
amitriptyline-induced mood disorder
AML (Automated Multitest Laboratory)
AMLB (Alternate Monaural Loudness
  Balance)
amnemonic agraphia
amnemonic aphasia
amnesia
  acute
  alcoholic
  antegrade
  anterograde
  asymmetrical
  auditory
  Broca
  childbirth
  chronic
  circumscribed
  complete
  concussion
  continuous

amnesia *(cont.)*
  degree of
  dissociative
  emotional
  episodic
  evidence of
  generalized
  global
  hippocampal
  hysterical
  ictal
  infantile
  Korsakoff
  lacunar
  localized
  nonpathological
  olfactory
  organic
  partial
  patchy
  postconcussive
  posthypnotic
  posttraumatic (PTA)
  profound
  psychogenic
  retroactive
  retrograde
  reversible
  selective
  shrinking retrograde
  subsequent
  systematized
  tactile
  toxin-provoked
  transient global (TGA)
  traumatic
  true
  verbal
  visual
amnesiac
amnesia after trance
amnesia for sleep and dreaming

amnesia for sleep-terror event
amnesia in children
amnesia loss of memory
amnesic amimia
amnesic amnesia
amnesic aphasia
amnesic syndrome
amnestic aphasia
amnestic apraxia
amnestic confabulatory alcoholic
   psychosis
amnestic confabulatory syndrome
amnestic disorder
   alcohol
   alcohol-induced persisting
   anxiolytic
   substance-induced persisting
amnestic psychosis
amnestic state
amnestic syndrome
   alcohol
   drug-induced
   posttraumatic
amobarbital (street names)
   blue angels
   bluebirds
   blue devils
   blues
   Christmas trees
   double trouble
   greenies
   lilly
   rainbows
   tooies
"amoeba" (phencyclidine)
amok (culture-specific syndrome)
   (also amuck)
amoral psychopathic personality
amotivated behavior
amotivation, denial of
amotivational syndrome
"amp" (amphetamine)

"amped-out" (re: amphetamine use)
ampere (A)
amphetamine (AMT) (street names)
   A
   A's
   aimies
   amp
   bam
   beans
   bennies
   Benz
   black beauties
   black birds
   black bombers
   black mollies
   blacks
   blue boy
   bottles
   brain ticklers
   browns
   bumblebees
   cartwheels
   chalk
   chicken powder
   chocolate
   Christina
   coast to coast
   copilots
   crisscross
   crossroads
   diet pills
   dominoes
   double crosses
   eye opener
   fives
   footballs
   forwards
   French blue
   glass
   greenies
   hanyak
   head drugs

amphetamine *(cont.)*
 hearts
 hiroppon
 horse heads
 ice
 in-betweens
 jam
 jam cecil
 jelly baby
 jelly beans
 jolly bean
 jugs
 L.A.
 leapers
 lid poppers
 lightning
 little bomb
 manufacturing
 marathons
 minibennie
 nugget
 oranges
 peaches
 pep pills
 pink hearts
 pixies
 powder
 purple hearts
 red phosphorus
 rhythm
 rippers
 road dope
 Rosa
 roses
 snap
 snow
 snow pallets
 snow seals
 sparkle plenty
 sparklers
 speed
 speedball

amphetamine *(cont.)*
 splash
 splivins
 sugar daddies
 sweets
 thrusters
 TR-6s
 truck drivers
 turkey
 turnabout
 uppers
 uppies
 ups
 white
 white cross
 whites
 X
amphetamine abuse or dependence
amphetamine challenge test
amphetamine-induced anxiety
 disorder
amphetamine-induced mood disorder
amphetamine-induced sexual disorder
amphetamine intoxication
amphetamine intoxication delirium
amphetamine/methamphetamine,
 analog of
amphetamine psychosis
amphetamine use disorder
amphetamine withdrawal
"amping" (accelerated heartbeat)
"amp joint" (narcotic-laced cannabis
 cigarette)
amplification
 binaural
 compression
 memory
amplifier
amplify
amplitude
 effective
 maximum

amplitude *(cont.)*
  peak
  peak-to-peak
  reflex
  zero
amplitude asymmetry
amplitude distortion
amplitude gradient
amplitude modulation (AM)
AMR (alternate motion rate)
AMS (Access Management Survey)
AMSAODD (American Medical
  Society on Alcohol and Other
  Drug Dependencies)
amt (amount)
AMT (amphetamine)
AMT (Anxiety Management Training)
"AMT" (dimethyltryptamine)
amuck (also amok)
amusia
amychophobia
amygdalofugal fiber
amyl nitrite (street names)
  aimies
  ames
  amys
  boppers
  pearls
  pears
  poppers
  snappers
amyl nitrate inhalant
amyloid angiopathy
amyloidosis, metabolic
amyotrophic lateral sclerosis (ALS;
  Lou Gehrig's disease)
"amys" (amyl nitrite)
Amytal interview
AN (anorexia nervosa)
ANA (American Nurses Association)
anabolic steroid
anaclitic depression

anaclitic psychotherapy
anaclitic relationship
anaclitic therapy
anacusis
ANAD (anorexia nervosa and associated disorders)
anadrol (oral steroid)
anal character
anal erotism
analgesic
  controlled
  non-narcotic
anal intercourse
analog
anlogic change
analog marking
anal phase
anal sex
anal stage
anal stage psychosexual development
analysand
analysis
  acoustic
  aerodynamic
  auditory
  behavioral
  cephalometric
  cerebrospinal fluid (CSF)
  chain
  child
  contrastive
  cost-benefit
  discriminant
  distal distinctive feature
  ego
  Fourier
  gait
  grammatical
  hierarchial regression
  in-depth
  kinesthetic
  kinetic

analysis *(cont.)*
latent class
morphometric
natural process
neurometric
perceptual
phonemic
phonetic
phonological
segmental
sequential multiple (SMA)
solution
sound
substitution
suprasegmental
task
toxicological
traditional phonetic
transactional (TA)
analysis and synthesis
Analysis of Coping Style
analysis of homonymy
Analysis of Readiness Skills
analysis of transference
analysis of variance (ANOV,
ANOVA)
analytical psychology (anal. psychol.)
Analytical Reading Inventory
analytic boundaries
analytic frame
Analytic Learning Disability Assessment
analytic method
analytic object
analytic psychiatry
analytic psychology
analytic psychotherapy
analyzer
noise
Time Use
anamnesis

anamnestic
anancasm
anancastic neurosis
anancastic personality
anaphoric pronoun
anaphors
anaptyxis (pl. anaptyxes)
anarithmia literalis
anarthria
anatomical site of pain
anatomy, biochemical
anatrofin (injectable steroid)
anavar (oral steroid)
anchor
collapsing
firing an
stacking
stealing an
anchor signs of withdrawal
anchor symptoms
anchors/responses, integrating
ancraophobia
Andresen Six-Basic-Factors-Model
(A-SBFM) Questionnaire
androgen insensitivity syndrome
androgynous individual
andromania
androphobia
anechoic chamber
anemometer, warm-wire
anemophobia
anergastic organic psychosis
anergastic psychosis
anergic schizophrenic
anergy, denial of
anesthesia
conversion
emotional
first stage of
halogenated inhalational
hysterical
laryngeal

anesthesia *(cont.)*
  sensory
  sexual
  stocking-glove
  traumatic
anesthetic conversion reaction
"angel" (phencyclidine)
"angel dust" (phencyclidine)
"angel hair" (phencyclidine)
"angel mist" (phencyclidine)
"Angel Poke" (phencyclidine)
anger
  constant
  difficulty controlling
  fit of
  ineffective
  intense
  marked
  outburst of
anger expression, passivity in
anger mallet
anger reaction
"Angie" (cocaine)
anginophobia
angiopathy, amyloid
angle, alveolar
Anglomania
Anglophobia
"Angola" (cannabis)
angry affect
angry reaction to minor stimuli
angry word exchange
anguish
angular gyrus
angulation
anhedonia
anhedonic
anhedonism
aniled sense of self
anima
"animal" (lysergic acid diethyl-amide)

Animal and Opposite Drawing Technique (AODT)
Animal House
animal phobia
animal psychology
"animal trank" (phencyclidine)
"animal tranquilizer" (phencyclidine)
animal-type specific phobia
animals, aggression to
animate
animus
ankyloglossia
ankylosis, cricoarytenoid
Ann Arbor Learning Inventory and Remediation Program
Annett's hand preference scale
anniversary reaction
anode
anomalous movement
Anomalous Sentences Repetition Test (ASRT)
anomaly (pl. anomalies)
  craniofacial
  laryngeal
anomia
  color
  finger
  tactile
anomic aphasia
anomic errors
anomie
Anorectic Attitude Questionnaire
anorexia nervosa (AN)
anorexia nervosa and associated disorders (ANAD)
Anorexic Behavior Scale
anorexic fast
anorgasmia
anosmia
anosognosia
ANOV or ANOVA (analysis of variance)

ANQ (Adult Neuropsychological
   Questionnaire)
ANS (autonomic nervous system)
ANSER System
ANSI (American National Standards
   Institute)
antagonism
antagonist, beta-adrenergic
antagonist medication
antagonistic muscle strength
antalgic gait
antecedent-consequence variables
antecedent event
antecedent variables
antegrade amnesia
antegrade amnesic
anterior, alexia
anterior digastric muscle
anterior feature English phoneme
anterior partial laryngectomy
anterior vertical canal
anterograde amnesia
anterograde loss of memory
anterograde memory
anthelix
anthomania
anthrophobia
anthropological linguistics
anthropomorphic face
anthropophobia
anti-expectancy
anti-parkinsonism
antianxiety agent; drug
anticholinergic delirium
anticholinergic effect
anticholinergic property
anticholinergic side effects
anticipatory and struggle behavior
   (theory in stuttering)
anticipatory anxiety
anticipatory coarticulation
anticonvulsant drugs

anticonvulsant intoxication
anticonvulsant medication-induced
   postural tremor
anticonvulsive
antidepressant
   heterocyclic
   monocyclic
   tricyclic (TCA, TCAD)
antidepressant agent
antidepressant medication-induced
   postural tremor
antidepressant-type (drug) abuse
antidipsotropic agent or drug
antidiuretic hormone (ADH) for bed-
   wetting
antidote drug
antiexpectancy speech
"antifreeze" (heroin)
antihallucinatory
antihelix
antimanic agent or drug
antimongolism
antipanic agent; drug
antiparkinsonism agent; drug
antipsychotic agent; drug
antipsychotic, tricyclic (TCA)
antiresonance
antiseizure drug
antisocial (AS) activity
antisocial behavior
   adolescent
   adult
   child
   pattern of
antisocial personality (ASP)
antisocial personality disorder
antisocial psychopathic personality
antisocial reaction
antisocial tendencies
antisocialism
antitragus
antlophobia

Anton Brenner Developmental
  Gestalt Test of School Readiness
antonym
anvil
anxietas presenilis
anxiety
  adjustment disorder with
  adolescent
  alcohol-induced
  amphetamine-induced
  anticipatory
  anxiolytic-induced
  basic
  caffeine-induced
  cannabis-induced
  castration
  catastrophic
  childhood
  clinically significant
  cocaine-induced
  debilitating
  dental
  desertion
  environmentally induced
  excessive
  excessive social
  extreme
  feelings of
  focus of
  free-floating
  frequency of
  gender differences in
  generalized (GAD)
  high (HA)
  hypnotic-induced
  hyposomnia associated with
  immediate
  insomnia associated with
  intense
  intercurrent
  level of
  low (LA)

anxiety (cont.)
  marked
  neutralized
  noetic
  nonpathological
  nonpsychotic
  panic-type
  performance
  pervasive
  physical concomitant of
  primary
  prominent
  provoked
  psychogenic
  reactive depression and
  reduction of
  sedative-induced
  separation (SAD)
  severe
  signal
  situation
  sleeplessness associated with
  social
  stranger
  substance-induced
  undue social
anxiety attack
  acute (AAA)
  dream (nightmare)
Anxiety Control Training (ACT)
anxiety-depressive disorder, mixed
anxiety disorder (see anxiety)
anxiety disorder due to GMC
  (general medical condition)
Anxiety Disorders Interview
  Schedule
anxiety disturbance
anxiety dream
anxiety due to potential evaluation by
  others
anxiety hysteria
anxiety index (AI)

anxiety-induced impaired social functioning
anxiety inventory (see *test*)
Anxiety Management Training (AMT)
anxiety neurosis
    generalized
    panic-type
anxiety psychoneurosis
anxiety psychoneurotic reaction
anxiety rating scale (see *test*)
anxiety reaction, mild (ARM)
anxiety-related mental disorder
anxiety response
anxiety scale (see *test*)
Anxiety Scale Questionnaire (ASQ)
Anxiety Scales for Children and Adults (ASCA)
anxiety sensitivity (AS)
Anxiety Sensitivity Index (ASI)
anxiety state (AS)
anxiety status inventory (ASI)
anxiety tension state (ATS, A.T.S.)
anxiolytic abuse
anxiolytic agent; drug
anxiolytic amnestic disorder
anxiolytic effect
anxiolytic-induced anxiety
anxiolytic intoxication
anxiolytic intoxication delirium
anxiolytic, serotonergic
anxiolytic use disorder
anxiolytic withdrawal delirium
anxious delirium
anxious-fearful cluster
anxious mood adjustment reaction
AO (avoidance of others)
AOA (American Orthopsychiatric Association)
AOB (alcohol on breath)
AODT (Animal and Opposite Drawing Technique)

AOT (Association of Occupational Therapists)
AOTA (American Occupational Therapy Association)
A+Ox3 (alert and oriented times three)
A+Ox4 (alert and oriented times four)
APA (American Psychiatric Association)
APA (American Psychoanalytic Association)
APA (American Psychological Association)
APA (American Psychopathological Association)
"Apache" (fentanyl)
apandria
apanthropia
apanthropy
APAT (Accounting Program Admission Test)
apathetic affect
apathetic thyrotoxicosis
apathetic-type personality disorder
apathetic withdrawal
apathic
apathism
apathy
A.P.C. (aspirin, phenacetin, caffeine tablets)
APDI (adult personal data inventory)
apeirophobia
APELL (Assessment Program of Early Learning Levels)
aperiodic wave
aperta, rhinolalia
aperture
apex (pl. apices) of tongue
APGAR (adaptability, partnership, growth, affection, and resolve)
    Score

aphagia, psychogenic
aphasia
  acoustic
  acoustic-amnestic
  acquired
  acquired epileptic
  acquired fluent
  afferent (kinesthetic) motor
  ageusic
  amnemonic
  amnesic
  amnestic
  anomic
  associative
  ataxic
  auditory
  Broca
  callosal disconnection syndrome
  central
  childhood
  combined
  commissural
  complete
  conduction
  cortical
  developmental
  dynamic
  efferent (kinetic) motor
  executive
  expressive
  expressive-receptive
  fluent
  frontocortical
  frontolenticular
  functional
  gibberish
  global
  graphic
  graphomotor
  Grashey
  hypophonic
  ideomotor

aphasia *(cont.)*
  impressive
  infantile
  intellectual
  isolation
  jargon
  Kussmaul
  lenticular
  Lichtheim
  major motor
  mixed
  motor
  nominal
  nonfluent
  optic
  parieto-occipital
  partial nominal
  pathematic
  pictorial
  pragmatic
  psychosensory
  pure
  receptive
  semantic
  sensory
  similarity disorder of
  simple
  speech reading
  subcortical
  subcortical motor
  syntactic
  tactile
  temporoparietal
  total
  transcortical mixed
  transcortical motor
  transcortical sensory
  true
  verbal
  visual
  Wernicke
Aphasia Clinical Battery

Aphasia Language Performance
  Scales (ALPS)
aphasia lethica
aphasia screening test
aphasic acalculia
aphasic agraphia
aphasic errors
aphasic impairment
aphasic migraine headache
aphasic phonological impairment
aphasic seizure
  fluent
  nonfluent
aphasiologist
aphasiology
aphemesthesia
aphemia, pure
aphemic
aphephobia
aphonia
  acute
  conversion
  functional
  hysteric
  intermittent
  syllabic
aphonia paranoica
aphonic
aphrasia
aphrodisiomania
API (Activity Pattern Indicators)
API (Adult Personality Inventory)
apicalization
apices (see *apex*)
apimania
apiphobia
aplasia
  cerebral
  cochlear
  labyrinthine
APLS (Adult Performance Level
  Survey)

APM (Academy of Psychosomatic
  Medicine)
APMR (Association for Physical and
  Mental Rehabilitation)
apnea
  central
  central sleep
  mixed sleep
  obstructive
  obstructive sleep
  sleep
  true
apnea syndrome
  adult obstructive sleep
  central sleep
  obstruction sleep
apneic period
apneic seizure
apneustic breathing
apneustic period
apocarteresis
apoplectic coma
apoplectiform convulsion
apoplexy
apostrophe (figure of speech)
APP (addiction-prone personality)
APP (Advanced Placement Program)
APP-R (Assessment of Phonological
  Processes—Revised)
apparent competence
appendicular ataxia
apperception test
apperceptive visual agnosia
appersonification
appetite disorder, psychogenic
appetitive drive
"apple jacks" (crack)
application, ritualized makeup
applied psychology
appositive
Appraisal of Language Disturbances
  (ALD)

apprehension state
apprehension test (see *test*)
apprehensive
apprehensiveness, social
approach
  adaptational
  categorical
  checklist
  descriptive
  dimensional
  fundamental
  here-and-now
  mixture
  nondirective
  psychodynamic
  regressive-reconstructive
  yawn-sign
approach-approach conflict
approach-avoidance conflict
approach-avoidance stance
appropriate affect
appropriate behavior
appropriate relationship
appropriate self-stimulatory behaviors in the young
"approximate answers" syndrome
approximation
  successive
  vocal fold
  word
APR (auropalpebral reflex)
apractic agraphia
apractic disorder
apractic dysarthria
apraxia
  akinetic
  amnestic
  buccofacial
  callosal
  cerebral mapping of
  classic
  constructional

apraxia *(cont.)*
  cortical
  developmental articulatory
  disconnection
  dressing
  ideational
  ideatory
  ideokinetic
  ideomotor
  innervation
  Liepmann
  magnetic
  motor
  ocular
  oculomotor
  oral
  sensory
  speech
  transcortical
  verbal
apraxia algera
Apraxia Battery for Adults (ABA)
apraxic agraphia
apraxic behaviors
apraxic disorder
apraxic dysarthria
aprophoria
aprosexia
aprosody
APS (Adult Protective Services)
APS (American Psychological Society)
APS (American Psychosomatic Society)
apsychia
apsychosis
APT (Age Projection Test)
aptitude (see also *test*)
  numerical (N)
  spatial (S)
aptitude battery (see *test*)
Aptitude-Intelligence Test Series, I.P.I.

Aptitude Interest Measurement
Aptitude Survey and Interest
    Schedule, Second Edition–Interest
    Survey (OASIS-2 IS)
aptitude test (see *test*)
Aptitude Tests for School Beginners
    (ASB)
AQ (achievement quotient)
aquaphobia
arachnophobia
arc
    reflex
    sensorimotor
arch
    alveolar
    glossopalatine
    pharyngopalatine
archaic-paralogical thinking
architecture of brain
architecture, sleep
Archive of General Psychiatry (AGP)
arcuate fasciculus (AF)
arcuate movement
area
    acoustic
    alveolar
    articulation
    auditory
    bilabial
    Broca's (Brodmann's 44)
    Brodmann's 41
    callosal (parolfactory nerve)
    catchment
    conflict-free
    glottal
    labiodental
    language
    lingua-alveolar
    linguodental
    motor
    olfactory
    palatal

area *(cont.)*
    parietal association
    parietotemporal
    premotor
    sclerotic
    sclerotome
    septal
    skill
    somesthetic
    velar
    visual
    watershed
    Wernicke's 22, 39, 40
area consonant placement
    bilabial
    glottal
    labiodental
    lingua-alveolar
    linguadental
    palatal
    velar
areata, alopecia
argentophilic Pick inclusion bodies
arginine vasopressin
argot
argument, semantic (communication
    pattern)
argumentative
"Aries" (heroin)
arithmetical skills learning retardation
Arithmetic Grade Equivalent
Arithmetic Grade Rating
arithmetic problems
arithmetic signs
arithmetic subtest
arithmomania
Arizona Articulation Proficiency
    Scale (AAPS), Revised
Arizona Battery for Communication
    Disorders of Dementia (ABCD)
Arlin Test of Formal Reasoning
ARM (anxiety reaction, mild)

Armed Services Vocational Aptitude
Battery (ASVAB)
ARMH (Academy of Religion and
Mental Health)
arm swing, decreased
ARNMD (Association for Research
in Nervous and Mental Disease)
"aroma of men" (isobutyl nitrite)
around-the-clock observation
arousability factors
arousal
  affective
  autonomic
  conditional
  confusional
  erotic
  increased
  intense autonomic
  oxygen-deprived sexual
  sense of
  sexual
  sleep
arousal disorder
  acquired-type female sexual
  female sexual
  generalized-type female sexual
  lifelong-type female sexual
  male erectile
  sexual
  situational-type female sexual
arousal dysfunction
arousal from sleep
arousal mechanism
arresting consonant
arrest of development
arrest of speech
arrest reaction
arrogant behavior
arson, "communicative"
art therapy
arteriosclerosis, cerebral
arteriosclerotic brain disease

arteriosclerotic cardiovascular
disease (ASCVD)
arteriosclerotic dementia or psychosis
  acute confusional state
  delirium
  delusional-type
  depressed-type
  paranoid-type
  simple-type
  uncomplicated
artery occlusion
artery stenosis
articulate speech
articulation
  addition
  deviant
  distortion
  manner of
  omission
  place of
  point of
  secondary
  speech
articulation curve
articulation disorder
  developmental
  functional
  organic
articulation error
  phonemic
  phonetic
articulation index
articulation programming
articulation test (see also *test*)
  deep
  diagnostic
  screening
articulators
articulatory apraxia
articulatory basis
articulatory disorder
articulatory output

articulatory phonetics
articulatory slowness
articulatory tic
artificial ear
Artificial Intelligence in Medicine
(AIM)
artificial larynx
electrical
electronic
pneumatic
reed
artificial mastoid
"artillery" (re: drug equipment)
aryepiglottic folds
aryepiglottic muscle
arytenoid cartilages
arytenoid muscle
arytenoideus obliquus
arytenoideus transversus
AS (antisocial)
AS (anxiety sensitivity)
AS (anxiety state)
ASA (aspirin)
as a general rule
A Sales Potential Inventory for Real
Estate (ASPIRE)
as desired (ad lib)
as necessary (p.r.n.)
as soon as possible (ASAP)
ASAP (American Society for Adolescent Psychiatry)
ASAP (as soon as possible)
asaphia
asapholalia
ASB (Anxiety Scale for the Blind)
ASCA (Anxiety Scales for Children
and Adults)
ascending pitch break
ascending technique
ascertainment, method of
asceticism
ASCH (American Society of
Clinical Hypnosis)

ASDA (American Sleep Disorders
Association)
ASDC (Association of Sleep
Disorders Centers)
asemasia
asemia graphica
asemia mimica
asemia verbalis
ASHA (American Speech-Language-
Hearing Association)
"ashes" (cannabis)
ASI (Addiction Severity Index)
ASI (Anxiety Sensitivity Index)
ASI (anxiety status inventory)
A-SICD (Adapted Sequenced
Inventory of Communication
Development)
ASIQ (Adult Suicidal Ideation
Questionnaire)
ASL (American Sign Language)
asocial acting out
asociality
asocial personality
asocial psychopathic personality
ASP (antisocial personality)
aspartate
aspect (pl. aspects)
executive
integrative
linguistic
speech
ASPECT (Ackerman-Schoendorf
Scales for Parent Evaluation of
Custody)
Asperger syndrome
aspermia, psychogenic (PA)
asphyctic syndrome
aspirate consonant
aspirated sounds
aspiration
aspirations, level of
ASPIRE (A Sales Potential Inventory
for Real Estate)

aspirin (ASA)
aspirin, phenacetin, caffeine tablets
(A.P.C.)
ASQ (Anxiety Scale Questionnaire)
ASQ (Attitude to School Questionnaire)
ASRT (The Anomalous Sentences
Repetition Test)
assaultative behavior
assaulter, serial
assaultive acts
assaultive behavior
assay (see *test*)
assembly
object (OA) (subtest)
picture
assertive behavior
assertive therapy
systematized (SAT)
systemic (SAT)
assertiveness skills
assertiveness training
Assessing Specific Competencies
Assessing Specific Employment Skill
Competencies
assessment (see *test*)
behavior-oriented
cultural
disorganized speech
environmental
functional
neurophysiological
neuropsychological
personality
quality of life rehabilitation
quantified cognitive
specialized language
written language
assessment battery (see *test*)
Assessment in Mathematics
assessment inventory (see *test*)
Assessment Link Between Phonology and Articulation

assessment of affect
Assessment of Basic Competencies
Assessment of Career Decision Making
(ACDM)
Assessment of Career Development
(ACT)
Assessment of Chemical Health Inventory
Assessment of Children's Language
Comprehension (ACLC)
Assessment of Conceptual Organization
(ACO)
Assessment of Core Goals (ACG)
Assessment of Intelligibility of Dysarthric
Speech
Assessment of Phonological Processes,
Revised (APP-R)
Assessment of Suicide Potential
Assessment Program of Early Learning
Levels (APELL)
assessment questionnaire (see *test*)
assessment scale (see *test*)
assigned sex
assimilated nasality
assimilating information
assimilation
double
information
progressive
reciprocal
regressive
velar
vowel
assimilation rules
assistant, psychiatric (PA)
assisted suicide
association (pl. associations) (see
also *association, professional*)
auditory-vocal
characteristic
clang
direct
etiological
free

association *(cont.)*
  frequency encountered
  loose
  looseness of
  loosening of (LOA)
  phoneme/grapheme
  sound-symbol
  tangential
  temporal
  word
association, professional (also called
  academy, board, center, college,
  conference, council, foundation,
  institute, organization, registry, or
  society)
  Acoustic Society of America
  Alexander Graham Bell Association for the Deaf
  American Academy of Audiology
  American Academy of Otolaryngology
  American Academy of Private Practice in Speech Pathology and Audiology
  American Association for Marriage and Family Therapy (AAMFT)
  American Association of Chairmen of Departments of Psychiatry (AACDP)
  American Association of Directors of Psychiatric Residency Training (AADPRT)
  American Association of Psychiatric Administrators (AAPA)
  American Association of Teachers of Spanish and Portuguese National Spanish Examinations
  American Association on Mental Deficiency (AAMD)
  American Auditory Society
  American Board of Family Practice (ABFP)

association, professional *(cont.)*
  American Board of Psychiatry and Neurology (ABPN)
  American College of Neuropsychiatrists (ACN)
  American College of Physicians (ACP)
  American Council on Education (ACE)
  American Dialect Society
  American Group Psychotherapy Association (AGPA)
  American Health Information Management Association (AHIMA)
  American Hearing Research Foundation
  American Medical Association (AMA)
  American Medical Society on Alcohol and Other Drug Dependencies (AMSAODD)
  American National Standards Institute (ANSI)
  American Nurses Association (ANA)
  American Occupational Therapy Association (AOTA)
  American Orthopsychiatric Association (AOA)
  American Psychiatric Association (APA)
  American Psychoanalytic Association (APA)
  American Psychological Association (APA)
  American Psychological Society (APS)
  American Psychopathological Association (APA)
  American Psychosomatic Society (APS)

association *(cont.)*
 American Sleep Disorders Association (ASDA)
 American Society for Adolescent Psychiatry (ASAP)
 American Society of Clinical Hypnosis (ASCH)
 American Society for Deaf Children
 American Speech-Language-Hearing Association (ASHA)
 American Tinnitus Association
 Association for Advancement of Behavior Therapy (AABT)
 Association for Persons with Severe Handicaps
 Association for Physical and Mental Rehabilitation (APMR)
 Association for Research in Nervous and Mental Disease (ARNMD)
 Association for Research in Otolaryngology
 Association for the Advancement of Gestalt Therapy (AAGT)
 Association of Academic Psychiatry (AAP)
 Association of Departments of Family Medicine (ADFM)
 Association of Gay and Lesbian Psychiatrists (AGLP)
 Association of Mental Health Clergy (AMHC)
 Association of Sleep Disorders Centers (ASDC)
 British Society of Audiology
 Canadian Association of Speech-Language Pathologists & Audiologists
 Canadian Association of the Deaf
 Center for Mental Health Services

association *(cont.)*
 Center for Stress and Anxiety Disorders
 Conference of Educational Administrators Serving the Deaf
 Convention for American Instructors of the Deaf
 Council for Exceptional Children
 Deafness & Rehabilitation Association
 Deafness Research Foundation
 Ear Foundation
 Educational Audiology Association
 Helen Keller National Center for Deaf-Blind Youths & Adults
 International Association for the Study of Pain (IASP)
 International Hearing Society
 International Phonetic Association
 International Society for General Semantics
 International Society for the Study of Dissociation
 International Society for Traumatic Stress Studies
 International Society for the Study of Dissociation
 International Society for Traumatic Stress Studies
 Linguistic Society of America
 Mental Health Association
 National Association for the Deaf
 National Association for the Visually Handicapped
 National Association of Social Workers (NASW)
 National Association of Veterans Affairs Chiefs of Psychiatry (NAVACP)
 National Board of Certification of Hearing Instrument Sciences

association *(cont.)*
   National Captioning Institute
   National Center for Health
      Statistics (NCHS)
   National Center for Law &
      Deafness
   National Center on Employment
      of the Deaf
   National Council of Community
      Mental Health Centers
      (NCCMHC)
   National Cued Speech Associ-
      ation
   National Depressive and Manic
      Depressive Association
      (NDMDA)
   National Foundation for Chil-
      dren's Hearing Education &
      Research
   National Hearing Aid Society
   National Information Center for
      Children & Youth with Dis-
      abilities
   National Information Center on
      Deafness
   National Institute of Alcohol
      Abuse and Alcoholism
   National Institute of Drug Abuse
   National Institute of Mental
      Health (NIMH)
   National Institute of Neurological
      and Communicative Disorders
      and Stroke (NINCDS)
   National Institute on Aging (NIA)
   National Institute on Alcohol
      Abuse and Alcoholism
      (NIAAA)
   National Institute on Deafness &
      Other Communication Dis-
      orders
   National Institute on Drug Abuse
      (NIDA)

association *(cont.)*
   National Mental Health Associ-
      ation (NMHA)
   National Multiple Sclerosis
      Society (NMSS)
   National Student Speech-Lan-
      guage-Hearing Association
   National Technical Institute for
      the Deaf
   Registry of Interpreters for the
      Deaf
   Society for Psychotherapy
      Research (SPR)
   Society of Teachers of Family
      Medicine (STFM)
Association Adjustment Inventory
association area
association characteristics
association cortex
Association for Advancement of
   Behavior Therapy (AABT)
Association for the Advancement of
   Gestalt Therapy (AAGT)
Association for Physical and Mental
   Rehabilitation (APMR)
Association for Research in Nervous
   and Mental Disease (ARNMD)
association learning
association mechanism
association neurosis
Association of Academic Psychiatry
   (AAP)
Association of Departments of
   Family Medicine (ADFM)
Association of Gay and Lesbian
   Psychiatrists (AGLP)
Association of Mental Health Clergy
   (AMHC)
Association of Sleep Disorders
   Centers (ASDC)
association of sounds and symbols
associative aphasia

associative visual agnosia
assonance
astasia-abasia, hysterical
astereocognosy
astereognosis
asteric seizure
asterixis
asthenia
 neurocirculatory
 psychogenic
asthenic neurosis
asthenic personality
asthenic reaction
asthenophobia
astomia
astraphobia
astrapophobia
astrocytic gliosis
astrophobia
astrotraveling
asyllabia
asymbolia
asymmetrical amnesia
asymmetry
 abnormal
 amplitude
 facial
 interhemispheric
 reflex
 skull
asymptomatic seizure
asyndesis
asynergia
asynergic
asynergy
AT (Activities Therapist)
atactic agraphia
atactic ataxia
atactica, agraphia
ataractic drug
ataraxia
ataraxic

ataraxy
ataxia
 absent
 alcoholic
 appendicular
 Briquet
 Broca
 Bruns
 cerebellar
 crural
 equilibratory
 hysterical
 intrapsychic
 ipsilateral cerebellar
 kinesigenic
 locomotor
 mild
 moderate
 moral
 psychogenic
 sensory
 severe
ataxia conversion
ataxiamnesic
ataxiaphasia
ataxic amimia
ataxic aphasia
ataxic cerebral palsy (CP)
ataxic dysarthria
ataxic gait
ataxic speech
ataxiophobia
ataxophobia
ATDP (Attitudes Toward Disabled
 Persons)
atelophobia
atephobia
atherosclerosis, cerebral
atherosclerotic heart disease
athetoid cerebral palsy (CP)
athetoid movements
athetosic idiocy

athetosis
Athletic Motivation Inventory (AMI)
ATMS (Attitudes Toward Main-
    streaming Scale)
"atom bomb" (cannabis and heroin)
atomistic psychology
atonia
atonic absence seizure
atonic cerebral palsy (CP)
atoxic speech
ATR (Activities Therapist, Regis-
    tered)
atresia
    aural
    laryngeal
    oral
atrophic dementia
atrophy
    brain
    cerebral
    frontotemporal brain
    structural
ATS, A.T.S. (anxiety tension state)
"atshitshi" (cannabis)
attachment
    Bowlby theory of
    mother-infant
    object
    oscillations of
    selective
    social
    suffocating
    symbiotic
    theory of
    unstable
attachment/commitment, emotional
attachment disorder
attachment figures
attachment-separation disorder
attack
    acute anxiety (AAA)
    anxiety

attack *(cont.)*
    character
    dream anxiety (nightmare)
    glottal
    limited-symptom
    nocturnal panic
    panic
    physical
    psychotic
    rage
    refreshing sleep
    schizophreniform
    sleep
    transient ischemic
    uncontrollable sleep
    vocal
    word
attacker role
attainment, emotional
attempt
    failed suicide
    history of suicide
    reconciliation
    risk of suicide
    suicide or suicidal (SA)
attend to task
attention
    auditory
    center of
    disturbance in
    fix and focus
    focus of
    focus of clinical
    heightened
    need for constant
    raptus of
    state of heightened
attentional ability
attentional control
attentional set of disturbances
attentional skills
attention and concentration

attentional
attention-deficit disorder (A DD)
Attention Deficit Disorder Behavior
Rating Scales (ADDBRS)
Attention Deficit Disorders Evaluation Scale (ADDES)
attention-deficit hyperactivity
disorder (ADHD)
combined-type
predominantly hyperactive-
impulsive
predominantly inattentive-type
attention-seeking behavior
attention shift ability
attention skills
attention span
attention to sounds
attentive
attenuation, intra-aural
attitude
categorical
complacent
cultural
do-not-care
gender-based
hyperdefensive
inappropriate
inflexible
over-dependent
primary oppositional
rigid
self-centered
sexual
attitude inventory (see *test*)
attitude questionnaire (see *test*)
attitude reassessment
attitude restructuring
attitude scale (see *test*)
attitude survey (see *test*)
Attitude Survey Program for Business and Industry
Attitude to School Questionnaire
(ASQ)

Attitudes Toward Disabled Persons
(ATDP)
Attitudes Toward Mainstreaming
Scale (ATMS)
attonita
amentia
melancholia
attributable risk
attribute-entity
Attributional Style Questionnaire
atypical absence seizure
atypical affective disorder
atypical bipolar disorder
atypical childhood psychosis
atypical clefts
atypical delusional experience
atypical depressive disorder
atypical depressive psychosis
atypical features
atypical manic disorder
atypical manic psychosis
atypical schizophrenia
atypical somatoform disorder
audiation
audibility threshold
audible blocking in speech
audible field
audible pressure
audible range
audible reaction time
audible speech blocking
audiogenic seizure
audiological evaluation
audiologist
audiology
clinical
educational
experimental
geriatric
pediatric
rehabilitative
audiometer (see *audiometry*)

audiometric tests
audiometric zero
audiometry
  auditory brainstem response
    (ABR)
  automatic
  average evoked response (AERA)
  behavioral observation (BOA)
  Békésy
  brain stem evoked response
    (BSER)
  brief tone (BTA)
  cardiac evoked response (CERA)
  conditioned orientation reflex
    (COR)
  crib-o-gram
  delayed feedback (DFA)
  diagnostic
  electric response (ERA)
  electrocochleography (ECoG,
    ECochG)
  electrodermal (EDA)
  electrodermal response test
    (EDRA)
  electrophysiologic
  evoked response (ERA)
  galvanic skin response (GSRA)
  group
  high-frequency (HF)
  identification
  industrial
  limited range
  live voice
  monitoring
  narrow range
  neonatal auditory response cradle
  play
  psychogalvanic skin response
  pure-tone (AC or BC)
  screening
  speech
  speech discrimination

audiometry *(cont.)*
  speech reception
  tangible reinforcement operant
    conditioning (TROCA)
  visual reinforcement
  wide range
audition, central
auditory abilities
auditory acuity
auditory adaption
auditory agnosia
  generalized
  selective
  verbal
auditory alexia
auditory amnesia
Auditory Analysis Test
auditory aphasia
auditory area
auditory attention
auditory aura
auditory brain stem response (ABR)
  audiometry
auditory canal
auditory closure
auditory comprehension of language
auditory cortex
auditory cue
auditory differentiation
Auditory Discrimination and
  Attention Test
auditory disorder
auditory event-related potential
auditory evoked potential (AEP),
  brain stem (BAEP)
auditory evoked response, brain
  stem (BAER)
auditory fatigue
auditory feedback
  delayed (DAF)
  electronic
auditory flutter

auditory flutter fusion
auditory function
auditory hallucinations
auditory illusions
auditory imperception
auditory localization
auditory meatus
  external
  internal
auditory memory span
auditory method
auditory neglect
auditory nerve (cranial nerve VIII)
auditory oculogyric reflex
auditory pathways
auditory pattern
auditory perception
auditory phonetics
auditory physiology
Auditory Pointing Test
auditory processing of language
auditory recall
auditory reflex
auditory response cradle audiometry
auditory screening test
auditory seizure
auditory sensory modality
auditory sequencing
auditory shock
auditory skills
auditory stimulation
auditory stimulus
auditory storage
auditory symptom
auditory synthesis
auditory system
auditory teeth
Auditory Test W-22
Auditory Test W-1/W-2
auditory threshold
auditory trainer
  desk-type
  frequency-modulation

auditory trainer *(cont.)*
  hard-wire
  loop-induction
auditory training units
auditory tube
auditory-verbal dysgnosia
auditory-vocal association
augmentative communication
AUI (Alcohol Use Inventory)
aulophobia
"Aunt Hazel" (heroin)
"Aunt Mary" (cannabis)
aura
  auditory
  déjà vu
  epigastric
  epileptic
  gustatory
  hysterical
  intellectual
  jamais vu
  kinesthetic
  migraine
  motor
  olfactory
  reminiscent
  sensory
  status
  visual
aura hysterica
aural atresia
aural pathology
aural rehabilitation
  combined
  lipreading
  simultaneous
  speech reading
aura procursiva
auropalpebral reflex (APR)
aurophobia
auroraphobia
Austin Spanish Articulation Test
authoritarianism

authoritarian personality
authority figure
authority principle
autism
  akinetic
  childhood
  infantile
  primary
  secondary
  semantics of
Autism Screening Instrument for
  Educational Planning
Autistic Behavior Composite
  Checklist and Profile
autistic disorder
autistic fantasy
autistic proband
autistic thinking
autobiographical information
autochthonous idea
autoclitic operant
autoerogenous
autoerotic
autoeroticism
autoerotism
autogenic training
autogenous depression
autognosis
autognostic
autohypnosis
autohypnotic
autohypnotism
auto-immune disease
autokinesis
autokinetic effect
automania
Automated Child/Adolescent Social
  History
Automated Multitest Laboratory
  (AML)
automatic audiometry
automatic behavior

automatic epilepsy
automatic gain control
automatic language
automatic phrase level
automatic psychological process
automatic speech
automatic volume control (AVC)
automatism
  ambulatory
  chewing
  command
  epileptic
  facial expression
  gestural
  ictal
  mumbling
  swallowing
automnesia
automysophobia
autonomic activity
autonomic activity-reactivity
autonomic arousal
autonomic conversion reaction
autonomic denervation
autonomic disorder
autonomic dysfunction
autonomic dysnomia
autonomic hyperactivity
autonomic hyperarousal
autonomic hyperreflexia
autonomic hyperventilation
autonomic nervous system (ANS)
autonomic neuropathy
autonomic response
autonomic signs
autonomous psychotherapy
autonomy, loss of
autonomy scale
autophagia
autophagic
autophagy
autophilia

autophobia
autophonia
autophonomania
autoplastic change
autoplasty
autopsy, brain
autopsychosis
autopunition
autosexualism
autosomal dominant pattern
autosomatognosis
autosomatognostic
autosuggestibility
autosuggestion
autosynnoia
autotherapy
autotopagnosia agnosia
auxiliary ego
auxiliary therapist
auxiliary verb
AVC (automatic volume control)
Avellis syndrome
average evoked response audiometry
    (AERA)
average SSPL (saturation sound
    pressure level) 90 output, HF
    (high-frequency)
aversion-covert conditioning
aversion disorder
    acquired-type sexual
    generalized-type sexual
    lifelong-type sexual
    sexual
    situational-type sexual
aversion, occasional sexual
aversion therapy
aversive conditioning
aversive control
aversive drive
aversive incentive
aversive stimulus
aviators' effort syndrome

avoidance-avoidance conflict
avoidance behavior
avoidance learning
avoidance of speech dysfluencies
avoidance pattern
avoidance speaking
avoidance syndrome
avoidant-attached behavior
avoidant behavior
avoidant personality disorder
avolition
awake, alert, and oriented (AAO)
awake state
awareness
    conscious
    emotional
    environmental
    heightened
    interoceptive
    lack of
    lack of interoceptive
    lapse of
    leisure
    phonemic
    postural
    sensory (SA)
    state of heightened
    subconscious
awareness threshold
awkwardness, social
AWOL (absent without leave)
    ideation
axonal idiocy
axonapraxia
axon degeneration
axon flare
axon loss
axonometer
axonopathy
axon terminal
Aztec idiocy

B, b

B (behavior; behavioral)
babbling
  non-reduplicated
  reduplicated
  social
"babe" (drug used for detoxification)
Babinski reflex
Babinski sign
"baby" (cannabis)
"baby bhang" (cannabis)
"baby habit" (re: drug use)
"babysit" (re: drug use)
"Baby T" (crack)
Bachelor of Social Work (BSW)
bacillophobia
backache, psychogenic
"backbreakers" (lysergic acid diethylamide and strychnine)
"back door" (re: drug equipment)
back-formation word
background activity
background noise
backing to velars
"backjack" (re: opium use)
back phoneme
backslide
backsliding

"back to back" (re: heroin and crack use)
"backtrack" (re: drug injection)
"backup" (re: drug injection)
back vowel
backward coarticulation
backward masking
"backwards" (barbiturate)
backwards from 100 test, count
bacterial meningitis
bacteriophobia
"bad" (crack)
"bad bundle" (re: poor quality heroin)
bad conduct discharge (BCD)
"bad go" (re: drug reaction)
"bad seed" (cannabis; heroin;
  mescaline)
"bad trip" (re: hallucinogens)
BAEP (brain stem auditory evoked
  potential)
BAER (brain stem auditory evoked
  response)
baffle effect, body (hearing aid)
BaFPE (Bay Area Functional Performance Evaluation), Second Edition
"bag" (re: drug container)
"bag bride" (re: crack user)
"bagging" (re: inhalant use)

"bag lady"
"bag man" (re: drug dealing)
bailout behavior
balance (pl. balances)
  acid-base
  core body
  dynamic ambulatory
  dynamic standing
  homeostatic
  impaired
  sitting
  spacial
  standing
balance mechanism
balanced words, phonetically (PB
  words)
"bale" (cannabis)
"ball" (crack)
"balling" (re: cocaine concealment)
ballistic movement
ballistomania
ballistophobia
"balloon" (re: heroin supplier)
"ballot" (heroin)
Balthazar Scales for Adaptive
  Behavior I: Scales of Functional
  Independence
Balthazar Scales for Adaptive
  Behavior II: Scales of Social
  Adaptation
"bam" (amphetamine; barbiturate)
"Bambalacha" (cannabis)
"bambs" (barbiturate)
band (pl. bands), vocal
band analyzer, octave
band frequency
band-like headache
B&O (belladonna and opium)
band-pass filter
band spectrum
bandwidth
"bang" (re: drug injection; inhalant)

"bank bandit pills" (barbiturate)
"bank deposit pills" (barbiturate)
Bankson-Bernthal Test of Phonology
  (BBTOP)
Bankson Language Screening Test
  (BLST)
Bankson Language Test-2 (BLT-2)
BAP (Behavior Activity Profile)
BAP (Behavioral Assessment of Pain
  Questionnaire)
"bar" (cannabis)
"Barb" (barbiturate)
barbaralalia
Barber Scales of Self-Regard for
  Preschool Children
"Barbies" (barbiturate)
barbiturate (street names)
  backwards
  bam
  bambs
  bank bandit pills
  bank deposit pills
  Barb
  Barbies
  barbs
  beans
  black beauties
  block busters
  blue
  blue bullets
  blue dolls
  blue heavens
  blue tips
  busters
  candy
  chorals
  Christmas rolls
  coral
  courage pills
  disco biscuits
  dolls
  downers

barbiturate *(cont.)*
  downie
  drowsy high
  fender benders
  gangster pills
  G.B.
  golf balls
  goofballs
  goofers
  gorilla pills
  green frog
  idiot pills
  in-betweens
  jellies
  joy juice
  King Kong pills
  lay back
  lib (Librium)
  little bomb
  love drug
  luding out
  luds
  M&M
  marshmallow reds
  Mexican reds
  Mickey
  Mickey Finn
  Mighty Joe Young
  mother's little helper
  nemmies
  nimbies
  peanuts
  peth
  purple hearts
  Q
  quad
  quas
  red and blue
  red bullets
  red devil
  seggy
  sleeper

barbiturate *(cont.)*
  sleeping pills
  softballs
  sopers
  stoppers
  strawberries
  stumbler
  tooles
  tooties
  tranq
  tuie
  Uncle Milty
  ups and downs
  yellow jackets
  yellows
"barbs" (barbiturate; cocaine)
Barclay Classroom Climate Inventory (BCCI)
Barclay Learning Needs Assessment Inventory (BLNAI)
Bardet-Biedl syndrome
"barf tea" (mescaline)
barophobia
barotrauma
Barranquilla Rapid Survey Intelligence Test (BARSIT)
"barrels" (lysergic acid diethylamide)
barrenness, inner
barrier (pl. barriers)
  blood-brain
  communication
  language
barriers to interventions
Barron-Welsh Art Scale (BWAS)
Barry Five Slate System
Barthel ADL Index
BARSIT (Barranquilla Rapid Survey Intelligence Test)
BAS (British Ability Scales: Spelling Scale)
BASA (Boston Assessment of Severe Aphasia)

basal age
basal fluency
basal ganglia
basal pitch
BASE (Brief Aphasia Screening
　Examination)
"base" (cocaine; crack)
"baseball" (crack)
base component
"base crazies" (re: crack acquisition)
basedowian insanity
"base head" (re: freebaser)
base impulse
baseline (BL)
baseline monitoring
baseline symptoms
base rule
base structure
base word
"bash" (cannabis)
Basic Achievement Skills Individual
　Screener
basic anxiety
Basic Concept Inventory
Basic Educational Skills Test
Basic Inventory of Natural Language
Basic Language Concepts Test
Basic Occupational Literacy Test
Basic Personality Inventory (BPI)
Basic Reading Inventory, Fifth Edition
　(BRI)
Basic School Skills Inventory (BSSI)—
　Diagnostic
Basic School Skills Inventory (BSSI)—
　Screen
Basic Screening and Referral Form for
　Children with Suspected Learning
　and Behavioral Disabilities
Basic Skills Assessment Program
basilar insufficiency
basilar membrane
basilar migraine headache

basilect
basophobia
basophobic
"basuco" (cigarette laced with coca
　paste; cocaine)
Batelle Developmental Inventory
bathophobia
bathmophobia
bathroom privileges (BRP)
"bathtub speed" (methcathinone)
batophobia
batrachophobia
"batt" (re: drug equipment)
battacca bat
Battelle Developmental Inventory
battered child syndrome
battery (pl. batteries) (see also test)
"battery acid" (lysergic acid diethyl-
　amide)
battery clusters, inner
battery of tests, neuropsychologic
battle fatigue
battle neurosis
"batu" (smokable methamphetamine)
Bay Area Functional Performance
　Evaluation (BaFPE), Second
　Edition
Bayley Scales of Infant Development
"bazooka" (cocaine; crack)
"bazulco" (cocaine)
BBT (Bingham Button Test)
BBTOP (Bankson-Bernthal Test of
　Phonology)
BC (behavior control)
BC (bone conduction)
BCCI (Barclay Classroom Climate
　Inventory)
BCR (behavior control room)
BCRS (Brief Cognitive Rating Scale)
BD (behavior disorder)
BDAC (Bureau of Drug Abuse
　Control)

BDAE (Boston Diagnostic Aphasia
  Examination)
BDD (body dysmorphic disorder)
BDI (Beck Depression Inventory)
BDID (bystander dominates initial
  dominant)
BDIS (Behavior Disorders
  Identification Scale)
BDRS (Blessed Dementia Rating
  Scale)
BEAM (brain electrical activity map)
"beam me up Scottie" (crack dipped
  in phencyclidine)
"beamer" or "beemer" (crack user)
"beans" (amphetamine sulfate;
  barbiturate; mescaline)
Beard disease
Beard, George M. (1839-1883)
"beast" (heroin; lysergic acid diethylamide)
"beat artist" (dealer of bogus drugs)
"beat vials" (re: fake crack)
"beautiful boulders" (crack)
"Bebe" (crack)
Beck Depression Inventory (BDI)
Beck Hopelessness Scale (BHS)
Beck Questionnaire
Beckwith-Wiedeman syndrome
beclouded dementia
"bedbugs" (fellow drug addicts)
bed crisis
bedlam
bedpartners
bedridden
Bedside Evaluation and Screening
  Test of Aphasia
bedtime (BT; h.s.)
bed wetter, bed-wetting
"beemers" or "beamers" (crack)
Beers, Clifford W. (1876-1943)
Beery-Buktinica Developmental Test
  of Visual Motor Integration

Beery Picture Vocabulary Test (PVT)
  and Beery Picture Vocabulary
  Screening (PVS) Series
before (a)
before meals (a.c.)
before noon (A.M., AM, a.m.)
beh. (behavior; behaviorism)
behavior (pl. behaviors)
  aberrant
  abusive vocal
  acceptable
  accident prone
  acting-out
  activity and
  adaptive
  addictive
  adient
  adolescent
  adolescent antisocial
  adolescent cross-gender
  adolescent risk-taking
  adult antisocial
  adult criminal
  adult cross-gender
  adultomorphic
  age-appropriate
  age-level
  aggressive
  agitated
  agnostic
  aimless
  alleviating aggressive
  ambient
  amoral
  amotivated
  angry
  anticipatory
  antisocial
  appetitive
  appropriate
  apraxic
  arrogant

behavior *(cont.)*
  assaultative
  assertive
  attention-seeking
  automatic
  aversive
  avoidance
  avoidant
  avoidant attached
  bad
  bailout
  binge-eating
  binge-eating/purging
  bizarre
  borderline
  catatonic
  catatonic motor
  ceremonial
  child
  child antisocial
  childhood cross-gender
  choice
  clinging
  compensatory
  competitive
  complex motor
  compulsive
  compulsive drug-taking
  contractual
  countertransference
  courtship
  cooperative
  covert
  criminal
  cross-dressing
  cunning and hiding
  de-escalating aggressive
  defensive
  defiant
  delusional
  demanding
  dementia-related

behavior *(cont.)*
  dependent
  direct self-destructive (DSDB)
  disinhibited
  disobedient
  disorganized
  disruptive
  disturbed eating
  dominant-subordinate
  drinking
  driven motor
  driving (automobile)
  drug-seeking
  dysarthric
  dyssocial
  eccentric
  ego-dystonic
  ego-syntonic
  empathic
  envious
  eroticized
  erratic
  ethical
  ethnic relational (ERB)
  evasive
  excitable
  exhibitionistic
  exploratory
  explosive
  extramarital
  feeding
  felony
  fidgeting
  flirtatious
  gambling
  goal-directed
  grossly disorganized
  hair-pulling
  hallucinatory
  haughty
  head-banging
  health

behavior *(cont.)*
help-seeking
helping
high-risk
homicidal
hostile
hyperactive
hyperactive-impulsive combined
illness
imitative
impulsive
inappropriate
inattentive
incoherent
indirect self-destructive (ISDB)
incompatible
infant
infantile
ingratiating
initiation of goal-directed
intense sexual
interictal
intermittent explosive
interpersonal
intimidating
irrational
irresponsible work
isolative
lawful
leadership
learned dysfunctional
limit-testing
maladaptive
manipulative
masochistic sexual
mass
maternal
mercurial
mischievous
modeled
moral
motor

behavior *(cont.)*
murderous predation
negative
negativistic
nonfunctional and repetitive motor
nonfunctional motor
nonparaphilic
nonverbal
normative
obedient
obsessive
odd
on-task
operant
out-of-control
overt
pacing
pain
paranoid
paraphiliac
parasuicidal
passive-aggressive
paternal
pathological
pattern of antisocial
peculiar
pedophilic
phobic
pressured
promiscuous sexual
provocative
psychomotor
purposeful
reckless
regressive
rehabilitation
REM sleep
repetitive
repetitive checking
repetitive pattern of
repetitive restricted
repressive

behavior *(cont.)*
 respondent
 restless
 risk-taking
 ritualistic
 seductive
 self-damaging
 self-defeating
 self-destructive
 self-dramatizing
 self-injurious (SIB)
 self-mutilating
 self-punishing
 self-stimulatory
 semipurposeful
 sensory/motor
 sex-role
 sexual
 sexually addictive
 sexually arousing
 sexually seductive
 sexual predation
 "sissyish"
 sleepwalking
 social
 social phobic-like
 social stereotypical
 spatial
 speech and language
 splitting
 stalking
 stereotyped
 stereotyped restricted
 stereotypic
 stereotypical
 stereotypic sex-role
 struggle
 subliminal
 submissive
 substance-seeking
 substituting
 sucking

behavior *(cont.)*
 suicidal
 superstitious
 target
 terminal
 terminal achievement
 terrorism
 threatening
 ticlike
 tomboy
 trancelike
 transference
 unacceptable
 uncued
 unethical
 unexpected
 unlawful
 unpurposeful
 unusual
 variable
 verbal
 violent
 voyeuristic
 voyeuristic sexual
 wild
Behavior Activity Profile (BAP)
behavioral (B)
Behavioral Academic Self-Esteem
behavioral analysis
Behavioral Assessment of Pain
 Questionnaire (BAP; P-BAP)
behavioral avoidance tests (BATs) for
 OCD (obsessive-compulsive
 disorder)
behavioral changes, maladaptive
Behavioral Checklist
behavioral criterion
Behavioral Deviancy Profile
behavioral disorganization in schizophrenia
behavioral disturbance
behavioral dyscontrol

behavioral dysfunction
behavioral flexibility
behavioral genetics
behavioral hearing tests
Behavioral Inattention Test (BIT)
behaviorally oriented assessment
behavioral management
behavioral manifestation
behavioral mapping
behavioral marital therapy (BMT)
behavioral medicine
behavioral memory
behavioral monitoring
    distortion of inferential
    exaggeration of inferential
behavioral neurobiology
behavioral neurology
behavioral objective
behavioral observation audiometry
    (BOA)
Behavioral Observation Scale for
    Autism
behavioral outbursts
behavioral psychotherapy
behavioral reaction brain syndrome
behavioral research orientation
behavioral sciences
behavioral semantics
behavioral set of disturbances
behavioral sensitization
behavioral syndrome
behavior-altering substance
behavioral transgressions
behavioral undercontrol
behavior characteristics, child (CBC)
behavior checklist (see *test*)
behavior control (BC)
behavior control room (BCR)
Behavior Disorders Identification
    Scale (BDIS)
behavior disorders of childhood
behavior disturbance

Behavior Evaluation Scale–2 (BES-2)
behavior inventory (see *test*)
behaviorism (beh.)
behaviorist
behavioristic psychology
behavior modification (B-mod)
    program
behavior pattern
Behavior Problem Checklist (BPC),
    Revised
Behavior Rating Instrument for
    Autistic and Other Atypical
    Children
Behavior Rating Profile, Second
    Edition (BRP-2)
behavior reaction
behavior role
behavior therapy
Behaviour Assessment Battery, 2nd
    Edition
behind-the-ear hearing aid
"behind the scale" (re: cocaine value)
"beiging" (re: cocaine purity)
Békésy audiometer
Békésy audiometry
bel (logarithmic unit)
belief
    cultural
    culture-bound
    delusional
    deviant
    erroneous
    exaggerated
    false
    fixed
    internal world of
    loss of
    odd
    shared delusional
    sustained
    traditional
    true

belief *(cont.)*
  unreasonable
  unshakable
belief system, paranoid
belittling
"belladonna" (phencyclidine)
belladonna and opium (B&O)
Bell disease
belle indifférence (also, la belle indif-
  férence)
Bellevue Index of Depression
belligerent
Bell mania
Bell Object Relations-Reality Testing
  Inventory
Bell palsy
Bell paralysis
Bell phenomenon
bell-shaped curve
Bell Visible Speech
belonephobia
"belt" (intoxication)
"Belushi" (cocaine and heroin)
"Belyando spruce" (cannabis)
Bem Sex-Role Inventory
benchmarks
Bender Visual Gestalt drawings
Bender Visual-Motor Gestalt Test
  (BVMGT)
Bender Visual Retention Test
"bender" (drug party)
Bennett Mechanical Comprehension
  Test
"bennies" (amphetamine sulfate)
Benson-Geschwind classification of
  aphasia
Benton Revised Visual Retention Test
Benton Visual Retention Test (BVRT)
bent-over neck
bent posture
"Benz" (amphetamine)

benzamide
benzocaine (street names)
  flat chunks
  potato chips
benzodiazepine-GABA-receptor
  complex
benzodiazepine receptor binding
benzoylecgonine
berate
bereavement disorder
bereavement-related depression
Bergeron disease
"Bernice" (cocaine)
"Bernie" (cocaine)
"bernie's flakes" (cocaine)
"bernie's gold dust" (cocaine)
Bernoulli law
berserk
BES-2 (Behavior Evaluation Scale–2)
bestiality (zoophilia)
beta activity
beta-adrenergic antagonist
beta-adrenergic medication
beta-adrenergic medication-induced
  postural tremor
beta-adrenergic receptor
beta-amyloid protein
beta blocker
beta-carboline
beta-endorphin
beta index
beta pattern on EEG
beta wave on EEG
bewildered
Bexley-Maudsley Automated
  Psychological Screening
Beziehungswahn, sensitizer
BFQ (Big Five Questionnaire)
BG (Bender Gestalt)
BGT (Bender Gestalt Test)
"bhang" (cannabis)

BHS (Beck Hopelessness Scale)
bias (pl. biases)
  experimenter
  evaluator
  free recall
  memory
  selection
  societal
  volunteer
BIB (brought in by)
bibliokleptomania
bibliomania
bibliophobia
bibliotherapeutic strategies
bibliotherapy
bicircadian rhythm
BICROS (bilateral contralateral
  routing of signals)
bicuspid teeth
b.i.d. (twice a day)
bidirectional selection study
Bielschowsky idiocy
bifid tongue
bifrontal headache
bifurcation
bigamist
bigamy
"big B" (1/8 kilogram of crack)
"big bag" (heroin)
"big bloke" (cocaine)
"big C" (cocaine)
"big chief" (mescaline)
"big D" (lysergic acid diethylamide)
Big Five Questionnaire (BFQ)
"big flake" (cocaine)
"big H" (heroin)
"big Harry" (heroin)
"big man" (re: drug supplier)
"big O" (opium)
"big rush" (cocaine)
bilabial area consonant placement

bilingualism
  active
  passive
Bilingual Syntax Measure (BSM) II
  Test
"Bill Blass" (crack)
"billie hoke" (cocaine)
binary principle
binaural amplification
binaural CROS (contralateral routing
  of signals)
binaural fusion
binaural hearing aid
binaural integration
binaural resynthesis
binaural separation
binaural summation
binders, breast
binding
  benzodiazepine receptor
  in vivo benzodiazepine receptor
"bindle" (re: drug quantity)
Binet age
binge and purge
binge eater
binge-eating pattern
binge-eating/purging behavior
bingeing (also binging)
Bingham Button Test (BBT)
Binswanger dementia
Binswanger disease
bioacoustics
bioavailability
bioccipital headache
biochemical anatomy
biochemical imbalance
biodynamics
bioenergetic therapy
bioequivalence
biofeedback
  EEG (electroencephalograph)
  electrodermal response (EDR)

biofeedback *(cont.)*
    electromyography
    galvanic skin response (GSR)
    temperature
biofeedback computer
biofeedback meter
biofeedback tones
biogenic amine hypothesis
Biographical Inventory Form U
biographical memory, loss of
biolinguistic language theory
biologic age
biological act
biological basis
biological causation
biological children
biological dysfunction
biological factors
biological orientation
biological parents
biological predisposition
biological sex
biologic psychiatry
biologic rhythms
biologic sign depression
biology of deceit
biophysical life change
biopsy, brain
biopsychosocial model
BIP (Canter Background Interference
    Procedure for the Bender Gestalt
    Test)
biphasic potential
bipolar affective psychosis
    atypical
    depressed
    manic
    mixed
bipolar depression
bipolar disorder
    affective
    alternating
    atypical

bipolar disorder *(cont.)*
    depressed
    manic
    mixed
bipolar I disorder
    major depressive episode
        chronic
        in full remission
        in partial remission
        mild
        moderate
        severe without psychotic features
        severe with psychotic features
        with atypical features
        with catatonic features
        with melancholic features
        with postpartum onset
        with rapid cycling
        with seasonal pattern
    manic type
        in full remission
        in partial remission
        mild
        moderate
        severe without psychotic features
        severe with psychotic features
        with catatonic features
        with postpartum onset
        with rapid cycling
    mixed type
        in full remission
        in partial remission
        mild
        moderate
        severe without psychotic features
        severe with psychotic features
        with catatonic features
        with postpartum onset
        with rapid cycling
bipolar II disorder
    depressed episode
    hypomanic episode
    major depressive episode

bipolar II disorder *(cont.)*
  chronic
  in full remission
  in partial remission
  mild
  moderate
  severe without psychotic features
  severe with psychotic features
  with atypical features
  with catatonic features
  with melancholic features
  with postpartum onset
  with rapid cycling
  with seasonal pattern
Bipolar Psychological Inventory
bipolar psychosis
birth cry
birth order
Birth to Three Assessment and
  Intervention System
Birth to Three Developmental Scale
birth trauma
birth, year of (YOB)
bisensory method
bisexuality, theory of constitutional
bisexual libido
bisexual orientation
bisyllable
BIT (Behavioral Inattention Test)
bite, closed
bite marks
bitemporal hemianopsia
biting, nail
biundulant viral encephalitis
bizarre behavior
BL (baseline)
black-and-white thinking
"black bart" (cannabis)
"black beauties" (barbiturate)
"black birds" (amphetamine)
"black bombers" (amphetamine)
Black English (Ebonics)

"black ganga" (cannabis resin)
"black gold" (cannabis)
"black gungi" (cannabis)
"black gunion" (cannabis)
"black hash" (cannabis and opium)
"black mo" (cannabis)
"black moat" (cannabis)
"black mollies" (amphetamine)
"black mote" (cannabis and honey)
blackout (pl. blackouts)
black-patch syndrome
"black pearl" (heroin)
"black pill" (opium pill)
"black rock" (crack)
"Black Russian" (cannabis; opium)
"black star" (lysergic acid diethylamide)
"black stuff" (heroin)
"black sunshine" (lysergic acid
  diethylamide)
"black tabs" (lysergic acid diethylamide)
"black tar" (heroin)
"black whack" (phencyclidine)
"blacks" (amphetamine)
Blacky Pictures, The
blade of tongue
BLADES (Bristol Language Development Scales)
"blahs," the
blame-placing (communication
  pattern)
blameworthy
"blanco" (heroin)
bland affect
"blanket" (cannabis cigarette)
"blanks" (re: low-quality drugs)
blank screen
blank stare
blasphemous thoughts
"blast" (re: cannabis use; crack use)
"blast a joint" (re: cannabis use)

"blast a roach" (re: cannabis use)
"blast a stick" (re: cannabis use)
"blasted" (re: drug influence)
blast, stoma
blend (pl. blends), consonant
blended family
blending
   auditory
   sound
blennophobia
Blessed Behavior Scale
Blessed Dementia Rating Scale (BDRS)
Blessed Information-Memory-
   Concentration Test
Bleuler, Eugen (1857-1939)
BLHI (Brief Life History Inventory)
blind, double
blindfolding (sensory bondage)
blind headache
Blind Learning Aptitude Test
blindness
   conversion
   hysterical
   object
   word
blind spot, figurative (scotoma)
blinking, eye
"blizzard" (re: cocaine smoke)
BLNAI (Barclay Learning Needs
   Assessment Inventory)
bloating
"block" (cannabis)
block
   atrioventricular
   clonic (in stuttering)
   left bundle branch
   tonic (in stuttering)
blockade
   audible speech
   emotional
   muscarine
   muscarinic receptor

blockade *(cont.)*
   nicotinic
   nicotinic receptor
   silent speech
   thought
"block busters" (barbiturate)
block design subtest
blocked speech
blocking drugs, narcotic
blocking in speech
   audible
   silent
Block Survey and SLIDE
Blom-Singer tracheoesophageal fistula
"blonde" (cannabis)
blood alcohol level
blood-brain barrier
blood disorder, psychogenic
blood drug screen
blood flow, cerebral (CBF)
blood-injection-injury type
blood level (of drug)
blood screen for drugs test
Bloods and Crips (gangs)
Bloom Analogies Test
"blotter" (cocaine; lysergic acid
   diethylamide)
"blotter acid" (lysergic acid diethylamide)
"blotter cube" (lysergic acid diethylamide)
"blow" (cocaine)
"blow a fix" (re: drug injection)
"blow a shot" (re: drug injection)
"blow a stick" (re: cannabis use)
"blow blue" (re: cocaine use)
"blowcaine" (crack diluted with
   cocaine)
"blow coke" (re: cocaine use)
"blowing smoke" (cannabis)
"blow one's roof" (re: cannabis use)
"blowout" (crack)

"blow smoke" (re: cocaine use)
"blow the vein" (re: drug injection)
"blow up" (crack cut with lidocaine)
BLST (Bankson Language Screening Test)
BLT-2 (Bankson Language Test-2)
"blue" (barbiturate; crack)
"blue acid" (lysergic acid diethylamide)
"blue angels" (amobarbital)
"blue barrels" (lysergic acid diethylamide)
"bluebirds" (amobarbital)
"blue boy" (amphetamine)
"blue bullets" (barbiturate)
"blue caps" (mescaline)
"blue chairs" (lysergic acid diethylamide)
"blue cheers" (lysergic acid diethylamide)
"blue de hue" (cannabis)
"blue devils" (amobarbital)
"blue dolls" (barbiturate)
"blue heaven" (lysergic acid diethylamide)
"blue heavens" (barbiturate)
"blue madman" (phencyclidine)
"blue microdot" (lysergic acid diethylamide)
"blue mist" (lysergic acid diethylamide)
"blue moons" (lysergic acid diethylamide)
"blues" (amobarbital; oxymorphine)
"blue sage" (cannabis)
"blue sky blond" (cannabis)
"blue tips" (barbiturate)
"blue velvet" (cough preparations with codeine)
"blue vials" (lysergic acid diethylamide)
blueness

"blunt" (cannabis inside a cigar)
blunted affect
blunting, emotional
blurring of vision
BMI (body mass index)
B-mod (behavior modification)
BMT (behavioral marital therapy)
BNDD (Bureau of Narcotics and Dangerous Drugs)
BNMSE (Brief Neuropsychological Mental Status Examination)
BOA (behavioral observation audiometry)
board
    conversation
    direct selection communication
    encoding communication
    scanning communication
board-certified psychiatrist
board-eligible psychiatrist
"boat" (phencyclidine)
"bobo" or "bo-bo" (cannabis; crack)
"bobo bush" (cannabis)
Boder Test of Reading-Spelling Patterns
bodies, intraneuronal argentophilic Pick inclusion
bodily change, sense of
bodily illusion
bodily injury, self-inflicted
bodily movement
bodily orifices, nonfunctional and repetitive picking at
body appearance
body baffle effect (hearing aid)
body balances, core
body contact-exploration maneuver
body dipping
body dissatisfaction
body dysgnosia
body dysmorphic defect
body dysmorphic disorder

body dysphoria
body dystonia
body functioning
body gestures
body hearing aid
body image
  changed
  distorted
  disturbed
  negative
Body Image and Eating Questionnaire
body-image perception
body-image recall
body language
body mass index (BMI)
body mechanics
body memory
body movements
  complex whole
  stereotyped
body odor
body orifices
"body packer" (re: cocaine or crack
  concealment)
body position
body posture
body-rocking
body shape
body size
"body stuffer" (re: crack concealment)
body swaying
body temperature, core
body tics
Boehm Test of Basic Concepts—
  Revised
"Bogart a joint" (re: cannabis use;
  refuse to share)
bogyphobia
"bohd" (cannabis; phencyclidine)
bolasterone (injectable steroid)
"Bolivian marching powder" (cocaine)
"bolo" ($50 piece of crack)

"bolt" (butyl nitrite)
bombarding (speech technique)
"bombit" (methamphetamine hydrochloride)
bond (bonding)
  emotional
  human-pet
  male
  mother-child
  parent-offspring
bondage, physical (restraint)
bone (pl. bones) (speech therapy)
  alveolar supporting
  ethmoid
  frontal
  hyoid
  lacrimal
  malar
  mandibular
  maxillary
  nasal concha
  palatine
  sphenoid
  temporal
  turbinate
  zygomatic
bone conduction (BC)
  compression
  distortional
  inertial
  pure tone
bone-conduction hearing aid
bone-conduction oscillator
bone-conduction receiver
bone-conduction threshold, pure tone
bone-conduction vibrator
"bonecrusher" (crack)
bonelet
bone marrow suppression
"bones" (crack)
"bong" (cannabis equipment)
"bonita" (heroin)

bony labyrinth
"boo" (cannabis)
"boom" (cannabis)
"boomers" (psilocybin/psilocin)
"boost" (re: drug injection; also, to
    steal)
"boost and shoot" (steal to support a
    habit)
"booster" (re: cocaine use)
"boot" (re: drug injection)
"booted" (re: drug influence)
"boot the gong" (re: cannabis use)
"boppers" (amyl nitrite)
borderline behavior
borderline intellectual functioning
borderline personality disorder (BPD)
borderline psychosis
    childhood
    prepubertal
borderline range
borderline retardation
borderline schizophrenia (BS)
borderline state
border, vermillion
boredom, tendency toward
bore hole
borrowing, linguistic
bossy
Boston Assessment of Severe Aphasia
    (BASA)
Boston Classification System
Boston Diagnostic Aphasia
    Examination (BDAE)
Boston Naming Test
Boston opium
Boston University Speech Sound
    Discrimination Test
Botel Reading Inventory
"botray" (crack)
"bottles" (amphetamine; crack vials)
botulinum neurotoxin, therapeutic
"boubou" (crack)

bouffée delirante
"boulder" (crack; $20 worth of crack)
"boulya" (crack)
bounce technique (stuttering)
"bouncing powder" (cocaine)
bound (cued) panic attacks
bound morpheme
bound pronoun
boundaries and gender
boundaries in postanalytic supervision
boundaries in psychoanalysis
boundary (p. boundaries)
    analytic
    ego
    lack of
    language
    little sense of other people's
    loose
    loss of ego
    poorly defined
    posttermination
    problems with
    role
    subsystem
boundary violations
boundless energy
bouts of insomnia
bowed vocal folds
bowel control, loss of
Bowlby's theory of attachment
"boxcar ventricles"
"boxed" (in jail)
"boy" (cocaine)
"bozo" (heroin)
BP (British Pharmacopoeia)
BPC (Behavior Problem Checklist)
BPC (British Pharmaceutical Codex)
BPD (borderline personality disorder)
B.Ph. (British Pharmacopoeia)
BPI (Basic Personality Inventory)
BPRS (brief psychiatric rating scale)
BPRS (brief psychiatric reacting scale)

Bracken Basic Concept Scale
brackets, square
bradyarthria
bradyesthesia
bradyglossia
bradykinesia
bradykinetic syndrome
bradylalia
bradylexia
bradylogia
bradyphasia
bradyphrasia
bradyphrenia
bradypsychia
bradyteleokinesis
braggadocio
brain
  architecture of
  concussion of (grades 1-3)
  glucose metabolism in
  hemangioma of the
  mapping of language areas of
brain abnormalities, structural
brain atrophy
brain autopsy
brain cell damage
brain concussion
brain contusion
brain convulsion
brain damage
brain death
brain degeneration
brain depressant
brain disease
brain disease-type organic psychosis,
  arteriosclerotic
brain dysfunction
  diffuse
  mid
  minimal (MBD)
  organic
  severe diffuse

brain electrical activity map (or mapping) (BEAM)
brain function
  integrity of
  semi-autonomous systems concept
    of
brain imaging, functional
brain infection organic psychosis
  acute
  chronic
  subacute
brain injury
  dementia due to traumatic
  traumatic (TBI)
brain involvement, subcortical
brain lesion
brain map
brain-mind dichotomy
brain neoplasm
  benign
  malignant
brain pathology
brain regions
brain spectin
brain stem auditory evoked potential
  (BAEP)
brain stem auditory evoked response
  (BAER)
brain stem evoked potential
brain stem evoked response
  audiometry (BSER)
brain stem function
brain stem reflex
brain stem response audiometry,
  auditory (ABR)
brain stem reticular formation
brain stem signs
brain stem stroke
brain stem tumor
brain syndrome
  acute organic
  behavioral reaction

brain syndrome *(cont.)*
  chronic (CBS)
  chronic alcoholic (CABS)
  neurotic reaction
  nonpsychotic
  organic (OBS)
  postcontusional
  posttraumatic
  psycho-organic
  psychotic
  senile
brain test
"brain ticklers" (amphetamine)
"brain tiredness"
brain trauma organic psychosis
  acute
  birth
  chronic
  electrical current
  subacute
  surgical
brainwashing
brake, descending pitch
branching steps in therapy
branching tree diagram
Bravais-jacksonian epilepsy
bravura
Brawner decision
break
  ascending pitch
  phonation
  pitch
break down (verb)
breakdown
  nervous
  speech
breakdown theory in stuttering
"breakdowns" ($40 crack rock sold
  for $20)
"break night" (re: pulling an all-
  nighter)
break state

breakthrough tearfulness
break with reality
breast binders
breath chewing
breathiness
breathing
  apneustic
  crescendo-decrescendo
  daytime mouth
  diaphragmatic
  opposition
breathing disorder
breathing method of esophageal
  speech
breathing-related sleep disorder
breathing speech
breathing tic
breath stream
bredouillement
Breuer, Josef (1842-1925)
"brewery" (drug-making place)
BRI (Basic Reading Inventory), Fifth
  Edition
bribe
bribery
"brick" (crack; 1 kilogram of
  cannabis)
"brick gum" (heroin)
"bridge up" (re: drug injection)
Brief Aphasia Screening Examination
  (BASE)
Brief Cognitive Rating Scale (BCRS)
Brief Drinker Profile
Brief Life History Inventory (BLHI)
Brief Neuropsychological Mental
  Status Examination (BNMSE)
brief psychiatric rating scale (BPRS)
brief psychiatric reacting scale (BPRS)
brief pulse bilateral ECT
brief pulse ECT
brief pulse unilateral ECT
brief pulse waveform

brief stimulus therapy (BST)
Brief Symptom Inventory
brief tone audiometry (BTA)
Brigham, Amariah (1798-1849)
bright normal range
Brill, A. A. (1874-1948)
"bring up" (re: drug injection)
Briquet ataxia
Briquet syndrome
Brissaud-Marie syndrome
Bristol Language Development Scales
    (BLADES)
Bristol Social Adjustment Guides
Bristowe syndrome
British Ability Scales: Spelling Scale
    (BAS)
British Pharmaceutical Codex (BPC)
British Pharmacopoeia (BP, B.Ph.)
British Stammering Association (BSA)
"britton" (mescaline)
broadcasting, thought
broad heritability
broad phonemic transcription
broad transcription
Broca amnesia
Broca aphasia
Broca area (Brodmann area 44)
Broca ataxia
"broccoli" (cannabis)
Brodmann area 41
Brodmann area 44 (Broca area)
broken words
"broker" (go-between in a drug deal)
bromidrosiphobia
bromine compound
bromism (due to bromide intoxication)
bronchial respiration
bronchus (pl. bronchi)
brontophobia
brooding compulsion
Brook Reaction Test (BRT)
brother complex

brought in by (BIB)
"brown" (cannabis; heroin)
"brown bombers" (lysergic acid
    diethylamide)
"brown crystal" (heroin)
"brown dots" (lysergic acid diethyl-
    amide)
brownian motion
"brownies" (dextroamphetamine
    sulfate)
"brown rhine" (heroin)
"browns" (amphetamine)
"brown sugar" (heroin)
BRT (Brook Reaction Test)
Bruininks-Oseretsky Standardized Test
Bruininks-Oseretsky Test of Motor
    Proficiency
Bruns ataxia
Brushfield-Wyatt disease
brusque
bruxism
bruxomania
Bryant-Schwan Design Test (BSDT)
BS (borderline schizophrenia)
BSA (British Stammering Association)
BSDT (Bryant-Schwan Design Test)
BSER (brain stem evoked response)
    audiometry
BSSI (Basic School Skills Inventory)
BST (brief stimulus therapy)
BSW (Bachelor of Social Work)
BT (bedtime)
BTA (brief tone audiometry)
B_{12} deficiency, vitamin
"bubble gum" (cocaine; crack)
buccal cavity
buccal speech
buccal whisper
buccofacial apraxia
buccolabial
buccoversion of teeth
"buck" (shoot someone in the head)

"bud" (cannabis)
"buda" (crack-laced cannabis cigarette)
"buffer" (crack prostitute; crack user)
"bugged" (annoyed; re: drug injection)
building restrictions
bulbar paralysis
bulimia nervosa
bulimic purge
"bull" (narcotics agent or police officer)
"bullet" (butyl nitrite)
"bullet bolt" (inhalant)
"bullia capital" (crack)
"bullion" (crack)
bullying
"bullyon" (cannabis)
"bumblebees" (amphetamine)
"bummer trip" (re: bad PCP experience)
"bump" (crack; $20 worth of ketamine; fake crack)
"bundle" (heroin)
bundle of isoglosses
"bunk" (fake cocaine)
Bureau of Drug Abuse Control (BDAC)
Bureau of Narcotics and Dangerous Drugs (BNDD)
"Burese" (cocaine)
Burks' Behavior Rating Scale
"burned" (purchase fake drugs)
"burnout," "burned out" (drug user; re: drug use; drug injection)
burnout (exhaustion), professional
"Burnese" (cocaine)
"burnie" (cannabis)
Burns/Roe Informal Reading Inventory (IRI): Preprimer to Twelfth Grade, Third Edition
"burn the main line" (drug injection)

Buros Institute
Burrow, Trigant L. (1875-1951)
Buschke Short-Term Recall Test
"bush" (cannabis; cocaine)
"businessman's acid" (psilocin/psilocybin)
"businessman's LSD" (dimethyltryptamine)
"businessman's special" (dimethyltryptamine)
"businessman's trip" (dimethyltryptamine)
Buss-Durkee Hostility Inventory
"busted" (arrested)
"busters" (barbiturate)
"busy bee" (phencyclidine)
butane (lighter fluid)
butane sniffing dependence
"butch" (lesbian)
"butter" (cannabis; crack)
"butter flower" (cannabis)
"butt naked" (phencyclidine)
"buttons" (mescaline)
"butu" (heroin)
butyl nitrite (street names)
    bolt
    bullet
    climax
    locker room
    rush
butyrophenone-based neuroleptic drugs
"buzz" (re: drug influence)
"buzz bomb" (nitrous oxide)
buzzing sensation
Bzoch-League Receptive-Expressive Emergent Language Scale
BVMGT (Bender Visual-Motor Gestalt Test)
BVRT (Benton Visual Retention Test)
BWAS (Barron-Welsh Art Scale)
bystander dominates initial dominant (BDID)

C, c

C (classes)
"C" (cocaine)
"the C" (methcathinone)
CA (chronological age)
CA (Cocaine Anonymous)
CAAS (Children's Attention and
Adjustment Survey)
CAB (Comprehensive Ability Battery)
CABS (chronic alcoholic brain
syndrome)
cachinnation
cacodemonomania
"cactus" (mescaline)
CADL (Communicative Abilities in
Daily Living)
CADT (Communication Abilities
Diagnostic Test)
caffeine-induced anxiety disorder
caffeine-induced postural tremor
caffeine-induced sleep disorder
caffeine withdrawal
CAGE alcohol use questionnaire
(CAGE, *cutting* down on drinking,
annoyance at others' concern about
drinking, feeling *guilty* about
drinking, using drinking as an
eye-opener in the morning).

CAI (Cultural Attitude Inventories)
CAIN (Computer Anxiety Index)
(Version AZ)
Cain complex
"caine" (cocaine; crack)
Cain-Levine Social Competency Scale
cainophobia
cainotophobia
calcification, basal ganglia
calculation skills
calibrate
calibrated loop
California Achievement Tests (CAT),
Fifth Edition (CAT/5)
California Child Q-Set
California Consonant Test
"California cornflakes" (cocaine)
California Critical Thinking
Dispositions Inventory (CCTDI)
California Critical Thinking Skills
Test (CCTST)
California Life Goals Evaluation
Schedules
California Marriage Readiness
Evaluation (CMRE)
California Motor Accuracy Test,
Southern (Revised)

California Occupational Preference Survey (or System) (COPS)
California Personality Inventory (CPI)
California Phonics Survey
California Preschool Social Competency Scale (CPSCS)
California Psychological Inventory (CPI) test (CPIT)
California Q-Sort
California Relative Value Studies (CRVS)
California Short-Form Test of Mental Maturity (CTMM-SF)
"California sunshine" (lysergic acid diethylamide)
California Test of Basic Skills (CTBS)
California Test of Personality (CTP)
California Verbal Learning Test
Callier-Azusa Scale: G Edition
callomania
callosal apraxia
callosal (parolfactory nerve) area
callosal commissurotomy
callosal disconnection syndrome
callosal gyrus
callosal sulcus
callosum, corpus
callous
callousness
caloric stimulation test for vestibular function
Caloric Test
CALS (Checklist of Adaptive Living Skills)
"Cambodian red" (cannabis)
Cambridge battery
"came" (cocaine)
Camelot Behavioral Checklist (CBC)
CAML (Coarticulation Assessment in Meaningful Language)
camouflage the defect
cAMP (cyclic adenosine monophosphate)

Campbell Leadership Index (CLI)
Campbell Organizational Survey (COS)
camptocormia
camptocormy
"Cam red" (cannabis)
"Cam trip" (cannabis)
"can" (cannabis)
Canadian Association for People Who Stutter (CAPS)
"Canadian black" (cannabis)
Canadian Cognitive Abilities Test, Form 7 (CCAT)
Canadian Neurological Scale
Canadian Tests of Basic Skills (CTBS)
canal
    alveolar
    alveolodental
    anterior vertical
    auditory
    cochlear
    craniopharyngeal
    ear
    Guyon
    horizontal
    internal auditory
    intramedullary
    lateral
    medullary
    posterior vertical
    semicircular
    vestibular
canal caps hearing protection device
canal hearing aid
"canamo" (cannabis)
"canappa" (cannabis)
cancellation test, letter
"cancelled stick" (cannabis cigarette)
cancerophobia
cancerphobia
"candy" (barbiturate)
"candy C" (cocaine)

Canfield Instructional Styles Inventory
canine hysteria
canine teeth
cannabinoids, cross-reacting (CRC)
cannabinol (CBN)
cannabis (street names)
    Acapulco gold
    Acapulco red
    ace
    Afghanistan black
    African black
    African bush
    African woodbine
    airplane
    Alice B. Toklas
    amp joint
    Angola
    ashes
    atom bomb
    atshitshi
    Aunt Mary
    baby
    baby bhang
    bad seed
    bale
    Bambalacha
    bar
    bash
    Belyando spruce
    bhang
    black bart
    black ganga
    black gold
    black gungi
    black gunion
    black hash
    black mo
    black moat
    black mote
    Black Russian
    blanket
    block

cannabis *(cont.)*
    blonde
    blowing smoke
    blue de hue
    blue sage
    blue sky blond
    blunt
    bo-bo
    bobo bush
    bohd
    boo
    boom
    broccoli
    brown
    bud
    buda
    bullyon
    burnie
    bush
    butter
    butter flower
    Cambodian red
    Cam red
    Cam trip
    can
    Canadian black
    canamo
    canappa
    cancelled stick
    cartucho
    catnip
    Cavite all star
    charas
    charge
    cheeba
    cheeo
    chiba chiba
    Chicago black
    Chicago green
    chira
    chronic
    churus

cannabis *(cont.)*
Cid
cochornis
coli
coliflor tostao
Colorado cocktail
Colombian marijuana
Columbus black
cosa
crack back
crazy weed
cripple
cubes
culican
dagga
dawamesk
dew
diambista
dimba
ding
dinkie dow
dirt grass
ditch
ditch weed
djamba
domestic
don jem
Dona Juana
Dona Juanita
doobie/dubbe/duby
dope
doradilla
drag weed
dry high
Durog
Duros
earth
el diablito
el diablo
endo
Esra
Fallbrook redhair

cannabis *(cont.)*
fatty
fine stuff
finger
fir
flower
flower tops
fraho/frajo
frios
fry daddy
fu
fuel
fuma D'Angola
gage/guage
gange
gangster
ganja
gash
gasper
gasper stick
gauge butt
geek
Ghana
giggle smoke
gimmie
gold
gold star
golden leaf
gong
good butt
good giggles
goof butt
grass
grass brownies
grata
green
green goddess
greeter
Greta
griefo
griff
griffa

cannabis *(cont.)*
griffo
G-shot
gungun
gyve
hanhich
happy cigarette
hash
hash oil
Hawaiian marijuana
hay
hay butt
hemp
Herb
Herb and Al
herba
hit
hocus
homegrown marijuana
honey blunts
hooch
hooter
hot stick
Indian boy
Indian hay
Indica
Indo
Indonesian bud
J
Jane
jay
jay smoke
Jim Jones
jive
jive stick
joint
jolly green
joy smoke
joy stick
ju-ju
Juan Valdez
Juanita

cannabis *(cont.)*
juice joint
Kali
kaya
Kentucky blue
KGB (killer green bud)
kick stick
kif
killer
killer weed
kilter
kind
Kumba
L.L.
lace
lakbay diva
Latin lettuce
laughing grass
laughing weed
leaf
Lebanese red
light stuff
Lima
little smoke
llesca
loaf
lobo
locoweed
log
love boat
lovelies
love weed
lubage
M
M.J.
M.O.
M.U.
machinery
Macon
maconha
magic smoke
Manhattan silver

cannabis *(cont.)*
Mari
marijuana (also marihuana)
Mary
Mary and Johnny
Mary Ann
Mary Jane
Mary Jonas
Mary Warner
Mary Weaver
Maui wauie
Meg
Megg
Meggie
messorole
Mexican brown
Mexican red
mighty mezz
modams
mohasky
monte
mooca/moocah
mooster
moota/mutah
mooters
mootie
mootos
mor a grifa
mota/moto
mother
muggie
mutha
nail
number
O.J.
P.R. (Panama Red)
pack
pack of rocks
Pakalolo
Pakistani black
Panama cut
Panama gold

cannabis *(cont.)*
Panama red
panatella
parsley
Pat
pin
pocket rocket
pod
poke
pot
potten bush
prescription
pretendica
pretendo
primo
Queen Anne's lace
ragweed
railroad weed
rainy day woman
Rangood
rasta weed
red cross
red dirt
reefer
righteous bush
righteous weed
rocket
root
rope
Rose Marie
ruderalis
Salmon River Quiver
salt and pepper
Santa Marta
sasfras
sativa
scissors
seeds
sen
sess
sezz
shake

cannabis *(cont.)*
  Siddi
  sinse
  sinsemilla
  sinsemillan marijuana
  skunk
  Skunk Number 1
  smoke
  smoke Canada
  snop
  splim
  square mackerel
  stack
  stems
  stick
  stink weed
  straw
  sugar weed
  supergrass
  Sweet Lucy
  T
  taima
  Takkouri
  Texas pot
  Texas tea
  Tex-Mex
  Thai marijuana
  Thai sticks
  THC
  thirteen
  thumb
  tops
  torch
  torpedo
  turbo
  Turkish green
  twist
  twistum
  viper's weed
  wac
  wacky weed
  weed

cannabis *(cont.)*
  weed tea
  wheat
  white-haired lady
  X
  yeh
  yellow submarine
  yen pop
  yerba
  yerba mala
  yesca
  yesco
  Zacatecas purple
  zambi
  zig zag man
  zol
  zoom
cannabis-induced anxiety disorder
cannabis intoxication delirium
cannabis tea
cannabis use disorder
cannula
Canter Background Interference
  Procedure (BIP) for the Bender
  Gestalt Test
"cap" (crack; lysergic acid diethylamide)
capacitance
capacitor
capacity
  diminished
  dissociative
  functional
  functional residual (FRC)
  hedonic
  inspiratory (IC)
  intellectual
  lung
  measured
  mental
  nonverbal intellectual
  orgasmic

capacity *(cont.)*
  oxygen-carrying
  potential intellectual
  respiratory
  self-regulatory
  speaking
  testamentary
  vital (VT)
capacity for independent living
CAP Assessment of Writing
Capgras syndrome
"capital H" (heroin)
CAPP (Clinical Appraisal of Psychological Problems)
CAPPS (Current and Past Psychopathology Scales)
"caps" (crack; heroin; psilocybin/psilocin)
caps, canal
CAPS (Canadian Association for People Who Stutter)
captation
captive, indoctrination while
"cap up" (re: drug containers)
CAQ (Change Agent Questionnaire)
CAQ (Classroom Atmosphere Questionnaire)
CAQ (Clinical Analysis Questionnaire)
carbamazepine for mood disorders
carbon dioxide intoxication
carbon dioxide therapy
carbonic anhydrase inhibitors
carbon monoxide intoxication
carbonyl modification
"carburetor" (re: crack equipment)
carcinophobia
cardiac disorder, psychogenic functional
cardiac evoked response audiometry (CERA)
cardiac neurosis

cardinal ocular movement
cardinal vowels
cardiophobia
cardiospasm, psychogenic
cardiovascular disorder, psychogenic
cardiovascular neurosis
cardiovascular seizure
care
  ambulatory
  clinical
  continuum of
  excessive need for
  foster
  grossly pathogenic
  inappropriate dependent
  individual
  medical
  need for
  pastoral
  pathogenic
  pathological
  personal
  primary
care and protection proceedings
Career Assessment Inventories: For the Learning Disabled
Career Assessment Inventory, The Enhanced Version
Career Beliefs Inventory (CBI)
Career Decision-Making (CDM)
Career Decision Scale
Career Development Inventory
Career Maturity Inventory (CMI)
Career Planning Program (CPP)
Career Problem Check List
caregiver
  adoptive
  primary
Caregiver School Readiness Inventory (CSRI)
Caregiver Strain Index
care organization

caretaker
caretaking role
CARF (Commission on Accreditation
    of Rehabilitation Facilities)
"carga" (heroin)
Caring Relationship Inventory (CRI)
Carlson Psychological Survey
"carmabis" (cannabis)
carnal
"carne" (heroin)
"carnie" (cocaine)
carnophobia
carouse
carouser
"carpet patrol" (re: crack acquisition)
carphologia
carphology
Carrell Discrimination Test
"Carrie" (cocaine)
"Carrie Nation" (cocaine)
Carrow Auditory-Visual Abilities Test
Carrow Elicited Language Inventory
    (CELI)
carryover coarticulation
CARS (childhood autism rating scale)
CARS (Children's Affective Rating
    Scale)
cartilage
    arytenoid
    corniculate
    cricoid
    cuneiform
    thyroid
cartilage shaving, thyroid
"cartucho" (package of cannabis ciga-
    rettes)
"cartwheels" (amphetamine sulfate)
CAS (Concept-Specific Anxiety Scale)
CAS (Creativity Attitude Survey)
CAS (Cultural Attitude Scales)
case-control (experimental study
    designs)

case management
case study
CASH (Comprehensive Assessment of
    Symptoms and History)
"Casper the ghost" (crack)
CAST (Children of Alcoholism
    Screening Test)
CAST (Children's Apperceptive Story-
    Telling Test)
castrate
castration anxiety
castration complex
CAT (California Achievement Test)
CAT (Children Apperception Test)
CAT (Children Articulation Test)
CAT (Cognitive Abilities Test)
CAT (computerized axial tomography)
    scan
"cat" (methcathinone)
cataclysmic headache
catalepsy, schizophrenic
cataleptic
cataleptiform
cataleptoid
catalogia
cataphasia
cataphoria
cataphoric
cataphrenia
cataplectic
cataplexis
cataplexy, episode of
cataracts, traumatic
catarrh
catarrhal deafness
catastrophic ancataplexy syndrome,
    narcolepsy
catastrophic anxiety
catastrophic stress
catastrophic reaction
catastrophic response
catathymia

catathymic
catatonia
  lethal
  schizophrenic
catatonic behavior
catatonic disorder due to general
  medical condition
catatonic excitation
catatonic excitement
catatonic features, mood disorders with
catatonic motor behaviors
catatonic mutism
catatonic negativism
catatonic posturing
catatonic presentation
catatonic rigidity
catatonic schizophrenia
  acute
  agitation
  excited
  stupor
  withdrawn
catatonic state
catatonic stupor
catatonic symptom
catatonic-type schizophrenia
catatony
catch, glottal
catchment area
cat cry syndrome (cri du chat)
catecholamine neurotransmitter
  (norepinephrine)
categelophobia
categorical classification
categorical model
categorical thought
category (pl. categories)
  checklist of problem
  grammatical
  lexical
  phrasal
  syntactic

catenation
CAT/5 (California Achievement Tests,
  Fifth Edition)
CAT-H (Children's Apperception
  Test-Human)
cathard
catharsis, conversational
cathartic method, Freud
cathectic
cathexis
cathisophobia
cathode (C or Ca)
"catnip" (cannabis cigarette)
catoptrophobia
Cattell Infant Intelligence Scale
Cattell Personality Factor Questionnaire
"cat valium" (ketamine)
caudal
caudate nucleus
causal factor
causalgia
causality
  direct
  presumed
causal link
causal relationship
caudate nucleus
causation, biological
causative agent
causative pathophysiological mechanism, direct
causative stress
cause and effect, laws of
caustic ingestion
cautionary
CAVD (completion, arithmetic
  [problems], vocabulary [following]
  directions)
cavernosography
"caviar" (crack)
"Cavite all star" (cannabis)

cavity
  buccal
  oral
CAVLT-2 (Children's Auditory Verbal Learning Test-2)
CBC (Camelot Behavioral Checklist)
CBC (child behavior characteristics)
CBF (cerebral blood flow)
CBI (Career Beliefs Inventory)
CBN (cannabinol)
CBS (chronic brain syndrome)
CBS (culture-bound syndrome)
CBT (cognitive behavior therapy)
cc (cubic centimeter)
CC (chief complaint)
CCAE (Checklist for Child Abuse Evaluation)
CCAS (Comprehensive Career Assessment Scale)
CCAT (Canadian Cognitive Abilities Test), Form 7
CCC-SLP (Certificate of Clinical Competence Speech-Language Pathologist)
CCQ (Chronicle Career Quest)
CCSEQ (Community College Student Experiences Questionnaire)
CCTDI (California Critical Thinking Dispositions Inventory)
CCTST (California Critical Thinking Skills Test)
CCW (Central Colony in Wisconsin)
CD (chemical dependency)
CD (chemically dependent)
C/D, C/d (cigarettes per day)
CDC (Chemical Dependency Counselor)
CDI (Children's Diagnostic Inventory)
CDM (Career Decision-Making)
CDM-R (Harrington-O'Shea Career Decision-Making System, Revised)
CDR (Chronological Drinking Record)

CDR (Clinical Dementia Rating Scale)
CDRS-R (Children's Depression Rating Scale—Revised)
CDS (Children's Depression Scale), Second Research Edition
CE (cocaethylene assay)
ceaseless pacing
"Cecil" (cocaine)
cecocentral scotoma
CEFT (Children's Embedded Figures Test)
CELF-R (Clinical Evaluation of Language Functions—Revised)
CELI (Carrow Elicited Language Inventory)
cell
  Golgi
  hair
  nerve
  Purkinje
cell body
cellular effects of lithium
Celtophobia
cenesthopathic schizophrenia
cenophobia
censor
  freudian
  psychic
centeredness
Center for Epidemiologic Studies Depression Scale (CES-D Scale)
Center for Mental Health Services
Center for Stress and Anxiety Disorders
center of attention
center of gravity (CG)
central alexia
central alveolar hypoventilation syndrome
central aphasia
central apnea
central audition

central auditory processing disorder
Central Colony in Wisconsin (CCW)
central convulsion
central deafness
central drive for respiration
Central European viral encephalitis
central excitatory state
central gray matter (CGM)
central hearing
central incisor teeth
Central Institute for the Deaf (CID)
Central Institute for the Deaf Preschool
　Performance Scale
central language disorder (CLD)
central language imbalance
central masking
central motor pathways disease
central nervous system (CNS)
central neurogenic hyperventilation
central scotoma
central sleep apnea syndrome
central speech range
central vowel
centration
centrencephalic seizure
centripetal
centrotemporal epilepsy
cephalalgia
cephalic seizure
cephalometric
cephalometric analysis
CER (conditioned emotional response)
CERA (cardiac evoked response
　audiometry)
CERAD (Consortium to Establish a
　Registry for Alzheimer Disease)
　Assessment Battery
ceraunophobia
cerea, flexibilitas
cerebellar ataxia, ipsilateral
cerebellar cortex
cerebellar degeneration

cerebellar fits (seizures)
cerebellar pathway
cerebellar scanning quality speech
cerebellar signs
cerebellar tremor
　essential
　progressive
cerebelli, ala
cerebellum (pl. cerebella)
cerebral agraphia
cerebral asymmetry
cerebral blood flow (CBF)
cerebral convulsion
cerebral cortex
cerebral cortical functions
cerebral disorder
cerebral dominance, mixed
cerebral dysfunction
　bilateral
　higher (HCD)
cerebral fissure, longitudinal
cerebral gait
cerebral glucose metabolism
cerebral hemisphere
cerebral lipidosis
cerebral mal
cerebral mapping of apraxia
cerebral outflow tremor
cerebral palsy (CP)
　ataxic
　athetoid
　atonic
　choreoathetoid
　clonic
　dyskinetic
　dystonic
　extrapyramidal
　flaccid
　hypotonic
　pyramidal
　rigid
　spastic
　tremulous

cerebral potential
cerebral syndrome, posttraumatic
cerebral thumb
cerebral tremor, essential
cerebral, zero
cerebri
   pseudotumor
   status post commotio
cerebrospinal convulsion
cerebrospinal fluid (CSF) analysis
cerebrovascular accident (CVA)
cerebrovascular disease-type organic
   psychosis
cerebrum (pl. cerebri)
ceremonial behavior
CERS (Crisis Evaluation Referral
   Service)
certificate
   dependent adult's
   detention
Certificate of Clinical Competence
   Speech-Language Pathologist
   (CCC-SLP)
certificate of incompetency
Certified Social Worker (CSW)
ceruloplasmin
cerumen, impacted
CES (Classroom Environmental
   Scale)
CES-D Scale (Center for Epidemio-
   logic Studies Depression Scale)
cessation
CF (Coalition for the Family)
C-factor (cleverness factor)
CFBRS (Cooper-Farran Behavioral
   Rating Scales)
C-fibers
CFIT (Culture Fair Intelligence Test)
CFIT (Culture Free Intelligence Test)
CFQ-for-others assessment
CFSEI-2 (Culture-Free Self-Esteem
   Inventories, Second Edition)

CFT (Complex Figure Test)
CG (center of gravity)
CGIC (Clinical Global Impression of
   Change)
CGM (central gray matter)
CGP (Comparative Guidance and
   Placement) Program
CGRS (Clinician's Global Rating
   Scale)
chaetophobia
chain analysis
chaining responses
chain, ossicular
"chalk" (amphetamine; methamphetamine)
"chalked up" (re: cocaine influence)
"chalking" (chemically whitening
   cocaine)
challenge, neuroendocrine
challenge test
chamber
   anechoic
   echo
   no-echo
   pure
chameleon
CHAMPUS (Citizen Health and Medical Program of the Uniformed
   Services)
chance-response parameter
"chandoo/chandu" (opium)
change (pl. changes)
   agent of
   age-related pharmacodynamic
   age-related pharmacokinetic
   age-related physical
   analogic
   behavioral
   conditioned sound
   conversion sensory
   digital
   job

change *(cont.)*
   language
   life
   life cycle
   major life
   maladaptive behavioral
   maladaptive psychological
   mental
   mental status
   personality
   psychomotor
   psychophysiological
   reflex
   sense of bodily
   time-zone
   transitional
   unpredictable mood
changeability
Change Agent Questionnaire (CAQ)
change events, life
change in activity, rapid
change in mentation
changes in mood
changes of consciousness, episodic
change units, life (LCU)
changing sleep-wake pattern
"channel" (re: drug injection)
channel flux assay, chloride
channel, membrane ion
"channel swimmer" (re: heroin
   injection)
chaotic
character analysis
character attack
character defense
characteristic age
characteristic association
characteristic features
characteristic paraphiliac focus
characteristic pattern
characteristic sign
characteristic syndrome

characteristic withdrawal syndrome
characteristics
   change in personality
   child behavior (CBC)
   clang association
   demand‾
   primary sex
   psychometric performance
   secondary sex
   sex
characteristics of cleft palate, speech
   and language
character neurosis
character pathology
"charas" (cannabis)
Charcot, Jean M. (1825-1893)
"charge" (cannabis)
"charged up" (re: drug influence)
charisma
charismatic
"Charley" (heroin)
"Charlie" (cocaine)
charm, superficial
Charteris Reading Test
"chase" (re: cannabis or cocaine use)
chase (gambling), long-term
"chaser" (re: crack user)
"chasing the dragon" (crack and
   heroin)
"chasing" one's losses
"chasing the tiger" (re: heroin use)
chastise
chastisement
"cheap basing" (crack)
"check" (personal supply of drugs)
checklist (also check list) (see *test*)
checklist approach
"cheeba" (cannabis)
cheeking medication
"cheeo" (cannabis)
cheerlessness
cheiloschisis

cheimaphobia
cheimatophobia
cheirognostic feeling
"chemical" (crack)
chemical abuse
chemical dependency (CD)
Chemical Dependency Counselor
(CDC)
chemically dependent (CD)
chemical messengers
chemistry, psychiatric
chemotherapeutic
chemotherapy
cheromania
cherophobia
chest pulse
chest voice
"chewies" (crack)
chewing automatism
chewing, breath
Cheyne-Stokes psychosis
Cheyne-Stokes respiration
CHF (congestive heart failure)
CHI (closed head injury)
"chiba chiba" (cannabis)
chibih
"Chicago black" (cannabis)
"Chicago green" (cannabis)
Chicano English
"chicken powder" (amphetamine)
"chicken scratch" (re: crack acquisition)
"chicle" (heroin)
"chief" (lysergic acid diethylamide;
mescaline)
chief complaint (CC)
"chieva" (heroin)
child abuse, adult survivor of
Child Abuse Potential Inventory
child abuse syndrome
child analysis

Child and Adolescent Adjustment
Profile
Child and Adolescent Fear and
Anxiety Treatment Program
child antisocial behavior
Child Anxiety Scale
Child Assessment Schedule
Child "At Risk" for Drug Abuse
Rating Scale (DARS)
Child Autism Rating Scale
child behavior characteristics (CBC)
Child Behavior Checklist
childbirth amnesia
childbirth-type organic psychosis
Child Care and Guidance (NOCTI
Teacher Occupational Competency
Test)
Child Care Inventory
child counselor
Child Depression Inventory
child dyssocial behavior
child group therapies
child guidance
childhood aphasia
childhood autism, neuroleptic treatment of
childhood autism rating scale (CARS)
childhood cross-gender behavior
childhood disintegrative disorder
childhood disorder
childhood encephalopathy
childhood epilepsy
childhood figure
childhood illnesses, usual (UCI)
childhood-onset type conduct disorder
childhood psychosexual identity
disorder
childhood psychosis
atypical
disintegrative
interactional

childhood schizophrenia, neuroleptic
treatment of
childhood sexual abuse
childhood Tourette syndrome
childhood trauma
childhood truancy
socialized
unsocialized
childhood-type schizophrenia
childish emotion
child issues, inner
child language development
childlike silliness
child maltreatment
child molestation
child neglect
Child Neuropsychological Questionnaire (CNQ)
child(ren) of alcoholic (CoA)
Child Personality Scale (CPS)
child psychiatrist
child psychiatry (CHP, CP), psychopharmacology in
child psychology (CP)
child psychosis
Children's Academic Intrinsic Motivation Inventory
Children's Adaptive Behavior Scale—
Revised
Children's Affective Rating Scale
(CARS)
Children's Apperception Test (CAT)
Children's Apperception Test—Human
(CAT-H)
Children's Apperceptive Story-Telling
Test (CAST)
Children's Articulation Test (CAT)
Children's Attention and Adjustment
Survey (CAAS)
Children's Auditory Verbal Learning
Test-2 (CAVLT-2)
Children's Coma Score

Children's Depression Inventory
Children's Depression Scale, Revised
(RCDS)
Children's Depression Scale [Second
Research Edition] (CDS)
Children's Depression Rating Scale—
Revised (CDRS-R)
Children's Diagnostic Inventory (CDI)
Children's Embedded Figures Test
(CDFT)
Children's Hypnotic Susceptibility
Scale
Children's Inventory of Self-Esteem
(CISE)
Children's Language Battery
Children's Language Processes
Children's Manifest Anxiety Scale,
Revised (RCMAS)
Children of Alcoholism Screening
Test (CAST)
Children of Deaf Adults
Children's Perception of Support
Inventory (CPSI)
Children's Personality Questionnaire
(CPQ)
Children's Psychiatric Rating Scale
(CPRS)
Children's Self-Concept Scale (CSCS)
Children's Version/Family Environ-
mental Scale
child sexual abuse
child support
"China cat" (heroin)
"China girl" (fentanyl)
Chinamania
"China town" (fentanyl)
"China white" (heroin; analog of
fentanyl)
"Chinese molasses" (opium)
"Chinese red" (heroin)
"Chinese tobacco" (opium)
chink glottal

chionomania
chionophobia
"chip" (heroin)
"chipper" (re: drug user)
"chipping" (re: drug use)
"chippy" (cocaine)
"chira" (cannabis)
chlamydia
chloral hydrate
chloride channel flux assay
chlorohydrocarbon (inhalation) dependence
chlorpromazine
chlorthiazides
"chocolate" (amphetamine; opium)
"chocolate chips" (lysergic acid diethylamide)
"chocolate ecstasy" (crack processed with chocolate milk powder)
choice behavior
choice reaction time test, visual
choking during sleep
cholerophobia
cholesteatoma
choline acetyltransferase
cholinergic neurons
cholinergic receptor
    muscarinic
    nicotinic
"cholly" (cocaine)
choral reading
choral speaking
"chorals" (barbiturate)
chorditis nodosa
chorditis tuberosa
chorea
    Huntington (HC)
    senile
    Sydenham
choreal
choreic insanity
choreiform movements

choreoathetoid movement
choreoid
choreoathetoid cerebral palsy (CP)
choreoathetosis
choreomania
choreophrasia
ChP (child psychiatry)
chrematomania
chrematophobia
"Christina" (amphetamine)
"Christmas rolls" (barbiturate)
"Christmas trees" (amobarbital/ secobarbital; dextroamphetamine sulfate)
chromatophobia
chromophobia
chromosomal
chromosome 21-trisomy syndrome
chromosomes, sex
"chronic" (cannabis and crack)
chronic alcoholic brain syndrome (CABS)
chronic brain syndrome (CBS)
Chronic Family Invalid—Depressed
chronic fatigue syndrome
chronic feelings of emptiness
Chronicle Career Quest (CCQ)
chronic mania
    single episode
    recurrent episode
chronic phase of stable sleep difficulty
chronic schizophrenia
chronic stress disorder
chronic tissue damage
chronic toxic effects
chronobiological disorder
chronological age (CA)
Chronological Drinking Record (CDR)
chronological relationship
chronology
chronophobia
"chucks" (re: heroin withdrawal)

chunking
"churus" (cannabis)
"CIBA's" (glutethimide)
cibophobia
"Cid" (cannabis cigarette)
CID (Central Institute for the Deaf)
CID Preschool Performance Scale
cigarettes per day (C/D, C/d)
cigarette-related pathology
CIMS (Conflict in Marriage Scale)
cinefluorography
cinefluoroscopy
cineradiography
cineroentgenography
cingulate gyrus
cingulotomy
cingulum
CIP (Comprehensive Identification
    Process)
cipher method, numerical
circadian pacemaker, endogenous
circadian period, endogenous
circadian phase of sleep
circadian rhythm phase, endogenous
circadian rhythm sleep disorder
circle of thoughts, wide
circuit
    convergence
    divergence
    neuronal
circular insanity
circular psychosis
circular thinking
circular-type manic-depressive
    psychosis
circumaural hearing protection devices
circumfix morpheme
circumflex
circumlocution of speech
circumlocutory
circumscribed amnesia
circumscribed delusion

circumstantial migraine headache
circumstantial speech
circumstantiality
CIRP (Cooperative Institutional
    Research Program)
CISE (Children's Inventory of Self-
    Esteem)
cisternography, isotope
citalopram
Citizen Health and Medical Program
    of the Uniformed Services
    (CHAMPUS)
city and state test
"C joint" (cocaine-buying place)
clairaudience
clairsentience
clairvoyance
clairvoyant dream
clammy extremities
clammy skin
clang associations
clanging
clarity of language
Clarke Reading Self-Assessment
    Survey
Clark-Madison Test of Oral Language
Clark Picture Phonetic Inventory
clasp-knife phenomenon
class
    closed
    social
CLASSI (Cornell Learning and Study
    Skills Inventory)
classical conditioning
classical migraine headache
classic apraxia
Classroom Atmosphere Questionnaire
    (CAQ)
Classroom Environmental Scale
    (CES)
Classroom Environment Index
class word

claustrophilia
claustrophobia
Claude hyperkinesis sign
Claude syndrome
claudication, neurogenic
clausa, rhinolalia
clause
    constituent
    dependent
    embedded
    independent
    main
    principal
    subordinate
clause terminal
clavicular respiration
Claybury Selection Battery
clay-eating (pica)
CLCS (Comprehensive Level of
    Consciousness Scale)
CLD (central language disorder)
clearly demarcated relationships
clear sensorium
cleft (pl. clefts)
    atypical
    labial
    nose
    rare
cleft lip
    bilateral
    median
    unilateral
cleft palate
    bilateral
    complete
    incomplete
    occult
    partial
    submucous
    subtotal
    total
    unilateral

cleft palate fistula
clenching, fist
CLEP (College-Level Examination
    Program General Examination)
cleptophobia
Clerambault erotomania syndrome
clerical perception
clerical response
cleverness factor (C factor, C-factor)
CLI (Campbell Leadership Index)
click, glottal
Clifton Assessment Procedure for the
    Elderly
climacophobia
climacteric insanity
climacteric melancholia
climacteric neurosis
climacteric paranoid psychosis
climacteric paraphrenia
climacteric psychoneurosis
climacteric psychosis
climate, emotional
"climax" (butyl nitrite)
climax, sexual
cling
clinging dependency
Clinical Analysis Questionnaire (CAQ)
Clinical Appraisal of Psychological
    Problems (CAPP)
clinical audiology
Clinical Dementia Rating Scale (CDR)
Clinical Evaluation of Language
    Functions—Revised (CELF–R)
clinical features
Clinical Global Impression of Change
    (CGIC)
Clinical Global Improvement Scale
clinical interview
clinical management
clinical performance score (CPS)
Clinical Probes of Articulation
    Consistency (C-PAC)

clinical psychobiology
clinical psychologist
clinical psychology
clinical psychopharmacology
Clinical Rating Scale (CRS)
clinical scale
Clinical Scales (MMPI)
clinical setting
clinical status
Clinical Support System Battery
clinically significant anxiety
Clinician's Global Rating Scale
  (CGRS)
Clinician Rated Anxiety Scale (CRAS)
Clinician Rated Overall Life Impairment Scale
clinic patient populations
clinomania
clinophobia
clipped speech
clipped word
clipping, peak
"clips" (re: drug vials)
clithrophobia
clitoris
clock face test, draw a
"clocking paper" (re: drug profits)
clomipramine
clonic block (in stuttering)
clonic cerebral palsy (CP)
clonic seizure
clonic-tonic-clonic seizure
clonus
closed bite
closed bite malposition of teeth
closed class
closed head injury (CHI)
closed juncture
closed syllable
close phonetic transcription
closet alcoholic
"closet baser" (re: crack user)

closet homosexual
close transcription
close vowel
close watch restrictions
closure
  auditory
  grammatic
  perceptual
  velopharyngeal
  visual
closure task, sentence
Closure Test, Sentence
"cloud" (crack)
clouded state, epileptic
clouding of consciousness
"cloud nine" (crack)
cloudy sensorium
clozapine for mood disorders
CLS (confused language syndrome)
CLS (Consultation-Liaison Service)
"cluck" (re: crack user)
clucking, tongue
clumsiness syndrome
clumsy gesture
Clunis inquiry forensic psychiatry
cluster
  anxious-fearful
  consonant
  dramatic-emotional
  odd-eccentric
  situation
cluster characteristics in personality
  disorder
cluster headache
cluster of situations
cluster reduction
cluster suicides
cluttering
Clyde Mood Scale (CMS)
Clymer-Barrett Readiness Test
Cm (communality)
CMA (Conflict Management Appraisal)

CMAS (Children's Manifest Anxiety
   Scale)
CME (continuing medical education)
CME (crude marijuana extract)
CMEE (Content Mastery Examinations
   for Educators)
CMI (Career Maturity Inventory)
CMI (chronically mentally ill)
CMII (College Major Interest Inven-
   tory)
CMMS (Columbia Mental Maturity
   Scale)
CMRE (California Marriage Readiness
   Evaluation)
CMS (Clyde Mood Scale)
CMS (Conflict Management Survey)
CMT (Concept Mastery Test)
cnidophobia
CNQ (Child Neuropsychological
   Questionnaire)
CNS (central nervous system)
CNS depressant
CNS disease group
CNS insult
CNS stimulant
CNS syphilis
CNS trauma
CNT ("could not test")
CNV (conative negative variation)
c/o (complaints of; complains of)
CoA (child[ren] of alcoholic)
COAB (Computer Operator Aptitude
   Battery)
coalescence
Coalition for the Family (CF)
coarctated personality
coarse tremor
coarticulation
   anticipatory
   backward
   carryover
   forward

Coarticulation Assessment in
   Meaningful Language (CAML)
"coasting" (re: drug influence)
"coasts to coasts" (amphetamine)
"coca" (cocaine)
cocaethylene (CE) assay
cocaine (street names)
   all-American drug
   Angie
   barbs
   base
   basuco
   bazooka
   Bazulco
   Belushi
   Bernice
   bernies
   Bernie's flakes
   Bernie's gold dust
   big bloke
   big C
   big flake
   big rush
   billie hoke
   blotter
   blow
   blowcaine
   Bolivian marching powder
   bouncing powder
   boy
   bubble gum
   Burnese
   bush
   C
   caine
   California cornflakes
   came
   candy C
   carnie
   Carrie
   Carrie Nation
   Cecil

cocaine *(cont.)*
   Charlie
   chippy
   cholly
   coca
   coconut
   coke
   cola
   Corrinne
   cotton brothers
   crack
   dama blanca
   double bubble
   dream
   duct
   dynamite
   el diablito
   el diablo
   flake
   flamethrower
   Florida snow
   foo-foo dust
   foo foo stuff
   foolish powder
   free base
   freebase rocks
   freeze
   Frisco special
   Frisco speedball
   friskie powder
   G-rock
   gift-of-the-sun
   gin
   girlfriend
   glad stuff
   gold dust
   green gold
   H & C
   happy dust
   happy powder
   happy trails
   have a dust

cocaine *(cont.)*
   heaven dust
   Henry VIII
   her
   hooter
   hunter
   ice
   icing
   Inca message
   jam
   jelly
   joy powder
   king's habit
   lace
   lady
   lady caine
   lady snow
   leaf
   line
   love affair
   mama coca
   mayo
   merk
   Mojo
   mosquitos
   movie star drug
   mujer
   nose candy
   nose powder
   nose stuff
   number one
   number 3
   paradise
   paradise white
   pearl
   Perico
   Peruvia
   Peruvian
   Peruvian flake
   Peruvian lady
   pimp
   polvo blanco

cocaine *(cont.)*
  powder diamonds
  press
  quill
  racehorse charlie
  rane
  ready rock
  rock
  Roxanne
  schmeck
  schoolboy
  scorpion
  Scottie or Scotty
  Serpico 21
  Seven-up
  she
  smoking gun
  snow
  snowball
  snowbirds
  snowcones
  snow seals
  Snow White
  society high
  soda
  speedball
  stardust
  star-spangled powder
  sugar
  sweet stuff
  T
  teeth
  thing
  toot
  toxic effects of
  turkey
  tutti-frutti
  white
  white girl
  white horse
  white lady
  white mosquito

cocaine *(cont.)*
  white powder
  whiz bang
  wild cat
  wings
  wired on
  witch
  yeyo
  zip
Cocaine Anonymous (CA)
cocaine binge
"cocaine blues" (re: cocaine use)
cocaine "crash"
cocaine delusion
cocaine-laced cigarette (street names)
  cocktail
  coolie
  monkey
  monos
  primos
cocaine run
cocainism
cocainization
cocainize
cochlea, fenestra
cochlear aplasia
cochlear canal
cochlear duct
cochlear implant device
cochlear implant hearing aid
cochlear microphonia
cochlear nerve
cochlear nucleus
  dorsal
  ventral
cochlear reflex
cochlear window
cochleo-orbicular reflex
cochleopalpebral reflex (CPR)
"cochornis" (cannabis)
"cocktail" (cocaine- or crack-laced
  cigarette)

cocktail party paradigm
"cocoa puff" (re: cocaine and
  cannabis use)
co-conscious
co-consciousness
"coconut" (cocaine)
"coco rocks" (crack processed with
  chocolate pudding)
"coco snow" (benzocaine used as
  cutting agent for crack)
"cod" (re: currency)
CODA (Codependency Anonymous)
codeine dependence
codeine, schoolboy
codependency
Codependency Anonymous (CODA)
codependent
coefficient
  alternate forms reliability
  comparable forms reliability
  odd-even method reliability
  split half reliability
  test-retest reliability
coenesthesiopathic schizophrenia
coercion, sexual
coercive communication
coeundi, impotentia
coexist
coexistent culture
coexisting disorders
"coffee" (lysergic acid diethylamide)
COG (Cognitive Observation Guide)
Cog Disorg (cognitive disorganization)
cognate confusion
cognates
cognition
  dysfunctional
  empiric
Cognitive Abilities Test (CAT)
cognitive approaches to dreaming and
  repression
cognitive assessment, quantified

cognitive assessment techniques,
  standardized
cognitive/attitudinal factors
cognitive-behavioral technique
Cognitive Behavior Rating Scales
cognitive behavior therapy (CBT)
Cognitive Control Battery
cognitive decline, age-related
cognitive deficit
  global
  multiple
cognitive development stages (Period
  I-IV)
Cognitive Diagnostic Battery
cognitive disorganization (Cog Disorg)
cognitive dissonance
cognitive distancing
cognitive distortion
cognitive dysfunction
cognitive function
  higher level
  impairment of
cognitive functioning
  impaired
  impairment in
cognitive mapping
Cognitive Observation Guide (COG)
cognitive personality traits
cognitive psychology
cognitive psychotherapy
cognitive rehabilitation
cognitive science
cognitive self-hypnosis training
Cognitive Skills Assessment (CSA)
  Battery
cognitive variables
cognizant
cogwheel rigidity
cohabit
cohabitant
cohabitation
coherent stream of thought

cohesion, group
cohesive devices
cohesive family
cohesiveness, level of
cohort (experimental study designs)
COIB (Crowley Occupational Interests
    Blank)
coil, induction
coinage, word
coin new words
coital orgasm
coitophobia
coitus interruptus
coitus, psychogenic painful
"coke" (cocaine)
"coke bar" (re: cocaine use)
"cola" (cocaine)
coldness, emotional
Cold-Running Speech Test
"cold turkey" (drug withdrawal)
"coli" (cannabis)
"coliflor tostao" (cannabis)
colitis, mucous
collaboration
Collaborative Study Psychotherapy
    Rating Scale
collapse delirium
collapsing anchors
collar, shower
collateral sources
collective experience
collective monologue
collective unconscious
College and University Environment
    Scales (CUES)
College Basic Academic Subjects
    Examination
College-Level Examination Program
    General Examination (CLEP)
College Major Interest Inventory
    (CMII)
College Student Questionnaires (CSQ)

College Student Satisfaction Question-
    naire (CSSQ)
Collet-Sicard syndrome
Collis-Romberg Mathematical Problem
    Solving Profiles
colloquial
colloquialism
Colombian marijuana
"Colorado cocktail" (cannabis)
Colorado Educational Interest
    Inventory
color agnosia
color anomia
color perception
color responses
color therapy
Coloured Progressive Matrices
Columbia Mental Maturity Scale
    (CMMS)
"Columbo" (phencyclidine)
"Columbus black" (cannabis)
columella (pl. columellae)
coma
    alcoholic
    apoplectic
    irreversible
    metabolic
coma therapy, insulin (ICT)
comatose patient
coma vigil
combat exhaustion
combat fatigue
combative patient
combat neurosis
combat stress exposure
combination-drug dependence
combination, fabulized
combination headache
combinations, frequency
combinative thinking
combined aphasia
combined aural rehabilitation

combined behavior, hyperactive-
impulsive
combined therapy
combined-type attention-deficit/hyper-
activity disorder
combined-type personality disorder
combining power test (CPT)
"comeback" (re: adulteration of
cocaine)
"come home" (re: lysergic acid
diethylamide use)
cometophobia
comfortable loudness, most (MCL)
comfortable loudness range, most
(MCLR)
comitial mal
command
embedded
negative
command automatism
command hallucination
command negativism
command test, three-stage
commensalism
comment
derogatory
threatening
commentary, running
Commission on Accreditation of
Rehabilitation Facilities (CARF)
commissural aphasia
commissure
commissurotomy, callosal
commitment, involuntary
commitment of mentally ill
committee, utilization review
common experience
common migraine headache
common objects test, naming
common precipitant exposure
common sense
common shared features

common theme
communality (Cm)
communicated insanity
communicating epilepsy
communicating hydrocephalus
communication
coercive
distortion of language and
exaggeration of language and
illogic
impaired
impaired effective
irreverent
language and
manual
nonverbal
nonvocal
pathological
persuasive
privileged
problem-solving
qualitative impairment in
reciprocal
total
unaided augmentative
vague
vehicle for
verbal
Communication Abilities Diagnostic
Test (CADT) and Screen
communication ability
communication barriers
communication board
direct selection
encoding
scanning
communication/cognition treatment
communication pattern
blame-placing
gesturing
intellectualization
interpersonal spacing

communication pattern *(cont.)*
  language spoken at home
  language spoken outside home
  manipulation
  monopolization
  scapegoating
  semantic argument
  silence
  touching
  validation
Communication Screen: A Pre-school
  Speech-Language Screening Tool
Communication Sensitivity Inventory
communication skills, positive
Communicative Abilities in Daily
  Living (CADL)
"communicative" arson
communicative disorder
Communicative Evaluation Chart
  from Infancy to Five Years
communicative interaction
community
  dialect speech
  speech
  therapeutic
Community College Student Experiences Questionnaire (CCSEQ)
community mental health center
  (CMHC)
Community-Oriented Programs
  Environment Scale (COPES)
community resources
comorbid Axis II diagnoses
comorbidity, psychiatric
comorbid personality disorder
compact phoneme
comparable forms reliability coefficient
Comparative Guidance and Placement
  Program (CGP)
comparative linguistics
comparative psychology

comparative research
comparative, superlative
compartmentalize
compensation psychoneurosis
compensatory behavior
compensatory mood swing
compensatory movement
compensatory technique
competence
  apparent
  communicative
  facade of
  linguistic
  mental
  social
  velopharyngeal
competency to stand trial
competent relational functioning
competing messages integration
Competing Sentence Test
competition
competitive behavior
complacent attitude
complaining, help-rejecting
complaint (pl. complaints)
  chief (CC)
  pain
  primary
  sleep
  somatic
  subjective insomnia
complaints of (c/o)
complement, objective
complemental air
complementarity of interaction
complementary distribution
complementary role
complete amnesia
complete aphasia
complete cleft palate
completed suicide
complete predicate

complete subject
completion
  arithmetic (problems), vocabulary, (following) directions (CAVD)
  picture (PC) (subtest)
  sentence
  task
complex
  AIDS dementia (ADC)
  benzodiazepine-GABA-receptor
  brother
  Cain
  castration
  Diana
  Electra
  father
  femininity
  God
  homosexual
  hypersexual
  inferiority
  Jocasta
  K
  Lear
  martyr
  messiah
  Mother Superior
  Oedipus
  persecution
  PTSD (posttraumatic stress disorder)
  spike and wave
  superiority
complex equivalence
complex hallucination
complex motor behavior
complex motor tics
complex multistep task
complex noise
complex partial seizure (CPS)
complex seizure, partial
complex sentence

Complex Speech Sound Discrimination Test
complex syllabics
complex task
complex thematic pictures test
complex tone
complex vocal tics
complex wave
complex whole body movements
complex word
compliance masking covert resistance, overt
compliance, patient
complicated grief disorder
complicated migraine headache
complications, psychosocial
complimentizer
component
  base
  grammatical
  morphological linguistic
  morphophonemic
  phonological linguistic
  pragmatic linguistic
  semantic linguistic
  syntactic linguistic
Composite Psycholinguistic Age
Composite Risk Index (CRI)
compound-complex sentence
compound consonant
compound sentence
compound word
Comprehending Oral Paragraphs
comprehension and production, language
comprehension deficit
comprehension factor, verbal (V factor)
comprehension impairment, reading
comprehension span
comprehension subtest
Comprehensive Ability Battery (CAB)

Comprehensive Assessment of
   Symptoms and History (CASH)
Comprehensive Assessment Program:
   Achievement Series
Comprehensive Career Assessment
   Scale (CCAS)
Comprehensive Developmental
   Evaluation Chart
Comprehensive Drinker Profile
Comprehensive Identification Process
   (CIP)
Comprehensive Level of Conscious-
   ness Scale (CLCS)
Comprehensive Psychiatric Rating
   Scale (CPRS)
Comprehensive Psychopathological
   Rating Scale
Comprehensive Test of Adaptive
   Behavior
Comprehensive Test of Basic Skills,
   Forms U and V
Comprehensive Test of Visual
   Functioning (CTVF)
compressed speech
compression amplification
compression bone conduction
compression, brain stem
compromise, cerebral
compromised function
compromise formation
Compton Speech and Language
   Screening Evaluation
compulsion neurosis
compulsion-obsession
compulsion psychoneurosis
compulsive action
compulsive behavior
compulsive disorder
compulsive disturbance
compulsive drug-taking behavior
compulsive eating
compulsive gambling

compulsive idea
compulsive insanity
compulsive mania
compulsive masturbation
compulsive neurosis
compulsive personality
compulsive psychasthenia, mixed
compulsive psychogenic tic
compulsive psychoneurotic reaction
compulsive reaction
compulsive substance use
   pattern of
   signs of
compulsive swearing
compulsive thoughts
compulsive tic
compulsive water drinking
computational process
computed tomography (CT) scan
computed tomography, single-photon
   emission (SPECT)
Computer Anxiety Index (Version
   AZ) (CAIN)
computer, biofeedback
computerized axial tomography
   (CAT) scan
Computer Operator Aptitude Battery
   (COAB)
Computer Programmer Aptitude
   Battery (CPAB)
Comrey Personality Scales
con-artists
conation
conative negative variation (CNV)
concatenation
conceit
conceited
concentrate
concentration
concentration ability, impaired
concentration and attention
concentration camp syndrome

concentration performance test (CPT)
concept (pl. concepts)
  abstract
  concrete
  critical band
  grandiose
  lexical
  medicine
  mental
  object
  self-derogatory
  self-role
concept formation
conception
Concept Mastery Test (CMT)
concept of brain function, semi-
  autonomous systems
Concept-Specific Anxiety Scale (CAS)
conceptual ability
conceptual disorder
conceptualization
conceptual skills
Conceptual Systems Test (CST)
conceptual thinking
concha (pl. conchae)
  inferior nasal
  medial nasal
  nasal
concomitant of anxiety, physical
concordance
concrete abstractive abilities
concrete concept
concreteness
concrete operations period
concrete representation
concrete thought processes
concretism
concurrent psychiatric problems
concurrent validity
concussion, brain
concussion amnesia

concussion of brain (grades 1-3)
condensation
condenser
condescending evaluation
condescension
conditioned emotional response (CER)
conditioned orientation reflex audiometry (COR)
Conditioned Place Preference (CPP)
conditioned response
conditioned sound change
conditioned stimulus
conditioning
  aversion-covert
  aversive
  classical
  counter
  eyelid
  instrumental
  negative (for sleep)
  operant
  pavlovian
  phonological
  respondent
conduct discharge, bad (BCD)
conduct disorder (pl. disorders)
  adjustment reaction
  adolescent
  adult-onset type
  childhood-onset type
  compulsive
  group-type
  hyperkinetic
  impulse control
  mixed conduct/emotions
  neuroleptic treatment of childhood
  socialized
  solitary aggressive type
  undersocialized
  undifferentiated
conduct-disordered child

conduction
air (AC)
bone (BC)
compression bone
distortional bond
ephaptic
inertial bone
motor nerve
pure tone air
pure tone bone
conduction aphasia
conduction studies, nerve
conductive deafness
conductive hearing loss
conductivity
"conductor" (lysergic acid diethylamide)
cone of light
confabulans, paraphrenia
confabulate
confabulated detail response
confabulation of speech
confabulatory alcoholic psychosis,
amnestic
confessions, false
confidence, facade of competence and
confidentiality
confident status
configuration
conflict (pl. conflicts)
approach-approach
approach-avoidance
avoidance-avoidance
emotional
extrapsychic
family
increased interpersonal
internal
interpersonal
intrafamilial
intrapsychic

conflict (cont.)
level of
marital
oedipal
parent-child
role
unconscious
conflicted (adj.)
conflict-free area
conflicting motives
Conflict in Marriage Scale (CIMS)
Conflict Management Appraisal
(CMA)
Conflict Management Survey (CMS)
conflict-resolution strategies
Conflict Tactics Scale
conflict theory, focal
conflictual relationship
conflictual situation
conforming
conformity, social
confront
confrontation naming test
confrontive
confused delusion
confused language syndrome (CLS)
confused speech
confusion
cognate
episodic
gender identity
identity
mental
nocturnal
postictal
postoperative
psychogenic
reactive
right-left
confusional arousals from sleep
confusional episode

confusional insanity
  acute
  subacute
confusional migraine headache, acute
confusional psychosis
  acute
  subacute
confusional psychotic reaction
confusional schizophrenic psychosis
confusional schizophreniform
  psychosis
confusional seizure, ictal
confusional state
  acute (ACS)
  alcoholic
  arteriosclerotic dementia
  arteriosclerotic psychosis
  drug-induced
  epileptic (ECS)
  postoperative
  presenile dementia
  reactive
  senile dementia
  subacute (SCS)
  twilight
confusion reactive psychosis
congenital deafness
congenital intersex condition
congenital syphilitic paralytic dementia
congruent affect
congruent, mood
conjoiner (parts of speech)
conjoint therapy
conjunction (parts of speech)
"connect" (drug supplier; to purchase
  drugs)
connectedness, family
connected speech
connective tissue
Conners Abbreviated Symptom Questionnaire
Conners Hyperkinesis Index, Parent
  Form

Conners Hyperkinesis Index, Teacher
  Form
Conners Parent and Teacher Symptom
  Questionnaire
Conners Parent Questionnaire (CPQ)
Conners Parent Rating Scale
  (CPRS-48, CPRS-93)
Conners Teacher Questionnaire
  (CTQ)
Conners Teacher Rating Scale
  (CTRS-28, CTRS-39)
connotation
consanguineous marriage
consanguinity
conscience
conscientious
conscientiousness
conscious awareness
consciousness (CS, Cs, cs)
  change in level of
  clouding of
  crude
  declining
  depression of
  discrimination
  disturbance in
  effect of trauma on
  episodic changes of
  impaired
  impairment of
  level of (LOC)
  loss of
  parasomniac
  state of (SOC)
consciousness disturbance stress
  reaction
conscious state, parasomniac
consensual validation
consent, informed
consenting adult
consenting partner
consequated

consequences of actions
conservation
  hearing
  speech
conservatorship
considered thought
consolidated sleep
consonance
consonant (pl. consonants)
  abutting
  arresting
  aspirate
  compound
  double
  final
  flap
  flat
  formation of
  fortis
  initial
  lax
  lenis
  nasal
  placement of
  position of
  releasing
  syllabic
  velarized
  vibrant
  voiced
  voiceless
  voicing of
consonantal alliteration
consonantal sound
consonantal writing
consonant blend
consonant cluster
consonant formation
  affricate
  continuant
  dark lateral
  fricative

consonant formation *(cont.)*
  frictionless
  glide
  groove fricative
  implosive
  light lateral
  liquid
  nasal
  obstruent
  plosive
  retroflex
  semi-vowel
  sibilant
  sonant
  spirant
  stop
  trill
consonant-injection method
consonant placement
  alveolar
  bilabial area
  glottal area
  labiodental area
  lingua-alveolar area
  linguadental area
  palatal area
  velar area
consonant position
  final
  initial
  intervocalic
  medial
  postvocalic
  prevocalic
consonant voicing
consonant-vowel (C-V)
consonant-vowel-consonant (C-V-C)
consonant-vowel-consonant syllable
consonant-vowel preference
consonant-vowel syllable
consort
conspiracy

conspirator
conspiratorial
conspire
constancy, object
constellation of signs and symptoms
constipation, psychogenic
constituent clause
constituent sentence
constituents
  immediate sentence
  sentence
constitution
  ideo-obsessional
  posttraumatic psychopathic
  psychopathic
constitutional psychology
constitutional psychopathia inferiority
  (CPI)
constitutional psychopathic state (CPS)
constitutional type
  asthenic
  athletic
  choleric
  dysplastic
  ectomorphic
  endomorphic
  melancholic
  mesomorphic
  phlegmatic
  pyknic
  sanguine
constraints, semantic
constricted activity
constricted affect
constricted, emotionally
constricted pupils
constricted vocal production
constriction
  emotional
  nares
  vocal
constriction of affect

constriction of thought
constrictor muscle
  inferior pharyngeal
  middle pharyngeal
  superior pharyngeal
construction
  endocentric
  exocentric
  phrase (PC)
  visual field
constructional ability
constructional apraxia
constructional dyspraxia
construction of femininity
construction of phrases
  absolute
  endocentric
  exocentric
construction, phrase (PC)
construct theory, personal
construct validity
consultation liaison psychiatry
Consultation-Liaison Service (CLS)
consumption
contact-exploration maneuver, body
contact, eye
"contact lens" (lysergic acid diethylamide)
contact ulcer
contact with reality, inconsistent
contagion
contamination
contemporaneity
contempt
contemptuous
content
  dream
  grandiose
  language
  latent
  manifest
  paucity of speech

content *(cont.)*
  positive speech
  poverty of
  self-derogatory
  speech
  thought
Content Mastery Examinations for
  Educators (CMEE)
Content Scales (on MMPI)
content speech, serial
content validity
content word
context, phonetic
context reframing
contextual therapy
contiguity aphasia
contiguity disorder aphasia
continence, fecal
contingency management
continuant consonant formation
continuing medical education (CME)
continuity disturbance, sleep
Continuous Performance Testing (CPT)
continuous reinforcement (CR)
Continuous Visual Memory Test
  (CVMT)
continuum of care
continuum theory
contour (pl. contours)
  equal loudness
  intonation
contour tones
contract (pl. contracts)
  formal
  formalized
  group
  informal
  legal
  quasi
contraction, rhythmic
contractual behavior
contractual psychiatry

contractual psychotherapy
contradictory information
contralateral neglect syndrome
contralateral parietal lobe dysfunction
contralateral routing of signals
  (CROS)
  bilateral (BICROS)
  focal (FOCALCROS)
contralateral routing of signals hearing
  aid (CROS)
contrast sensitivity
contrastive analysis
contrastive distribution
contrastive linguistics
contrastive stress
contrasts
  maximal
  minimal
contrasts processes, feature
contributing role
control
  attentional
  automatic gain
  automatic volume (AVC)
  aversive
  brain stem
  degree of
  delusion of
  diminished
  ego
  executive
  external
  feedback
  feeling out of
  image
  impaired
  impulse
  internal-external
  interpersonal
  island of
  lack of
  locus of (LOC)

control *(cont.)*
  losing
  loss of
  manual volume
  mental
  mind
  need to
  neurological
  not in
  one's own
  out of (OOC)
  outside
  personal
  psycho-optical reflex
  rate
  social
  stimulus
  superego
  swing phase
  taking
  thought
  tone
  ventilatory
control feedback
control frustration
control group
controlled analgesics
controlled, delusion of being
controlled emotion
controlled environment
controlled release drug (CR)
controlling external entities
controlling external spirits
controlling identity
contusion
  brain
  cerebral
convergence circuit
conversation board
conversational catharsis
conversational postulates
conversational speech

conversion anesthesia
conversion aphonia
conversion ataxia
conversion blindness
conversion deafness
conversion disorder
conversion hysteria psychoneurosis
conversion neurosis
conversion paralysis
conversion reaction
  anesthetic
  autonomic
  hyperkinetic
  hysterical (HCR)
  mixed paralytic
  paresthetic
  psychoneurotic
conversion seizure
conversion sensory change
conversion symptoms
conversion-type hysterical neurosis
conversion unconsciousness
conviction, delusional
convolution
convulsant
convulsibility
convulsion (see *seizure*)
convulsive disorder
convulsive equivalent
convulsive melancholia
convulsive seizure
convulsive state
convulsive status epilepticus
convulsive therapy
convulsive tic
co-occurrence of depression
co-occurring mental disorders
cooing
"cook" (re: drug injection)
"cook down" (re: heroin use)
"cooker" (re: drug injection)
"cookies" (crack)

"cooler" (drug-laced cigarette)
"coolie" (cocaine-laced cigarette)
Cooperation Institutional Research
    Program (CIRP)
Cooperation Preschool Inventory—
    Revised
cooperative behavior
Cooperative Primary Tests (CPT)
Cooper-Farran Behavioral Rating
    Scales (CFBRS)
Cooper-MacGuire Diagnostic Word
    Analysis Test
coordinate convulsion
coordination disorder, developmental
"cop" (to obtain drugs)
COPD (chronic obstructive pulmonary
    disease)
COPE (Coping Operations Preference
    Enquiry)
cope, inability to
COPES (Community-Oriented Pro-
    grams Environment Scale)
"copilots" (amphetamine)
coping
    ideational style of
    rational/cognitive
coping ability
Coping Inventory, Early
coping mechanisms
Coping Operations Preference Enquiry
    (COPE)
Coping Resources Inventory (CRI)
coping strategies
coping style
    analysis of
    extratensive
Coping with Stress test
copodyskinesia
"copping zone" (re: drug-buying area)
co-presence
coprolagnia
coprolalia

coprolalomania
coprophagia
coprophagous
coprophagy
coprophilia
coprophobia
coprostasophobia
COPS (California Occupational
    Preference Survey or System)
COPSystem Interest Inventory
copula
copy geometric designs test
copy intersecting pentagons test
coquettish
COR (conditioned orientation reflex
    audiometry)
"coral" (barbiturate)
cordectomy
cords, vocal
core body temperature measurement
core gender identity
core mindfulness skills
core vocabulary
"coriander seeds" (re: currency)
"cork the air" (re: cocaine use)
Cornell Critical Thinking Tests,
    Level X and Level Z
Cornell Learning and Study Skills
    Inventory (CLASSI)
Cornell Medical Index
Cornell Word Form (CWF)
corniculate cartilage
coronal orientation
coronal plane
coronal sounds
corporal agnosia
corporal punishment
corpus (pl. corpora)
corpus callosum
Correctional Institutions Environment
    Scale
Correctional Officers' Interest Blank

correctional transfer (C.T.)
correction, speech
corrective emotional experience
corrective feedback
corrective therapy
correlates, psycho-physiologic
correlation
   coefficient of
   negative
   positive
"Corrinne" (cocaine)
corroborative
cortex (pl. cortices)
   association
   auditory
   cerebellar
   cerebral
   deep
   motor
   primary auditory
   sensory
cortical alexia
cortical aphasia
cortical apraxia
cortical deafness
cortical epilepsy
cortical evoked potential
cortical function, mapping of
cortical gray matter deficit
cortical lateralization
cortical mapping
cortical network
cortical sensory loss
cortical testing
cortical thumb position
cortices (see *cortex*)
corticoadrenal insufficiency
cortisol, plasma
cortisol secretion
COS (Campbell Organizational Survey)
"cosa" (cannabis)
cosine wave

cosmic identification
Costa/McCrae factors
cost-benefit analysis
Costen syndrome
Cotard syndrome
co-therapy
"cotics" (heroin)
cotinine
"cotton" (re: currency)
"cotton brothers" (cocaine, heroin,
   and morphine)
cough preparations with codeine
   (street names)
   blue velvet
   Robby
   schoolboy
cough, psychogenic
coulomb
counseling psychology
counselor
   camp
   Chemical Dependency (CDC)
   child
   couples
   disability
   drug
   family
   genetic
   grief
   individual
   legal
   marital
   marriage
   pastoral
   personal
   professional
   rehabilitation
   school
   spiritual
   substance abuse
   youth
count backwards from 100 test

counter conditioning
counterhostility
counterphobia
counterphobic
countertransference
counting-money tremor
coupler
couples counselor
Couples Pre-Counseling Inventory
couples therapy
coupling, nasal
"courage pills" (barbiturate; heroin)
course
    atypical
    clinical
    continuous
    deteriorating
    episodic
    global
    rapid-cycling
"course note" (re: currency)
course of abuse, long-term
course of action
course of illness
course of treatment
course patterns, prototypical
courtship behavior
co-variance
covert behavior
covert feelings
covert message
covert resistance, overt compliance
    masking
covert response
"Cozmo's" (phencyclidine)
CP (child psychiatry, child psychology)
CPAB (Computer Programmer
    Aptitude Battery)
C-PAC (Clinical Probes of Articulation Consistency)
CPI (California Personality Inventory)

CPI (California Psychological
    Inventory)
CPI (constitutional psychopathia
    inferiority)
CPIT (California Psychological
    Inventory Test)
CPP (Career Planning Program)
CPP (Conditioned Place Preference)
CPQ (Children's Personality
    Questionnaire)
CPQ (Conners Parent Questionnaire)
CPRS (Children's Psychiatric Rating
    Scale)
CPRS (Comprehensive Psychiatric
    Rating Scale)
CPRS-48, CPRS-93 (Conners Parent
    Rating Scale)
CPS (Child Personality Scale)
CPS (clinical performance score)
CPS (complex partial seizure)
CPS (constitutional psychopathic state)
CPS (cumulative probability of
    success)
cps (cycle per second) tremor
CPSCS (California Preschool Social
    Competency Scale)
CPSI (Children's Perception of
    Support Inventory)
CPT (combining power test)
CPT (concentration performance test)
CPT (continuous performance task or
    test)
CPT (Cooperative Primary Tests)
CR (continuous reinforcement)
CR (controlled release)
crack (processed cocaine) (street
    names)
    apple jacks
    Baby T
    bad
    ball
    base

crack *(cont.)*

baseball
bazooka
beam me up Scottie
beautiful boulders
Bebe
beemers
Bill Blass
black rock
blowcaine
blowout
blow up
blue
bobo
bonecrusher
bones
botray
boubou
boulder
boulya
brick
bubble gum
bullia capital
bullion
bump
butter
caine
cap
caps
Casper the ghost
caviar
chasing the dragon
cheap basing
chemical
chewies
chocolate ecstasy
cloud
cloud nine
coco rocks
cookies
crack back
crack cooler

crack *(cont.)*

crib
croak
demolish
devil's dandruff
devilsmoke
dime
dip
dirty basing
DOA
double rock
Eastside player
egg
eightball
eye opener
famous dimes
fat bags
fifty-one
fire
fish scales
flat chunks
freebase
French fries
fries
fry
fry daddy
garbage rock
geek
gimmie
glo
gold
golf ball
gravel
grit
groceries
hail
half track
hamburger helper
hard line
hard rock
hit
hotcakes

crack *(cont.)*
How do you like me now?
Hubba, I am back
hubbas
I am back
ice cube
issues
jelly beans
Johnson
kangaroo
Kokomo
Kryptonite
love
missile basing
mist
moonrock
nuggets
one-fifty-one
outerlimits
parachute
parlay
paste
patico
pebbles
Pee Wee
P-funk
piedras
piles
pony
potato chips
press
primo
raw
ready rock
red caps
regular P
roca
rock attack
rocks of hell
Rocky III
rooster
rox

crack *(cont.)*
Roxanne
Roz
schoolcraft
Scotty
scramble
scruples
Seven-up
sheet rocking
sherms
sightball
slab
sleet
smoke
snow soke
space base
space cadet
space dust
square time Bob
stones
sugar block
swell up
teeth
tension
the devil
tissue
top gun
torpedo
tragic magic
troop
turbo
ultimate
uzi
wave
white ball
white ghost
white sugar
white tornado
wrecking crew
yahoo/yeaho
Yale
yimyom

"crack attack" (crack craving)
"crack back" (crack and cannabis)
"crack cooler" (crack smoked in wine cooler)
"cracker jacks" (re: crack users)
"crackers" (lysergic acid diethylamide)
"crack gallery" (crack-buying place)
crack-laced cigarette (street names)
  cocktail
  crimmie
  fry daddy
"crack spot" (crack-buying place)
cradle audiometry, neonatal auditory response
cradle, neonatal auditory response
craft neurosis
cranial aneurysm
cranial nerve I (olfactory)
cranial nerve II (optic)
cranial nerve III (oculomotor)
cranial nerve IV (trochlear)
cranial nerve V (trigeminal)
cranial nerve VI (abducens)
cranial nerve VII (facial)
cranial nerve VIII (auditory)
cranial nerve IX (glossopharyngeal)
cranial nerve X (vagus)
cranial nerve XI (spinal accessory)
cranial nerve XII (hypoglossal)
cranial nerve deficit
cranial nerve palsy
craniocerebral trauma
craniofacial anomalies
craniopharyngeal canal
"crank" (methamphetamine hydrochloride)
"cranking up" (re: drug injection)
cranky mood
"crap/crop" (low-quality heroin)
CRAS (Clinician Rated Anxiety Scale)

"crash" (re: drug use)
cravings
"crazy coke" (phencyclidine)
"Crazy Eddie" (phencyclidine)
"crazy weed" (cannabis)
CRC (cross-reacting cannabinoids)
creativeness
Creativity Assessment Packet
Creativity Attitude Survey (CAS)
Creativity Checklist
Creativity Tests for Children (CTC)
credible
credibility
"credit card" (re: crack equipment)
creeping-crawling sensation
cremnomania
cremnophobia
Creole English
crepuscular state
crescendo-decrescendo breathing
cresomania
cretin
cretinism
cretinistic
cretinoid idiocy
cretinous
Creutzfeldt-Jakob disease
CRI (Caring Relationship Inventory)
CRI (Composite Risk Index)
CRI (Coping Resources Inventory)
"crib" (crack)
crib-o-gram
crib-o-gram audiometer
cricoarytenoid ankylosis
cricoarytenoid joint
cricoarytenoid muscle
  lateral
  posterior
cricoid cartilage
cricothyroid muscle
cricothyroid paralysis
cri-du-chat syndrome

criminal behavior
criminal insanity
criminality
criminaloid
criminal psychology
criminal sexual psychopath (CSP)
"crimmie" (crack-laced cigarette)
"crink" (methamphetamine)
"cripple" (cannabis cigarette)
cripple, social
"cris" (methamphetamine)
crisis (pl. crises)
  adolescent
  bed
  emotional
  financial
  hypertensive
  identity
  midlife
  oculogyric
  parkinsonian
  precipitating
  psychogenic oculogyric
  psychosexual identity
  therapeutic
crisis center, rape
Crisis Evaluation Referral Service
  (CERS)
crisis intervention
crisis-intervention group psychotherapy
"crisscross" (amphetamine)
"Cristina" (methamphetamine)
"Cristy" (smokable methamphetamine)
criteria (sing. criterion)
  abuse
  behavioral
  equivalent
  equivalent intoxication
  equivalent withdrawal
  evaluation of
  impairment
  full symptom

criteria *(cont.)*
  method of defining
  relevant diagnostic
  von Knorring
criteria set, single
criterion (singular) (see *criteria*)
criterion B for dysthymic disorder,
  alternative
criterion-referenced test
criterion-related validity
Criterion Test of Basic Skills
criterion variable
critical age
critical band concept
critical period of learning
critical ratio
Critical Reasoning Tests (CRT)
critical submodalities
criticism
  constructive
  destructive
  objective
  parental
  peer
  professional
  self-
  overt
criticize
Crk protein
"croak" (crack and methamphetamine)
crocidismus
crooked
CROS (contralateral routing of signals)
  binaural
  high (HICROS) frequency
CROS hearing aid
cross-bite malposition of teeth
cross-consonant injection method
cross-cultural psychiatry
cross-dressing
  complete
  forced

cross-dressing *(cont.)*
  motivation for
  partial
crossed laterality
cross-gender behavior
  adolescent
  adult
  childhood
cross-gender identification
cross hearing
cross-modality perception
cross-over mirroring
cross-reacting cannabinoids (CRC)
"crossroads" (amphetamine sulfate)
cross-sectional (experimental study
  designs)
cross-sex roles
cross-talk
cross-tolerance
cross validation
croupous laryngitis
crowd behavior
crowd consciousness
crowd control
Crowley Occupational Interests Blank
  (COIB)
CRS (Clinical Rating Scale)
CRT (Critical Reasoning Tests)
crude consciousness
crude marijuana extract (CME)
crural ataxia
crus (pl. crura)
CRVS (California Relative Value
  Studies)
crying jags
crying spells
cryomania
cryophobia
cryptococcal meningitis
cryptogenic epilepsy
cryptogenic seizure
cryptomnesia

cryptomnesic
cryptopsychic
cryptopsychism
"crystal" (methamphetamine hydrochloride)
"crystal joint" (phencyclidine)
crystallized grandiose delusion
"crystal meth" (methamphetamine
  hydrochloride)
crystallophobia
"crystal T" (phencyclidine)
"crystal tea" (lysergic acid diethyl-
  amide)
CS, Cs, cs (conscious, consciousness)
CSA (Cognitive Skills Assessment)
CSCS (Children's Self-Concept Scale)
CSF (cerebrospinal fluid)
CSF cytomegalovirus antibody
CSP (criminal sexual psychopath)
CSQ (College Student Questionnaires)
CSRI (Caregiver's School Readiness
  Inventory)
CSSQ (College Student Satisfaction
  Questionnaire)
CST (Conceptual Systems Test)
CSW (Certified Social Worker)
CT (computed tomography) scan
CT (correctional transfer)
CT (corrective therapy)
CTBS (California Test of Basic Skills)
CTBS (Canadian Tests of Basic
  Skills)
CTC (Creativity Tests for Children)
CTMM-SF (California Short-Form
  Test of Mental Maturity)
CTP (California Test of Personality)
CTQ (Conners Teacher Question-
  naire)
CTRS-28, CTRS-39 (Conners
  Teacher Rating Scale)
CTVF (Comprehensive Test of Visual
  Functioning)

"cube" (lysergic acid diethylamide;
   1 ounce)
"cubes" (cannabis tablets)
cubic centimeter (cc)
cuckold
cuddling behavior
cue (pl. cues)
   accessing
   auditory
   eye accessing
   kinesthetic
   learning
   visual
cued speech
cue-elicited craving
cueing
CUES (College and University
   Environment Scales)
cul-de-sac voice disorder
"culican" (cannabis)
culpable
cult
cult of personality
cults, killer
cultural adjustment following migration
cultural assessment
cultural assimilation
Cultural Attitude Inventories (CAI)
Cultural Attitude Scales (CAS)
cultural deprivation
cultural discrimination
cultural-familial mental retardation
cultural identity
Cultural Literacy Test
culturally appropriate avoidant
   behavior
culturally bound syndromes
culturally deprived
culturally disadvantaged
culturally sanctioned

culturally unsanctioned
cultural norms
cultural reference group
cultural-related standards of sexual
   behavior
cultural subgroup
culture
   coexistent
   drug
   host
   individual's
   industrialized
   person's
   street-drug
culture-bound belief
culture-bound syndrome (CBS)
Culture Fair Intelligence Test (CFIT)
Culture Free Intelligence Test (CFIT)
Culture-Free Self-Esteem Inventories,
   Second Edition (CFSEI-2)
Culture-Free Self-Esteem Inventories
   for Children and Adults
culture of origin
Culture Shock Inventory
culture-specific syndrome
   amok
   koro
   latah
   piblokto
   windigo
cumulative probability of success
   (CPS)
cuneiform cartilage
cunnilingus
cunning and hiding behavior
"cupcakes" (lysergic acid diethylamide)
"cura" (heroin)
curled into fetal position (posture)
current
   alternating (AC)
   direct (DC)

Current and Past Psychopathology
    Scales (CAPPS)
cursing
cursive epilepsy
Curtis Completion Form
Curtis Interest Scale
curve
    articulation
    bell-shaped
    discrimination
    falling
    frequency response
    gaussian
    learning
    normal probability
    probability
cushingoid facies
Cushing syndrome
custodial care
custody, joint
customs, foreign
"cushion" (re: drug injection)
cuspid teeth
Custody Quotient, The
"cut" (adulterate drugs)
cutaneous disorder, psychogenic
"cut-deck" (heroin mixed with
    powdered milk)
cut, visual field
CV or C-V (consonant-vowel)
CVA (cerebrovascular accident)
CVC, C-V-C (consonant-vowel-
    consonant)
CVMT (Continuous Visual Memory
    Test)
CWF (Cornell Word Form)
cyad
cybernetic theory in stuttering
cybernetics
cyclazocine

cycle
    basic rest-activity (BRAC)
    desire phase of sexual response
    duration duty
    excitement phase of sexual
        response
    glottal
    life
    menstrual
    orgasmic phase of sexual response
    perceptual
    phase shift of sleep-wake
    resolution phase of sexual response
    sexual response
    short
    sleep
    sleep-wake
    sleep-wakefulness
    vibratory
    vicious
cycle noise hum, sixth
cycler, rapid
cycles per second (CPS) tremor
cyclic abulia
cyclic adenosine monophosphate
    (cAMP)
cyclical pattern of symptoms
cyclical vomiting, psychogenic
cyclic depression
cyclic headache
cyclic history
cyclic insanity
cyclic mood disorder
cyclic schizophrenia
"cycline" (phencyclidine)
cycling, mood disorder with rapid
cycloid personality
"cyclones" (phencyclidine)
cycloplegia
cyclothyme

cyclothymia
cyclothymiac
cyclothymic personality disorder
cymophobia
cynomania

cynophobia
cypridophobia
cypriphobia
cystic fibrosis
cysts of the larynx

D, d

/d (daily, per day)
    1/d (once a day; q.d.)
    2/d (twice a day; b.i.d.)
    3/d (three times a day; t.i.d.)
    4/d (four times a day; q.i.d.)
D (divergent production)
"D" (lysergic acid diethylamide;
    phencyclidine)
DA (drug addict)
DAB-2 (Diagnostic Achievement
    Battery, Second Edition)
"dabble" (re: drug use)
Daberon Screening for School
    Readiness
DACA (Drug Abuse Control Amend-
    ments)
DACL (Depression Adjective Check
    List)
DaCosta syndrome
dactylology
dactyl speech
DAD (dispense as directed)
DAF (delayed auditory feedback)
"dagga" (ethnic term, cannabis)
daily (see /d)

daily living
    activities of (ADLs)
    simulated activities of (SADL)
daily living skills, activities of
    (ADLS)
daily symptom ratings
DALE (Developmental Assessment
    of Life Experiences) System
dam, dental
"dama blanca" (cocaine)
damped wave
damping
"dance fever" (fentanyl)
dance therapy
dancing disease
dancing mania
dangerous behavior reaction
danger to others/self
Dantomania
DAP (Diversity Awareness Profile)
DAP:SPED (Draw A Person: Screen-
    ing Procedure for Emotional
    Disturbance)
DAR (Diagnostic Assessments of
    Reading)

dark environment
dark lateral consonant formation
darkening of vision
DARS (The Child "At Risk" for Drug
   Abuse Rating Scale)
DART (Diagnostic and Achievement
   Reading Tests) Phonics Testing
   Program
DAS (Death Anxiety Scale)
DASE, D.A.S.E. (Denver Articulation
   Screening Examination)
DASI (Developmental Activities
   Screening Inventory)
DAT (dementia of the Alzheimer type)
DAT (Differential Aptitude Tests),
   Fifth Edition
data
   empirical
   epidemiological
   field
   long-term
   NIMH
   normative
   reanalyzed
   survey
data reanalysis strategy
data sets, unpublished
date of birth (DOB)
DAT for PCA (Differential Aptitude
   Tests for Personnel and Career
   Assessment)
dative case (parts of speech)
DATTA (Diagnostic and Therapeutic
   Technology Assessment)
daughter language
"dawamesk" (cannabis)
day (see /d)
day of month test
day residue
day terrors (pavor diurnus)
daytime mouth breathing
daytime somnolence

day-to-day function
day treatment center (DTC)
dB (decibel)
DBD (Dementia Behavior
   Disturbance) Scale
DBT (dialectical behavior therapy)
DC (direct current; discharge)
D/C (discontinue; discharge)
DCD (Dennis Test of Child Develop-
   ment)
DD (developmental disability)
DD (developmentally disabled)
DD (dysthymic disorder)
DDD (Division of Developmental
   Disabilities)
DDS (disability determination service)
DDST (Denver Developmental
   Screening Test)
DEA (Drug Enforcement
   Administration)
DEA # (Drug Enforcement Administration number)
deadness, emotional
"dead on arrival" (heroin)
dead room (no-echo chamber)
deaf mute
deaf speech
deafness
   acoustic trauma
   Alexander
   boilermaker's
   catarrhal
   central
   conductive
   congenital
   conversion
   cortical
   functional
   HF (high frequency)
   hysterical
   industrial
   labyrinthine

deafness *(cont.)*
  low-tone
  midbrain
  mixed
  Mondini
  nerve
  neural
  noise-induced
  nonorganic
  occupational
  organic
  perceptive
  postlingual
  prelingual
  prevocational
  psychogenic
  pure word
  retrocochlear
  Scheibe
  sensorineural
  tone
  toxic
  word
dealing drugs
death
  attitude to
  brain
  cause of
  cerebral
  cerebral brain
  expected
  expectation of
  fear of
  hypoxyphilia-caused
  impending
  nerve cell
  news of
  premature
  preoccupation with
  reaction to
  sudden sniffing
  suffering

death *(cont.)*
  survivors of
  thoughts of
  threat of
  unexpected
  untimely
  violent
Death Anxiety Scale (DAS)
deathbed
death instinct (Thanatos)
Death Personification Exercise (DPE)
death syndrome, brain
death wish, Klein's
debilitating anxiety
debility, nervous
"decadence" (methylenedioxymethamphetamine)
Deca-Durabolin (injectable steroid)
decanoate injection
decay
  reflex
  tone
decay period
decay rate
deceitfulness, therapeutic approaches
  for
deceive, intention to
decentration
deception, effects of
decibel (dB)
deciduous teeth
decision
  Brawner
  Gault
  Tarasoff
Decision-Making (test)
  Assessment of Career (ACDM)
  Career (CDM)
Decision Making Inventory
Decision-Making Organizer
decision-making process
decision theory

decision trees
decisive
"deck" (1 to 15 grams of heroin;
  packet of drugs)
declarative sentence
decline, age-related cognitive
decline in academic functioning
declining consciousness
decoder
decoding skills
Decoding Skills Test
decompensating
decompensation, impending
decomposition
deconditioning
decussation
deduction
"deeda" (lysergic acid diethylamide)
deep articulation test
deep cortex
deep nasolabial folds
deep sleep
deep structure
deep tendon reflexes (DTRs),
  exaggeration of
deep trance identification
de-escalating aggressive behavior
defecalgesiophobia
defect
  body dysmorphic
  camouflage the
  developmental
  exaggerated
  excessive concern for
  high-grade
  imagined
  learning
  physical
  preoccupation with
  slight
  speech
  visual field

defenestrated
defense
  character
  ego
  egomechanism of
  hysteroid
  insanity
  perceptual
  stormed
Defense Functioning Scale (DFS)
defense level
defense mechanism
  acting-out
  compensation
  conversion
  denial
  displacement
  dissociation
  idealization
  identification
  incorporation
  introjection
  projection
  rationalization
  reaction formation
  regression
  sublimation
  substitution
  symbolization
  undoing
Defense Mechanism Inventory (DMI)
defensive adultomorphic stance
defensive behavior
defensive dysregulation, level of
defensive functioning axis
Defensive Functioning Scale (DFS)
defiant behavior
deficiency (pl. deficiencies)
  dementia due to vitamin
  environmental
  familial
  hearing

deficiency *(cont.)*
  hereditary
  iron
  mental (MD)
  moral
  nutritional
  vitamin
  vitamin B$_{12}$
deficit
  attention
  central language
  central sensory
  cognitive
  comprehension
  cortical gray matter
  cranial nerve
  emotional
  gaze
  global cognitive
  gross motor
  gross neurologic
  gross sensory
  language
  linguistic
  memory
  mental
  motor
  multiple cognitive
  neural
  neurologic
  sensory
  speech-motor
  speech perception
deficit symptoms
defining criteria, method of
definition
  categorical
  operational
deflected eyes
deflection

degeneration
  axon
  brain
  cerebellar
  granulovascular
  neuronal
  olivopontocerebellar
  spinocerebellar
degeneration of true folds, polypoid
degenerative dementia
degenerative encephalopathy
degenerative insanity
degenerative primary dementia
degenitalize
deglutition
degrading ritual
degree of amnesia
degree of control
degree of disability
degree of impairment
Degrees of Reading Power (DRP)
dehumanization
dehumanizing
deictic
deinstitutionalization
deity
deixis
  person
  place
  time
déjà éntendu (already heard)
déjà eprouvé (already tested)
déjà fait (already done)
déjà pensé (already thought)
déjà raconté (already told)
déjà vécu (already lived)
déjà voulu (already desired)
déjà vu (already seen) aura
dejected mood
Dejerine syndrome
de Lange syndrome
delatestryl (injectable steroid)

delay, developmental
delayed auditory feedback (DAF)
delayed development
delayed feedback audiometry (DFA)
delayed gratification
delayed grief
delayed language
delayed memory
delayed posttraumatic stress disorder
delayed reflex
delayed response
delayed sleep phase dyssomnia
delayed speech
delayed toilet training
deleterious
deletion
    final consonant
    initial consonant
    stridency
    syllable
    thought
    unstressed syllable
    weak syllable
deliberate fire-setting
deliberate therapy
delineation
delinquency
    adolescent neurotic
    group
    juvenile neurotic
    neurotic
    recovery from
delinquent, juvenile
delirante, bouffée
deliriant
delirifacient
delirious mania
delirium (pl. deliria)
    acute
    alcoholic
    alcohol intoxication
    alcohol withdrawal

delirium *(cont.)*
    amphetamine intoxication
    anticholinergic
    anxiolytic intoxication
    anxiolytic withdrawal
    anxious
    cannabis intoxication
    chronic
    cocaine intoxication
    collapse
    digitalis-induced
    drug-induced
    eclamptic
    exhaustion
    febrile
    frank
    full-blown
    grave
    hallucinogen intoxication
    hypnotic intoxication
    hypnotic withdrawal
    hypoglycemic
    hysterical
    inhalant intoxication
    low
    manic
    melancholia with
    muttering
    opioid intoxication
    organic
    phencyclidine intoxication
    posttraumatic
    puerperal
    sedative intoxication
    sedative withdrawal
    senile
    subacute
    substance-induced
    substance intoxication
    substance withdrawal
    superimposed
    thyroid

delirium *(cont.)*
  toxic
  trauma-induced
  traumatic
delirium alcoholicum
delirium in presenile dementia
delirium in senile dementia
delirium-like state
delirium mussitans
delirium-related mental disorder
delirium schizophrenoides
delirium sine delirio
delirium tremens (DT, DTs, Dts, dt's)
delirium verborum
Del Rio Language Screening Test
  (DRLST), English/Spanish
delta activity, EEG
delta index
delta-9-THC
delta opiate receptors
delta receptors
delta rhythm
delta waves (on EEG)
delusion (pl. delusions)
  affect-laden
  alcohol-induced psychotic disorder
    with
  amphetamine-induced psychotic
    disorder with
  bizarre
  cannabis-induced psychotic
    disorder with
  circumscribed
  cocaine
  cocaine-induced psychotic disorder
    with
  confused
  control
  depression
  depressive
  disorganized
  encapsulated

delusion *(cont.)*
  erotomanic-type
  established
  expansive
  expressive
  first rank symptoms of
  fixed
  focus of the
  fragmentary
  grandeur
  grandiose
  grandiose-type
  infidelity
  influence
  jealous-type
  mixed-type
  mood-congruent
  mood-incongruent
  negation
  nihilistic
  non-bizarre
  nonsystematized
  object of a
  paranoid
  passivity
  persecution
  persecutory type
  persistent
  poverty
  reference
  referential
  religious
  somatic-type
  systematized
  unspecified-type
  unsystematized
  well-formed
delusional behavior
delusional belief
  dominant
  shared
delusional conviction

delusional depression
delusional disorder
delusional equivalent
delusional experience
  atypical
  brief
delusional, floridly
delusional insanity
delusional jealousy
delusional network
delusional projection
delusional proportions
delusional syndrome
  drug-induced organic
  drug psychosis with
delusional system
  fixed
  focus of
  persecutory
delusional thought patterns
delusional-type arteriosclerotic
  dementia
delusion of being controlled
demanding behavior
demandingness
demands of society
demarcated relationships
demarcation in sensory testing
demented
dementia
  acute
  advanced
  alcoholic
  alcohol-induced persisting
  Alzheimer
  arteriosclerotic
  atrophic
  beclouded
  Binswanger
  catatonic
  chronic
  congenital

dementia *(cont.)*
  developmental
  dialysis
  drug-induced
  early
  early phase of
  epileptic
  familial
  frontal lobe
  global
  hebephrenic
  Heller
  HIV-based
  impairments of
  infantile
  lacunar
  language disorder in
  legal aspects of
  multi-infarct
  old-age
  paralytic
  paranoid
  paraphrenic
  paretic
  persisting
  Pike
  post-traumatic
  preexisting
  pre-senile
  primary
  primary degenerative
  progressive
  psychobiological process of
  puerperal
  remitting
  repeated infarct
  schizophrenic
  secondary
  semantic
  senile (Alzheimer type) (SDAT)
  severe
  simplex type

dementia *(cont.)*
  stages of
  static
  subcortical
  substance-induced
  substance-induced persisting
  terminal
  toxic
  traumatic
  vascular
  Wernicke
dementia-aphonia syndrome of childhood
Dementia Behavior Disturbance Scale
  (DBD)
dementia complex, AIDS (ADC)
dementia due to:
  Alzheimer disease
  anoxia
  brain tumor
  endocrine conditions
  hepatic conditions
  Huntington disease
  immune disorders
  infectious disorders
  metabolic conditions
  neurological conditions
  normal-pressure hydrocephalus
  Parkinson disease
  Pick disease
  prion diseases
  traumatic brain injury
  vitamin deficiencies
dementia in:
  arteriosclerotic brain disease
  cerebral lipidoses
  epilepsy
  general paralysis of the insane
  hepatolenticular degeneration
  Huntington chorea
  Jakob-Creutzfeldt disease
  multiple sclerosis

dementia in:
  neurosyphilis
  Pelizaeus-Merzbacher disease
  Pick disease
  polyarteritis nodosa
  Wilson disease
Dementia Mood Assessment Scale
  (DMAS)
dementia myoclonica
dementia of the Alzheimer type (DAT)
dementia paralytica
dementia paralytica juvenilis
dementia paranoides
dementia praecox
dementia presenilis
dementia pugilistica
dementia-related mental disorder
dementing illness, progressive
"demo" (a sample-size quantity of
  crack)
democratic (leadership pattern)
"demolish" (crack)
demomania
demonomania
demonophobia
demonstrative article
demonstrative entity
demophobia
demyelinating encephalopathy
denarcotized opium
denasal
denasality voice disorder
denasalization
dendrite
dendrophobia
denervation
  autonomic
  level of
denial of anhedonia, amotivation or
  anergy
denial, psychotic
denial visual hallucination syndrome

denigrate
denigrated self-esteem
denigration
Dennie-Marfan syndrome
Dennis Test of Child Development
(DCD)
denotation
dense scotoma
dense sensory loss
density, REM
dental anxiety
dental arch
dental caries
dental dam
dental erosion
dental lisp
dentition
denuding, hair
Denver Articulation Screening
Examination (DASE, D.A.S.E.)
Denver Developmental Screening Test
(DDST)
Denver Prescreening Development
Questionnaire, Revised (R-PDQ)
Denver II test
deodorized opium
depalatalization
Department of Health and Human
Services, U.S. (DHHS)
Department of Mental Health (DMH)
dependence (substance)
absinthe
acemorphan
acetanilid(e)
acetophenetidin
acetorphine
acetyldihydrocodeinone
aerosol spray
airplane glue (sniffing)
alcohol
allobarbitone
alphaprodine

dependence *(cont.)*
Alurate
amethocaine
amidone
amidopyrine
aminopyrine
amobarbital
amphetamine
amphetamine analog
amylene hydrate
amyl nitrite
amylobarbitone
amylocaine
Amytal
analgesic drug
anesthetic (agent)
anileridine
antipyrine
aprobarbital
atropine
Avertin
barbenyl
barbital
barbitone
barbiturate
barbituric acid
benzedrine
benzine
bindweed
biphetamine
Brevital
bromal
bromide
bromine compounds
bromisovalum
bromoform
Bromo-Seltzer
butabarbital
butabarpal
butallylonal
butane (sniffing)
butethal

dependence *(cont.)*
  buthalitone
  Butisol
  butyl chloral
  butyl nitrate
  caffeine
  cannabis
  carbamazepine
  carbon tetrachloride
  carbromal
  carisoprodol
  Catha (C. edulis)
  chloral betaine
  chloralformamide
  chloral hydrate
  chloralose
  chlordiazepoxide
  Chloretone
  chlorobutanol
  chloroform
  chlorprothixene
  cleaning fluid (sniffing)
  coca leaf
  cocaine
  codeine
  cough preparations with codeine
  croton
  cyclobarbital
  cyclobarbitone
  Cylert
  d-lysergic acid diethylamide
  Dalmane
  Darvon
  Demerol
  desocodeine
  desomorphine
  desoxyephedrine
  dexamphetamine
  Dexamyl
  Dexedrine
  dextroamphetamine
  dextromethorphan

dependence *(cont.)*
  dextromoramide
  dextronorpseudoephedrine
  diacetylmorphine
  Dial
  diallylbarbituric acid
  diamorphine
  diazepam
  dibucaine
  dichloroethane
  Didrex
  diethyl barbituric acid
  difencloxazine
  dihydrocodeine
  dihydrocodeinone
  dihydrohydroxycodeinone
  dihydroisocodeine
  dihydromorphine
  dihydromorphinone
  dihydroxycodeinone
  Dilaudid
  dimenhydrinate
  dimethylmeperidine
  dimethyltryptamine
  dionin
  diphenoxylate
  dipipanone
  DMT
  Dolophine
  DOM
  Doriden
  dormiral
  drug
  duboisine
  ectylurea
  emotional
  Empirin
  Endocaine
  Equanil
  Eskabarb
  ethchlorvynol
  ether

dependence *(cont.)*
ethinamate
ethoheptazine
ethyl alcohol
ethyl bromide
ethyl carbamate
ethyl chloride
ethylene
ethylene dichloride
ethylidene chloride
ethyl morphine
etilfen
etorphine
etoval
eucodal
euneryl
fentanyl
fentanyl analog
flurazepam
14-hydroxy-dihydromorphinone
gardenal
gasoline (sniffing)
GBH (amino acid concoction)
gelsemine
gelsemium
glue sniffing
glutethimide
hashish
headache powder
hemp
heptabarbital
heptabarbitone
Heptalgin
heroin
hexethal
hexobarbital
Hycodan
hydrocarbon
hydrocodone
hydromorphine
hydromorphinol
hydromorphone

dependence *(cont.)*
hydroxycodeine
Indian hemp
inhalant
Ionamin
Kemithal
ketobemidone
lactucarium
laudanum
Levanil
Levo-Dromoran
levorphanol
Librium
lighter fluid (sniffing)
Lomotil
long-term
Lotusate
LSD (lysergic acid diethylamide)
Luminal
lysergic acid
lysergic acid diethylamide (LSD)
marijuana (also marihuana)
Mebaral
medinal
megahallucinogenics
Mepergan
meperidine
meperidine analog
mephobarbital
meprobamate
mescaline
methadone
methamphetamine
methamphetamine analog
methaqualone
metharbital
methedrine
methitural
methohexital
methopholine
methyl alcohol
methylated spirit

dependence *(cont.)*
    methyl bromide
    methylbutinol
    methyldihydromorphinone
    methyldimethoxyamphetamine
    methylene chloride
    methylene dichloride
    methylenedioxyamphetamine
    methyl morphine
    methylparafynol
    methylphenidate
    methyprylon
    metopon
    Miltown
    morning glory seeds
    morphine
    morpholinylethylmorphine
    muscarine
    myristicin
    nealbarbital
    nealbarbitone
    Nembutal
    Neraval
    nicotine
    Nisentil
    nitrous oxide
    Noctec
    Noludar
    normorphine
    noscapine
    Novocain
    Numorphan
    Nupercaine
    nutmeg
    opiate
    opium
    ortal
    oxazepam
    oxycodone
    oxymorphone
    Panadol
    Pantopon

dependence *(cont.)*
    papaverine
    paracetamol
    paracodin
    Paral
    paraldehyde
    paregoric
    Parepectolin
    PCP
    pentazocine
    pentobarbital
    pentobarbitone
    Pentothal
    percaine
    Percocet
    Percodan
    pethidine
    petrichloral
    peyote
    phenacetin
    phenadoxone
    phenaglycodol
    phenazocine
    phencyclidine
    phencyclidine analog
    phenmetrazine
    phenobarbital
    phenobarbitone
    phenomorphan
    phenoperidine
    pholcodine
    physiological
    piminodine
    Placidyl
    Plegine
    Pondimin
    Pontocaine
    pornography
    potassium bromide
    Preludin
    Prinadol
    probarbital

dependence *(cont.)*
   procaine
   propoxyphene
   psilocin
   psilocybine
   psychedelic agent
   psychoactive substance
   psychological
   psychostimulant
   psychotomimetic agent
   Quaalude
   quinalbarbitone
   racemoramide
   racemorphan
   Rela
   reward
   Ritalin
   Robitussin A-C
   scopolamine
   secobarbital
   Seconal
   Serax
   sernyl
   sodium bromide
   solvent (inhalation)
   Soma
   Sominex
   Somnos
   Soneryl
   stramonium
   substance
   sulfonethylmethane
   sulfonmethane
   Surital
   synthetic heroin
   talbutal
   Talwin
   Taractan
   tendency for
   Tenuate
   Tepanil
   terpin hydrate elixir

dependence *(cont.)*
   tetracaine
   tetrahydrocannabinol
   tetronal
   THC
   thebacon
   thebaine
   thiamylal
   thiopental
   tobacco
   toluene
   Tranxene
   tribromethanol
   tribromomethane
   trichloroethanol
   triclofos
   trional
   Tuinal
   Tussionex
   Tylenol with codeine
   urethane
   Valium
   Valmid
   veramon
   veronal
   versidyne
   vinbarbital
   vinbarbitone
   vinylbitone
   Voranil
   wine
   Zactane
dependence-independence, field
dependence on therapy
dependence syndrome
dependence-type organic psychosis
dependency
   chemical (CD)
   clinging
   hypnotic
   interpersonal
   long-term

dependency needs
dependent adult's certificate
dependent character
dependent clause
dependent personality disorder
dependent variable
depersonalization disorder
depersonalization experience
depersonalization neurosis
depersonalization psychoneurotic
reaction
depersonalization syndrome
depletion, metabolic volume
depolarizing muscle relaxants
Depo-Testosterone (injectable steroid)
depraved
depreciated subsystem
depr., depress. (depressed, depression)
deprementia
depressed affect
depressed bipolar disorder
depressed manic-depressive reaction
depressed mood
adjustment disorder with
adjustment disorder with mixed
anxiety and
depressed mood adjustment reaction
brief
conduct disturbance
prolonged
depressed reflex
depressed schizoaffective schizophrenia
depressed-type arteriosclerotic
dementia
depressed-type presenile dementia
depressed-type senile dementia
depressiform
depression
acute
agitated
anaclitic
anxiety

depression *(cont.)*
atypical
autogenous
bereavement-related
biologic sign
bipolar
clinical
co-occurrence of
delusional
double
endogenous
episodes of
exogenous
history of
hypersomnia associated with
hyposomnia associated with
hysterical
insomnia associated with
involutional
major
manic
marked
masked
mental
moderate
monopolar
nervous
neurotic
opticochiasmatic
overwhelming
periods of
posthysterectomy
postictal
postpartum major
postpsychotic
poststroke
psychoanalysis and
psychogenic
psychoneurotic
psychotic (PD)
reactive
recurrent

depression *(cont.)*
  resistant
  retarded
  risk for
  secondary
  senile
  severe
  situational
  sleeplessness associated with
  somatic treatment for
  somatizing clinical
  symptoms of
  syndromal
  unipolar
  winter
Depression Adjective Check List
  (DACL)
depression and anxiety, reactive
depression delusion
depression in epilepsy
depression inventory (see *test*)
depression of consciousness
depression phase of seizure, postictal
depression questionnaire (see *test*)
Depression Rating Scale
depression-related mental disorder
depression scale (see *test*)
depression sine depression (DSD)
Depression "2" Scale
depressive affect
depressive atypical psychosis
depressive character
depressive delusion
depressive disorder
  Abraham view of
  atypical
  Beck view of
  Bibring view of
  Cohen view of
  Freud view of
  Jacobson view of
  Klein view of

depressive disorder *(cont.)*
  major (MDD)
  minor
  postpsychotic
  Rado view of
  recurrent brief
  Sandler view of
  Seligman view of
Depressive Experiences Questionnaire
  (DEQ)
depressive hallucination
depressive neurotic reaction
depressive personality disorder
depressive phase
depressive psychoneurotic reaction
depressive psychosis
  atypical
  emotional stress
  involutional
  psychogenic
  psychological trauma
  reactive
  recurrent episode
  single episode
depressive reaction
  acute
  adjustment
  affective
  brief
  manic
  neurotic
  prolonged
  psychoneurotic
  psychotic
  situational
  transient
depressive spectrum disorder
depressive symptomatology
depressive syndrome
depressive-type manic-depressive
  psychosis
depressive-type psychoneurosis

depressive-type psycho-organic
    syndrome
depressive-type psychosis, reactive
depressors
deprivation
    cultural
    emotional
    environmental
    food
    maternal
    paternal
    psychosocial
    sensory
    severe environmental
    sleep
    social
    thought
    water
deprivation syndrome, sensory (SDS)
depth of sleep
depth perception
depth psychology
DEQ (Depressive Experiences
    Questionnaire)
derailment
    actual
    frequent
    speech
deranged, mentally
derangement
    mental
    metabolic
dereism
dereistic thinking
derelict, skid row
deride
derivational morphemes
derived adjective
derived sentence
dermatitis, psychogenic
dermatopathophobia
dermatophobia

dermatosiophobia
derogatory comment
DES (Dissociative Experiences Scale)
De Sanctis-Cacchione syndrome
DESBRS-II (Devereux Elementary
    School Behavior Rating Scale II)
description questionnaire (see *test*)
descriptive psychiatry
descending pitch brake
descending technique
descent through non-REM to REM
Description of Body Scale
descriptive approach
descriptive features
descriptive grammar
descriptive linguistics
descriptor (see *test*)
desensitization
    psychologic
    reciprocal inhibition and
    systematic
    systemic
desertion anxiety
deserved punishment
design
    block
    experimental
    geometric
    human
    study
designer drugs
desirability, social
desire
    absent sexual
    active
    deficient sexual
    disturbance in sexual
    hyperactive sexual
    hypoactive sexual
    impaired
    inhibited sexual
    intense

desire *(cont.)*
  lack of
  levels of
  loss of
  "low"
  low sexual
  sexual
  stated
desired effect
desire disorder
  hypoactive sexual
  sexual
desire for personal gain
desire for revenge
desire phase of sexual response cycle
desk-type auditory trainer
despair, feelings of
despondent
destruction, nerve cell
destructive relationship
destructive tendencies
DET (dimethyltryptamine)
detachment
  feeling of
  pattern of
  sense of
  social
detachment from social relationships
detail (pl. details)
  minimization of emotional
  preoccupation with
detailed dream
detailed history
detail response
  confabulated
  rare
  unusual rare
detectability threshold, speech (SDT)
detection
  deceit
  lie
  signal

detection threshold
  noise (NDT)
  speech (SDT)
detention certificate
deteriorating course
deteriorating function
deterioration
  age-related
  alcoholic
  appearance
  functioning
  grooming
  hygiene
  intellectual
  irradiation-induced mental
  language function
  manners
  mental
  mood
  motivation
  neurologic
  progressive
  prominent
  radiation-induced mental
  significant
  social skills
  status
  stepwise
  uniformly progressive
deterioration epilepsy
deteriorative disorder, simple
determinants of deceit
determination service, disability (DDS)
Determining Needs in Your Youth
  Ministry
determining risk
determinism
  linguistic
  psychic
detox (detoxification)
detoxification (detox, DTX)
detoxified alcoholic

detrimental
"Detroit pink" (phencyclidine)
Detroit Test of Learning Aptitude—
    Adult (DTLA-A)
Detroit Test of Learning Aptitude,
    Third Edition (DTLA-3)
detumescence
"deuce" (heroin; $2 worth of drugs)
devaluation
devalue
Developing Skills Checklist (DSC)
development
    abnormal
    anal stage psychosexual
    arrest of
    child
    child language
    cognitive
    delayed
    expressive language
    gender identity psychosexual
    growth and
    human
    impaired
    intellectual
    language
    late speech
    latency period psychosexual
    moral
    motor
    normal
    optimal
    oral stage psychosexual
    perinatal
    pervasive impairment of
    phallic stage psychosexual
    psychomotor
    psychosexual
    psychosocial
    receptive
    receptive language
    slow rate of language

development *(cont.)*
    speech sound
    subsequent
Developmental Activities Screening
    Inventory (DASI)
developmental age
developmental agraphia
developmental aphasia
developmental articulation disorder
Developmental Articulation Test
    (DAT)
developmental articulatory apraxia
Developmental Assessment of Life
    Experiences (DALE System)
developmental coordination disorder
developmental defect
developmental delay disorder (see also
    developmental disorder)
    arithmetical
    articulation
    coordination
    language
    mixed development
    motor retardation
    reading
    retardation
    speech
developmental disability (DD)
developmental disorder
    disinhibited type of passive
    expressive language
    expressive writing
    learning
    pervasive
    pervasive disinhibited type of
    specific (SDD)
    speech
developmental disorder associated with
    hyperkinesia
developmental dyslexia
developmental experimentation in
    childhood

developmental expressive language
disorder
developmental expressive writing
disorder
developmental idiocy
developmental imbalance
Developmental Indicators for Assessment of Learning (DIAL),
Revised/AGS Edition (DIAL-R)
developmental learning problems
(DLP)
developmentally appropriate avoidant
behavior
developmentally appropriate self-stimulatory behaviors in the young
developmentally appropriate shy
behavior
developmentally disabled (DD)
developmentally expected speech
sounds
developmentally inappropriate social
relatedness
developmental metaphor
developmental milestones
developmental model
Blos
Bowlby
Erickson
Gesell
Kohlberg
developmental period
developmental phase
developmental phonological processes
developmental profiles (see *test*)
developmental psychology
developmental reading disorder
developmental retardation
developmental roots
developmental scale (see *test)*
developmental schedule (see *test*)
developmental screening (see *test*)

Developmental Sentence Scoring
developmental skills
developmental stage
developmental stuttering
Developmental Test of Visual-Motor
Integration (VMI), Third Edition
Developmental Test of Visual
Perception (DTVP)
developmental word deafness
development inventory (see *test*)
development language scale (see *test*)
development profile (see *test*)
development program
development questionnaire (see *test*)
development scale (see *test*)
development stages
cognitive (Period I-IV)
Piaget cognitive
development test (see *test*)
Devereux Adolescent Behavior Rating
Scale
Devereux Child Behavior Rating Scale
Devereux Elementary School Behavior
Rating Scale II (DESBRS-II)
deviance
psychiatric
role
sexual
social
deviance disorder, sexual
deviant articulation
deviant behavior
deviant language
deviant pathway of development
deviant pattern of inner experience and
behavior
deviant, sexual
deviant speech
deviant swallowing
deviated septum
deviate, psychopathic (PD)

deviation
  mean
  primary sexual
  sexual
  standard (SD)
  statistical
deviation from physiological norm
deviation quotient (see *test*)
device (pl. devices)
  canal caps hearing protection
  circumaural hearing protection
  cochlear implant
  cohesive
  earmuffs hearing protection
  earplugs hearing protection
  hearing protection (HPD)
  insert hearing protection
  interrupter
  language acquisition (LAD)
  semiaural hearing protection
device for the deaf, telephone (TDD)
"devil" (crack)
"devil's dandruff" (crack)
"devil's dick" (re: crack equipment)
"devil's dust" (phencyclidine)
"devilsmoke" (crack)
Devine Inventory, The
devious manner
devoicing of final consonants
"dew" (cannabis)
"dews" ($10 worth of drugs)
dexamethasone nonsuppression
dexamethasone suppression test (DST)
"dexies" (dextroamphetamine sulfate)
dexterity
  finger (F)
  manual (M)
dexterity test (see also *test*)
dextral
dextrality
dextroamphetamine (street names)
  brownies
  Christmas trees

dextroamphetamine *(cont.)*
  dexies
  hearts
  wakeups
dextrophobia
DFA (delayed feedback audiometry)
DFS (Defense Functioning Scale)
DFS (Defensive Functioning Scale)
DFTT (Digital Finger Tapping Test)
DHHS (U.S. Department of Health
  and Human Services)
DI (drug information; drug interactions)
Diabetes Opinion Survey and Parent
  Diabetes Opinion Survey
diabetic ketoacidosis
diabetophobia
diachronic linguistics
diacritic
diadochokinesis
diagnosis (pl. diagnoses)
  comorbid Axis II
  differential
  DSM-IV
  dual
  equivalent
  focus of
  principal
  psychiatric
  rule in a
  rule out a
Diagnostic Achievement Battery,
  Second Edition (DAB-2)
Diagnostic Achievement Test for
  Adolescents
Diagnostic Analysis of Reading Errors
Diagnostic and Statistical Manual of
  Mental Disorders (DSM)
Diagnostic and Statistical Manual of
  Mental Disorders IV (DSM-IV)
Diagnostic and Therapeutic Technology
  Assessment (DATTA)
diagnostic articulation test

Diagnostic Assessments of Reading
  (DAR)
diagnostic audiometry
diagnostic battery (see *test*)
Diagnostic Checklist for Behavior-
  Disturbed Children Form E-2
diagnostic criteria
Diagnostic Employability Profile
diagnostic features
diagnostic information
diagnostic interview (see *test)*
Diagnostic Interview Schedule (DIS)
diagnostic inventory (see *test*)
diagnostic judgment
Diagnostic Mathematics Inventory
  (DMI)
Diagnostic Mathematics Profiles
Diagnostic Reading Scales: Revised
Diagnostic Skills Battery
diagnostic subtypes
diagnostic teaching
Diagnostic Tests and Self-Helps in
  Arithmetic
diagnostic therapy
diagnostic use of hypnosis
diagram, branching tree
dialectical behavior therapy
dialectical dilemmas
dialect leveling
dialect
  regional
  social
dialect speech community
dialogue
DIAL-R (Developmental Indicators
  for the Assessment of Learning,
  Revised/AGS Edition)
dialysis dementia
"diambista" (cannabis)
dianabol (veterinary steroid)
Diana complex

diaphragm
diaphragmatic-abdominal respiration
diaphragmatic breathing
diarrhea, psychogenic
diary, symptom
diathesis
diatribe
dibenzodiazepine
DIC (drug information center)
Dichotic Consonant-Vowel Test
Dichotic Digits Test
dichotic listening tasks
dichotic messages
dichotomy
diction
DID (dissociative identity disorder)
diencephalic seizure
diencephalon
diet
  aspartame-restricted
  improper
  limited
  low-tyramine
  reduced sodium
  restricted
diet foods, low-calorie
"diet pills" (amphetamine)
diet pills
difference (pl. differences)
  age
  cultural
  just noticeable (JND)
  language
  noticeable
  qualitative
  significant
difference limen (DL)
differences in interpretation
difference tone
Differential Ability Scales
Differential Aptitude Test (DAT),
  Fifth Edition (DAT)

Differential Aptitude Test for Personnel and Career Assessment (DAT for PCA)
differential diagnosis
differential function
differential reinforcement
differential relaxation
differential response
differential, semantic
Differential Test of Conduct and Emotional Problems (DT/CEP)
differential threshold
differentiation, auditory
differentiation scale, sexual (SDS)
difficult life circumstances
difficulty (pl. difficulties)
  academic
  concentration
  emotional
  interpersonal
  language
  learning
  memory
  multiple life
  protracted
  speech
  tactile sensory
  word-finding
difficulty adapting
difficulty in changing response set
diffidence (culturally appropriate)
diffracted wave
diffuse brain dysfunction, severe
diffuse encephalopathy
diffuse function
diffuse Lewy body disease
diffuse phoneme
digastric muscle
  anterior
  posterior
digestive disorder, psychogenic

digital change
Digital Finger Tapping Test (DFTT)
digital hearing aid
digitalis-induced delirium
digital manipulation
digital (or digit) span recall test
  forward
  reverse
digit recall
digit repetition test
digit reversal test
digit stamp
digit symbol (DS) test
digits test
diglossia
digraph
digressive speech
dihydroindolone
dihydrolone (injectable steroid)
dikephobia
DIL (drug information log)
dilated pupils
dilated ventricle (of brain)
dilemma (pl. dilemmas), dialectical
"dimba" (cannabis)
"dime" (crack)
"dime bag" ($10 worth of drugs)
dimensional approach
dimensional descriptors for schizophrenia, alternative
dimensional model of schizophrenia, 3-factor
dimethyltryptamine (street names)
  AMT
  businessman's LSD
  businessman's special
  businessman's trip
  DET
  DMT
  DPT
  Fantasia
  45-minute psychosis

"dime's worth" (amount of heroin to
cause death)
diminished capacity
diminished control
diminished effect
diminished libido
diminished pleasure in everyday
activities
diminished reality testing
diminished recall
diminished reflex
diminished response to pain
diminished responsibility
diminished responsiveness
diminished sensation
diminished sexual interest
diminution of affect
diminution of goal-directed behavior
diminution of thoughts
diminutive
DIMS (disorder of initiating and
maintaining sleep)
"ding" (cannabis)
"dinkie dow" (cannabis)
dinomania
dinophobia
diode
diotic listening
diotic messages
"dip" (crack)
diphasic spike
diphasic wave
diphenylbutyl
diphthong
diplacucis
echoica
binauralis
dysharmonica
monauralis
diplegia
diplegic idiocy
Diploma in Psychological Medicine
(DPM)

diplopiaphobia
"dipper" (phencyclidine)
dipping, body
"dipping out" (re: crack dealing)
dipsomania
DIR (disturbed interpersonal relationships)
direct association
direct causality
direct causative pathophysiological
mechanism
direct current (DC)
directional microphone
direction profile, neurotic
direction, psychotic
directive psychotherapy
directivity
direct laryngoscopy
direct motor system
direct object
direct observation
direct physiological effect
direct selection communication board
direct self-destructive behavior
direct suggestion under hypnosis
(DSUH)
"dirt" (heroin)
"dirt grass" (cannabis)
dirtiness, feelings of
"dirty" (re: drug-injecting equipment)
"dirty basing" (crack)
DIS (Diagnostic Interview Schedule)
disability (pl. disabilities)
associated
chronic
cognitive
degree of
developmental (DD)
emotional
functional
hearing
language

disability *(cont.)*
    learning
    manifested
    mental
    mild
    mobility
    neurologic
    observable
    partial
    partial permanent
    permanent
    posttraumatic chronic
    progressive
    psychiatric
    residual
    severe
    social
    speech
    temporary
    total
    work
disability counselor
disability determination service (DDS)
disability pension (DP)
disability status scale (DSS)
disable
disabled
    developmentally (DD)
    learning (LD)
    partially
    psychiatrically
    temporarily
    totally
disabling headache
disabling pattern, chronically
disabling stress
disaccharide malabsorption
disadvantage
disapproval, fear of
disassimilation
disassociation
disavow

disavowal level
disbelief
discipline problem, school
disclosure
"disco biscuits" (barbiturate)
discomfort threshold
discomfort with emotion
discomfort with gender role
disconjugate gaze
disconjugate movement
disconnected ideas
disconnected speech
disconnected thoughts
disconnection apraxia
disconnection syndrome aphasia,
    callosal
disconnection syndrome, callosal
disconnection thought disorder
disconnection with reality
discontinuation
discontinue (D/C)
discordance
discordant facial expression
discord, marital
discourse
discrepancy scale (see *test*)
discriminant analysis
discriminant validity
discrimination
    auditory
    oral sensory
    pitch
    speech (SD)
    speech sound
    visual
discrimination audiometry, speech
discrimination consciousness
discrimination curve
discrimination learning
discrimination loss
discrimination of sounds
discrimination score, word

discrimination test
discrimination training
disdain
"disease" (drug of choice)
disease
  advanced
  Alzheimer
  auto-immune
  Beard
  Bell
  Bergeron
  Binswanger
  biology of affective
  bodily
  brain
  brain stem
  Brushfield-Wyatt
  central motor pathways
  Creutzfeldt-Jakob
  dancing
  degenerative
  diffuse Lewy body
  Down
  feared
  Friedmann
  Gaucher
  Gilles de la Tourette
  Guinon
  Heidenhain
  Hirschsprung
  HIV
  Huntington (chorea)
  inherited
  inherited progressive degenerative
  Jakob-Creutzfeldt
  Janet
  Kanner
  kinky hair
  Korsakoff
  Krabbe
  Kufs
  Lasègue

disease *(cont.)*
  laughing
  life-threatening
  Lou Gehrig (ALS, amyotrophic lateral sclerosis)
  Meniere
  mental
  nervous
  neurodegenerative
  Niemann-Pick
  organic
  Parkinson
  Pelizaeus-Merzbacher
  Pick
  primary Parkinson
  prion
  progressive degenerative
  psychiatric
  psychotic
  Sander
  sexually transmitted (STD)
  suspected
  Tay-Sachs
  white matter
  Wilson hepatolenticular degeneration
disequilibrium (or dysequilibrium)
disequilibrium state
disfluency dyskinesia
disfluent speech
disgust, feeling of
disharmony
disheveled
dishonesty
dishonorable discharge
disinhibited-type pervasive developmental disorder
disinhibited-type reactive attachment disorder
disinhibition
  emotional
  motor

disintegration, speech
disintegrative disorder
disintegrative psychosis
disobedient behavior
disorder (pl. disorders)
  abnormal involuntary movement
    (AIMD)
  academic underachievement
  acquired-type female orgasmic
  acquired-type female sexual
    arousal
  acquired-type hypoactive sexual
    desire
  acquired-type male erectile
  acquired-type male orgasmic
  acquired-type sexual aversion
  acute labyrinthine
  acute stress
  addictive
  adjustment
  adjustment interface
  adolescence
  adolescent conduct
  adult-life psychosexual identity
  adult-onset type conduct
  affective
  aggressive
  aggressive-type personality
  alcohol amnestic
  alcohol-induced anxiety
  alcohol-induced persisting amnestic
  alcohol-induced psychotic
  alcohol-induced sleep
  alcohol-related
  alcohol use
  alpha-methyldopa-induced mood
  amitriptyline-induced mood
  amnestic
  amphetamine-induced anxiety
  amphetamine-induced mood
  amphetamine-induced psychotic
  amphetamine use

disorder (cont.)
  antisocial personality
  anxiety
  anxiety-related mental
  anxiolytic amnestic
  anxiolytic-related
  anxiolytic use
  apathetic-type personality
  aphasia
  apractic
  apraxic
  articulatory
  Asperger
  associated
  associated personality
  attachment-separation
  attention-deficit (ADD)
  attention-deficit hyperactivity
    (ADHD)
  auditory
  auditory processing
  autistic
  autonomic
  avoidant
  avoidant personality
  behavior
  bereavement
  binge-eating
  bipolar
  bipolar I
  bipolar II
  body dysmorphic
  borderline personality
  brain
  breathing
  breathing-related sleep
  Briquet
  caffeine-induced anxiety
  caffeine-induced sleep
  caffeine-related
  caffeine withdrawal
  cannabis-induced anxiety

disorder *(cont.)*
   cannabis-induced psychotic
   cannabis use
   catatonic
   central auditory processing
   central language (CLD)
   cerebral
   character
   childhood
   childhood disintegrative
   childhood-onset-type conduct
   childhood psychosexual identity
   chronic motor tic
   chronic vocal tic
   chronobiological
   circadian rhythm sleep
   cocaine-induced
   cocaine-induced anxiety
   cocaine-induced mood
   cocaine-induced psychotic
   cocaine-induced sleep
   cocaine-related
   coexisting
   cognitive
   combined-type personality
   communication
   communicative
   comorbid personality
   complicated grief
   conceptual
   conduct
   contiguity
   conversion
   convulsive
   co-occurring mental
   coordination
   cul-de-sac voice
   cyclothymic
   delirium-related
   delirium-related mental
   delusional
   dementia-related mental

disorder *(cont.)*
   denasality voice
   dependent personality
   depersonalization
   depression-related mental
   depressive
   depressive personality
   depressive spectrum
   developmental coordination
   developmental expressive language
   developmental expressive writing
   disinhibited-type of pervasive
     developmental
   disinhibited-type personality
   disruptive behavior
   dissociative
   dissociative identity (DID)
   dissociative interface
   dissociative trance
   dream anxiety
   drug-related
   dyssocial personality
   dysthymic (DD)
   eating
   electroconvulsive therapy-induced
   elimination
   emancipation
   emotional
   endocrine
   evidence of dissociation
   explosive
   expressive language
   factitious
   factitious interface
   false role
   familial
   feeding and eating
   female orgasmic
   female sexual arousal
   fluency
   formal thought
   functional

disorder *(cont.)*
functional articulation
gait
gender identity (GID)
generalized anxiety (GAD)
generalized-type female orgasmic
generalized-type female sexual
    arousal
generalized-type hypoactive sexual
    desire
generalized-type male erectile
generalized-type male orgasmic
generalized-type sexual aversion
geriatric depressive
GIDAANT (Gender Identity Dis-
    order of Adolescence or Adult-
    hood, Nontranssexual Type)
hallucinogen persisting perception
hallucinogen-related
histrionic personality
homosexual conflict
hyperactivity
hyperrhinolalia voice
hyperrhinophonia voice
hypnotic-related
hypnotic use
hypoactive sexual desire
hypomanic
identity
impulse
impulse-control interface
inadequate personality
induced psychotic
inhalant-related
insomnia-type caffeine-induced
    sleep
insomnia-type substance-induced
    sleep
intermittent explosive disorder
labile-type personality
labyrinthine
language

disorder *(cont.)*
late luteal phase dysphoric
learning
lifelong-type sexual aversion
light-therapy-induced mood
limbic system
major depressive (MDD)
male erectile
male erectile arousal
male orgasmic
malingering
manic
manic-depressive
mathematics
medical/psychiatric sleep
medication-induced movement
mental
mental subnormality
mild neurocognitive
minor depressive
mixed anxiety-depressive
mixed nasality voice
mixed receptive-expressive
    language
mood
motor skills
motor tic
motor-verbal tic
multiple personality (MPD)
narcissistic personality
negativistic personality
neuroleptic-induced acute
    movement
neuropsychiatric
neuropsychiatric movement
neuropsychologic
neurotic
nicotine-related
nicotine use
nightmare
non-substance-induced
non-substance-induced mental

disorder *(cont.)*

   not otherwise specified (NOS)
   obsessive-compulsive personality
   opioid-related
   oppositional
   oppositional-defiant
   organic
   organic articulation
   orgasmic
   other type personality
   overanxious
   over-the-counter drug-related
   pain
   panic
   paranoid
   paranoid personality
   parasomnia-type substance-induced
     sleep
   passive-aggressive personality
   PCP use
   perception
   perceptual
   personality
   pervasive
   pervasive developmental
   phencyclidine-related
   phobic
   phonation
   phonatory
   phonological
   pica
   polysubstance-related
   postconcussional
   postpsychotic depressive
   posttraumatic stress (PTSD)
   predominantly hyperactive-impulsive
     attention-deficit/hyperactivity
   predominantly inattentive-type
     attention-deficit/hyperactivity
   premenstrual dysphoric
   prescription drug-related
   primary affective (PAD)

disorder *(cont.)*

   primary anxiety
   primary mental
   primary mood
   primary psychotic
   primary sleep
   processing
   psychiatric
   psychiatric system interface
   psychic
   psychoactive
   psychoactive substance-induced
   psychoactive substance-induced
     organic mental
   psychoaffective (PAD)
   psychogenic
   psychogenic pain
   psychomotor
   psychoneurotic
   psychophysiological
   psychosexual
   psychosomatic
   psychotic
   reactive attachment
   reading
   receptive language
   recurrent brief depressive
   related sleep
   REM sleep behavior
   repetitive impulse
   resonance
   respiratory
   Rett
   rhinolalia aperta voice
   rhinolalia clausa voice
   rumination
   schizoaffective
   schizoid personality
   schizoid-schizotypal personality
     (SSPD)
   schizophrenic spectrum
   schizophrenic speech and language

disorder *(cont.)*
  schizophreniform
  schizotypal personality
  seasonal affective (SAD)
  sedative-related
  sedative use
  semantic pragmatic
  separation anxiety (SAD)
  sexual
  sexual and gender identity
  sexual arousal
  sexual aversion
  sexual desire
  sexual deviance
  sexual identity
  sexual pain
  sexual response
  shared psychotic
  simple deteriorative
  situational-type
  sleep
  sleep terror
  sleepwalking
  social anxiety
  somatization
  somatoform
  somatoform interface
  somatoform pain
  specific developmental (SDD)
  speech
  speech and language
  stereotypic movement
  stress
  substance abuse
  substance-induced
  substance-induced sleep
  substance-related
  substance use
  substitution
  thought
  thought process
  tic

disorder *(cont.)*
  tobacco use
  Tourette
  transient tic
  unaggressive
  undersocialized
  unipolar
  unknown substance-induced mood
  unsocialized
  visceral
  voice phonation
  voice resonance
  unspecified bipolar I
  unspecified-type personality
  visual
  visuospatial
  voice
  voice resonance
disorder affecting general medical
  condition (GMC)
disorder aphasia, contiguity
disorder by proxy, factitious
disorder due to combined factors
disordered mentally
disordered thinking
disorganization
  cognitive (Cog Disorg)
  linguistic
  psychotic
  spatial
disorganization dimension of positive
  schizophrenic symptoms
disorganization in discourse
disorganization in schizophrenia
  behavioral
  linguistic
  psychotic
disorganized behavior, grossly
disorganized factor in schizophrenia
disorganized speech assessment
disorganized speech in schizophrenia
disorganized thinking

disorganized-type schizophrenia
disorientation
  graphic
  right-left
  spatial
  visuospatial
disparity
  phase
  vision
dispense as directed (DAD)
dispersonalization
displaceability
displaced speech
displacement
  affect
  brain stem
  geographic
  guilt
displacement of emotive energy,
  active
display, emotional
display of emotion, public
disposition, placid
disproportionate impairment
disregard for rights of others,
  pattern of
disrupted relational functioning
disrupted sleep organization
disruption, speech
disruptive behavior disorder
disruptive emotion
disruptive environment, socially
disruptive family functioning
dissimilation rules
dissociated sensory loss
dissociation
  peritraumatic
  syndrome of sensory
dissociative amnesia
dissociative capacity
dissociative disorder
Dissociative Disorders Interview Scale

Dissociative Disorders Interview
  Schedule
dissociative episode
Dissociative Experiences Scale (DES)
dissociative fugue
dissociative hysteria psychoneurosis
dissociative hysterical reaction
dissociative identity disorder (DID)
dissociative interface disorder
dissociative phenomenon
dissociative psychoneurotic reaction
dissociative reaction
dissociative state
dissociative symptoms
dissociative trance disorder
dissociative-type hysterical neurosis
dissolution
dissonance, cognitive
  distal distinctive feature analysis
  distal renal tubular acidosis
distance perception
distancing, cognitive
distinct identities, multiple
distinctive feature analysis
distoclusion of teeth
distort
distorted body image
distorted communication in schizophrenia
distorted grief
distorted inferential thinking
distorted language in schizophrenia
distorted perception
distorter
distortion
  amplitude
  body image
  cognitive
  figure-ground
  harmonic
  inferential behavioral monitoring
  inferential perception

distortion *(cont.)*
  language and communication
  memory
  nonlinear
  parataxic
  perceptual
  psychotic
  spatial
  speech
  transient
  visual-spatial
  waveform
distortional bone conduction
distortion articulation
distoversion of teeth
distractibility
distractible, easily
distraction
distress
  clinically significant
  emotional
  intense psychological
  intrapsychic
  no acute (NAD)
  psychological
  significant subjective
  social avoidance and (SAD)
distressed
distressing dream
distressing thoughts
distributed memories
distribution
  complementary
  contrastive
  gaussian
  noncontrastive
  normal
  parallel
  stocking-glove
distribution of power
distributive analysis and synthesis

distrust
  interpersonal
  malevolent
  pervasive
distrust of others' motives, pattern of
disturbance (pl. disturbances)
  activity and attention
  acute situational
  adjustment reaction
  affective
  analyzing new information
  anxiety
  assimilating information
  attentional
  behavior
  behavioral
  body image
  breathing-related sleep
  chronic sleep
  chronobiological
  cognitive
  compulsive
  concentration
  conduct
  consciousness
  domestic
  electrolyte
  emotional
  executive functioning
  explosive
  fluctuating mood
  fluency
  fluid
  focal neurologic
  frequency
  functioning
  gait
  high level perceptual
  hyperkinetic
  identity
  infancy and early childhood

disturbance *(cont.)*
  language
  learning new information
  linguistic
  memory
  mental
  metabolic
  mixed conduct/emotional
  mixed symptom picture with
    perceptual
  motor skill
  normal fluency of speech
  oculomotor
  perception
  perceptual
  perceptual motor abilities
  personality
  planning
  predominant mood
  psychiatric
  psychic
  psychographic
  psychomotor
  psychotic
  rate of fluency
  reasoning
  recalling new information
  sexual desire
  sleep
  sleep continuity
  sociopathic
  socialized
  social relatedness
  speech
  speed of information processing
  stocking-and-glove anesthetic
  stress-related
  thought
  time patterning of speech
  visual
  visual field
  word-finding ability

disturbance adjustment reaction,
  conduct
disturbance in integrating:
  auditory information with motor
    activity
  tactile information with motor
    activity
  visual information with motor
    activity
disturbances in feeding and eating,
  infancy and early childhood
disturbed body image
disturbed eating behavior
disturbed home environment
disturbed interpersonal relationships
  (DIR)
disturbed orientation
disturbed personality
disturbed sense of self
disturbed sleep pattern
disturbed social relatedness
disturbing the peace
disturbing thoughts
disyllabic
disyllable
"ditch" (cannabis)
"ditch weed" (cannabis)
Ditthomska syndrome
diurnal enuresis
diurnal epilepsy
diurnal variation
diurnus, pavor (day terrors)
divagation
divergence circuit
divergent production
diverse group
diversion
Diversity Awareness Profile (DAP)
diversity, group
Division of Developmental Disabilities
  (DDD)
divisive

divorce as major childhood stressor
Dix, Dorothea Lynde (1802-1887)
dizygotic twins
dizzy, feeling
dizzy spell
"djamba" (cannabis)
DL (difference limen)
DLP (developmental learning problems)
DMAS (Dementia Mood Assessment Scale)
DMH (Department of Mental Health)
DMI (Defense Mechanism Inventory)
DMI (Diagnostic Mathematics Inventory)
DMI Mathematics Systems Instructional Objectives Inventory
"DMT" (dimethyltryptamine)
"DOA" (crack; phencyclidine)
"do a joint" (re: cannabis use)
"do a line" (re: cocaine use)
DOB (analog of amphetamine/ methamphetamine)
DOB (date of birth)
"doctor" (methylenedioxymethamphetamine)
Doctor of Philosophy (Ph.D.)
doctor-patient relationship
doctrine, usage
Dodd Test of Time Estimation
"dog" (good friend)
"dog food" (heroin)
"dogie" (heroin)
dogma, dogmatic
"do it Jack" (phencyclidine)
Dole Vocational Sentence Completion Blank
"dollar" ($100 worth of drugs)
"dolls" (barbiturate)
doll's eye reaction
doll's eyes
"dollys" (methadone hydrochloride)

DOM (analog of amphetamine/ methamphetamine)
domain of information
domains, adaptive skill
domatophobia
"domes" (lysergic acid diethylamide; phencyclidine and amphetamine/ methamphetamine)
"domestic" (locally grown cannabis)
domestic aggression
domestic disturbance
domestic environment
domestic violence (DV)
"domex" (methylenedioxymethamphetamine and phencyclidine)
domicile
domiciliary
dominance
  cerebral
  lateral
  left hemisphere
  left/right hemisphere
  mixed cerebral
  right hemisphere
  social
  theory of social
  X-linked
dominance and handedness, cerebral (theory in stuttering)
dominance-subordination
dominant delusional belief
dominant features
dominant gene, autosomal
dominant hand
dominant idea, permanent
dominant language
dominant pattern, autosomal
dominant person
dominant-subordinate behavior
dominant trait
dominant waking frequency
dominate

dominates initial dominant, bystander
　(BDID)
domination
dominatrix
domineer
domineering
"dominoes" (amphetamine)
"Dona Juana" (cannabis)
"Dona Juanita" (cannabis)
"don jem" (cannabis)
Don Juanism
do-not-care attitude
"doobie/dubbe/duby" (cannabis)
"doogie/doojee/dugie" (heroin)
"dooley" (heroin)
doom, sense of impending
dopamine and homovanillic acid
dopamine-beta-hydroxylase
dopamine hypothesis
dopamine metabolite
dopamine reuptake
dopaminergic medication-induced
　postural tremor
"dope" (cannabis; morphine)
"dope fiend" (crack addict)
"dope smoke" (re: cannabis use)
"dopium" (opium)
Doppler effect
Doppler phenomenon
Doppler shift
"doradilla" (cannabis)
doramania
doraphobia
Doren Diagnostic Reading Test of
　Word Recognition Skills
dorsal cochlear nucleus
dorsal dorsum (pl. dorsa)
dorsal gray matter
dorsum of tongue
dosage, equivalent
dosage reduction, trial of
Dos Amigos Verbal Language Scales

dose-dependent effect
dose, maintenance
dosing, need for frequent drug
"dots" (lysergic acid diethylamide)
"doub" ($20 worth of rock cocaine)
double assimilation
double-blind clinical trial
double-blind messages (communica-
　tion pattern)
double blind theory
"double bubble" (cocaine)
double consonant
"double crosses" (amphetamine)
double depression
"double dome" (lysergic acid diethyl-
　amide)
double entendre
double insanity
double meaning
double personality
"double rock" (crack diluted with
　procaine)
"double trouble" (amobarbital/
　secobarbital)
"double ups" (re: drug value)
double vision
"double yoke" (morphine)
doubling
doubting insanity
doubting mania
doubt, morbid
doubts of loyalty
doubts of trustworthiness
"Dover's powder" (opium)
dovetail
Down disease
downdrift pitch
"downers" (barbiturate)
down from overdose
"downie" (barbiturate)
down in the dumps
downs, ups and

Down syndrome
downward drift
DP (disability pension)
DPE (Death Personification Exercise)
DPI (Dynamic Personality Inventory)
DPM (Diploma in Psychological
    Medicine)
DPP (Dropout Prediction and
    Prevention)
DPT (dimethyltryptamine)
dr (dram)
Dr (rare detail response)
"draf weed" (cannabis)
"drag weed" (cannabis)
dram (dr)
drama
dramatic affect
dramatic-emotional cluster
dramatic interpersonal style
dramatism
dramatization
dramatize
drapetomania
drastic
Draw-a-Clock-Face test
Draw-A-Family test
Draw-a-House test
Draw A Person: Screening Procedure
    for Emotional Disturbance
    (DAP:SPED)
Draw-a-Picture-from-Memory test
drawing (pl. drawings)
drawing ability
drawing test
dread, feeling of
dread of insanity
dreaded situation
dream
    anxiety
    clairvoyant
    detailed

dream (cont.)
    distressing
    erotic
    recurring
    vivid
    wet
"dream" (cocaine)
dream anxiety attack (nightmare)
dream anxiety disorder
dream content
"dreamer" (morphine)
dream experience
"dream gum" (opium)
dream image
    fragmentary
    vivid
dreaming and repression, cognitive
    approaches to
dream interpretation
dreamland
dreamless sleep
dreamlike hallucination
dream pain
dream recall, vivid
"dreams" (opium)
dream sequence
    elaborate
    storylike
dream state
"dream stick" (opium)
dream symbolism
dream-work
dreamy state
dreariness
dreary
"dreck" (heroin)
dressing apraxia
DRI (Driver Risk Inventory)
drift, downward
"drink" (phencyclidine)
drinker

drinking
  aftereffects of
  alcohol
  binge
  compulsive water
  continued
  controlled
  early-onset
  evening
  heavy
  light
  morning
  nonproblematic
  persistent
  problem
  recreational
  repeated heavy
  social
  state markers of heavy (GGT)
  volitional
  weekend
drinking behavior, out-of-control
drinking history
drinking pattern
drinking syndrome, nocturnal
drive
  aggressive
  appetitive
  aversive
  exploratory
  hedonic
  hunger
  innate
  internal
  learned
  primary
  repressed instinctual
  secondary
  sexual
  stimulus (SD, Sd)
  subjective
  thirst

driven motor behavior
driver's license
  revocation of
  suspension of
driver's rage
Driver Risk Inventory (DRI)
driving (automobile) behavior
driving habits, reckless
driving under the influence (DUI)
driving while intoxicated (DWI)
DRLST (Del Rio Language Screening
  Test)
dromomania
dromophobia
droning speech
drooping eyelids
"drop acid" (re: lysergic acid diethylamide use)
drop curve audiogram configurations,
  sudden
Dropout Prediction and Prevention
  (DPP)
dropouts, student
"dropper" (re: drug injection)
drowsiness, marked
"drowsy high" (barbiturate)
DRP (Degrees of Reading Power)
drug (pl. drugs) (see also *dependence*;
  drugs, street; *medication*)
  absorption of
  abuse of nonprescription
  addictive potential of
  amphetamine
  antianxiety
  antidepressant
  antidote
  antimanic
  antipanic
  antiparkinsonism
  antipsychotic
  antiseizure
  anxiolytic

drug *(cont.)*
  ataractic
  barbiturate
  barbiturate hypnotic
  benzodiazepine
  bromine compound
  butyrophenone-based tranquilizer
  chloral hydrate
  controlled release (CR)
  craving for
  designer
  frequency of self-administration of
  glutethimide group
  hallucinogen
  heterocyclic antidepressant
  high-dose
  hypnotic
  inhalation of
  illegal
  illicit
  intranasal
  intravenous
  long-acting (LA)
  methaqualone compound
  mixed sedative
  monamine oxidase inhibitor
    (MAO)
  monocyclic antidepressant
  narcotic
  narcotic agonist
  narcotic blocking (narcotic
    antagonists)
  negative effect of
  neuroleptic
  nonprescription
  paraldehyde
  peak level of
  phenothiazine-based tranquilizer
  prescription
  psychiatric
  psychoactive
  psychodysleptic

drug *(cont.)*
  psychostimulant
  psychotic
  psychotomimetic
  psychotropic (PTD)
  recreational
  sedative
  sedative/hypnotic
  self-administration of psychoactive
    (SAPD)
  sex for
  slow release (SR)
  street
  sublingual (SL)
  sympathomimetic
  toxic effect of
  tranquilizer
  tricyclic antidepressant
  wearing-off effect of
drug abstinence syndrome
Drug Abuse Control Amendments
  (DACA)
drug abuse, mixed
drug abuser
Drug Abuse Resistance Education
drug action, duration of
drug addict (DA)
drug addiction
drug binge
drug consumption
drug counselor
drug craving
drug dealing
drug dependence
  analgesic
  anesthetic
  cannabis-type
  combination
  hallucinogenic
  hypnotic
  multiple
  narcotic

drug dependence *(cont.)*
  opioid type
  psychostimulant
  sedative
  soporific
  synthetic
  tranquilizer
  withdrawal
drug-dependent insomnia
drug dosing
drug effect
Drug Enforcement Administration (DEA)
Drug Enforcement Administration number (DEA #)
"druggie" (re: drug user)
drug habit
drug holiday, therapeutic
drug-induced confusional state
drug-induced depressive state
drug-induced hallucinatory state
drug-induced mental disorder
drug-induced organic personality syndrome
drug-induced paranoid state
drug-induced parkinsonism (pseudo-parkinsonism)
drug-induced seizure
drug information (DI)
drug information center (DIC)
drug information log (DIL)
drug ingestion
drug-injecting equipment
  "dirty"
  used
drug insanity
drug interactions (DI)
drug intolerance
drug intoxication
  organic psychosis
  pathological
drug level

drug maintenance treatment
drug names (slang), see *drugs, street*
drug-negative urine
drug of abuse (see *dependence* and *drugs, street*)
drug of choice
drug paraphernalia, shared
drug possession
drug problem
drug psychosis
  amnestic syndrome
  delirium state
  delusional syndrome
  dementia state
  depressive state
  hallucinatory state
  organic affective syndrome
  organic delusional syndrome
  organic personality syndrome
  paranoid state
  pathological drug intoxication
  withdrawal syndrome
drug-related disorder
drug-related insomnia
drug-related violence
drug screen test
  blood
  urine
drug-seeking behavior
drug supplies
drug-taking behavior, compulsive
drug tolerance
drug toxicity
drug treatment for personality disorders
drug trip
drug use
  high frequency of
  low frequency of
  recreational
Drug Use Index
drug use review (DUR)

drug users, injection
drug withdrawal
drug withdrawal seizure
drug withdrawal syndrome
drugs, street (slang terms)
   A's (lysergic acid diethylamide;
     amphetamine sulfate)
   Acapulco red (cannabis)
   Acapulco gold (cannabis)
   ace (cannabis; phencyclidine)
   acid (lysergic acid diethylamide)
   AD (phencyclidine)
   Adam (analog of amphetamine/
     methamphetamine)
   Afghanistan black (cannabis)
   African black (cannabis)
   African bush (cannabis)
   African woodbine (cannabis)
   ah-pen-yen (opium)
   aimies (amphetamine; amyl nitrite)
   AIP (herion)
   air blast (inhalant)
   airplane (cannabis)
   Alice B. Toklas (cannabis)
   all-American drug (cocaine)
   alpha-ET (alpha-ethyltryptamine)
   ames (amyl nitrite)
   amoeba (phencyclidine)
   amp (amphetamine)
   amp joint (cannabis)
   AMT (dimethyltryptamine)
   amys (amyl nitrite)
   angel (phencyclidine)
   angel dust (phencyclidine)
   angel hair (phencyclidine)
   angel mist (phencyclidine)
   Angel Poke (phencyclidine)
   Angie (cocaine)
   Angola (cannabis)
   animal (lysergic acid diethylamide)
   animal trank (phencyclidine)
   animal tranquilizer (phencyclidine)

drugs, street (cont.)
   antifreeze (heroin)
   Apache (fentanyl)
   apple jacks (crack)
   Aries (heroin)
   aroma of men (isobutyl nitrite)
   ashes (cannabis)
   atom bomb (cannabis and heroin)
   atshitshi (cannabis)
   Aunt Hazel (heroin)
   Aunt Mary (cannabis)
   baby (cannabis)
   baby bhang (cannabis)
   Baby T (crack)
   backbreakers (lysergic acid diethyl-
     amide and strychnine)
   backwards (barbiturate)
   bad (crack)
   bad seed (mescaline; heroin;
     cannabis)
   bale (cannabis)
   ball (crack)
   ballot (heroin)
   bam (barbiturate; amphetamine)
   Bambalacha (cannabis)
   bambs (barbiturate)
   bank bandit pills (barbiturate)
   bank deposit pills (barbiturate)
   bar (cannabis)
   Barb, barbs (barbiturate)
   Barbies (barbiturate)
   barbs (barbiturate; cocaine)
   barf tea (mescaline)
   barrels (lysergic acid diethylamide)
   base (cocaine; crack)
   baseball (crack)
   bash (cannabis)
   basuco (cocaine)
   bathtub speed (methcathinone)
   battery acid (lysergic acid diethyl-
     amide)
   batu (methamphetamine)

drugs, street *(cont.)*
  bazooka (cocaine; crack)
  Bazulco (cocaine)
  beam me up Scottie (crack and
    phencyclidine)
  beans (amphetamine sulfate;
    barbiturate; mescaline)
  beast (heroin; lysergic acid diethyl-
    amide)
  beautiful boulders (crack)
  Bebe (crack)
  beemers (crack)
  belladonna (phencyclidine)
  Belushi (cocaine and heroin)
  Belyando spruce (cannabis)
  bennies (amphetamine sulfate)
  Benz (amphetamine)
  Bernice (cocaine)
  bernies (cocaine)
  Bernie's flakes (cocaine)
  Bernie's gold dust (cocaine)
  bhang (cannabis)
  big bag (heroin)
  big bloke (cocaine)
  big C (cocaine)
  big chief (mescaline)
  big D (lysergic acid diethylamide)
  big flake (cocaine)
  big H (heroin)
  big Harry (heroin)
  big O (opium)
  big rush (cocaine)
  Bill Blass (crack)
  billie hoke (cocaine)
  black bart (cannabis)
  black beauties (amphetamine;
    barbiturate)
  black birds (amphetamine)
  black bombers (amphetamine)
  black ganga (cannabis resin)
  black gold (cannabis)
  black gungi (cannabis)

drugs, street *(cont.)*
  black gunion (cannabis)
  black hash (cannabis and opium)
  black mo (cannabis)
  black moat (cannabis)
  black mollies (amphetamine)
  black mote (cannabis)
  black pearl (heroin)
  black pill (opium)
  black rock (crack)
  Black Russian (cannabis and
    opium)
  blacks (amphetamine)
  black star (lysergic acid diethyl-
    amide)
  black stuff (heroin)
  black sunshine (lysergic acid
    diethylamide)
  black tabs (lysergic acid diethyl-
    amide)
  black tar (heroin)
  black whack (phencyclidine)
  blanco (heroin)
  blanket (cannabis)
  block (cannabis)
  block busters (barbiturate)
  blonde (cannabis)
  blotter (lysergic acid diethylamide;
    cocaine)
  blotter acid (lysergic acid diethyl-
    amide)
  blotter cube (lysergic acid diethyl-
    amide)
  blow (cocaine)
  blowcaine (crack and cocaine)
  blowing smoke (cannabis)
  blowout (crack)
  blow up (crack and lidocaine)
  blue (barbiturate; crack)
  blue acid (lysergic acid diethyl-
    amide)
  blue angels (amobarbital)

drugs, street *(cont.)*
blue barrels (lysergic acid diethylamide)
bluebirds (amobarbital)
blue boy (amphetamine)
blue bullets (barbiturate)
blue caps (mescaline)
blue chairs (lysergic acid diethylamide)
blue cheers (lysergic acid diethylamide)
blue de hue (cannabis)
blue devils (amobarbital)
blue dolls (barbiturate)
blue heaven (lysergic acid diethylamide)
blue heavens (barbiturate)
blue madman (phencyclidine)
blue microdot (lysergic acid
diethylamide)
blue mist (lysergic acid diethylamide)
blue moons (lysergic acid diethylamide)
blues (amobarbital or oxymorphine)
blue sage (cannabis)
blue sky blond (cannabis)
blue tips (barbiturate)
blue velvet (cough preparations
with codeine)
blue vials (lysergic acid diethylamide)
blunt (cannabis)
boat (phencyclidine)
bo-bo (cannabis)
bobo (crack)
bobo bush (cannabis)
bohd (cannabis; phencyclidine)
Bolivian marching powder
(cocaine)
bolt (butyl nitrite)

drugs, street *(cont.)*
bombit (methamphetamine hydrochloride)
bonecrusher (crack)
bones (crack)
bonita (heroin)
boo (cannabis)
boom (cannabis)
boomers (psilocybin/psilocin)
boppers (amyl nitrite)
botray (crack)
bottles (amphetamine)
boubou (crack)
boulder (crack)
boulya (crack)
bouncing powder (cocaine)
boy (cocaine)
bozo (heroin)
brain ticklers (amphetamine)
brick (crack)
brick gum (heroin)
britton (mescaline)
broccoli (cannabis)
brown (heroin; cannabis)
brown bombers (lysergic acid
diethylamide)
brown crystal (heroin)
brown dots (lysergic acid diethylamide)
brownies (dextroamphetamine
sulfate)
brown rhine (heroin)
browns (amphetamine)
brown sugar (heroin)
bubble gum (cocaine; crack)
bud (cannabis)
buda (cannabis and crack)
bullet (butyl nitrite)
bullet bolt (inhalant)
bullia capital (crack)
bullion (crack)
bullyon (cannabis)

drugs, street *(cont.)*

bumblebees (amphetamine)
bump (crack)
bundle (heroin)
Burese (cocaine)
Burnese (cocaine)
burnie (cannabis)
bush (cocaine; cannabis)
businessman's acid (psilocin/
   psilocybin)
businessman's LSD (dimethyltryptamine)
businessman's special (dimethyltryptamine)
businessman's trip (dimethyltryptamine)
busters (barbiturate)
busy bee (phencyclidine)
butt naked (phencyclidine)
butter (cannabis; crack)
butter flower (cannabis)
buttons (mescaline)
butu (heroin)
buzz bomb (nitrous oxide)
C (cocaine; methcathinone)
cactus (mescaline)
caine (cocaine; crack)
California cornflakes (cocaine)
California sunshine (lysergic acid
   diethylamide)
Cambodian red (cannabis)
came (cocaine)
Cam red (cannabis)
Cam trip (cannabis)
can (cannabis)
Canadian black (cannabis)
canamo (cannabis)
canappa (cannabis)
cancelled stick (cannabis)
candy (barbiturate)
candy C (cocaine)
cannabis tea (cannabis)

drugs, street *(cont.)*

cap (crack; lysergic acid diethylamide)
capital H (heroin)
caps (crack; heroin; psilocybin/
   psilocin)
carga (heroin)
carmabis (cannabis)
carne (heroin)
carnie (cocaine)
Carrie (cocaine)
Carrie Nation (cocaine)
cartucho (cannabis)
cartwheels (amphetamine sulfate)
Casper the ghost (crack)
cat (methcathinone)
catnip (cannabis)
cat valium (ketamine)
caviar (crack)
Cavite all star (cannabis)
Cecil (cocaine)
chalk (methamphetamine; amphetamine)
chandoo/chandu (opium)
charas (cannabis)
charge (cannabis)
Charley (heroin)
Charlie (cociane)
chasing the dragon (crack and
   heroin)
cheap basing (crack)
cheeba (cannabis)
cheeo (cannabis)
chemical (crack)
chewies (crack)
chiba chiba (cannabis)
Chicago black (cannabis)
Chicago green (cannabis)
chicken powder (amphetamine)
chicle (heroin)
chief (lysergic acid diethylamide;
   mescaline)

drugs, street *(cont.)*
chieva (heroin)
China cat (heroin)
China girl (fentanyl)
China town (fentanyl)
China white (analog of fentanyl)
Chinese molasses (opium)
Chinese red (heroin)
Chinese tobacco (opium)
chip (heroin)
chippy (cocaine)
chira (cannabis)
chocolate (opium; amphetamine)
chocolate chips (lysergic acid
    diethylamide)
chocolate ecstasy (crack)
cholly (cocaine)
chorals (barbiturate)
Christina (amphetamine)
Christmas rolls (barbiturate)
Christmas trees (amobarbital/
    secobarbital or dextroampheta-
    mine sulfate)
chronic (cannabis; cannabis and
    crack)
churus (cannabis)
CIBAs (glutethimide)
Cid (cannabis)
climax (butyl nitrite)
cloud (crack)
cloud nine (crack)
coasts to coasts (amphetamine)
coca (cocaine)
cochornis (cannabis)
cocktail (cannabis)
coco rocks (crack)
coco snow (benzocaine and crack)
coconut (cocaine)
coffee (lysergic acid diethylamide)
coke (cocaine)
cola (cocaine)
coli (cannabis)

drugs, street *(cont.)*
coliflor tostao (cannabis)
Colombian marijuana (cannabis)
Colorado cocktail (cannabis)
Columbo (phencyclidine)
Columbus black (cannabis)
conductor (lysergic acid diethyl-
    amide)
contact lens (lysergic acid diethyl-
    amide)
cookies (crack)
coolie (cocaine)
copilots (amphetamine)
coral (barbiturate)
Corrinne (cocaine)
cosa (cannabis)
cotics (heroin)
cotton brothers (cocaine, heroin
    and morphine)
courage pills (heroin; barbiturate)
Cozmo's (phencyclidine)
crack (processed cocaine)
crack back (crack and cannabis)
crack cooler (crack)
crackers (lysergic acid diethyl-
    amide)
crank (methamphetamine hydro-
    chloride)
crap/crop (heroin)
crazy coke (phencyclidine)
Crazy Eddie (phencyclidine)
crazy weed (cannabis)
crib (crack)
crimmie (crack)
crink (methamphetamine)
cripple (cannabis)
cris (methamphetamine)
crisscross (amphetamine)
Cristina (methamphetamine)
Cristy (methamphetamine)
croak (crack and methampheta-
    mine)

drugs, street *(cont.)*
crossroads (amphetamine sulfate)
crystal (methamphetamine
  hydrochloride)
crystal joint (phencyclidine)
crystal meth (methamphetamine
  hydrochloride)
crystal T (phencyclidine)
crystal tea (lysergic acid diethylamide)
cube (lysergic acid diethylamide)
cubes (cannabis)
culican (cannabis)
cupcakes (lysergic acid diethylamide)
cura (heroin)
cut-deck (heroin)
cycline (phencyclidine)
cyclones (phencyclidine)
D (lysergic acid diethylamide;
  phencyclidine)
dagga (cannabis)
dama blanca (cocaine)
dance fever (fentanyl)
dawamesk (cannabis)
dead on arrival (heroin)
decadence (methylenedioxymethamphetamine)
deeda (lysergic acid diethylamide)
demolish (crack)
DET (diemethyltryptamine)
Detroit pink (phencyclidine)
deuce (heroin)
devil (crack)
devil's dandruff (crack)
devil's dust (phencyclidine)
devilsmoke (crack)
dew (cannabis)
dexies (dextroamphetamine sulfate)
diambista (cannabis)
diet pills (amphetamine)
dimba (cannabis)

drugs, street *(cont.)*
dime (crack)
ding (cannabis)
dinkie dow (cannabis)
dip (crack)
dipper (phencyclidine)
dirt (heroin)
dirt grass (cannabis)
dirty basing (crack)
disco biscuits (barbiturate)
ditch (cannabis)
ditch weed (cannabis)
djamba (cannabis)
DMT (dimethyltryptamine)
DOA (phencyclidine; crack)
DOB (analog of amphetamine/
  methamphetamine)
doctor (methylenedioxymethamphetamine)
dog food (heroin)
dogie (heroin)
do it Jack (phencyclidine)
dolls (barbiturate)
dollys (methadone hydrochloride)
DOM (analog of amphetamine/
  methamphetamine)
domes (lysergic acid diethylamide;
  phencyclidine and amphetamine/
  methamphetamine)
domestic (cannabis)
dominoes (amphetamine)
Dona Juana (cannabis)
Dona Juanita (cannabis)
don jem (cannabis)
doobie/dubbe/duby (cannabis)
doogie/doojee/dugie (heroin)
dooley (heroin)
dope (cannabis or morphine)
dopium (opium)
doradilla (cannabis)
dots (lysergic acid diethylamide)
double bubble (cocaine)

drugs, street *(cont.)*
double crosses (amphetamine)
double dome (lysergic acid diethylamide)
double rock (crack)
double trouble (amobarbital/secobarbital)
double yoke (morphine)
Dover's powder (opium)
downers (barbiturate)
downie (barbiturate)
draf weed (cannabis)
drag weed (cannabis)
dream (cocaine)
dreamer (morphine)
dream gum (opium)
dream stick (opium)
dreams (opium)
dreck (heroin)
drink (phencyclidine)
drowsy high (barbiturate)
dry high (cannabis)
duct (cocaine)
duji (heroin)
dummy dust (phencyclidine)
Durog (cannabis)
Duros (cannabis)
dust (phencyclidine)
dusted parsley (phencyclidine)
dust joint (phencyclidine)
dust of angels (phencyclidine)
dynamite (heroin and cocaine)
dyno (heroin)
dyno-pure (heroin)
earth (cannabis)
easing powder (opium)
Eastside player (crack)
ecstasy (also, XTC) (methylenedioxymethamphetamine)
egg (crack)
eightball (crack and heroin)
eighth (heroin)

drugs, street *(cont.)*
el diablito (cannabis, cocaine, heroin and phencyclidine)
el diablo (cannabis, cocaine and heroin)
Electric Kool Aid (lysergic acid diethylamide)
elephant (phencyclidine)
elephant tranquilizer (phencyclidine)
embalming fluid (phencyclidine)
emsel (morphine)
endo (cannabis)
energizer (phencyclidine)
ephedrone (methcathinone)
erth (phencyclidine)
Esra (cannabis)
essence (analog of amphetamine/methamphetamine)
estuffa (heroin)
ET (alpha-ethyltryptamine)
Eve (MDEA)
eye opener (crack; amphetamine)
fairy dust (heroin; phencyclidine)
fake STP (phencyclidine)
Fallbrook redhair (cannabis)
famous dimes (crack)
Fantasia (dimethyltryptamine)
fat bags (crack)
fatty (cannabis)
fender bender (barbiturate)
fi-do-nie (opium)
fields (lysergic acid diethylamide)
fifty-one (crack)
fine stuff (cannabis)
finger (cannabis)
fir (cannabis)
fire (crack and methamphetamine)
first line (morphine)
fish scales (crack)
fives (amphetamine)
fizzies (methadone)
flake or flakes (cocaine; phencyclidine)

drugs, street *(cont.)*

flamethrower (cocaine and heroin)
flash (lysergic acid diethylamide)
flat blues (lysergic acid diethylamide)
flat chunks (crack and benzocaine)
flea powder (heroin)
Florida snow (heroin; cocaine)
flower (cannabis)
flower power (morning glory
seeds)
flower tops (cannabis)
fly (muscarine)
foo-foo dust (cocaine)
foo-foo stuff (heroin; cocaine)
foolish powder (heroin; cocaine)
footballs (amphetamine)
45-minute psychosis (dimethyltryptamine)
forwards (amphetamine)
fraho/frajo (cannabis)
freebase (crack)
freebase rocks (rock cocaine)
freeze (cocaine)
French blue (amphetamine)
French fries (crack)
fresh (phencyclidine)
friend (fentanyl)
fries (crack)
frios (cannabis and phencyclidine)
Frisco special (cocaine, heroin, and
lysergic acid diethylamide)
Frisco speedball (cocaine, heroin,
and lysergic acid diethylamide)
friskie powder (cocaine)
fry (crack)
fry daddy (crack and cannabis)
fu (cannabis)
fuel (cannabis; phencyclidine)
fuma D'Angola (cannabis)
gag (heroin)
gage/gauge (cannabis)

drugs, street *(cont.)*

gagers or gaggers (methcathinone)
galloping horse (heroin)
gamot (heroin)
gange (cannabis)
gangster (cannabis)
gangster pills (barbiturate)
ganja (cannabis)
garbage rock (crack)
gash (cannabis)
gasper (cannabis)
gasper stick (cannabis)
gato (heroin)
gauge butt (cannabis)
G.B. (barbiturate)
gee (opium)
geek (crack and cannabis)
George smack (heroin)
Ghana (cannabis)
GHB (gamma hydroxybutyrate)
ghost (lysergic acid diethylamide)
gift-of-the-sun (cocaine)
giggle smoke (cannabis)
gimmie (crack and cannabis)
gin (cocaine)
girl (heroin)
girlfriend (cocaine)
glad stuff (cocaine)
glancines (heroin)
glass (amphetamine)
glo (crack)
God's drug (morphine)
God's flesh (psilocybin/psilocin)
God's medicine (opium)
go-fast (methcathinone)
gold (cannabis; crack)
gold dust (cocaine)
golden Dragon (lysergic acid
diethylamide)
golden girl (heroin)
golden leaf (cannabis)
gold star (cannabis)

drugs, street *(cont.)*
  golf ball (crack)
  golf balls (barbiturate)
  golpe (heroin)
  goma (opium; heroin)
  gondola (opium)
  gong (cannabis; opium)
  goob (methcathinone)
  good (phencyclidine)
  good and plenty (heroin)
  good butt (cannabis)
  goodfellas (fentanyl)
  good giggles (cannabis)
  good H (heroin)
  goofball (barbiturate)
  goof butt (cannabis)
  goofers (barbiturate)
  goofy (lysergic acid diethylamide)
  goon (phencyclidine)
  goon dust (phencyclidine)
  Goric (opium)
  gorilla biscuits (phencyclidine)
  gorilla pills (barbiturate)
  gorilla tab (phencyclidine)
  gram (cannabis)
  grape parfait (lysergic acid diethylamide)
  grass (cannabis)
  grass brownies (cannabis)
  grata (cannabis)
  gravel (crack)
  gravy (heroin)
  great bear (fentanyl)
  great tobacco (opium)
  green (cannabis; phencyclidine; ketamine)
  green double domes (lysergic acid diethylamide)
  green dragon (lysergic acid diethylamide)
  green frog (barbiturate)
  green goddess (cannabis)

drugs, street *(cont.)*
  green gold (cocaine)
  greenies (amphetamine sulfate/amobarbital)
  green leaves (phencyclidine)
  green single domes (lysergic acid diethylamide)
  green tea (phencyclidine)
  green wedge (lysergic acid diethylamide)
  greeter (cannabis)
  Greta (cannabis)
  grey shields (lysergic acid diethylamide)
  griefo (cannabis)
  griff (cannabis)
  griffa (cannabis)
  griffo (cannabis)
  grit (crack)
  groceries (crack)
  G-rock (cocaine)
  G-shot (cannabis)
  gum (opium)
  guma (opium)
  gungun (cannabis)
  gyve (cannabis)
  H (heroin)
  hache (heroin)
  hail (crack)
  hairy (heroin)
  half moon (mescaline)
  half track (crack)
  hamburger helper (crack)
  H & C (heroin and cocaine)
  hanhich (cannabis)
  hanyak (amphetamine)
  happy cigarette (cannabis)
  happy dust (cocaine)
  happy powder (cocaine)
  happy trails (cocaine)
  hard candy (heroin)
  hard line (crack)

drugs, street *(cont.)*

hard rock (crack)
hard stuff (heroin)
hardware (isobutyl nitrite)
Harry (heroin)
hash (cannabis)
hashish (cannabis)
hash oil (cannabis)
hats (lysergic acid diethylamide)
have a dust (cocaine)
Hawaiian marijuana
Hawaiian sunshine (lysergic acid
   diethylamide)
hawk (lysergic acid diethylamide)
hay (cannabis)
hay butt (cannabis)
haze (lysergic acid diethylamide)
Hazel (heroin)
H Caps (heroin)
HCP (phencyclidine)
head drugs (amphetamine)
headlights (lysergic acid diethylamide)
heart-on (inhalant)
hearts (amphetamine sulfate or
   dextroamphetamine sulfate)
heaven and hell (phencyclidine)
heaven dust (heroin; cocaine)
heavenly blue (lysergic acid diethylamide; morning glory seeds)
Helen (heroin)
hell dust (heroin)
he-man (fentanyl)
hemp (cannabis)
Henry (heroin)
Henry VIII (cocaine)
her (cocaine)
Herb (cannabis)
herba (cannabis)
Herb and Al (cannabis and alcohol)
herms (phencyclidine)
hero (heroin)

drugs, street *(cont.)*

heroina (heroin)
herone (heroin)
hero of the underworld (heroin)
hessle (heroin)
hikori (mescaline)
hikuli (mescaline)
him (heroin)
Hinkley (phencyclidine)
hippie crack (inhalant)
hiroppon (methamphetamine)
hit (crack; cannabis)
hocus (opium; cannabis)
hog (phencyclidine)
hombre (heroin)
hombrecitos (psilocybin)
homegrown marijuana (cannabis)
honey blunts (cannabis)
honey oil (ketamine; inhalant)
hong-yen (heroin)
hooch (cannabis)
hooter (cocaine; cannabis)
hop/hops (opium)
horning (heroin)
horse (heroin)
horse heads (amphetamine)
horse tracks (phencyclidine)
horse tranquilizer (phencyclidine)
hotcakes (crack)
hot dope (heroin)
hot ice (methamphetamine)
hot stick (cannabis)
How do you like me now? (crack)
hows (morphine)
HRN (heroin)
Hubba, I am back (crack)
hubbas (crack)
huff (inhalant)
hunter (cocaine)
hyatari (mescaline)
I am back (crack)
ice (cocaine; amphetamine;
   phencyclidine)

drugs, street *(cont.)*
ice (methamphetamine hydrochloride)
ice cube (crack)
icing (cocaine)
idiot pills (barbiturate)
in-betweens (amphetamine; barbiturate; lysergic acid diethylamide)
Inca message (cocaine)
Indian boy (cannabis)
Indian hay (cannabis)
Indica (cannabis)
Indo (cannabis)
Indonesian bud (cannabis; opium)
instant zen (lysergic acid diethylamide)
Isda (heroin)
issues (crack)
J (cannabis)
jackpot (fentanyl)
jam (amphetamine; cocaine)
jam cecil (amphetamine)
Jane (cannabis)
jay (cannabis)
jay smoke (cannabis)
jee gee (heroin)
jellies (barbiturate; temazepam)
jelly (cocaine)
jelly baby (amphetamine)
jelly beans (amphetamine sulfate;
  crack)
jet (ketamine)
jet fuel (phencyclidine)
Jim Jones (cannabis, cocaine, and
  phencyclidine)
jive (heroin; cannabis)
jive doo jee (heroin)
jive stick (cannabis)
Johnson (crack)
joint (cannabis)
jojee (heroin)
jolly bean (amphetamine)

drugs, street *(cont.)*
jolly green (cannabis)
Jones (heroin)
joy flakes (heroin)
joy juice (barbiturate)
joy plant (opium)
joy powder (heroin; cocaine)
joy smoke (cannabis)
joy stick (cannabis)
Juanita (cannabis)
Juan Valdez (cannabis)
jugs (amphetamine)
juice (steroids, phencyclidine)
juice joint (cannabis)
ju-ju (cannabis)
junk (heroin)
K (phencyclidine)
kabayo (heroin)
Kaksonjae (methamphetamine)
Kali (cannabis)
kangaroo (crack)
kaps (phencyclidine)
Karachi (heroin)
kaya (cannabis)
K-blast (phencyclidine)
Kentucky blue (cannabis)
KGB (killer green bud) (cannabis)
kick (inhalant)
kick stick (cannabis)
kif (cannabis)
killer (cannabis; phencyclidine)
killer weed (cannabis; phencyclidine)
kilter (cannabis)
kind (cannabis)
king ivory (fentanyl)
King Kong pills (barbiturate)
king's habit (cocaine)
KJ (phencyclidine)
Kleenex (methylenedioxymethamphetamine)
Kokomo (crack)

drugs, street *(cont.)*
koller joints (phencyclidine)
kools (phencyclidine)
Kryptonite (crack)
krystal (phencyclidine)
krystal joint (phencyclidine)
Kumba (cannabis)
KW (phencyclidine)
L (lysergic acid diethylamide)
L.A. (amphetamine)
lace (cocaine and cannabis)
lady (cocaine)
lady caine (cocaine)
lady snow (cocaine)
L.A. glass (methamphetamine)
L.A. ice (methamphetamine)
lakbay diva (cannabis)
las mujercitas (psilocybin)
lason sa daga (lysergic acid
diethylamide)
Latin lettuce (cannabis)
laughing gas (nitrous oxide)
laughing grass (cannabis)
laughing weed (cannabis)
lay back (barbiturate)
LBJ (lysergic acid diethylamide;
phencyclidine; heroin)
leaf (cannabis; cocaine)
leaky bolla (phencyclidine)
leaky leak (phencyclidine)
leapers (amphetamine)
Lebanese red (cannabis)
lemonade (heroin)
lemon 714 (phencyclidine)
lens (lysergic acid diethylamide)
lethal weapon (phencyclidine)
lib (Librium) (barbiturate)
licorice (tincture of opium)
lid poppers (amphetamine)
lightning (amphetamine)
light stuff (cannabis)
lilly (amobarbital)

drugs, street *(cont.)*
Lima (cannabis)
lime acid (lysergic acid diethylamide)
line (cocaine)
little bomb (amphetamine; heroin;
barbiturate)
little ones (phencyclidine)
little smoke (cannabis; psilocybin/
psilocin)
live ones (phencyclidine)
L.L. (cannabis)
llesca (cannabis)
loaf (cannabis)
lobo (cannabis)
locker room (butyl nitrite)
locoweed (cannabis)
log (phencyclidine; cannabis)
Logor (lysergic acid diethylamide)
lords (hydromorphine)
love (crack)
love affair (cocaine)
love boat (cannabis; phencyclidine)
love drug (methylenedioxymethamphetamine; barbiturate)
lovelies (cannabis and phencyclidine)
lovely (phencyclidine)
love pearls (alpha-ethyltryptamine)
love pills (alpha-ethyltryptamine)
love trip (amphetamine/metham-
phetamine and mescaline)
love weed (cannabis)
LSD (lysergic acid diethylamide)
lubage (cannabis)
Lucy in the sky with diamonds
(lysergic acid diethylamide)
ludes (methaqualone)
luding out (barbiturate)
luds (barbiturate)
M (cannabis; morphine)
machinery (cannabis)

drugs, street *(cont.)*
Macon (cannabis)
maconha (cannabis)
mad dog (phencyclidine)
madman (phencyclidine)
magic (psilocin/psilocybin)
magic dust (phencyclidine)
magic mushroom (psilocybin/
psilocin)
magic smoke (cannabis)
mama coca (cocaine)
M&M (barbiturate)
Manhattan silver (cannabis)
marathons (amphetamine)
Mari (cannabis)
marijuana (cannabis)
marshmallow reds (barbiturate)
Mary (cannabis)
Mary and Johnny (cannabis)
Mary Ann (cannabis)
Mary Jane (cannabis)
Mary Jonas (cannabis)
Mary Warner (cannabis)
Mary Weaver (cannabis)
Matsakow (heroin)
Maui wauie (cannabis)
Max (gamma hydroxybutyrate and
amphetamines)
mayo (cocaine; heroin)
MDA (methylenedioxyampheta-
mine)
MDM (analog of amphetamine/
methamphetamine)
MDMA (analog of amphetamine/
methamphetamine; methylene-
dioxymethamphetamine)
mean green (phencyclidine)
Meg or Megg (cannabis)
Meggie (cannabis)
mellow yellow (lysergic acid
diethylamide)
merk (cocaine)

drugs, street *(cont.)*
mesc (mescaline)
mescal (mescaline)
mese (mescaline)
messorole (cannabis)
meth (methamphetamine hydrochloride)
methylphenidate (methamphetamine)
Mexican brown (heroin; cannabis)
Mexican horse (heroin)
Mexican mud (heroin)
Mexican mushroom (psilocybin/
psilocin)
Mexican red or reds (cannabis)
mezc (mescaline)
Mickey or Mickey Finn (barbiturate)
microdot (lysergic acid diethylamide)
midnight oil (opium)
Mighty Joe Young (barbiturate)
mighty mezz (cannabis)
Mighty Quinn (lysergic acid
diethylamide)
mind detergent (lysergic acid
diethylamide)
minibennie (amphetamine)
mint leaf (phencyclidine)
mint weed (phencyclidine)
mira (opium)
Miss Emma (morphine)
missile basing (crack and phencyclidine)
mist (phencyclidine; crack smoke)
mister blue (morphine)
M.J. (cannabis)
M.O. (cannabis)
modams (cannabis)
mohasky (cannabis)
Mojo (cocaine; heroin)
monkey (cocaine and tobacco)

drugs, street *(cont.)*

monkey dust (phencyclidine)
monkey tranquilizer (phencyclidine)
monos (cocaine and tobacco)
monte (cannabis)
mooca/moocah (cannabis)
moon (mescaline)
moonrock (crack and heroin)
mooster (cannabis)
moota/mutah (cannabis)
mooters (cannabis)
mootie (cannabis)
mootos (cannabis)
mor a grifa (cannabis)
more (phencyclidine)
morf (morphine)
Morotgara (heroin)
morpho (morphine)
mortal combat (heroin)
mosquitos (cocaine)
mota/moto (cannabis)
mother (cannabis)
mother's little helper (barbiturate)
movie star drug (cocaine)
MPPP (analog of meperidine)
MPTP (analog of meperidine)
M.S. (morphine)
M.U. (cannabis)
mud (heroin)
muggie (cannabis)
mujer (cocaine)
murder 8 (fentanyl)
murder one (heroin and cocaine)
mushroom (psilocin/psilocybin)
musk (psilocybin/psilocin)
mutha (cannabis)
muzzle (heroin)
nail (cannabis)
nanoo (heroin)
nebbies (pentobarbital)
nemmies (barbiturate)

drugs, street *(cont.)*

new acid (phencyclidine)
New Jack Swing (heroin and morphine)
new magic (phencyclidine)
nice and easy (heroin)
nickel bag (heroin)
nickel deck (heroin)
niebla (phencyclidine)
nimbies (barbiturate)
nitrous (nitrous oxide)
noise (heroin)
nose (heroin)
nose candy (cocaine)
nose drops (heroin)
nose powder (cocaine)
nose stuff (cocaine)
nubs (mescaline)
nugget (amphetamine)
nuggets (crack)
number (cannabis)
number 3 (cocaine and heroin)
number 4 (heroin)
number 8 (heroin)
O (opium)
octane (phencyclidine and gasoline)
ogoy (heroin)
oil (heroin, phencyclidine)
O.J. (cannabis)
Old Steve (heroin)
one-fifty-one (crack)
one way (lysergic acid diethylamide)
O.P. (opium)
ope (opium)
O.P.P. (phencyclidine)
optical illusions (lysergic acid diethylamide)
orange barrels (lysergic acid diethylamide)
orange crystal (phencyclidine)
orange cubes (lysergic acid diethylamide)

drugs, street *(cont.)*
orange haze (lysergic acid diethylamide)
orange micro (lysergic acid diethylamide)
oranges (amphetamine)
orange sunshine (lysergic acid diethylamide)
orange wedges (lysergic acid diethylamide)
outerlimits (crack and lysergic acid diethylamide)
Owsley's acid (lysergic acid diethylamide)
Oz (inhalant)
ozone (phencyclidine)
P (peyote; phencyclidine)
pack (heroin; cannabis)
pack of rocks (cannabis)
Pakalolo (cannabis)
Pakistani black (cannabis)
Panama cut (cannabis)
Panama gold (cannabis)
Panama red (cannabis)
panatella (cannabis)
pancakes and syrup (glutethimide and codeine cough syrup)
pane (lysergic acid diethylamide)
Pangonadalot (heroin)
paper acid (lysergic acid diethylamide)
parachute (crack and phencyclidine; heroin)
paradise (cocaine)
paradise white (cocaine)
parlay (crack)
parsley (cannabis and phencyclidine)
paste (crack)
Pat (cannabis)
patico (crack)
paz (phencyclidine)

drugs, street *(cont.)*
PCE (analog of phencyclidine)
PCP (phencyclidine)
PCPA (phencyclidine)
PCPy (analog of phencyclidine)
peace (lysergic acid diethylamide and phencyclidine)
peace pills (phencyclidine)
peace tablets (lysergic acid diethylamide)
peace weed (phencyclidine)
peaches (amphetamine sulfate)
peanuts (barbiturate)
peanut butter (phencyclidine)
pearl; pearls (cocaine; amyl nitrite)
pearly gates (lysergic acid diethylamide; morning glory seeds)
pebbles (crack)
peep (phencyclidine)
Pee Wee (crack)
Peg (heroin)
pellets (lysergic acid diethylamide)
pen yan (opium)
pep pill (amphetamine)
Perfect High (heroin)
Perico (cocaine)
Peruvia (cocaine)
Peruvian (cocaine)
Peruvian flake (cocaine)
Peruvian lady (cocaine)
Peter Pan (phencyclidine)
peth (barbiturate)
peyote (mescaline)
P-funk (heroin; crack and phencyclidine)
PG (tincture of opium)
phennies (phenobarbital)
pheno (phenobarbital)
piedras (crack)
Pig Killer (phencyclidine)
piles (crack)
pimp (cocaine)

drugs, street *(cont.)*
pin (cannabis)
pin gon (opium)
pink blotters (lysergic acid diethylamide)
pink hearts (amphetamine)
pink lady (secobarbital)
Pink Panther (lysergic acid diethylamide)
pink robots (lysergic acid diethylamide)
pinks (secobarbital)
pink wedges (lysergic acid diethylamide)
pink witches (lysergic acid diethylamide)
pin yen (opium)
pit (phencyclidine)
pixies (amphetamine)
PMA (analog of amphetamine/
methamphetamine)
pocket rocket (cannabis)
pod (cannabis)
poison (heroin; fentanyl)
poke (cannabis)
polvo (heroin; phencyclidine)
polvo blanco (cocaine)
polvo de angel (phencyclidine)
polvo de estrellas (phencyclidine)
pony (crack)
poor man's pot (inhalant)
poppers (amyl nitrite)
poppy (heroin)
pot (cannabis)
potato (lysergic acid diethylamide)
potato chips (crack and benzocaine)
potten bush (cannabis)
powder (heroin; amphetamine)
powder diamonds (cocaine)
pox (opium)
P.R. (Panama Red) (cannabis)

drugs, street *(cont.)*
prescription (cannabis)
press (cocaine; crack)
pretendica (cannabis)
pretendo (cannabis)
primo (crack; cannabis and crack)
primos (cocaine and heroin)
puffy (phencyclidine)
pulborn (heroin)
pure (heroin)
pure love (lysergic acid diethylamide)
purple (ketamine)
purple barrels (lysergic acid
diethylamide)
purple flats (lysergic acid diethylamide)
purple haze (lysergic acid diethylamide)
purple hearts (lysergic acid diethylamide; amphetamine; barbiturate;
phenobarbital)
purple microdot (lysergic acid
diethylamide)
purple ozoline (lysergic acid
diethylamide)
purple rain (phencyclidine)
Q (barbiturate)
quad (barbiturate)
quarter moon (cannabis)
quas (barbiturate)
Queen Anne's lace (cannabis)
quicksilver (isobutyl nitrite)
quill (methamphetamine; heroin;
cocaine)
racehorse charlie (cocaine; heroin)
ragweed (cannabis; heroin)
railroad weed (cannabis)
rainbows (amobarbital/secobarbital)
rainy day woman (cannabis)
Rambo (heroin)
rane (cocaine; heroin)

drugs, street *(cont.)*
Rangood (cannabis)
rasta weed (cannabis)
raw (crack)
ready rock (cocaine; crack; heroin)
recycle (lysergic acid diethylamide)
red and blue (barbiturate)
red bullets (barbiturate)
red caps (crack)
red cross (cannabis)
red chicken (heroin)
red devil (barbiturate, phencyclidine)
red devils (secobarbital)
red dirt (cannabis)
red dragon (lysergic acid diethylamide)
red eagle (heroin)
red phosphorus (smokable amphetamine)
reds (secobarbital)
reefer (cannabis)
regular P (crack)
reindeer dust (heroin)
Rhine (heroin)
rhythm (amphetamine)
righteous bush (cannabis)
righteous weed (cannabis)
rippers (amphetamine)
road dope (amphetamine)
Robby (cough preparations with codeine)
roca (crack)
roche (Rophynol)
rock (processed cocaine)
rock attack (crack)
rocket (cannabis)
rocket fuel (phencyclidine)
rocks of hell (crack)
Rocky III (crack)
rolling (methylenedioxymethamphetamine)

drugs, street *(cont.)*
roofies (Rophynol)
rooster (crack)
root (cannabis)
rope (cannabis)
roples (Rophynol)
Rosa (amphetamine)
Rose Marie (cannabis)
roses (amphetamine)
rox (crack)
Roxanne (cocaine; crack)
royal blues (lysergic acid diethylamide)
Roz (crack)
ruderalis (cannabis)
ruffles (Rophynol)
running (methylenedioxymethamphetamine)
rush (butyl nitrite)
rush snappers (isobutyl nitrite)
Russian sickles (lysergic acid diethylamide)
sack (heroin)
sacrament (lysergic acid diethylamide)
sacre mushroom (psilocybin)
Salmon River Quiver (cannabis)
salt (heroin)
salt and pepper (cannabis)
sandos (lysergic acid diethylamide)
Santa Marta (cannabis)
sasfras (cannabis)
satan's secret (inhalant)
sativa (cannabis)
scaffle (phencyclidine)
scag (heroin)
scat (heroin)
scate (heroin)
schmeck (cocaine)
schoolboy (cocaine; codeine; cough preparations with codeine)
schoolcraft (crack)

drugs, street *(cont.)*
  scissors (cannabis)
  scorpion (cocaine)
  Scott (heroin)
  Scottie (cocaine)
  Scotty (cocaine; crack)
  scramble (crack)
  scrubwoman's kick (naphtha)
  scruples (crack)
  scuffle (phencyclidine)
  seccy (secobarbital)
  seeds (cannabis)
  seggy (barbiturate)
  sen (cannabis)
  seni (mescaline)
  sernyl (phencyclidine)
  Serpico 21 (cocaine)
  sess (cannabis)
  Seven-up (cocaine; crack)
  sezz (cannabis)
  shabu (methamphetamine
    hydrochloride)
  shake (cannabis)
  she (cocaine)
  sheet rocking (crack and lysergic
    acid diethylamide)
  sheets (phencyclidine)
  shermans (phencyclidine)
  sherms (phencyclidine; crack)
  shmeck/schmeek (heroin)
  shoot the breeze (nitrous oxide)
  shrooms (psilocybin/psilocin)
  Siddi (cannabis)
  sightball (crack)
  Silly Putty (psilocybin/psilocin)
  Simple Simon (psilocybin/psilocin)
  sinse (cannabis)
  sinsemilla (cannabis)
  sinsemillan marijuana
  skag (heroin)
  skee (opium)
  skid (heroin)

drugs, street *(cont.)*
  skuffle (phencyclidine)
  skunk (cannabis)
  Skunk Number 1 (cannabis)
  slab (crack)
  sleeper (heroin; barbiturate)
  sleeping pill (barbiturate)
  sleet (crack)
  slick superspeed (methcathinone)
  slime (heroin)
  smack (heroin)
  smears (lysergic acid diethylamide)
  smoke (cannabis; heroin and crack;
    crack)
  smoke Canada (cannabis)
  smoking (phencyclidine)
  smoking gun (heroin and cocaine)
  snap (amphetamine)
  snappers (amyl nitrite)
  sniff (inhalant; methcathinone)
  snop (cannabis)
  snorts (phencyclidine)
  snow (cocaine; heroin;ampheta-
    mine)
  snowball (cocaine and heroin)
  snowbirds (cocaine)
  snowcones (cocaine)
  snow pallets (amphetamine)
  snow seals (cocaine and ampheta-
    mine)
  snow soke (crack)
  Snow White (cocaine)
  society high (cocaine)
  soda (cocaine)
  softballs (barbiturate)
  soles (cannabis)
  soma (phencyclidine)
  sopers (barbiturate)
  sopors (methaqualone)
  space base (crack and phencycli-
    dine)
  space cadet (crack and phencycli-
    dine)

drugs, street *(cont.)*

space dust (crack and phencyclidine)
sparkle plenty (amphetamine)
sparklers (amphetamine)
special "K" (ketamine)
special la coke (ketamine)
speed (amphetamine or methamphetamine hydrochloride)
speedballs (cocaine-heroin combination; amphetamine)
speed boat (cannabis, phencyclidine, and crack)
speed for lovers (methylenedioxymethamphetamine)
spider blue (heroin)
splash (amphetamine)
spliff (cannabis)
splim (cannabis)
splivins (amphetamine)
spores (phencyclidine)
spray (inhalant)
square mackerel (cannabis)
square time Bob (crack)
stack (cannabis)
star (methcathinone)
stardust (cocaine, phencyclidine)
star-spangled powder (cocaine)
stat (methcathinone)
stems (cannabis)
stick (cannabis, phencyclidine)
stink weed (cannabis)
stones (crack)
stoppers (barbiturate)
STP (phencyclidine; analog of amphetamine/methamphetamine)
straw (cannabis)
strawberries (barbiturate)
strawberry hill (lysergic acid diethylamide)
stuff (heroin)
stumbler (barbiturate)

drugs, street *(cont.)*

sugar (cocaine; lysergic acid diethylamide; heroin)
sugar block (crack)
sugar cubes (lysergic acid diethylamide)
sugar daddys (amphetamine)
sugar lumps (lysergic acid diethylamide)
sugar weed (cannabis)
sunshine (lysergic acid diethylamide)
super (phencyclidine)
super acid (ketamine)
super C (ketamine)
Super Grass (cannabis; phencyclidine)
super ice (methamphetamine)
super joint (phencyclidine)
super kools (phencyclidine)
super weed (phencyclidine)
surfer (phencyclidine)
Sweet Jesus (heroin)
Sweet Lucy (cannabis)
sweet stuff (heroin; cocaine)
sweets (amphetamine)
swell up (crack)
synthetic cocaine (phencyclidine)
synthetic heroin (analog of fentanyl/meperidine)
synthetic THT (phencyclidine)
T (cocaine; cannabis)
tabs (lysergic acid diethylamide)
tail lights (lysergic acid diethylamide)
taima (cannabis)
taking a cruise (phencyclidine)
Takkouri (cannabis)
Tango & Cash (fentanyl)
tar (opium; heroin)
tardust (cocaine)
taste (heroin)

drugs, street *(cont.)*

T-buzz (phencyclidine)
TCP (analog of phencyclidine)
tea (cannabis; phencyclidine)
tecate (heroin)
teeth (cocaine; crack)
tension (crack)
Texas pot (cannabis)
Texas tea (cannabis)
Tex-Mex (cannabis)
Thai marijuana (cannabis)
Thai sticks (cannabis)
THC (tetrahydrocannabinol)
thing (heroin; cocaine)
thirteen (cannabis)
thrust (isobutyl nitrite)
thrusters (amphetamine)
thumb (cannabis)
tic (phencyclidine)
ticket (lysergic acid diethylamide)
tic tac (phencyclidine)
tish (phencyclidine)
tissue (crack)
titch (phencyclidine)
TMA (analog of amphetamine/
    methamphetamine)
T.N.T. (heroin; fentanyl)
toilet water (inhalant)
toncho (octane booster which is
    inhaled)
tooies (amobarbital/secobarbital)
tooles (barbiturate)
toot (cocaine)
tooties (barbiturate)
Tootsie roll (heroin)
top gun (crack)
topi (mescaline)
tops (cannabis; mescaline)
torch (cannabis)
torpedo (crack and cannabis)
tout (opium)
toxy (opium)

drugs, street *(cont.)*

TR-6s (amphetamine)
tragic magic (crack and phencycli-
    dine)
trank (phencyclidine)
tranq (barbiturate)
trip (lysergic acid diethylamide;
    alpha-ethyltryptamine)
troop (crack)
truck drivers (amphetamine)
truth serum (scopolamine)
TT1 (phencyclidine)
TT2 (phencyclidine)
TT3 (phencyclidine)
tuie (barbiturate)
turbo (crack and cannabis)
turkey (cocaine; amphetamine)
Turkish green (cannabis)
turnabout (amphetamine)
tutti-frutti (cocaine)
tweek (methamphetamine-like
    substance)
tweeker (methcathinone)
twenty-five (lysergic acid diethyl-
    amide)
twist (cannabis cigarette)
twistum (cannabis cigarette)
2,5-DMA (analog of amphetamine/
    methamphetamine)
ultimate (crack)
Uncle Milty (barbiturate)
unkie (morphine)
uppers (amphetamine)
uppies (amphetamine)
ups (amphetamine)
ups and downs (barbiturate)
uzi (crack)
V (Valium)
viper's weed (cannabis)
vodka acid (lysergic acid diethyl-
    amide)
wac (phencyclidine and cannabis)

drugs, street *(cont.)*
wack (phencyclidine)
wacky weed (cannabis)
wakeups (dextroamphetamine sulfate)
water (methamphetamine; phencyclidine)
wave (crack)
wedding bells (lysergic acid diethylamide)
wedge (lysergic acid diethylamide)
weed (cannabis; phencyclidine)
weed tea (cannabis)
whack (phencyclidine and heroin)
wheat (cannabis)
when-shee (opium)
whippets (nitrous oxide)
white or whites (amphetamine; cocaine)
white ball (crack)
white boy (heroin)
white cross (methamphetamine; amphetamine)
white dust (lysergic acid diethylamide)
white ghost (crack)
white girl (cocaine; heroin)
white-haired lady (cannabis)
white horizon (phencyclidine)
white horse (cocaine)
white junk (heroin)
white lady (cocaine; heroin)
white lightning (lysergic acid diethylamide)
white mosquito (cocaine)
white nurse (heroin)
whiteout (isobutyl nitrite)
white Owsley's (lysergic acid diethylamide)
white powder (cocaine; phencyclidine)
white stuff (morphine)

drugs, street *(cont.)*
white sugar (crack)
white tornado (crack)
whiz bang (cocaine and heroin)
wild cat (methcathinone and cocaine)
window glass (lysergic acid diethylamide)
window panes (lysergic acid diethylamide)
wings (heroin; cocaine)
witch (heroin; cocaine)
witch hazel (heroin)
wobble weed (phencyclidine)
wolf (phencyclidine)
wollie (crack and cannabis)
worm (phencyclidine)
wrecking crew (crack)
X (cannabis; amphetamine/ methamphetamine)
X-ing (methylenedioxymethamphetamine)
XTC (analog of amphetamine/ methamphetamine; also, ecstasy)
yahoo/yeaho (crack)
Yale (crack)
yeh (cannabis)
yellow or yellows (lysergic acid diethylamide; barbiturate)
yellow bam (methamphetamine)
yellow bullets (pentobarbital)
yellow dimples (lysergic acid diethylamide)
yellow dolls (pentobarbital)
yellow jacket (barbiturate)
yellow fever (phencyclidine)
yellow submarine (cannabis)
yellow sunshine (lysergic acid diethylamide)
yen pop (cannabis)
Yen Shee Suey (opium)
yerba (cannabis)

drugs, street *(cont.)*
  yerba mala (phencyclidine and
    cannabis)
  yesca (cannabis)
  yesco (cannabis)
  yeyo (cocaine)
  yimyom (crack)
  Zacatecas purple (cannabis)
  zambi (cannabis)
  zen (lysergic acid diethylamide)
  zero (opium)
  zig zag man (lysergic acid diethyl-
    amide; cannabis)
  zip (cocaine)
  zol (cannabis)
  zombie (phencyclidine)
  zombie dust (phencyclidine)
  zombie weed (phencyclidine)
  zoom (phencyclidine; cannabis and
    phencyclidine)
drumhead
drum membrane
drunkenness
  acute
  chronic
  pathological
  simple alcoholic
  sleep
"dry" (without alcohol)
dry drunk
dry heaves
"dry high" (cannabis)
dry hoarseness
DS (digit span)
DS (digit symbol)
DSC (Developing Skills Checklist)
DSD (depression sine depression)
DSDB (direct self-destructive behavior)
DSM (*Diagnostic and Statistical
  Manual of Mental Disorders*)

DSM-IV (*Diagnostic and Statistical
  Manual of Mental Disorders,* IV)
DSM-IV, Structured Clinical Interview
  for Dissociative Disorders (SCID-D),
  Revised
DSS (disability status scale)
DST (dexamethasone suppression test)
DSUH (direct suggestion under
  hypnosis)
DT, DTs, Dt's, dt's (delirium tremens)
DTC (day treatment center)
DT/CEP (Differential Test of Conduct
  and Emotional Problems)
DTLA (Detroit Tests of Learning
  Aptitude)
DTLA-3 (Detroit Test of Learning
  Aptitude–Third Edition)
DTLA-A (Detroit Test of Learning
  Aptitude–Adult)
DTLA-P:2 (Detroit Test of Learning
  Aptitude–Primary, Second Edition)
DTRs (deep tendon reflexes)
DTVP (Developmental Test of Visual
  Perception)
DTVP-2 (Developmental Test of Visual
  Perception, Second Edition)
DTX (detoxification)
dual diagnosis
dual-earner household
dualism, mind/body
dual personality
dual-sex therapy
"duct" (cocaine)
duct, cochlear
"due" (re: base residue)
DUI (driving under the influence)
"duji" (heroin)
dull headache
dullness, emotional
dull normal range
dummy (placebo, British)

"dummy dust" (phencyclidine)
duodenal ulcer, psychogenic
duplication, syllable
DUR (drug use review)
durabolin (injectable steroid)
duration duty cycle
duration of drug action
duration of illness
duration of pain
duration of phonation, maximum
duration of sustained blowing, maxi-
    mum
durations of intoxication, characteristic
durations, syllable
Durham Rule
"Durog" (cannabis)
"Duros" (cannabis)
Durrell Analysis of Reading Difficulty:
    Third Edition
"dust" (phencyclidine)
"dusted parsley" (phencyclidine)
"dusting" (adding heroin to cannabis;
    adding phencyclidine to cannabis)
"dust joint" (phencyclidine)
"dust of angels" (phencyclidine)
duty cycle, duration
duty to warn
D-V (domestic violence)
dwarfism, psychosocial
DWI (driving while intoxicated)
Dx (diagnosis)
Dx (diagnostic therapy)
dyad
Dyadic Parent-Child Interaction Coding
    System
dyadic psychotherapy
dyadic session
dymethzine (injectable steroid)
dynamic ambulatory balance
dynamic aphasia
Dynamic Personality Inventory (DPI)
dynamic psychiatry

dynamic psychology
dynamic psychotherapy
dynamic range
dynamic reasoning
dynamics
    family
    infantile
    group
dynamic standing balance
dynamism, lust
"dynamite" (heroin and cocaine)
dynamometer, hand
dyne
"dyno" (heroin)
"dyno-pure" (heroin)
dysacusis
dysanagnosia
dysantigraphia
dysaphia
dysarthria
    apractic
    apraxic
    ataxic
    flaccid
    hyperkinetic
    hypokinetic
    laryngeal
    parkinsonian
    peripheral
    sensual
    somesthetic
    spastic
dysarthria literalis
dysarthria syllabaris spasmodica
dysarthric behaviors
dysautonomia
dyscalculia
dyschiria
dyscontrol
    affective
    behavioral
    emotional

dyscontrol *(cont.)*
    episodic
    impulsive
    temper
dysequilibrium (or disequilibrium)
dyserethesia
dyserethism
dysesthesia
dysesthesic sensation
dysesthetic
dysfluencies
    avoidance of speech
    emotional response to speech
    speech
dysfunction
    acquired sexual
    alcohol-induced sexual
    amphetamine-induced sexual
    arousal
    autonomic
    behavioral
    bilateral cerebral
    biological
    brain
    brain stem
    cerebral
    cocaine-induced sexual
    cognitive
    contralateral parietal lobe
    diffuse brain
    educational
    ejaculatory
    emotional
    erectile
    focal/lateralized
    frontal lobe
    generalized sexual
    hemispheral
    hemispherical
    higher cerebral (HCD)
    higher cortical

dysfunction *(cont.)*
    interpersonal
    language
    life-long sexual
    lingual airway
    male erectile
    mid brain
    minimal brain (MBD)
    neurological
    organic brain
    orgasmic
    parietal lobe
    posttraumatic cortical
    psychological
    psychosexual
    school
    self-care
    severe diffuse brain
    sexual
    situational sexual
    social
    substance-induced sexual
    swallowing
    sympathetic
    tongue
    vocal cord
    work
dysfunctional behavior, learned
dysfunctional cognitions
dysfunctional relational functioning
dysfunctional relationship
dysgeusia
dysgnosia
    auditory-verbal
    body
    visual letter
    visual number
dysgrammatism
dysgraphia
dysgraphicus, status
dysharmonica diplacusis

dyskinesia
  disfluency
  laryngeal
  neuroleptic-induced tardive
  tardive
  tardive oral
  tardive orobuccal
dyskinetic cerebral palsy (CP)
dyskinetic movement
dyskoimesis
dyslalia
dyslexia
  acquired
  developmental
Dyslexia Determination Test
Dyslexia Screening Survey, The
dyslexic
dyslogia
dysmenorrhea, psychogenic
dysmetric hand movements
dysmimia
dysmnesia
dysmnesic psychosis
dysmnesic syndrome
dysmorphic defect, body
dysmorphic disorder, body
dysmorphophobia
dysnomia, autonomic
dysosmia
dysostosis, mandibulofacial
dyspareunia
  acquired-type
  female
  functional
  generalized-type
  lifelong-type
  male
  psychogenic
  situational-type
dyspepsia, psychogenic
dysphagia nervosa
dysphagy

dysphasia
dysphemia
dysphonia
  adductor spasmodic
  hyperkinetic
  spastic
  ventricular
dysphonic
dysphoretic
dysphoria
dysphoriant
dysphoric affect
dysphoric disorder
  late luteal phase
  premenstrual
dysphoric mood
dysphrasia
dysphylaxia
dysplasia
dyspnea response
dyspneic disorder, psychogenic
dyspractic movement
dyspraxia
  constructional
  spelling
dyspraxia syndrome
dysprosody
dysregulation, defensive
dysrhythmia
dysrhythmic movement
dysrhythmic speech
dyssocial behavior
  adolescent
  adult
  child
dyssocial personality disorder
dyssocial reaction
dyssomnia
  jet lag-type
  shift work-type
  unspecified-type
dyssymbolia

dyssymboly
dysthymia
dysthymic adjustment reaction
dysthymic disorder (DD), alternative
  criterion B for
dystonia
  body
  idiopathic
  neuroleptic-induced acute
  nocturnal paroxysmal
  oropharyngeal
  substance-induced
  tardive

dystonic cerebral palsy (CP)
dystonic movements
dystonic tremor
dystrophy, muscular
dysuria, psychogenic

E, e

EA (educational age)
E&H (environment and heredity)
E&O (evaluation and observation)
EAP (Employee Assistance Program)
ear (pl. ears)
    artificial
    external
    glue
    inner
    low-set
    middle
    outer
    third
earhook
early-age trauma and PTSD
Early Child Development Inventory
early childhood disturbances in feed-
    ing and eating, infancy and
Early Coping Inventory
early dementia
Early Development Scale for
    Preschool Children
early environment, impoverished
early full remission
Early Language Milestone Scale
early latency potentials
early onset drinking

early phase
early relationship
Early School Assessment (ESA)
Early School Personality Question-
    naire (ESPQ)
Early Screening Inventory
early sign
Early Social Communication Scale
    (ESCS)
Early Speech Perception (ESP) Test
early traumatic epilepsy
Early Years Easy Screen (EYES)
earmold
    open
    nonoccluding
    perimeter
    shell
    skeleton
    standard
    vented
earmuffs (hearing protection device)
ear muscle reflex, middle
earphone
earplugs
earplugs hearing protection device
"earth" (cannabis cigarette)
ear training

earwax
ease of fatigue
EASIC (Evaluating Acquired Skills in
    Communication), Revised)
easily distractible
easily disturbed sleep
easily provoked
"easing powder" (opium)
eastern equine viral encephalitis
"Eastside player" (crack)
easy fatigability
"easy score" (easy drug acquisition)
EAT (Edinburgh Articulation Test)
EAT (Education Apperception Test)
"eating" (taking a drug orally)
eating binge
eating, compulsive
eating disorder, gender differences in
Eating Disorder Inventory for Children
Eating Disorder Inventory-2 (EDI-2)
eating hairs
Eating Inventory
eating syndrome, nocturnal
Ebonics (Black English)
EBPS (Emotional and Behavior
    Problem Scale)
ebullient
Eby Elementary Identification
    Instrument
ECA (Epidemiologic Catchment Area)
eccentricities of behavior, pattern of
eccentricity
eccentric personality
eccentric thinking
ecclesiophobia
ecdemiomania
ecdysiasm
ECES (Education and Career Explora-
    tion System)
echo chamber
echoic memory

echoic operant
echokinesis
echolalia
    immediate
    mitigated
    unmitigated
echolocation
echomatism
echomimia
echomotism
echopathy
echophrasia
echopraxia
echopraxis
echo speech
eclamptic convulsion
eclamptic delirium
eclamptic idiocy
eclecticism
ECochG or ECoG (electrocochle-
    ography)
ecological validity
ecomania
economic self-sufficiency
economy reward, token
ecophobia
ecopsychiatry
"ecstasy" (aka XTC) (methylenedioxy-
    methamphetamine)
ecstasy, religious
ecstatic
ECT (electroconvulsive therapy;
    treatment)
    bilateral
    brief pulse
    sine wave
    suprathreshold
    unilateral
eczema, psychogenic
EDEN (Evaluation Disposition
    [Toward the] Environment)

edeomania
Edinburgh Articulation Test (EAT)
Edinburgh Functional Communication
   Profile, Revised (EFCP)
Edinburgh Handedness Inventory
Edinburgh Picture Test
Edinburgh Reading Tests
Edinburgh Rehabilitation Status Scale
Edinburgh-2 Coma Scale
EDI-2 (Eating Disorder Inventory-2)
ED/LD (emotionally disturbed/learn-
   ing disabled)
EDPA (Erhardt Developmental Prehension Assessment)
EDR (electrodermal response biofeedback)
EDRA (electrodermal response
   audiometry) test
EDS (Ego Development Scale)
educable mentally retarded (EMR)
education
   age-appropriate
   continuing medical (CME)
   speech
   vocational rehabilitation and
      (VR&E)
educational age (EA)
educational audiology
Educational Development Series
educational dysfunction
educational functioning
educational history
educational level
educationally mentally handicapped
   (EMH)
educationally mentally retarded
   (EMR)
educational psychology
educational quotient (EQ)
educational setting
educational situations
Educational Testing Service (ETS)

educational tool
Education and Career Exploration
   System (ECES)
Education Apperception Test (EAT)
education quotient (EQ)
EDVA (Erhardt Developmental Vision
   Assessment)
Edwards Personal Preference Schedule
   (EPPS)
EE (expressed emotion)
EEG (electroencephalogram;
    electroencephalograph)
   beta pattern on
   beta rhythm on
   beta wave on
   diffuse slowing of
   nonspecific abnormality on
   phase lag on
   phase reversal on
   phase spike on
   sleep deprived
   sleep spindle on
   waking
EEG activity measurement
EEG activity, slow-frequency (delta)
EEG alpha activity
EEG delta activity
EEG potential
EEG theta activity
EEG tracing
EEG with NP leads
EFCP (Revised Edinburgh Functional
   Communication Profile)
effect (pl. effects)
   acute toxic
   adaptation
   adverse
   anticholinergic
   anxiolytic
   autokinetic
   body baffle (hearing aid)
   cellular

effect *(cont.)*
    central nervous system
    chronic toxic
    cocaine
    consistency
    deception
    desired
    diminished
    direct physiological
    Doppler
    dose-dependent
    drug
    electrocardiographic
    Féré
    fetal alcohol (FAE)
    frequency
    hallucinogen
    halo
    head shadow
    "hit and run"
    laws of cause and
    lithium
    long-term
    major
    maximal
    medication
    medication side
    narcotic
    occlusion
    off
    on-off (of L-dopa)
    parkinsonism-like
    peripheral sympathomimetic
    placebo
    possible
    potential adverse
    practice
    psychoactive
    sedative
    side
    spiral
    stimulant

effect *(cont.)*
    Stroop
    suggestibility
    sympathomimetic
    therapeutic
    toxic
    trauma
    treatment
    treatment side
    unintended
    wearing off
    Wever-Bray
effective action
effective amplitude
effective communication, impaired
effective masking
effectiveness, decreased
Effective Reading Tests
Effective School Battery, The (ESB)
effect of trauma
effector operation
effeminacy
effeminate
effemination
efferent aphasia
efferent feedback
efferent (kinetic) motor aphasia
efferent nerve
efficiency
    good sleep
    lack of
    masking
    sleep
    vocal
effort
    new-work
    vocal
effort level
effort syndrome
    aviators
    psychogenic
effusion ego egocentric

EFT (Embedded Figures Test)
EFT (extended family therapy)
"egg" (crack)
ego
ego-alien
ego analysis
ego, auxiliary
ego boundaries, loss of
egocentric, effusion ego
egocentricity
Egocentricity Index
egocentric language
egocentric speech
egocentric thought processes
egocentrism
ego control, weak
ego-coping skills
ego defense
ego-defense mechanism
Ego Development Scale (EDS)
ego-dystonia
ego-dystonic behavior
ego-dystonic homosexuality
ego-dystonic intrusions
egodystonicity
ego-dystonic orientation
ego-dystonic pseudohallucination
ego egocentric, effusion
Ego Function Assessment
ego function, executive
ego-ideal
Ego-Ideal and Conscience
    Development Test (EICDT)
ego identity
ego instinct
ego integration
egoism
egoïsme à deux
ego libido
egomania
egomechanism of defense
ego model

ego psychology
Ego State Inventory (ESI)
ego state, multiple
ego-state therapy
ego strength
ego structure, stable
ego-syntonic behavior
egosyntonicity
ego-syntonic traits
egotism
egotistical
egotropic
EH (emotional handicap)
EICDT (Ego-Ideal and Conscience
    Development Test)
eidetic imagery
Eidetic Parents Test (EPT)
"eightball" (1/8 ounce of drugs;
    (crack and heroin)
"eighth" (heroin)
eighth nerve tumor
Eight State Questionnaire
eisoptrophobia
Eitingon, Max (1881-1943)
EIWA (Escala de Inteligencia
    Wechsler para Adultos)
ejaculation
    premature
    retrograde
ejaculatory dysfunction
ejaculatory incompetence (impotence)
ejaculatory inevitability, sensation of
EL (elopement)
elaborate dream sequence
elaboration, symbolic
elasticity
elated affect
elation
elder abuse
elderly
elder maltreatment and PTSD (post-
    traumatic stress disorder)

"el diablito" (cannabis, cocaine, heroin, and phencyclidine)
"el diablo" (cannabis, cocaine, and heroin)
El Dx (electrodiagnosis)
elective mutism adjustment reaction
elective mutism, relative
Electra complex
electrical activity map (mapping), brain (BEAM)
electrical artificial larynx
electrical measurement of speech production
electrical potential
electrical shock
electric field
electric irritability
electricity, feeling of
"Electric Kool Aid" (lysergic acid diethylamide)
electric response audiometry (ERA)
electric shocks
electric shock sensation
electrocardiographic effect
electrocochleography (ECochG; ECoG)
electrocochleography audiometry (ECoG; ECochG)
electroconvulsive shock therapy
electroconvulsive therapy-induced mood disorder
electrode
electrodermal audiometry (EDA)
electrodermal response audiometry (EDRA) test
electrodermal response biofeedback (EDR)
electrodiagnosis (El Dx)
electrodiagnostic studies
electroencephalograph (EEG) biofeedback
electroencephalography

electrolyte abnormalities
electrolyte disturbance
electrolyte imbalance
electromagnetic wave
electromotive force (EMF)
electromyogram (EMG)
electromyographic activity, peripheral
electromyographic perineometer
electromyographic speech analysis
electromyography biofeedback
electron
electronarcosis (EN)
electronic artificial larynx
electronic auditory feedback
electronics
electronystagmography (ENG)
electrooculographic activity
electrophobia
electrophysiologic audiometry
electrophysiology
electroshock, maximal (MES)
electroshock seizures, maximal (MES)
electroshock therapy (or treatment) (EST)
electroshock treatment, regressive (REST)
electrostimulation
elements, cultural
elements of performance objective
"elephant" (phencyclidine)
"elephant tranquilizer" (phencyclidine)
eleutheromania
eleutherophobia
elevated mood
elevated risk
elevation screen, THC
elevator muscle of soft palate
elevators, mood
ELI (Environmental Language Inventory)
Elicited Articulatory System Evaluation

elicited imitation
eligibility, benefit
Elihorn Maze Test
elimination disorder
elision
Elizur Test of Psycho-Organicity:
    Children & Adults
ellipsis (pl. ellipses)
elopement (EL)
elopement ideation
elopement status (ES)
ELP (Estimated Learning Potential)
ELU (extended length of utterance)
elurophobia
emancipated minor
emancipation disorder of adolescence
EMAS; EMAS-P; EMAS-S; EMAS-T
    (Endler Multidimensional Anxiety
    Scales)
emasculation
"embalming fluid" (phencyclidine)
embedded clause
embedded command
Embedded Figures Test (EFT)
embedded sentence
embedded sound
embezzlement
embolism
embololalia
embolophrasia
embryo
embryonic
EMDR (eye movement densitization
    reprocessing)
"emergency gun" (re: drug injection)
emergent language
emetophobia
EMF (electromotive force)
EMH (educationally mentally handi-
    capped)
emission, nasal

emission tomography scan, positron
    (PET)
emotion (pl. emotions)
    childish
    controlled
    defensive
    diminished feeling of
    discomfort with
    disruptive
    disturbance of
    effect of trauma on
    exaggerated expression of
    expressed (EE)
    expression of
    impaired
    intense
    lack of
    negative
    nocturnal
    positive
    powerful
    public display of
    rapidly shifting
    rapid shifting of
    restricted range of
    roller-coaster
    shallow expression of
    strong
emotional abandonment, perceived
emotional/activation factors
emotional activity
emotional age
emotional agitation
emotional amnesia
Emotional and Behavior Problem
    Scale (EBPS)
emotional anesthesia
emotional atmosphere
emotional attachment/commitment
emotional attainment
emotional awareness

emotional blackmail
emotional blocking
emotional blunting
emotional bond
emotional cause of seizure
emotional climate
emotional coldness
emotional conflict
emotional constriction
emotional crisis
emotional deadness
emotional deficit
emotional dependence
emotional deprivation
emotional disability
emotional disinhibition
emotional disorder
emotional distress
emotional disturbance of adolescence
emotional disturbance of childhood
emotional disturbance stress reaction
emotional dullness
emotional dyscontrol
emotional dysfunction
emotional emptiness
emotional explosivity
emotional handicap (EH)
emotional handicap, severe (SEH)
emotional illness
emotional impairment
emotional incontinence
emotional inhibition
emotional insight
emotional instability personality
   disorder
emotionalism
emotionality
   excessive
   labile
   negative
   pathological
   positive

emotional lability
emotionally constricted
emotionally disturbed/learning
   disabled (ED/LD)
emotionally impaired
emotionally isolated
emotionally laden topics
emotionally provoking stimulus
emotionally stable
emotionally ungiving
emotionally unstable
emotionally unstable immaturity
   reaction
emotionally unstable personality
emotionally upset
emotional maltreatment of children
emotional manipulation
emotional modulation
emotional modulation skills
emotional needs
emotional numbing
emotional overlay
emotional overreaction
emotional reaction
emotional reaction/conflict
emotional reciprocity
emotional repression
emotional response, conditioned (CER)
emotional response to speech
   dysfluencies
emotional responsiveness
emotional shading
emotional state
emotional stimulus
emotional stress
emotional stress depressive psychosis
emotional stress precipitating tremor
emotional support
emotional symptoms
emotional tone
emotional turmoil
emotional undercontrol

emotional vulnerability
emotion-cognition interface
emotion-laden situations
emotion-related feedback stimuli
emotions/conduct adjustment reaction,
     mixed
Emotions Profile Index
emotive energy, active displacement of
emotive language
emotive speech
emotive therapy, rational (RET)
empathic behavior
empathize
empathy
     communicating
     generative
empirical data
empirical evidence
empirical process
empirical review
empirical support
empiric cognition
empleomania
Employability Inventory
Employee Aptitude Survey Tests
Employee Assistance Program (EAP)
Employee Attitude Inventory
Employee Effectiveness Profile
Employee Reliability Inventory (ERI)
Employment Inventory, PDI
empowered families
empowerment
emptiness
     chronic feelings of
     feelings of deep
     feelings of emotional
     sense of
emptiness of affect
empty nest syndrome
empty stare
EMR (educable mentally retarded)
EMR (educationally mentally retarded)

"emsel" (morphine)
emulate peers, to
emulation
EN (electronarcosis)
encapsulated delusion
encephalopathy
     AIDS
     allergic
     anoxic
     childhood
     degenerative
     demyelinating
     diffuse
     hepatic (HE)
     hypertensive
     hypoxic-ischemic (HIE)
     idiopathic
     metabolic
     neoplastic
     painter's
     postanoxic
     postcontusion syndrome
     posttraumatic
     progressive subcortical
     progressive traumatic
     punch-drunk
     static
     thiamine deficiency (TDE)
     toxic
     traumatic
     viral
     Wernicke
     Wernicke-Korsakoff
encoder
encoding communication board
encoding, impairment of new memory
encoding skills
encopresis
encotretic
encounter (pl. encounters)
     frequency of sexual
     indiscriminate sexual

encounter *(cont.)*
   patient
   types of sexual
encounter bats
encountered association, frequency
encounter group
endangered, physically
endangerment
endemic
endings, inflectional
Endler Multidimensional Anxiety Scales
   (EMAS; EMAS-P; EMAS-S;
   EMAS-T)
"endo" (cannabis)
endocentric construction
endocrine assessment
endocrine disorder, psychogenic
endocrine-type organic psychosis
endogenous abnormalities in sleep-wake
   timing mechanisms
endogenous circadian pacemaker
endogenous circadian period
endogenous circadian rhythm phase
endogenous depression
endogenous pain
endolymph
endolymphatic hydrops
end-organ of hearing
endorphin
endorsement of deviant thoughts and
   beliefs
endoscope
endoscopy
end-pleasure
end point tremor
enduring pattern of inflexibility
"energizer" (phencyclidine)
energy
   acoustic
   active displacement of emotive
   boundless
   decreased

energy *(cont.)*
   emotive
   excess
   increased
   kinetic
   lack of
   loss of
   low
   potential
   vital
energy expenditure, resting
energy level
enetophobia
ENG (electronystagmography)
engagement level
engineering, human
English
   African American vernacular
   Black
   Chicano
   Creole
   Hispanic
   pidgin Sign (PSE)
   signed
English Language Institute Listening
   Comprehension Test
English/Spanish Del Rio Language
   Screening Test
engram
engulfment
Enhanced ACT Assessment
enkaphalins
enmeshment
enoltestovis (injectable steroid)
enomania
ENT (ear, nose, throat)
entailment
entering problem, school
entheomania
entities, controlling external
entitlement, sense of
entity-locative

entomomania
entomophobia
entopic vision
entropy
enunciate
enuresis
  diurnal
  nocturnal
  psychogenic
enuretic events
envious behavior
environment
  academically understimulating
  awareness of
  complete unawareness of
  controlled
  dark
  decreased reactivity to
  distorted perception of
  disturbed home
  domestic
  home
  immediate
  impoverished early
  inadequate school
  inattention to the
  institutional
  invalidating
  low sensory
  low stimulation
  milieu
  multicultural
  natural
  nurturing
  response to
  perception of the
  physical
  problems related to the social
  scaffolded language-learning
  secure
  social
  socially disruptive

environment *(cont.)*
  stimulating
  vocational
environmental assessment
environmental deficiency
environmental deprivation, severe
environmental disturbances of sleep
Environmental Language Inventory
  (ELI)
environmentally induced anxiety
environmental neurosis
Environmental Pre-Language Battery
environmental pressure
environmental psychology
Environmental Response Inventory
  (ERI)
environmental stimulation
environmental stimuli, selective focusing on
environmental support
environmental understimulation
environment and heredity (E&H)
envy, penis
eosophobia
EOWPVT-R (Expressive One-Word
  Picture Vocabulary Test–Revised)
EP (evoked potential) brain test
EPAQ (Extended Personal Attributes
  Questionnaire)
ephaptic conduction
"ephedrone" (methcathinone)
EPI (Eysenck Personality Inventory)
epidemic hysteria
Epidemiologic Catchment Area (ECA)
epidemiological data
epidemiological study
epigastric aura
epigenesis
epiglottis
epilepsy
  absence
  acquired

epilepsy *(cont.)*
  activated
  alcoholic
  alcohol-precipitated
  automatic
  Bravais-jacksonian
  centrotemporal
  childhood
  chronic
  clouded state
  communicating
  cortical
  cryptogenic
  cursive
  deterioration
  diurnal
  early traumatic
  essential
  extrinsic
  focal
  gelastic
  generalized
  generalized flexion
  haut mal
  hippocampal
  hysterical
  idiopathic
  impulsive petit mal
  Jackson
  jacksonian
  Kojevnikoff
  Koshevnikoff
  larval
  laryngeal
  latent
  late traumatic
  localized
  major (grand mal)
  minor (petit mal)
  mixed type
  musicogenic
  nocturnal

epilepsy *(cont.)*
  organic
  partial
  pattern-induced
  perceptive
  peripheral
  photic
  photogenic
  photosensitive
  postanoxic
  posttraumatic
  procursive
  psychic
  psychomotor
  psychosensory
  reading
  reflex
  rolandic
  seizure
  senile
  sensorial
  sensory
  sensory-induced
  serial
  situation-related
  sleep
  sleep-related
  somatomotor
  somatosensory
  status
  symptomatic
  tardy
  television-induced
  temporal lobe
  thalamic
  traumatic
  twilight
  visual
epilepsy-type organic psychosis,
  transient
epileptica, absentia
epileptic aphasia, acquired

epileptic aura
epileptic automatism
epileptic clouded state
epileptic confusional state (ECS)
epileptic convulsion
epileptic dementia
epileptic equivalent
epileptic focus
epileptic fugue state
epileptic idiocy
epileptic mania
epileptic psychosis
epileptic twilight state
epileptic seizure
epileptic syndrome
epilepticus
    convulsive status
    nonconvulsive status
    status
epileptiform convulsion
epileptogenic stimulation
epileptogenic stimulus
epileptogenous
epileptoid personality
epileptologist
epileptology
epinephrine
episode (pl. episodes)
    acute schizophrenic
    aphonic
    cataplexy
    confusional
    current
    daytime sleep
    depersonalization
    depressed mood
    depression
    depressive
    first
    florid
    frequency of
    frequency of sleep terror

episode *(cont.)*
    gray-out
    hypomanic
    hypomanic-like
    hypomanic mood
    illneses
    intoxication
    major depressive (MDE)
    manic
    manic-like
    manic mood
    mixed
    mixed manic-depressive-like
    mixed mood
    mood
    most recent
    non-substance-induced
    non-substance-related
    prolonged
    prolonged nocturnal sleep
    prolonged sleep
    psychoepileptic
    psychotic
    psychotic schizophrenic
    recent
    recurrent
    recurrent mood
    recurring psychotic
    schizoaffective
    second
    single
    sleep onset
    sleep terror
    unintentional daytime sleep
    unspecified mood
    untreated
episodic amnesia
episodic changes of consciousness
episodic confusion
episodic course
episodic dyscontrol
epithelium (pl. epithelia)

epithets
  national
  racial
epochs, wakefulness
EPPS (Edwards Personal Preference
  Schedule)
EPQ (Eysenck Personality Questionnaire)
EPS (extrapyramidal syndrome)
EPS (extrapyramidal system)
EPT (Eidetic Parents Test)
EQ (education quotient)
equal frequency
equality, point of subjective (PSE)
equal loudness contours
equal sex ratio
equilibratory ataxia
equilibrium
equine viral encephalitis
  eastern
  western
equipment
  "dirty" drug-injecting
  used drug-injecting
equipose (veterinary steroid)
equivalence, complex
equivalent
  arithmetic grade
  convulsive
  delusional
  epileptic
  grammatical
  pharmaceutical
  psychic
  reading-grade
  spelling-grade
equivalent criteria
equivalent diagnosis
equivalent dosage
equivalent intoxication criteria
equivalent speech reception threshold
equivalent symptomatic presentation

equivalent symptoms
equivalent withdrawal criteria
ER (evoked response) brain test
ERA (electric response audiometry)
ERA (evoked response audiometry)
ERB (ethnic relational behavior)
Erb palsy
ERD (event-related desynchronization)
erectile arousal disorder, male
erectile disorder
  acquired-type male
  generalized-type male
  lifelong-type male
  male
  situational-type male
erectile disorder due to combined
  factors, male
erectile disorder due to psychological
  factors, male
erectile dysfunction
erectile functioning, vasculogenic loss
  of
erectile impotence
erection
  psychogenic painful
  sleeping
eremiomania
eremophobia
erethism, sexual
erethismic
erethistic idiocy
erethitic
ereuthrophobia
ergasia
ergasiomania
ergasiophobia
ergolid mesylate (for Alzheimer
  disease)
ergomania
ergometer
ergonomics
ergophobia

ergotism
Erhardt Developmental Prehension
    Assessment (EDPA)
Erhardt Developmental Vision
    Assessment (EDVA)
ERI (Employee Reliability Inventory)
ERI (Environmental Response
    Inventory)
ermitophobia
erogenous zone
eros
erosion, dental
erotically stimulating literature
erotic arousal
erotic dream
erotic feeling
eroticism
eroticize
eroticized behavior
erotic obsession
eroticomania
erotic stimulus (pl. stimuli)
erotism
    anal
    oral
erotization
erotize
erotogenesis
erotogenic
erotographomania
erotomania, Clerambault
erotomaniac
erotomanic-type delusion
erotomanic-type schizophrenia
erotopath
erotopathic
erotopathy
erotophobia
erotopsychic
erotosexual
errant thought

erratic behavior
erratic mood
erratic parenting
erratic rhythm of speech
erratic speech rhythm
erratic thinking
erroneous belief
erroneous impression
error (pl. errors)
    anomic
    aphasic
    paralexic
    phonemic articulation
    phonetic articulation
    standard
    type I; II
    vicarious trial and (VTE)
error signal, therapeutic (TES)
errors of metabolism, inborn
errors of ordering of sounds
errors of selection of sounds
"erth" (phencyclidine)
erudite
erudition
ERV (expiratory reserve volume)
erythromania
erythrophobia
ES (elopement status)
ESA (Early School Assessment)
ESB (Effective School Battery)
Escala de Inteligencia Wechsler para
    Adultos (EIWA)
escalating pattern of substance use
escalative process
escapade, sexual
escape learning
escape, nasal
escape reaction
ESCS (Early Social Communication
    Scale)
ESI (Ego State Inventory)

esophageal speech
  breathing method of
  inhalation method of
  injection method of
  methods of
  sniff method of
  suction method of
  swallow method of
esophageal tears
esophageal voice
esophagus disorder, psychogenic
ESP (Early Speech Perception Test)
ESP (extrasensory perception)
Español, MRT
ESPQ (Early School Personality
  Questionnaire)
"Esra" (cannabis)
ESS (The ACT Evaluation/Survey
  Service)
"essence" (analog of amphetamine/
  methamphetamine; methylenedioxymethamphetamine)
essential cerebellar tremor
essential cerebral tremor
essential convulsion
essential epilepsy
essential features
essential headache
essential tremor, benign
EST (electroshock therapy; treatment)
established delusion
esteem-enhancing
esthesic
Estimated Learning Potential (ELP)
"estuffa" (heroin)
"ET" (alpha-ethyltryptamine)
etat lacunaire (multiple small strokes)
ether dependence
etheromania
ethical aspects of assaultive client care
ethical aspects of dementia
ethical behavior

ethics, medical
ethmoid bone
ethnic background
ethnic reference group
ethnic relational behavior (ERB)
ethnocentrism
ethnopsychology
ethology
ethyl alcohol addiction
etiological agent
etiological association
etiological factor
etiological neurological condition
etiological relationship
etiology, generalized medical theories
  of
ETOH, EtOH (alcohol)
ETS (Educational Testing Service)
etymology
EU (expected utility)
eugnathia
eunoia
eunuch
eunuchism
eunuchoid
eunuchoidism
eunuchoid voice
euphemism
euphonic
euphoretic
euphoria
euphoriant
euphoric affect
euphoric, feeling
euphoric mood
euphorigenic
euphoristic
eupnea
eurotophobia
eustachian tube
euthanasia
euthymia

euthymic mood
euthymic state
evade
Evaluating Acquired Skills in Communication (EASIC), Revised
Evaluating Communicative Competence: A Functional Pragmatic Procedure
Evaluating Educational Programs for Intellectually Gifted Students
Evaluating Movement and Posture Disorganization in Dyspraxic Children
Evaluating the Participant's Employability Skills
evaluation (eval) (see also *test*)
  adolescents
  appropriate
  audiological
  clinical
  component of
  comprehensive
  condescending
  criterion
  cultural background
  cultural content of
  dementia
  educational background
  hearing aid (HAE)
  home
  indirect
  longitudinal
  mental capacity
  multiaxial
  need for continued
  negative
  neurological
  neuropsychologic
  process of clinical
  psychiatric
  psychoeducational
  psychological

evaluation *(cont.)*
  psychometric
  rehabilitation
  symptoms
  vocational (VE)
evaluation and observation (E&O)
Evaluation Disposition (Toward the) Environment (EDEN)
evaluator bias
evasion
evasive behavior
evasiveness
"Eve" (MDEA)
evening drinking
evening headache
event (pl. events)
  antecedent
  enuretic
  force of
  interpretation of
  life
  life change
  negative life
  past
  potential positive
  psychosocial
  recent life (RLE)
  reexperienced traumatic
  sense of reliving an
  traumatic
event-related desynchronization (ERD)
event-related potential
every (q)
every day (q.d.)
everyday activities, diminished pleasure in
everyday life
everyday memory questionnaire
every night (q.h.s.)
every other day (q.o.d.)
every two hours (q.2h.)

evidence
  amnesia
  blocking
  empirical
  incontrovertible
  interruption of
evidence-based process
evidence of intrusion of idiosyncratic
  material
evidence of intrusion of private
  material
eviration
evoked potential
  auditory (AEP)
  brain stem
  brain stem auditory (BAEP)
  visual (VEP)
evoked response (ER)
  brain stem auditory (BAER)
  visual (VER)
evoked response audiometry (ERA)
  average (AERA)
  brain stem (BSER)
  cardiac (CERA)
evoked response test, visual
evoked somatosensory response
evolutionary intervention
EWI (Experiential World Inventory)
exacerbated symptoms
exacerbation
  pain
  psychotic
  schizophrenic
ex-addict
exaggerated achievements
exaggerated belief
exaggerated communication in schizophrenia
exaggerated defect
exaggerated expression of emotions
exaggerated feeling of well being

exaggerated inferential thinking in
  schizophrenia
exaggerated language in schizophrenia
exaggerated negative qualities
exaggerated perception in schizophrenia
exaggerated startle response
exaggerated talent
exaggeration of:
  deep tendon reflexes
  inferential behavioral monitoring
  inferential perception
  inferential thinking
  language and communication
exaltation
exam or examination (see *test*),
examination phobia
Examining for Aphasia Test
exceptional child
excessive emotionality, pattern of
excessively impressionistic speech
excessively upset
excessive need
excitability
excitable behavior
excitant
excitation
  catatonic
  psychogenic
  reactive
  wave of
excitative psychosis
excitatory state, central
excited catatonic schizophrenia
excited schizoaffective schizophrenia
excitement
  adequate sexual
  caffeine-induced
  catatonic
  disturbance in
  inhibited sexual

excitement *(cont.)*
  manic
  psychomotor
  reactive
  sexual
excitement phase
excitement phase of sexual response
  cycle
excitement-seeking tendency
excitotoxicity, glutamate
exclamatory sentence
excoriation
excrescence
executive aphasia
executive aspect
executive control
executive ego function
executive functioning, disturbance in
executive language
Executive Profile Survey
executive speech
exercise (see *test*)
exertional headache, benign
exhalation muscles
exhaustion
  combat
  mental
  nervous
exhaustion delirium
exhaustion psychosis
exhaustion senile dementia
exhaustion syndrome
exhibitionism, shock
exhibitionistic behavior
exhilarant
ex-husband
existentialism
existential psychiatry
existential psychology
existential psychotherapy
existential therapy

Exner Scoring System (Rorschach
  test)
exocentric construction of phrases
exogenous depression
exogenous psychosis
exophoric pronoun
exorcism
expansion, perceptual
expansive delusion
expansiveness
expectable response
expectation, internal world of
expectation neurosis
expectation of death
expected death
expected speech sounds, developmentally
expected utility (EU)
expedient
expenditure, resting energy
experience (pl. experiences) (see also
  test)
  affective
  atypical delusional
  brief delusional
  clinical
  closed to
  collective
  common
  corrective emotional
  cultural
  culturally sanctioned
  depersonalization
  depressive
  dissociative episode
  disturbing
  dream
  external world
  fantasied sexual
  inner
  lack of

experience *(cont.)*
  life
  loss
  mystical
  narcolepsy
  openness to
  out-of-body (OBE)
  physical
  pleasure
  psychic
  repeated painful
  self
  sexual
  social phobia
  spiritual possession
  stimulating
  stressful life
  subjective
  success
  terrifying
  traumatic
  troubling
experience and behavior, deviant
  pattern of inner
experienced feeling state, subjectively
experience pleasure, inability to
experience sleep paralysis
experiential therapy
Experiential World Inventory (EWI)
experimental audiology
experimental design
experimental games
experimental group
experimental neurosis
experimental psychology
experimentation in childhood,
  developmental
experimenter bias
expert witness
expiation
expiration reserve volume (ERV)
expiratory volume, forced (FEV)

explanations for illness, cultural
expletive
explicit memory
explicit process
exploitation, interpersonal
exploitative
exploratory behavior
exploratory drive
exploratory therapy
"explorers club" (re: lysergic acid
  diethylamide users)
explosive behavior, intermittent
explosive personality disorder
explosive rage
explosive speech
explosivity, emotional
exposed, fear of being
exposure
  combat stress
  stress
exposure and response prevention
exposure-based therapy
exposure meter, noise
exposure to an object
exposure to toxins
expressed emotion (EE)
expressed feelings, freely
expressed motivation
expression
  affective
  discordant facial
  disorder of written
  emotional
  exaggerated
  facial
  nonverbal
  parenthetical
  passivity in anger
  sexual
  shallow
  staring facial
  verbal

expression of customs, acculturation problems with
expression of feelings
expressive aphasia
expressive delusion
expressive language development disorder
expressive language quotient
Expressive One-Word Picture Vocabulary Test, Revised (EOWPVT-R)
Expressive One-Word Picture Vocabulary Test, Upper Extension
expressive-receptive aphasia
expressive therapy, focused
expressive writing development disorder
extended family
extended family therapy (EFT)
extended jargon paraphasia
extended length of utterance (ELU)
Extended Merrill-Palmer Scale, The
Extended Personal Attributes Questionnaire (EPAQ)
extension semantics
extensor
extensor plantar response
exteriorized stuttering
external acoustic meatus
external auditory meatus
external awards, potential
external control
external ear
external entities, controlling
external force
external incentive motivation
external intercostal muscles
externalization
external memory aids
external reality, abnormal perceptions of
external rewards, potential

external scale, internal versus (I-E Scale)
external spirits, controlling
external stimulation
external stimulus
external stressor
external structure
external validity
external world
   experience of the
   perception of the
external world of reality
externalize blame, tendency to
exteroceptor
extinction, sensory
extracerebral aneurysm
extracranial aneurysm
extract, crude marijuana (CME)
extradural hemorrhage
extramarital affair
extramarital behavior
extramarital relations
extraneous movement
extraneous noise
extrapolation
extrapsychic conflict
extrapyramidal cerebral palsy (CP)
extrapyramidal effect
extrapyramidal medication side effect
extrapyramidal side effects
extrapyramidal syndrome (EPS)
extrapyramidal symptoms, prevention of
extrapyramidal system (EPS)
extrapyramidal tract
extrasensory perception (ESP)
extrasensory thought transference
extratensive coping style
extratensive personality style
extraversion
extravert

extreme hearing loss
extreme negativism
extreme stressor
extrinsic epilepsy
extrinsic muscles
    infrahyoid
    laryngeal
    suprahyoid
    tongue
extrovert
extroverted personality
ex-wife
eye (pl. eyes)
    defected
    fluttering of the
    lusterless
    narrow-set
    staring
    wide-set
eye accessing cues
eyeblink
eye contact
eye disorder, psychogenic

eyeglass hearing aid
eye gouging
eyelid conditioning
eyelids, drooping
eye memory
eye movement
    non-rapid (NREM)
    rapid (REM)
    reflex
    rhythmic slow
    saccadic
eye movement abnormality
eye movement densensitization and
    reprocessing (EMDR)
"eye opener" (amphetamine; crack)
EYES (Early Years Easy Screen)
eye scanning
eye teeth
Eysenck Personality Inventory (EPI)
Eysenck Personality Questionnaire
    (EPQ)
Eysenck Psychoticism Scale

F, f

F (figural)
F (finger dexterity)
F/A (Families Anonymous)
Fa (father)
fabulation
fabulized combination
fabulized response
facade of competence and confidence
face
 anthropomorphic
 staring
FACES III (Family Adaptability and
 Cohesion Evaluation Scales III)
face validity
Facial Action Coding System (FACS)
facial agnosia
facial asymmetry
facial expression
 discordant
 staring
facial expression automatism
facial grimace
facial nerve (cranial nerve VII)
facial paralysis
facial paresis, center of
facial reflex
facial responsiveness

facial sensation
facial tic
facial tremor
facial twitch; twitching
facies (pl. facies)
 mask (of parkinsonism)
 masklike
 myasthenic
 myopathic
 myotonic
 parkinsonian
facilitation, social
facioversion of teeth
FACS (Facial Action Coding System)
FACT (Flanagan Aptitude
 Classification Test)
factitious disorder
factitious disorder by proxy
factitious illness, chronic
factitious interface disorder
factitive case (parts of speech)
factor (pl. factors)
 arousability
 biological
 causal
 cleverness (C factor, C-factor)
 cognitive/attitudinal

207

factor *(cont.)*
  combined
  Costa/McCrae
  cultural
  disorganized
  emotional/activation
  etiological
  familial
  feedback inhibition (FIF)
  general (G factor)
  human growth (HGF)
  known organic
  method
  motivational/behavioral
  negative
  nerve growth (NGF)
  noise
  organic
  perpetuating
  physiological
  precipitating
  predisposing
  psychic
  psychological
  psychosocial
  psychotic
  risk
  schizophrenic
  significant risk
  suicide-risk
  trait
  unspecified psychological
  verbal comprehension (V factor)
factorial validity
factors for suicide, risk
"factory" (re: drug-making place)
faculty
  language
  mental
FAE (fetal alcohol effect)
Fagerstrom Tolerance Questionnaire
failed suicide attempt

failing grades, pattern of
failure
  communication
  fear of (FF)
"fairy dust" (heroin; phencyclidine)
faith conversion problem
"fake-bad"
"fake-good"
"fake STP" (phencyclidine)
faking feelings
"fall" (arrested)
"Fallbrook redhair" (cannabis)
false accusations
false belief
false confessions
false fluency
false folds, hyperkinesia of the
false hermaphroditism
false hope
false memories
false memory syndrome
false-negative response
false paracusis
false perceptions of movement
false-positive response
false role disorder
false threshold
false vocal folds
falsetto voice
falsifiable hypothesis
falsification, retrospective
fam. (family)
fam. hist. (family history)
familial aggregation
familial deficiency
familial dementia
familial disorder
familial factors
familial idiocy, amaurotic
familial migraine headache
familial pattern
familial seizure, benign neonatal

familial tendency
familial transmission of schizophrenia
familial tremor
familiarity
Families Anonymous (F/A)
family (fam.) (pl. families)
    blended
    cohesive
    dysfunctional
    empowered
    extended
    nuclear
    runs in
Family Adaptability and Cohesion
    Evaluation Scales III (FACES III)
family and systemic psychotherapy
Family Apperception Test (FAT)
Family Aptitudes Questionnaire
    (FAQ)
Family Attitudes Test (FAT)
family caregiver
family conflict
family connectedness
family counselor
family disruption
Family Drawing Depression Scale
    (FDDS)
family dynamics
Family Environment Scale, Second
    Edition (FES)
family functioning, disruptive of
family history (fam. hist., FH)
family idiocy
family instability
Family Inventory of Life Events and
    Changes (FILE)
family life
family medicine
family members
family neglect
family neurosis
family of health problems

family perception
family physician
family practice
family pursuits
family relations
Family Relationship Inventory
Family Relations Test (FRT),
    Children's Version
family routines
Family Satisfaction Scale
family separation
family situations
family stress
family support system
family/system research orientation
family therapy (FT), extended (EFT)
family treatments
family turbulence
family unit
family violence
"famous dimes" (crack)
Famous Sayings Test
fanatic personality
FANPT (Freeman Anxiety Neurosis
    and Psychosomatic Test)
"Fantasia" (dimethyltryptamine)
fantasized sexual experience
fantasy
    autistic
    bizarre
    grandiosity in
    intense sexual
    internal world of
    masochistic sexual
    nonpathological sexual
    paraphiliac
    pathological sexual
    romantic
    sexual
    sexually arousing
    voyeuristic sexually arousing
fantasy figure, female

fantasy life, impoverished
fantasy play
fantasy processes
FAQ (Family Aptitudes Question-
　naire)
farad (electrical capacity unit)
FAS Word Fluency Test
fasciculations of tongue
fasciculus (pl. fasciculi), arcuate (AF)
fashion, singsong
fast activity
fast, anorexic
FAST (Flowers Auditory Screening
　Test)
FAST (Frenchay Aphasia Screening
　Test)
fastidium
fasting, starvation
fast speech
FAT (Family Apperception Test)
FAT (Family Attitudes Test)
fatalistic
"fat bags" (crack)
father (Fa)
　primal
　surrogate
father complex
father fixation
fatigability (or fatigue)
　auditory
　battle
　chronic
　combat
　daytime
　ease of
　easy
　excessive
　marked
　mental
　nervous
　pseudocombat
　psychogenic

fatigability (continued)
　stimulation
　sustained
　symptoms of
　vocal
　voice
fatigue as cause of seizure
fatigued, feeling
fatigue neurosis
fatigue strength
fatigue stress
fatigue syndrome, chronic
fatness stimuli
FATSA (Flowers Auditory Test of
　Selective Attention)
"fatty" (cannabis cigarette)
fauces, isthmus of
fausse reconnaissance
faulty judgment
faute de mieux
favors, sexual
FB (feedback)
FCP (Functional Communication
　Profile)
FDA (Food and Drug Administration)
FDCT (Franck Drawing Completion
　Test)
FDDQ (Freedom from Distractibility
　Deviation Quotient)
FDDS (Family Drawing Depression
　Scale)
FDTVP (Frostig Developmental Test
　of Visual Perception)
fear, irrational (pl. fears) (also fear of)
　(see also *phobia*)
　abandonment
　acute
　agoraphobic
　air (aerophobia; pneumatophobia)
　alcoholism (alcoholophobia)
　aloneness (eremophobia; mono-
　　phobia)

fear, irrational *(continued)*
  angina pectoris attack (angino-
    phobia)
  animal skins (doraphobia)
  animals (zoophobia)
  anything new (neophobia)
  bacilli (bacillophobia)
  bacteria (bacteriophobia)
  barrenness (cenophobia;
    kenophobia)
  beards (pogonophobia)
  bearing a deformed child (terato-
    phobia)
  becoming deformed (dysmorpho-
    phobia)
  bees (apiphobia; melissophobia)
  being afraid (phobophobia)
  being alone (autophobia; mono-
    phobia; eremophobia)
  being beaten (rhabdophobia)
  being bound (merinthophobia)
  being buried alive (taphophobia;
    taphephobia)
  being dirty (automysophobia)
  being infected with syphilis
    (syphilophobia)
  being locked in (clithrophobia;
    claustrophobia)
  being on tall buildings (batophobia)
  being poisoned (iophobia)
  being scratched (amychophobia)
  being stared at (scopophobia)
  being touched (aphephobia; haphe-
    phobia; haphophobia; hapto-
    phobia)
  being weak (asthenophobia)
  birds (ornithophobia)
  black people (negrophobia)
  blood/bleeding (hemophobia;
    hematophobia)
  blushing (ereuthrophobia; erythro-
    phobia)

fear, irrational *(cont.)*
  body odors (osphresiophobia;
    bromidrosiphobia)
  books (bibliophobia)
  brain disease (meningitophobia)
  breathing (pneumatophobia)
  bulls (taurophobia)
  cancer (cancerophobia; carcino-
    phobia)
  cats (ailurophobia; elurophobia;
    felinophobia; gatophobia)
  celestial space (astrophobia)
  change (kainophobia)
  childbirth (tocophobia)
  children (pediophobia; pedophobia)
  choking (pnigophobia)
  choking/gagging on liquids
    (hydrophobia)
  cholera (cholerophobia)
  churches (ecclesiophobia)
  climate (meteorophobia)
  climbing (climacophobia)
  closed spaces (claustrophobia)
  clouds (nephophobia)
  cold temperatures (psychrophobia;
    frigophobia; cheimaphobia)
  color red (erythrophobia)
  colors (chromatophobia; chromo-
    phobia)
  comets (cometophobia)
  confinement (claustrophobia)
  confronting one's phobia (counter-
    phobia)
  contamination (molysmophobia;
    mysophobia)
  contamination by dirt (misophobia)
  corpses (necrophobia)
  criticism
  crossing a bridge (gephyrophobia)
  crossing streets (dromophobia)
  crowds (ochlophobia; demophobia)
  dampness (hygrophobia)

fear, irrational *(cont.)*
  danger
  darkness (nyctophobia; scotophobia;
    achluophobia)
  dawn (eosophobia; auroraphobia)
  daylight (phengophobia)
  dead, the (hadephobia)
  death (thanatophobia; necrophobia)
  deep spaces (bathophobia)
  defeat (kakorrhaphiophobia)
  defecation (rhypophobia)
  deformity (dysmorphophobia)
  demons and devils (demonophobia)
  demons and goblins (bogyphobia)
  deserted places (eremophobia)
  deserts (xerophobia)
  devil, the (satanophobia)
  diabetes (diabetophobia)
  dirt (mysophobia; rhypophobia;
    rupophobia)
  disapproval
  disease (nosophobia; pathophobia)
  disease, specific (monopatho-
    phobia)
  disorder (ataxiophobia; ataxophobia)
  dogs (cynophobia)
  dolls (pediophobia; pedophobia)
  drafts (aerophobia; anemophobia)
  dreams (oneirophobia)
  drinking, act of (hydrophobia;
    potophobia)
  drugs (pharmacophobia)
  dry places (xerophobia)
  dust (amathophobia; koniophobia)
  eating (phagophobia; sitiophobia;
    sitophobia)
  electricity (electrophobia)
  embarrassment
  empty room or space; emptiness
    (kenophobia; cenophobia)
  enclosed space (claustrophobia)

fear, irrational *(cont.)*
  England and things English
    (Anglophobia)
  environment (ecophobia)
  error (hamartophobia)
  everything (pantophobia)
  excessive
  excrement (coprophobia; scato-
    phobia)
  exposure
  eyes (ommatophobia)
  failure (kakorrhaphiophobia)
  family (oikophobia)
  fatigue (ponophobia; kopophobia)
  fearing (phobophobia)
  feathers (pteronophobia)
  feces (coprophobia; rhypophobia)
  female genitalia (eurotophobia)
  fever (pyrexiophobia; febriphobia)
  fibers (fibriphobia)
  filth (rhypophobia; mysophobia;
    rupophobia)
  filth, personal (automysophobia)
  fire (pyrophobia)
  fish (ichthyophobia)
  flavors (geumophobia)
  flesh (carnophobia)
  flood (antlophobia)
  flowers (anthophobia)
  flying (aerophobia)
  focus of
  fog (homichlophobia)
  food (cibophobia; sitiophobia;
    sitophobia)
  foreigners (xenophobia), English
    speaking/American (gringophobia)
  forests (hylephobia; hylophobia)
  France and things French (gallo-
    phobia)
  frogs and toads (batrachophobia)
  frost (cryophobia)

fear, irrational *(cont.)*
  functioning (ergasiophobia)
  fur (doraphobia)
  gagging (hydrophobia)
  gaiety (cherophobia)
  general anxiety (panphobia; panto-
    phobia; panophobia)
  Germany and things German
    (germanophobia)
  germs (bacillophobia; bacterio-
    phobia; microphobia; spermo-
    phobia)
  ghosts (phasmophobia)
  girls, young (parthenophobia)
  glare of light (photaugiaphobia)
  glass (crystallophobia; hyalophobia)
  God (theophobia)
  gold (aurophobia)
  graves (taphophobia; taphephobia)
  gravity (barophobia)
  hair (chaetophobia)
  hair (loose) on clothing (tricho-
    phobia)
  hair abnormalities and disease
    (trichopathophobia)
  harm
  heart disease (cardiophobia)
  heat (thermophobia)
  heights (acrophobia; altophobia;
    hypsophobia)
  hell (hadephobia; stygiophobia)
  helplessness
  hereditary disease (patriophobia)
  high objects (batophobia)
  home (domatophobia; oikophobia)
  home, returning to (nostophobia)
  homosexuality (homophobia)
  horses (hippophobia)
  human companionship (anthropo-
    phobia; phobanthropy)
  humiliation
  ice (cryophobia)

fear, irrational *(cont.)*
  ideas (ideophobia)
  illness (nosophobia)
  imperfection (atelophobia)
  incapacitating
  infection (molysmophobia; myso-
    phobia)
  injections (trypanophobia)
  injury (traumatophobia)
  innovation (neophobia)
  insanity (lyssophobia; maniaphobia)
  insects (entomophobia)
  intense
  iron (siderophobia)
  irrational
  itching (acarophobia)
  jealousy (zelophobia)
  knives (aichmophobia)
  large objects (megalophobia)
  left side of the body, objects on
    (levophobia)
  leprosy (lepraphobia)
  lice (pediculophobia; phthirio-
    phobia)
  light (photophobia; phengophobia)
  locked in, being (claustrophobia;
    clithrophobia)
  loneliness
  looked at, being (scopophobia)
  loose hair on clothing, etc. (tricho-
    phobia)
  loss of approval
  loss of support
  loss through thievery (kleptophobia;
    cleptophobia)
  loud talking (phonophobia)
  machinery (mechanophobia)
  malignancy (cancerophobia;
    carcinophobia)
  many things (polyphobia)
  marked
  marriage (gamophobia)

fear, irrational *(cont.)*
  maturity
  meat (carnophobia)
  medicines (pharmacophobia)
  men, males (androphobia)
  meningitis (meningitophobia)
  metal objects (metallophobia)
  meteors (meteorophobia)
  mice (musophobia)
  microbes (microbiophobia)
  microorganisms (microbiophobia)
  mind, the (phronemophobia;
    psychophobia)
  minute objects (microphobia)
  mirror, seeing oneself in the
    (spectrophobia)
  missiles (ballistophobia)
  mite or tick infestation (acaro-
    phobia)
  moisture (hygrophobia)
  morbid cruelty (tyrannophobia)
  motion (kinesophobia)
  movements (kinesophobia)
  music (musicophobia)
  myths (mythophobia)
  nakedness (gymnophobia)
  names (nomatophobia; onomato-
    phobia)
  needles (belonephobia)
  neglect of duty (paralipophobia)
  newness (kainophobia; neophobia)
  night (nyctophobia; noctiphobia)
  noise (phonophobia; acoustico-
    phobia)
  nonspecific fear (panphobia; panto-
    phobia; panophobia)
  northern lights (auroraphobia)
  novelty (cainophobia; caintophobia;
    neophobia; kainophobia)
  nudity (nudophobia)

fear, irrational *(cont.)*
  objects
    large (megalophobia)
    pointed (aichmophobia)
    small (microphobia)
  odor, personal body (automyso-
    phobia, bromidrosiphobia,
    osphresiophobia)
  odor (olfactophobia; osmophobia)
  omission of duty (paralipophobia)
  open spaces (agoraphobia; ceno-
    phobia; kenophobia)
  overwork (ponophobia)
  pain (algophobia; odynophobia)
  paranoid
  parasites (parasitophobia)
  people (anthropophobia; demophobia)
  perception (symbolophobia)
  performance
  persistent
  personal ruin (atephobia)
  phantoms (spectrophobia)
  philosophers (philosophobia)
  phobias (phobophobia)
  phobias, mild (paraphobia)
  physical love (erotophobia)
  pins and needles (belonephobia)
  places (topophobia)
  pleasure (hedonophobia)
  pointed objects (aichmophobia)
  poison (toxiphobia; toxicophobia;
    toxophobia)
  poisoned, being (iophobia)
  politicians (politicophobia)
  poverty (peniaphobia)
  precipices (cremnophobia)
  pregnancy (maieusiophobia)
  pseudorabies (cynophobia)
  punishment (poinephobia)
  punishment by rod (rhabdophobia)

fear, irrational *(cont.)*
  rabies (lyssophobia; hydrophobo-
    phobia)
  radiation (radiophobia)
  railways (siderodromophobia)
  rain (ombrophobia)
  rain storms (ombrophobia)
  rapid motion (hormephobia)
  reasonable
  reckless impulse (atephobia)
  rectal disease (proctophobia; recto-
    phobia)
  rectal excreta (coprophobia)
  rectum (proctophobia; rectophobia)
  rejection
  religious objects (hierophobia)
  reptiles (herpetophobia; ophidio-
    phobia)
  responsibility (hypengyophobia)
  ridicule (katagelophobia)
  right side of the body, objects on
    (dextrophobia)
  rivers (potamophobia)
  robbers (harpaxophobia)
  rod as an instrument of punishment
    (rhabdophobia)
  rough skin (pellagraphobia)
  ruin, personal (atephobia)
  Russia or things Russian (Russo-
    phobia)
  rusty objects (iophobia)
  sacred objects (hierophobia; hagio-
    phobia)
  saints (hagiophobia)
  satan, the devil (satanophobia)
  scabies (scabiophobia)
  scratches, being scratched (amycho-
    phobia)
  scrutiny
  sea, the (thalassophobia)
  self (autophobia)
  self-care

fear, irrational *(cont.)*
  semen, loss of (spermatophobia)
  sensations of
  separation
  sermons (homilophobia)
  sexual feelings (erotophobia)
  sexual intercourse (coitophobia;
    cypridophobia; genophobia)
  sexual perversion (paraphobia)
  shadows (sciophobia)
  shaking (thixophobia)
  shame
  sharpness (acerophobia)
  sharp objects (belonephobia)
  shock (hormephobia)
  sin (hamartophobia)
  sinning (peccatiphobia)
  sitting (thaasophobia)
  sitting down (kathisophobia;
    cathisophobia)
  skin disease (dermatophobia;
    dermatosiophobia; dermatopatho-
    phobia)
  skin of animals (doraphobia)
  skin, rough (pellagraphobia)
  sleep (hypnophobia)
  slime (myxophobia)
  small objects (microphobia)
  small organisms (microbiophobia)
  small things (tapinophobia)
  smells (olfactophobia; osmophobia)
  smothering (pnigerophobia)
  snakes (ophidiophobia)
  snake venom (ophiophobia)
  snow (chionophobia)
  solitude (eremophobia; autophobia;
    monophobia)
  sounds (acousticophobia; phono-
    phobia)
  sourness (acerophobia)
  speaking (lalophobia; glossophobia;
    laliophobia)

fear, irrational *(cont.)*
  speed (tachophobia)
  spiders (arachnephobia)
  spirits (demonophobia)
  stairs (climacophobia)
  stand and/or walk, attempting to
    (stasibasiphobia)
  standing still (stasiphobia)
  stars (astrophobia; siderophobia)
  stings (cnidophobia)
  stories (mythophobia)
  strangers (xenophobia)
  streets (agyiophobia)
  string (linonophobia)
  stuttering (laliophobia)
  subjective
  sudden
  sunlight or sun's rays (heliophobia)
  surgery (tomophobia)
  swallowing (phagophobia)
  sweat (bromidrosiphobia)
  symbolism (symbolophobia)
  syphilis (syphilophobia)
  talking (lalophobia; laliophobia;
    glossophobia)
  tapeworms (taeniophobia)
  taste (geumaphobia)
  teeth (odontophobia)
  teleology (teleophobia)
  telephone (telephonophobia)
  termites (isopterophobia)
  theaters (theatrophobia)
  things teutonic (teutonophobia)
  thinking (phronemophobia)
  thirteen (triskaidekaphobia; trideca-
    phobia)
  thoughts (phronemophobia)
  thunder (tonitrophobia; bronto-
    phobia)
  thunder and lightning (astraphobia;
    astrapophobia; keraunophobia;
    ceraunophobia)

fear, irrational *(cont.)*
  thunder storms (brontophobia)
  time (chronophobia)
  touching or being touched (aphe-
    phobia; haphephobia; hapto-
    phobia)
  trains (siderodromophobia)
  trauma (traumatophobia)
  traveling (hodophobia)
  trees (dendrophobia)
  trembling (tremophobia)
  trichinosis (trichinophobia)
  tuberculosis (tuberculophobia)
  tyrants (tyrannophobia)
  uncleanliness (automysophobia)
  unclothed (nudophobia)
  unreasonable
  urine, passing (urophobia)
  using obscene language (scato-
    phobia)
  vaccination (vaccinophobia)
  vehicles (amaxophobia; hamaxo-
    phobia; ochophobia)
  venereal disease (cypridophobia;
    venereophobia)
  voice, one's own (phonophobia)
  voices (phonophobia)
  voids (kenophobia)
  vomiting (emetophobia)
  wasps (sphecidophobia)
  wasting sickness (tabophobia)
  water (aquaphobia; hydrophobia)
  weakness (asthenophobia)
  wealth (chrematophobia)
  weather (meteorophobia)
  whirlpools (dinophobia)
  wind (anemophobia)
  women (gynephobia; gynophobia)
  wood (hylephobia)
  words (logophobia)
  words, certain (onomatophobia)
  work (ergophobia)

fear, irrational *(cont.)*
   working (ergasiophobia)
   worms (helminthophobia; vermi-
     phobia)
   wounds (traumatophobia)
   writing (graphophobia)
feared disease
feared object
feared single performance situation
feared situation
feared words
fearfulness disorder of adolescence
fearfulness disorder of childhood
fear reaction
Fear Survey Schedule (FSS) for
   Children, Revised
feature (pl. features)
   age
   age-related
   age-specific
   agitative
   associated
   atypical
   catatonic
   characteristic
   clinical
   common shared
   cultural
   culture-related
   culture-specific
   delusional
   depressive
   descriptive
   diagnostic
   dominant
   essential
   gender-specific
   hysteroid
   insomnia
   junctural
   manic
   melancholic

feature *(cont.)*
   mixed
   mood-congruent psychotic
   mood-incongruent psychotic
   neurotic
   nondistinctive
   obsessive-compulsive
   paranoid
   personality
   phonetic
   prosodic
   psychotic
   schizoid
   semantic
   shared phenomenological
   similar shared
   sociodemographic
   specific age
   specific gender
feature analysis, distal distinctive
feature contrasts processes
febrile convulsion
febrile delirium
febrile psychosis
febriphobia
fecal continence
fecal incontinence
feculent
Federn, Paul (1871-1950)
feebleminded
feeblemindedness
feedback (FB)
   acoustic
   afferent
   auditory
   biofeedback
   constructive
   control
   corrective
   delayed auditory (DAF)
   efferent
   haptic

feedback *(cont.)*
  inverse
  kinesthetic
  negative
  positive
  proprioceptive
  tactile
  whistle
feedback control
feedback inhibition factor (FIF)
feedback noise
"feed bag" (re: cannabis container)
feeding and eating disorder
feeding and eating, infancy and early
  childhood disturbances in
feeding behavior
feeding disorder, psychogenic
feeling (pl. feelings)
  absence of
  affected by
  ambivalent
  anxiety
  associated
  "blah"
  blue
  cheirognostic
  choking
  chronic
  covert
  danger
  deep emptiness
  dejection
  depressive
  derealization
  despair
  detachment
  diminished emotion
  dirtiness
  disgust
  disturbing
  dread
  dysphoria

feeling *(cont.)*
  electric
  emotional emptiness
  erotic
  euphoric
  exaggerated well-being
  excessive anger
  faking
  freely expressed
  futility
  guilt
  helplessness
  "high"
  hopelessness
  inadequacy
  incisiveness
  ineffectiveness
  inferiority to others
  intimate
  irritable
  keyed up
  knowing
  lack of self-confidence
  lethargic
  loneliness
  low self-worth
  loving
  maladaptive
  negative
  not fitting in
  numb
  numbness
  on edge
  out of control
  permanently damaged
  personal unappeal
  pessimism
  positive
  premorbid inferiority (PIF)
  rageful
  rejection
  repressed

feeling *(cont.)*
  restlessness
  sad
  sadness
  self-disgust
  separation of ideas from
  shame
  social ineptness
  state, subjectively experienced
  subjective
  suddenly fearful
  suddenly sad
  superior to others
  tense
  tension
  threatened
  threshold
  transference
  unacceptable
  unreality
  verbalization of
  "wired"
  worthlessness
feign
feigned symptoms
feigning
felinophobia
fellatio
felony behavior
female dyspareunia
female fantasy figure
female homosexuality
female language
female object of sexual fantasy
female orgasmic disorder
  acquired-type
  generalized-type
  lifelong-type
  situational-type
female orgasm, inhibited

female sexual arousal disorder
  acquired-type
  generalized-type
  lifelong-type
  situational-type
femaleness
female-to-male transgender identity
feminine clothing
feminine mannerisms
feminine speech patterns
femininity complex
femininity, construction of
feminism
feminization
fence, low
"fender bender" (barbiturate)
fenestra (pl. fenestrae)
fenestra cochlea
fenestra ovalis
fenestra rotunda
fenestra vestibuli
fenestration
fentanyl (street names)
  Apache
  China girl
  China town
  dance fever
  friend
  goodfellas
  great bear
  he-man
  jackpot
  king ivory
  murder 8
  poison
  Tango & Cash
  T.N.T.
Féré effect
Ferenczi, Sandor (1873-1933)
Fer-Will Object Kit

FES (Family Environment Scale,
   Second Edition)
festinant quality in parkinsonian
   speech
festinating gait
fetal alcohol effect (FAE)
fetal alcohol syndrome
fetal movement, subjective sensation
   of
fetal position, curled into (posture)
fetation
fetishism, transvestic
fetishist
fetish object
FEV (forced expiratory volume)
FF (fear of failure)
FH (family history)
FI (fixed internal)
fiber, nerve
fiberscope
fibriphobia
fibrosis, cystic
fickle
fickleness
fiddling with fingers, nonfunctional
   and repetitive
fidgeting behavior
"fi-do-nie" (opium)
field
   electric
   free
   minimum audible (MAF)
   sound
   visual
field construction, visual
field cut, visual
field data
field dependence-independence
field room, free
"fields" (lysergic acid diethylamide)
field theory

field-trial projects
field-trial results
field trials
Field Work Performance Report
"fiend" (re: cannabis user)
FIF (feedback inhibition factor)
"fifteen cents" ($15 worth of drugs)
15-Item Memorization Test
"fifty-one" (crack)
5150 (danger to others/self)
fights, recurrent physical
figural (F)
figural aftereffect
figural memory
figurative blind spot (scotoma)
Figurative Language Interpretation
   Test (FLIT)
figurative meaning
figure (pl. figures)
   attachment
   authority
   childhood
   female fantasy
   major attachment
   noise
   simple
figure-ground distortion
figure-ground perception
figure of speech
   allusion
   apostrophe
   hyperbole
   idiom
   irony
   litotes
   metaphor
   metonymy
   overstatement
   personification
   simile
   synecdoche
   understatement

FILE (Family Inventory of Life
   Events and Changes)
filial imprinting
filled pauses in speech
filler words
filter
   active
   band-pass
   high-pass
   octave-band
   pass-band
   perceptual
   rational
   wave
filtered speech
filter frequency
   high (HFF)
   low (LFF)
FIM (Functional Independence
   Measure)
finajet/finaject (veterinary steroid)
final consonant
   deletion of
   devoicing of
final consonant position
financial crisis
financial remuneration
findings
   neurophysiological
   neuropsychological
fine motor movements
fine postural tremor
"fine stuff" (cannabis)
fine tactile sensation
fine tremor
"finger" (cannabis cigarette)
finger agnosia
finger anomia
finger dexterity (F)
finger-flicking
Finger Localization Test (FLT)
Finger Oscillation Test

fingerspelling
finger-tapping score
Fingertip Number Writing Perception
finite grammar
"fir" (cannabis)
"fire" (crack and methamphetamine)
"fire it up" (re: cannabis use)
"fire plan"
fire setter (FS)
fire setting
   deliberate
   intentional
   juvenile
firing an anchor
FIRO-B (Fundamental Interpersonal
   Relations Orientation—Behavior)
FIRO-F (Fundamental Interpersonal
   Relations Orientation—Feelings)
first deciduous molar teeth
first-degree biological relatives
first language
"first line" (morphine)
first position
first premolar teeth
first-rank symptoms (FRS) of delusions (schneiderian)
first sentences first words
first-time drinkers
first words, first sentences
Fisher-Logemann Test of Articulation
   Competence (FLTAC)
"fish scales" (crack)
FISS (Flint Infant Security Scale)
fissure
   longitudinal cerebral
   rectal
   rolandic (Rolando)
   sylvian (Sylvius)
fissured tongue
fist clenching
FIT (Flanagan Industrial Tests)
fit (see *seizure*)

fitful sleep
Fitzgerald Key
five (5) items after 5 minutes test, recall
five-axis system
"five cent bag" ($5 worth of drugs)
"five C note" (re: currency)
"five dollar bag" ($50 worth of drugs)
5-HIAA (serotonin metabolite 5-hydroxyindoleacetic acid)
Five P's: Parent Professional Pre-school Performance Profile
"fives" (amphetamine)
"fix" (re: drug injection)
fix and focus attention
fixation
    father
    mother
fixation hysteria
fixation in stuttering
fixation neurosis
fixed belief
fixed delusion
fixed delusional system
fixed-ended session
fixed idea
fixed internal (FI)
"fizzies" (methadone)
F-JAS (Fleishman Job Analysis Survey)
flaccid cerebral palsy (CP)
flaccidity
flaccid speech
"flag" (re: drug injection)
flagellation
flagrante delicto
"flake" or "flakes" (cocaine; phency-clidine)
flamboyant
"flame cooking" (re: cocaine use)
flame, manometric

"flamethrower" (cocaine- and heroin-laced cigarette)
Flanagan Aptitude Classification Test (FACT)
Flanagan Industrial Tests (FIT)
flap consonant
flap, pharyngeal
flapping movement
flapping tremor
flare, axon
flare up
"flash" (lysergic acid diethylamide)
flashbacks, acid
flashes of color
flat affect
flat audiogram configurations
"flat blues" (lysergic acid diethyl-amide)
"flat chunks" (crack cut with benzo-caine)
flat consonant
flattened affectivity
flattening, affective
"flea powder" (heroin)
fleeting image
Fleishman Job Analysis Survey (F-JAS)
flexibilitas cerea schizophrenia
flexibility
    behavioral
    lack of
    waxy
flexion reflex
flexor
flicker fusion
Fliess, Wilhelm (1858-1928)
flight into health
flight of ideas (FOI)
flight or fight response
Flint Infant Security Scale (FISS)
flirtatious behavior
flirting and coquetting

FLIT (Figurative Language Interpretation Test)
floating sensation, drug-induced
floccillation
flooding (implosion)
florid episode
Florida International Diagnostic–Prescriptive Vocational Competency Profile
Florida Kindergarten Screening Battery
"Florida snow" (cocaine; heroin)
floridly delusional
floridly paranoid
florimania
flounder
"flower" (cannabis)
"flower power" (morning glory seeds)
Flowers Auditory Screening Test (FAST)
Flowers Auditory Test of Selective Attention (FATSA)
Flowers-Costello Tests of Central Auditory Abilities
"flower tops" (cannabis)
flow of ideas
FLT (Finger Localization Test)
FLTAC (Fisher-Logemann Test of Articulation Competence)
fluctuating affect
fluctuating level of consciousness
fluctuating mood disturbance
fluency
  basal
  disturbance in
  disturbance in rate of
  false
  reduced
  verbal
  word
fluency disorder

fluency of speech
  decreased
  disturbance in the normal
fluency of thought
fluency shaping therapy
fluent aphasia, acquired
fluent aphasic speech
fluent paraphasic speech
fluent speech
fluid disturbance
fluid overload
fluid retention
flutter
  alar
  auditory
fluttering of the eyes
"fly" (slang term, muscarine)
flying, sensation of
FM (frequency modulation)
FMSTB (Frostig Movement Skills Test Battery)
FNA (Functional Needs Assessment)
focal ability, impaired
focal conflict theory
focal contralateral routing of signals (focal CROS)
focal CROS (focal contralateral routing of signals)
focal dysfunction
focal epilepsy
focal neurologic disturbance
focal neurologic impairment
focal neurologic signs
focal nonextrapyramidal neurologic signs
focal twitch/twitching
focus
  activity
  anxiety
  attention
  avoidance

focus *(cont.)*
  body parts
  characteristic paraphiliac
  clinical attention
  concern
  delusional system
  diagnosis
  epileptic
  fear
  delusion
  mirror
  multiple
  principal
  somatic
  stationary
  thought
  treatment
  tone
  unilateral
  vocal
  worry
focus groups
focused expressive therapy (treatment
  modality)
focusing on environmental stimuli,
  selective
FOI (flight of ideas)
foibles, common human
folate-deficiency
fold
  aryepiglottic
  bowed vocal
  deep nasolabial
  false vocal
  true vocal
  ventriculus
  vestibular
fold approximation, vocal
fold paralysis, vocal
folic acid-deficiency
folie à deux (shared delusional belief)
folie circulaire

folie du doute
folie du pourquoi
folie gémellaire
folie raisonnante
folk illness
follower role
following movement
follow-up (FU, F/U)
Follow-up Drinker Profile
Folstein Mini-Mental Status
  Examination
fondle
fondling
Food and Drug Administration (FDA)
food cravings, marked specific
food deprivation
food habits
food intake abnormality
"foo-foo dust" (cocaine)
"foo-foo stuff" (cocaine; heroin)
"foolish powder" (cocaine; heroin)
"footballs" (amphetamine)
footplate
foot-pound
foot reflex, tonic
foramen, incisive
forbidden impulse
force
  electromotive (EMF)
  events
  external
  nerve
  outside
forced cross-gender
forced expiratory volume (FEV)
forced sex
forced sleep
forced vibration
forced whisper
forcibly
foreboding
forebrain, limbic

foreconscious
fore-glide
foreign customs
foreign standards
foreign values
forensic determinations
forensic psychiatrist
forensic psychiatry
forensic psychology
foreplay
fore-pleasure
Forer Structured Sentence Completion
    Test
foreshortened future, sense of a
foreskin, reduced sensation of the
forgery
forgetfulness
forked tongue
form (see also *test*)
    free
    language
    linguistic
    thought
formal contract
formal method
formal operations period
formal thought disorder
formal universals
formant frequency, singer's
formation
    brain stem reticular
    compromise
    concept
    consonant
    fricative consonant
    new identity
    omen
    personality
    reaction
    split fricative consonant
    symptom
    trill consonant

formed visual hallucination
former identity
form perception
form recognition, oral
formulate a plan
formulation
    cultural
    language
    psychodynamic
form word
fornication
fortification scotoma
fortis consonant
48-Item Counseling Evaluation Test
    (ICET)
"45-minute psychosis" (dimethyltrypt-
    amine)
forward coarticulation
forward digital span recall test
forward masking
"forwards" (amphetamine)
forward visual masking
fossa (pl. fossae)
foster care
Foster Mazes
Four Picture Test
four-point restraints
four-pointed, to be (restrained)
four times a day (q.i.d.; 4/d)
Fourier analysis
Fourier's law
foveal vision
FPI (Freiburger Personality Inventory)
FPR (Functional Performance Record)
fragile X syndrome
fragment
fragmentary delusions in schizo-
    phrenia
fragmentary dream image
fragmentary hallucinations in schizo-
    phrenia
fragmented nighttime sleep

"fraho/frajo" (cannabis)
frame, analytic
franca, lingua
Franceschetti's syndrome
Franck Drawing Completion Test
   (FDCT)
Francomania
Francophobia
frank delirium
frantic
fraternal twins
fraud
FRC (functional residual capacity)
free access to processes
free association
"freebase" (crack; re: cocaine use)
"freebase rocks" (crack/cocaine)
freebasing
Freedom from Distractibility Deviation Quotient (FDDQ)
free field
free field room
free-floating anxiety
free form
freely expressed feelings
Freeman Anxiety Neurosis and
   Psychosomatic Test (FANPT)
free mandibular movement
free morpheme
free radicals
free recall bias
free variation
free vibration
"freeze" (cocaine; to renege on a
   drug deal)
freezing of movement
freezing phenomenon
Freiburger Personality Inventory (FPI)
Frenchay Activities Index
Frenchay Aphasia Screening Test
   (FAST)
Frenchay Dysarthria Assessment

"French blue" (amphetamine)
"French fries" (crack)
frenetic
frenetically
freneticism
frenulum (pl. frenula)
frenum (pl. frena or frenums), lingual
frenzied
frenzy
frequency
   alpha
   anxiety
   anxiety symptoms
   band
   decreased
   depressive symptoms
   dominant waking
   drug use
   episodes
   equal
   formant
   fundamental
   headache
   high (HF)
   high drug use
   high filter (HFF)
   increased
   infrasonic
   low (LF)
   low drug use
   low filter (LFF)
   mean peak
   modal
   natural
   range of
   reinforcement
   resonant
   respiratory
   seizure (SF)
   self-administration of drugs
   sexual encounters
   singer's formant

frequency *(cont.)*
   sleep terror episodes
   speech
   treatment
   ultrasonic
   violent acts
frequency-amplitude gradient
frequency combinations
frequency CROS, high (HICROS)
frequency distribution
frequency effect
frequency encountered association
frequency filtering speech discrimination
frequency hearing theory
frequency jitter
frequency masking
frequency modulation (FM)
frequency-modulation auditory trainer
frequency range, maximum
frequency response curve
frequent derailment
frequent drug dosing, need for
"fresh" (phencyclidine)
Freud
   Anna (1896-1982)
   Sigmund (1856-1939)
Freud cathartic method
freudian censor
freudian psychoanalysis
freudian psychotherapy
freudian slip
freudian theory
Freud theory
fricative
   gliding of
   groove
   split
   stopping of
fricative consonant formation
fricative sounds
frictionless consonant formation

Friedmann disease
"friend" (fentanyl)
friendship, platonic
"fries" (crack)
frightening stimulus
fright, stage
frigid
frigidity
frigophobia
"frios" (cannabis laced with phencyclidine)
"Frisco special" (cocaine, heroin, and
   lysergic acid diethylamide)
"Frisco speedball" (cocaine, heroin
   and lysergic acid diethylamide)
"friskie powder" (cocaine)
frog in the throat
frontal bone
frontal gyri
frontal headache
frontal lisp
frontal lobe dementia
frontal lobe dysfunction
frontal lobe syndrome
frontal lobotomy
frontal plane
frontal release signs, positive
frontal routing of signals, ipsilateral
   (IFROS)
frontal sulcus (pl. sulci)
   inferior
   middle
   superior
fronting, palatal
frontocortical aphasia
frontolateral laryngectomy
frontolenticular aphasia
frontotemporal brain atrophy
frontotemporal hypometabolism
front phoneme
front routing of signals (FROS)
front vowel

FROS (front routing of signals)
Frostig Developmental Test of Visual
  Perception (FDTVP)
Frostig Movement Skills Test Battery
  (FMSTB)
Frost Self-Description Questionnaire
  (FSDQ)
frottage
frotteur
Frotteurism
FRS (first rank symptoms [schneider-
  ian])
FRT (Family Relations Test)
frustration tolerance
fry
  glottal
  vocal
"fry" (crack)
"fry daddy" (crack and cannabis;
  crack-laced cigarette)
FS (fire setter)
FS (Full Scale [I.Q.])
FSDQ (Frost Self-Description Ques-
  tionnaire)
FSI (Functional Status Index)
FSIQ (Full-Scale Intelligence
  Quotient)
FSQ (Functional Status Questionnaire)
FSS (Fear Survey Schedule)
FSST (Full-Scale Score Total)
FT (family therapy)
FTEQ (Functional Time Estimation
  Questionnaire)
FU or F/U (followup, follow up)
"fu" (cannabis)
"fuel" (cannabis mixed with insecti-
  cides; phencyclidine)
"fuete" (hypodermic needle)
fugue
  dissociative
  epileptic

fugue *(cont.)*
  hysterical
  psychogenic
Fuld Object-Memory Evaluation
fulfillment
full-blown delirium
Fullerton Language Test for Adolescents
full interepisode recovery
full of energy
full-on gain, HF (high-frequency) average
full panic attacks
Full-Range Picture Vocabulary Test
full remission, sustained
Full Scale Broad Cognitive Ability
Full-Scale Intelligence Quotient (FSIQ)
Full-Scale Score Total (FSST)
full-symptom criteria
full wakefulness, state of
"fuma D'Angola" (cannabis)
function (pl. functions)
  adequate sexual
  affective
  articulation-gain
  auditory
  brain
  brain stem
  central auditory
  cerebral cortical
  cognitive
  compromised
  cortical
  day-to-day
  deteriorating
  deterioration of language
  differential
  diffuse
  discrepant intellectual
  executive
  executive ego

function *(cont.)*
  generalized
  hepatic
  higher level
  higher level cognitive
  impaired
  impaired immune
  inability to
  intellectual
  interpersonal
  intrapsychical
  language
  marginal
  motor
  neuroendocrine
  occupational
  performance-intensity
  personal
  premorbid intellectual
  primary
  psychosocial
  referential
  reproductive
  role
  semi-autonomous systems concept
    of brain
  sensory
  social
  speech-motor
  spiritual
  unable to
  ventricular
  vestibular
functionability inventory, social stress
  and (SSFI)
functional age
Functional Ambulation Categories
functional aphasia
functional aphonia
functional articulation disorder
functional assessment
Functional Assessment Inventory

functional brain imaging
functional capacity
functional cardiac disorder
functional deafness
functional disability
functional dyspareunia
functional gain testing
functional headache
functional impairment
Functional Independence Measure
  (FIM)
Functional Limitation Profile
functional limitations (emotional
  problems)
functional loss
functionally impaired
functional movement
Functional Needs Assessment (FNA)
functional neurosis
Functional Performance Record (FPR)
Functional Pragmatic Procedure
  (Evaluating Communicative
  Competence)
functional psychosis
functional residual capacity (FRC)
functional shift
Functional Status Questionnaire (FSQ)
functional superego structure
Functional Time Estimation Questionnaire (FTEQ)
functional vaginismus
functional variation, physiological
functioning
  academic
  adaptive
  anxiety-induced impaired social
  body
  borderline intellectual
  cognitive
  competent relational
  daytime
  defensive

functioning *(cont.)*
   deterioration in
   discrepant intellectual
   disrupted relational
   disruptive of family
   disturbance in executive
   dysfunctional relational
   educational
   general intellectual
   hierarchical
   impairment of
   independent
   interepisode
   interpersonal
   level of
   level of intellectual
   level of occupational
   level of social
   long-term
   mental
   normal neurological
   occupational
   premorbid
   premorbid level of
   psychosocial
   receptor
   social
   social-emotional
   vocational
   voluntary motor
   voluntary sensory

functioning as a family
functioning in society
function words
fundamental approach
fundamental frequency
Fundamental Interpersonal Relations
   Orientation—Behavior (FIRO-B)
Fundamental Interpersonal Relations
   Orientation—Feelings (FIRO-F)
fund of information
fund of information test
fund of knowledge
fusion
   binaural
   flicker
futility, feelings of
futural outlook
future-oriented
future pace
future perfect progressive tense
future perfect tense
future progressive tense, simple
future shock
future tense, simple
futuristic thinking
F-zero

G, g

G (general learning ability)
"G" ($1000 or 1 gram of drugs; also,
   an unfamiliar male)
GA (Getting Along)
GABA (gamma aminobutyric acid)
GAD (generalized anxiety disorder)
GAEL (Grammatical Analysis of
   Elicited Language)
GAF (Global Assessment of Functioning) Scale score
"gaffel" (fake cocaine)
"gaffus" (hypodermic needle)
"gag" (heroin)
"gage/gauge" (cannabis)
"gaggers" (methcathinone)
gag reflex
GAI (guided affective imagery)
gain
   acoustic
   desire for personal
   high-frequency (HF) average full-on
   peak acoustic
   potential secondary
   primary
   secondary
gain control, automatic

gait
   abnormal
   antalgic
   ataxic
   cerebral
   disturbances of
   festinating
   hysterical
   narrow-based
   Parkinsonian
   retropulsion of
   shuffling
   slowed
   staggering
   stuttering
   swaying
   uncoordinated
   unsteady
   waddling
   wide-based
gait abnormalities
gait analysis
gait disorder
gait problem
galactorrhea
galactosemia

galeophobia
Gallaudet University
Gallomania
Gallophobia
"galloping horse" (heroin)
galvanic skin resistance
galvanic skin response (GSR)
galvanic skin response audiometry (GSRA)
galvanic skin response (GSR) biofeedback
galvanometer
Galveston Orientation and Awareness Test (GOAT)
gambling
  compulsive
  pathological
  professional
  social
gambling behavior, maladaptive
gambling strategy
games, experimental
game theory
gametophobia
gamma-aminobutyric acid (GABA)
gamma-glutamyltransferase (GGT)
gamma hydroxybutyrate (GHB)
gamma hydroxybutyrate and amphetamines
gamomania
gamophobia
"gamot" (heroin)
"gange" (cannabis)
ganglion (pl. ganglia or ganglions), basal
"gangster" (cannabis)
"gangster pills" (barbiturate)
"ganja" (cannabis)
"gank" (fake crack)
Ganser syndrome

gap
  air-bone
  lexical
  memory
GAP (Gardner Analysis of Personality Survey)
GAP (Group for the Advancement of Psychiatry)
gaping
"garbage" (poor quality drugs)
"garbage head" (multiple-drug user)
"garbage rock" (crack)
Gardner Analysis of Personality Survey (GAP)
GARF (Global Assessment of Relational Functioning) Scale
gargoylism
garrote
garrulous affect
GAS (general adaptational syndrome)
GAS (Global Assessment Scale)
"gash" (cannabis)
"gasper" (cannabis cigarette)
"gasper stick" (cannabis cigarette)
gasping during sleep
gastric disorder, psychogenic
gastric ruptures
gastric ulcer, psychogenic
gastritis, nervous
gastrointestinal functional disorder, psychogenic
gastrointestinal symptom, somatization
GAT (Gerontological Apperception Test)
GAT (group adjustment therapy)
GATB (General Aptitude Test Battery)
Gates-MacGinitie Reading Test, Third Edition
Gates-McKillop-Horowitz Reading Diagnostic Tests

Gate Theory of Pain
gathering, injustice
"gato" (heroin)
gatophobia
Gaucher disease
"gauge butt" (cannabis)
Gault Decision
gaussian curve
gaussian distribution
gaussian noise
gay
gaze deficit
gaze impairment
gaze palsy
gaze, tense
"G.B." (barbiturate)
GBCE (Grassi Basic Cognitive
    Evaluation)
GBH (amino acid concoction) depen-
    dence
GC (gonococcus)
GCDAS (The Gesell Child
    Development Age Scale)
GCI (General Cognitive Index)
GCS (Glasgow Coma Scale)
GCT (General Clerical Test)
"gee" (opium)
"geek" (crack and cannabis; strange
    person)
"geeker" (re: crack user)
"geeze" (re: cocaine use)
"geezer" (re: drug injection)
"geezin a bit of dee gee" (re: drug
    injection)
GEFT (Group Embedded Figures
    Test)
gegenhalten
GEI (The Grief Experience Inventory)
gelastic epilepsy
gender
    boundaries and
    multiple personality and

gender-based attitudes
gender confusion
gender differences
gender dysphoria
gender features
gender identity confusion
gender identity, core
gender identity disorder (GID)
Gender Identity Disorder of Adoles-
    cence or Adulthood, Nontrans-
    sexual Type (GIDAANT)
gender identity disorder of childhood
gender identity problem
gender identity psychosexual develop-
    ment
gender role
    persistent discomfort with
    social stereotypical
gender-sensitive psychopharmacology
gender-specific features
gene
    aberrant
    autosomal dominant
general adaptational syndrome (GAS)
General Aptitude Test Battery
    (GATB)
General Clerical Test (GCT)
General Cognitive Index (GCI)
general factor (G factor)
general grammar
General Health Questionnaire (GHQ)
general hospital consultation/liaison
    services
general intellectual functioning
generalization
    response
    stimulus
general learning ability
general linguistics
General Management In-Basket
    (GMIB)
general medical condition (GMC)

general semantics
generational responsibility
generative empathy
generative intervention
generative semantics
generative transformational grammar
generator
    new behavior
    noise
generic terms
genetic counseling
genetic counselor
genetic hearing loss
genetic linkage study
genetic marker
genetic material
genetic psychology
genetics, behavioral
genetic vulnerability
genetous idiocy
genic
geniohyoid muscle
genital contact
genital pain
genital phase
genital sexual contact
genital stimulation
genitalia, ambiguous
genitive case
genitourinary disorder, psychogenic
genophobia
genotype, schizophrenic
geographic displacement
geographic mobility
geometric design
"George smack" (heroin)
gephyromania
gephyrophobia
gerascophobia
geriatric audiology
Geriatric Depression Scale
geriatric depressive disorder

geriatric neuropsychiatry
geriatric psychiatry
geriatrics
Germanomania
Germanophobia
gerontological
Gerontological Apperception Test
    (GAT)
gerontology
gerontophobia
Gerstmann syndrome
gerund (parts of speech)
GES (Gifted Evaluation Scale)
GES (Group Encounter Survey)
GES (Group Environment Scale)
Gesell Child Development Age Scale
    (GCDAS)
Gesell Developmental Schedules
Gesell Preschool Test
Gesell School Readiness Test
gestalten
gestaltism
gestalt psychology
gestalt psychotherapy
gestalt theory
gestalt therapy marathon (treatment
    modality)
gestational psychosis
gestural automatism
gesture (pl. gestures)
    bizarre
    body
    clumsy
    kinesic
    suicidal
    suicide
gesture language
gesture speech, social
gesturing (communication pattern)
"get a gage up" (re: cannabis use)
"get a gift" (re: drug acquisition)
"get down" (re: drug injection)

"get high" (re: cannabis use; drug influence; drug intoxication)
"get lifted" (re: drug influence)
"get off" (re: drug injection; drug influence)
"get the wind" (re: cannabis use)
"get through" (re: drug acquisition)
geumatophobia
geumophobia
G (general) factor
GGT (state markers of heavy drinking)
GGT level
"Ghana" (cannabis)
"GHB" (gamma hydroxybutyrate)
ghetto, psychiatric
"ghost" (lysergic acid diethylamide)
"ghost busting" (re: crack acquisition; cocaine use)
GHQ (General Health Questionnaire)
Gi (good impression)
gibberish
gibberish aphasia
"gick monster" (re: crack user)
GID (gender identity disorder)
    GID of adolescence
    GID of adulthood
    GID of childhood
GIDAANT (Gender Identity Disorder of Adolescence or Adulthood, Nontranssexual Type)
giddy
Gifted and Talented Screening Form
gifted child
Gifted Evaluation Scale (GES)
Gifted Program Evaluation Survey
"gift-of-the-sun" (cocaine)
"giggle smoke" (cannabis)
giggling, nervous
Gilles de la Tourette syndrome
Gillingham-Childs Phonics Proficiency Scales: Series I and II
Gilmore Oral Reading Test

"gimmick" (re: drug injection)
"gimmie" (crack and cannabis)
"gin" (cocaine)
"girl" (heroin)
"girlfriend" (cocaine)
"give wings" (re: drug injection)
glabella tap reflex
"glading" (re: inhalant use)
"glad stuff" (cocaine)
"glancines" (heroin)
Glasgow Assessment Schedule
Glasgow Coma Scale (GCS)
Glasgow Outcome Scale
"glass" (amphetamine; hypodermic needle)
"glass gun" (hypodermic needle)
glide consonant formation
glide
    palatal
    vocalic
gliding of fricatives
gliding of liquids
gliosis, astrocytic
"glo" (crack)
global amnesia, transient (TGA)
global amnesic
global aphasia
Global Assessment of Functioning (GAF) Scale (Axis V)
Global Assessment of Relational Functioning (GARF) Scale
Global Assessment Scale (GAS)
global cognitive deficit
global course and outcome
global dementia
global loss of language
Global Sexual Satisfaction Index (GSSI)
globus hystericus
gloss
glossal catch
glossal word

glossectomy
glossitis
glossograph
glossokinetic potential
glossolalia
glossopalatine arch
glossopalatine muscle
glossopharyngeal (cranial nerve IX)
glossopharyngeal press
glossophobia
glossoptosis
glossosteresis
glottal area consonant placement
glottal attack, hard
glottal catch
glottal chink
glottal click
glottal cycle
glottal fry
glottal pulse
glottal stop
glottal stroke
glottal tone
glottal vibration
glottic
glottidospasm
glottis
glucose metabolism in brain
glue ear
glue sniffer's rash
glue sniffing dependence
"gluey" (person who sniffs glue)
glutamate excitotoxicity
glutethimide and codeine cough syrup
    ("pancakes and syrup")
glutethimide group
glutethimide intoxication
glycerol test
GMA (gross motor activities)
GMC (general medical condition)
GMIB (General Management In-Basket)
gnathic

gnawing
GnRH (gonadotropin-releasing
    hormone)
goal (see also *test*)
    long-term
    short-term (STG)
goal-directed activity
goal-directed behavior
    diminution of
    initiation of
goal orientation, lack of
goal-oriented processes
goal-setting, vocational
goals skills, negotiating
go-around
GOAT (Galveston Orientation and
    Awareness Test)
God complex
"God's drug" (morphine)
"God's flesh" (psilocybin/psilocin)
"God's medicine" (opium)
"go-fast" (methcathinone)
"go into a sewer" (re: drug injection)
"gold" (cannabis; crack)
"gold dust" (cocaine)
"gold star" (cannabis)
Goldberg Index
"golden dragon" (lysergic acid
    diethylamide)
"golden girl" (heroin)
"golden leaf" (cannabis)
Goldman-Fristoe Test of Articulation
Goldman-Fristoe-Woodcock Auditory
    Skills Test Battery
Goldman-Fristoe-Woodcock Test of
    Auditory Discrimination
Goldstein-Scheerer Tests of Abstract
    and Concrete Thinking
"golf ball" (crack)
"go loco" (re: cannabis use)
Golombok Rust Inventory of Marital
    State (GRIMS)

"golpe" (heroin)
"goma" (black tar heroin; opium)
gonad
gonadotropin-releasing hormone
(GnRH)
"gondola" (opium)
"gong" (cannabis; opium)
gonococcal (GC)
"goob" (methcathinone)
"good" (phencyclidine)
"good and plenty" (heroin)
"good butt" (cannabis cigarette)
Goodenough "Draw-A-Man" Test
Goodenough-Harris Drawings Test
"goodfellas" (fentanyl)
"good giggles" (cannabis)
"good go" (re: drug dealing)
"good H" (heroin)
good impression (Gi)
"good lick" (quality drugs)
Goodman Lock Box
good object
good relationship
good sleep efficiency
"goofballs" (barbiturate)
"goof butt" (cannabis cigarette)
"goofers" (barbiturate)
"goofy's" (lysergic acid diethylamide)
"goon" (phencyclidine)
"goon dust" (phencyclidine)
"gopher" (re: drug dealing)
Gordon Personal Inventory (GPI)
Gordon Personal Profile Inventory
"Goric" (opium)
"gorilla biscuits" (phencyclidine)
"gorilla pills" (barbiturate)
"gorilla tab" (phencyclidine)
GORT-3 (Gray Oral Reading Tests,
Third Edition)
"got it going on" (re: drug dealing)
gouging, eye
gown restrictions

GPI (Gordon Personal Inventory)
Graded Naming Test
Graded Word Spelling Test
grade equivalent
grade rating
gradient
amplitude
frequency-amplitude
gradual topic shift
"graduate" (re: ending drug usage)
Graduate and Managerial Assessment
Graduate Records Examination (GRE)
Graduate Records Examination Aptitude Test (GREAT)
"gram" (hashish)
grammar
descriptive
finite
general
generative
generative transformational
particular
pedagogical
phrase structure
pivot
prescriptive
scientific
teaching
traditional
universal
grammar case
grammar language quotient
Grammatical Analysis of Elicited
Language (GAEL)
grammatical categories
grammatical component
grammatical equivalent
grammaticality
grammatical meaning
grammatical morpheme
grammatical structure
grammatic closure

grandeur, delusion of
grandiose concepts
grandiose content
grandiose delusion
   crystallized
   paranoid
grandiose themes
grandiose-type delusions
grandiose-type schizophrenia
grandiosity in fantasy
grandiosity, pattern of
grand mal (tonic-clonic) seizure
grand mal status
granulated opium
granulovascular degeneration
"grape parfait" (lysergic acid diethylamide)
grapheme
grapheme/phoneme association
graphic aphasia
graphic disorientation
graphic impairment
graphomania
graphomotor aphasia
graphophobia
Grashey aphasia
grasp reflex
"grass" (cannabis)
"grass brownies" (cannabis)
Grassi Basic Cognitive Evaluation
   (GBCE)
Grassi Block Substitution Test
"grata" (cannabis)
gratification
   delayed
   immediate
   manipulative behavior for material
   sexual
gratify
gratifying
grave delirium
"gravel" (crack)

grave phoneme
gravel voice
gravis
   myasthenia
   oneirodynia
gravity perception
"gravy" (heroin)
gray matter (of CNS)
   center of
   central (CGM)
   cortical
   dorsal
Gray Oral Reading Tests, Third
   Edition (GORT-3)
gray-out syndrome
GRE (Graduate Records Examination)
"grease" (re: currency)
GREAT (Graduate Records Examination Aptitude Test)
"great bear" (fentanyl)
"great tobacco" (opium)
Grecomania
"green" (cannabis; ketamine; phencyclidine)
"green double domes" (lysergic acid
   diethylamide)
"green dragon" (lysergic acid diethylamide)
"green frog" (barbiturate)
"green goddess" (cannabis)
"green gold" (cocaine)
"green goods" (re: currency)
"greenies" (amphetamine sulfate/
   amobarbital)
"green leaves" (phencyclidine)
"greens/green stuff" (re: currency)
"green single domes" (lysergic acid
   diethylamide)
"green tea" (phencyclidine)
"green wedge" (lysergic acid diethylamide)
"greeter" (cannabis)

gregarious
Gregorc Style Delineator
"Greta" (cannabis)
"grey shields" (lysergic acid diethyl-
    amide)
"gridiron abdomen"
Grid Test of Schizophrenic Thought
    Disorder (GTSTD)
grief
    delayed
    distorted
    impacted
    prolonged
    unresolved
grief counselor
Grief Experience Inventory (GEI)
grief reaction
    acute
    brief
    prolonged
"griefo" (cannabis)
grieving, inhibited
"griff" (cannabis)
"griffa" (cannabis)
"griffo" (cannabis)
grimace
    facial
    ticlike facial
grimacing, prominent
GRIMS (Golombok Rust Inventory of
    Marital State)
grinding, teeth
gringophobia
Grip-Strength Test
"grit" (crack)
"groceries" (crack)
"G-rock" (1 gram of rock cocaine)
grommet
groomed
    neatly
    poorly
grooming, deterioration in

Grooved Pegboard Test
grooved tongue
groove fricative consonant formation
gross impairment
grossly disorganized behavior
grossly pathogenic care
gross neurologic deficit
gross motor activities (GMA)
gross motor deficit
gross sensory deficit
gross sound
gross stress reaction
"ground control" (re: hallucinogenic
    drug use)
ground rules
group (pl. groups)
    age
    CNS disease
    control
    diverse
    encounter
    experimental
    focus
    glutethimide
    heterogeneous
    high-risk
    matched
    natural
    peer
    primary support
    self-help
    sensitivity
    sensitivity-training (T-group)
    socioeconomic
    substance
    task-oriented
    therapeutic
    training (T-group)
    work
Group Achievement Identification
    Measure
group activities

group adjustment therapy (GAT)
group analytic psychotherapy
group audiometer
group audiometry
group cohesion
group contract
group delinquency
group delinquent reaction
group diversity
group dynamics
Group Embedded Figures Test
(GEFT)
Group Encounter Scale (GES)
Group Environment Scale (GES)
Group for the Advancement of
Psychiatry (GAP)
Group Inventory for Finding Creative
Talent
group living
group "means"
group norms
group of disorders
group-oriented
group phase
group play
group pressure
group psychotherapy
activity-interview (A-IGP)
crisis-intervention
marathon
psychoanalytic
repressive-inspirational
structured interactional
Group Reading Test (GRT), Third
Edition
group rules
group session
group setting
group stage
group stress reaction
group structure
Group Styles Inventory (GSI)

Group Tests of Musical Abilities
group therapy (therapies)
activity (AGT)
adolescent
adult
child
play (PGT)
group-type conduct disorder
growth chart, pediatric
growth factor
human (HGF)
nerve (NGF)
growth laboratory, personal
GRT (Group Reading Test, Third
Edition)
grudge bearing
grunting
"G-shot" (cannabis)
GSI (Group Styles Inventory)
GSR (galvanic skin response) biofeedback
GSR on EEG
GSRA (galvanic skin response
audiometry)
GSSI (Global Sexual Satisfaction
Index)
GTC (generalized tonic-clonic seizure)
GTSTD (Grid Test of Schizophrenic
Thought Disorder)
guarded manner
guardedness, adolescent
guardianship
guidance
child
vocational
guided affective imagery (GAI)
Guilford-Zimmerman Aptitude Survey
(GZAS)
Guilford-Zimmerman Interest Inven-
tory (GZII)
Guilford-Zimmerman personality test
(GZ)

Guilford-Zimmerman Temperament
  Survey (GZTS)
guilt
  feelings of
  pervasive proneness to
guilt displacement
guiltiness
guiltless
guilt obsession
guilty, feeling
Guinon disease
"gum" (opium)
"guma" (opium)
"gun" (needle)
"gungun" (cannabis)
gustatory aura
gustatory hallucination
gustatory sensory modality
"gutter" (re: drug injection)
"gutter junkie" (re: drug acquisition)
guttural voice
gutturotetany
Guyon canal
gymnomania
gymnophobia

gynecomania
gynecomastia
gynephobia
gynophobia
gyrectomy
gyrus (pl. gyri)
  angular
  callosal
  frontal
  Heschl
  postcentral
  precentral
  supramarginal
  temporal
  transverse temporal
"gyve" (cannabis cigarette)
GZ (Guilford-Zimmerman personality
  test)
GZAS (Guilford-Zimmerman Aptitude
  Survey)
GZII (Guilford-Zimmerman Interest
  Inventory)
GZTS (Guilford-Zimmerman
  Temperament Survey)

H, h

"H" (heroin)
h (hour)
HA (high anxiety)
habeas corpus
habit
   alcohol
   benign
   drug
   food
   temporary
   tongue
habit pattern
habit spasm
habit tic, transient disorder of childhood
habitual pitch
habituation
habromania
"hache" (heroin)
hadephobia
HAE (hearing aid evaluation)
hagiophobia
Hahnemann Elementary School Behavior
   Rating Scale
Hahnemann High School Behavior
   Rating Scale
HAIC (Hearing Aid Industry
   Conference)

"hail" (crack)
hair cells
hair denuding
hair follicles, damaged
hair loss
   nonnormative
   noticeable
   self-induced
hair-pulling behavior
hairs, eating
"hairy" (heroin)
"half" (1/2 ounce)
"half-a-C" (re: currency)
"half a football field" (50 rocks of
   crack)
"half G" (re: currency)
half-hearted attempt at suicide
half-life, mean (of a pharmaceutical)
"half load" (15 bags [decks] of heroin)
"half moon" (mescaline)
"half piece" (1/2 ounce of heroin or
   cocaine)
half reliability coefficient, split
"half track" (crack)
halfway house
Hall Occupational Orientation Inventory
   (HOOI)

hallucination
  accusatory
  alcoholic
  auditory
  command
  complex
  depressive
  dreamlike
  drug-induced
  fragmentary
  gustatory
  haptic
  hypnagogic
  hypnopompic
  kinesthetic
  lilliputian
  mood-congruent
  mood-incongruent
  nocturnal
  olfactory
  prominent
  reflex
  self-destructive
  simple
  sleep-related
  somatic
  structured
  stump
  tactile
  threatening
  transient auditory
  transient tactile
  transient visual
  unpleasant
  vestibular
  visual
  vivid
hallucination imagery, hypnagogic
hallucinative
hallucinatory behavior
hallucinatory experience, transient
hallucinatory mania

hallucinatory paranoia
hallucinatory state
  drug-induced
  drug psychosis
hallucinatory-type psycho-organic
  syndrome
hallucinogen abuse
hallucinogen dependence
hallucinogenesis
hallucinogenic drug dependence
hallucinogenic intoxication
hallucinogen intoxication delirium
hallucinogen persisting perception
  disorder
hallucinogen-related disorder
hallucinogen toxic effects
hallucinosis
  alcoholic
  alcohol withdrawal
  drug-induced
  organic
  peduncular
hallucinotic
halo around object
halo effect
halogenated inhalational anesthetics
Halstead and Reitan Batteries
Halstead Aphasia Test (HAT)
Halstead Category Test
Halstead-Reitan Neurological Battery
  and Allied Procedures
Halstead-Reitan Neuropsychologic
  Test Battery (HRNTB) for Adults
Halstead Russell Neuropsychological
  Evaluation System (HRNES)
Halstead-Wepman Aphasia Screening
  Test
HALT (Heroin Antagonist and Learning Therapy)
halting speech
HAMA (Hamilton Anxiety) scale
hamartomania

hamartophobia
hamaxophobia
"hamburger helper" (crack)
Hamburg-Wechsler Intelligence Test
for Children (HAWIC)
HAMD (Hamilton Depression [Scale])
Hamilton Anxiety (HAMA) scale
Hamilton Anxiety Rating Scale
(HARS)
Hamilton Depression (HAMD) (scale)
Hamilton Depression Rating Scale
(HDRS)
hammer
"H & C" (heroin and cocaine)
H&P (history and physical)
hand
dominant
nondominant
hand dynamometer
handedness, cerebral dominance and
(theory in stuttering)
handicap
emotional (EH)
severe emotional (SEH)
handicapped
educationally mentally (EMH)
perceptually
handle of malleus
handling of stressors
Hand Test (HT)
"hand-to-hand" (re: drug dealing)
"hand-to-hand man" (re: drug dealing)
hand tremor, increased
handwashing ritual
hand waving, nonfunctional and
repetitive
hand wringing
hangover (alcohol)
hangover effects, alcoholic intoxication
hangover headache

hang-up (noun)
"hanhich" (cannabis)
hanky-panky
"hanyak" (smokable amphetamine)
hapax legomenon
haphophobia
haplology
"happy cigarette" (cannabis cigarette)
"happy dust" (cocaine)
"happy powder" (cocaine)
"happy trails" (cocaine)
haptic feedback
haptic hallucination
Haptic Intelligence Scale (HIS)
haptic perception
haptic system
haptophobia
HAQ (Health Assessment Questionnaire)
harass
harassment
sexual (SH)
verbal
"hard candy" (heroin)
hard contacts
hard glottal attack
Harding W87 Test
"hard line" (crack)
hard-of-hearing
hard palate
"hard rock" (crack)
"hard stuff" (heroin)
"hardware" (isobutyl nitrite)
hard-wire auditory trainer
harelip
Hare Psychopathy Checklist, Revised
(PCL-R)
harm avoidance
harmonic distortion
harmonic motion, simple (SHM)
harmony processes
harm, prevention of physical

harpaxophobia
harpy (noun)
Harrington-O'Shea Career Decision-
Making System, Revised (CDM-R)
Harris-Lingoes Subscales–MMPI
"Harry" (heroin)
HARS (Hamilton Anxiety Rating
Scale)
harsh discipline
harshness
Harvard Group Scale of Hypnotic
Susceptibility (HGSHS)
HAS (high-amplitude sucking technique)
"hash" (cannabis)
hashish (street names)
gram
quarter moon
soles
hashish abuse
"hash oil" (cannabis)
HAT (Halstead Aphasia Test)
HATH (Heterosexual Attitudes
Toward Homosexuality [scale])
"hats" (lysergic acid diethylamide)
haughty behavior
haut mal epilepsy
"have a dust" (cocaine)
Hawaiian marijuana
"Hawaiian sunshine" (lysergic acid
diethylamide)
Hawaii Early Learning Profile
(HELP)
HAWIC (Hamburg-Wechsler Intelligence Test for Children)
"hawk" (lysergic acid diethylamide)
Haws Screening Test for Functional
Articulation Disorders
"hay" (cannabis)
Hay Aptitude Test Battery
"hay butt" (cannabis)
"haze" (lysergic acid diethylamide)

"Hazel" (heroin)
HBI (Hutchins Behavior Inventory)
HC (Huntington chorea)
"H Caps" (heroin)
HCD (higher cerebral dysfunction)
"HCP" (phencyclidine)
HCR (hysterical conversion reaction)
·HDH (Hostility and Direction of
Hostility)
HDHQ (Hostility and Direction of
Hostility Questionnaire)
HDRS (Hamilton Depression Rating
Scale)
HE (hepatic encephalopathy)
headache
aching
acute confusional migraine
alarm-clock
aphasic migraine
band-like
basilar migraine
benign exertional
bifrontal
bilateral migraine
biocipital
blind
cataclysmic
chronic
circumstantial migraine
classical migraine
cluster migraine
cocaine-related
combination
common migraine
complicated migraine
confusional migraine
disabling
dull
essential
evening
exertional
familial migraine

headache *(cont.)*
  frequency of
  frontal
  functional
  generalized
  hangover
  hemiparesthetic migraine
  hemiplegic migraine
  histamine
  ipsilateral
  late-life migraine
  migraine
  Monday morning
  morning
  muscle contraction
  nitrite
  nonpulsating
  ocular migraine
  paroxysmal migraine
  postconcussion
  posttraumatic
  psychogenic
  pulsating
  recurrent migraine
  seasonal migraine
  severe
  sex
  suboccipital
  sudden-onset
  temporal
  tension migraine
  tension-type
  tension-vascular
  throbbing
  traumatic
  unilateral migraine
  vascular
  vascular-type
  vasomotor
  vestibular migraine
  weekend
headache pain

headache syndrome
head banging, nonfunctional and
  repetitive
"head drugs" (amphetamine)
head injury, closed (CHI)
head jerking
"headlights" (lysergic acid diethylamide)
head shadow effect
head trauma
  closed
  occult
head turn technique
healing rituals
health
  attitude to
  flight into
  mental
  neglect of basic
  physical
  public
Health Assessment Questionnaire
  (HAQ)
health behavior, maladaptive
health care, patient acceptance of
Health Care Financing Administration
  (HCFA, "hick-fah")
health care provider
Health Care Questionnaire
health center, community mental
  (CMHC)
health clinic, mental (MHC)
health concern
health maintenance organization
  (HMO)
Health Problems C hecklist
health professional, allied
health-related consequence
health resource, mental
health risks
health systems agency (HSA)
healthy identification

Healy Pictorial Completion Test
hearing
  central
  cross
  end-organ of
  loss of
  speech and (S&H)
  visual
hearing aid
  air-conduction
  behind-the-ear
  binaural
  body
  bone-conduction
  canal
  cochlear implant
  contralateral routing of signals
    (CROS)
  digital
  eyeglass
  in-the-ear
  monaural
  programmable
  vibrotactile
  Y-cord
hearing aid assessment
hearing aid evaluation (HAE)
Hearing Aid Industry Conference
  (HAIC)
hearing aid systems
hearing conservation
hearing deficiency
hearing disability
hearing disorder
hearing God's voice
hearing impairment
  mild
  moderate
  moderately severe
  profound
  severe

hearing level (LH)
  threshold
  zero
hearing loss
  age-related
  conductive
  extreme
  genetic
  hereditary
  job-related
  mild
  mixed
  moderate
  moderately severe
  noise-induced
  nongenetic
  perceptive
  perinatal
  profound
  psychogenic
  sensorineural
  severe
  work-related
hearing protection device (HPD)
  canal caps
  circumaural
  earmuffs
  earplugs
  insert
  semiaural
hearing science, speech and
hearing sensation
hearing tests, behavioral
hearing theory
  frequency
  place
  telephone
  traveling wave
  volley
hearing threshold level (HTL)
hearing voices

heart disorder, psychogenic
"heart-on" (inhalant)
"hearts" (amphetamine sulfate;
    dextroamphetamine sulfate)
"heaven and hell" (phencyclidine)
"heaven dust" (cocaine; heroin)
"heavenly blue" (lysergic acid diethyl-
    amide; morning glory seeds)
heaves, dry
heavy metal screen
heavy use, long-term
hebephrenia
hebephrenic schizophrenia
    acute
    disorganized
hebetic
hebetude
hedonia
hedonic capacity
hedonic drive
hedonic response
hedonic volition
hedonism
hedonistic activity
hedonomania
hedonophobia
"heeled" (to have lots of money)
Heidenhain disease
heightened attention, state of
heightened awareness, state of
height, tongue
"Helen" (heroin)
heliomania
heliophobia
helium speech
helix
"hell dust" (heroin)
Heller syndrome
helminthophobia
HELP (Hawaii Early Learning
    Profile)
helper, inner self

helper role
helping behavior
helping verb
helpless, hopeless, and worthless
helplessness and hopelessness
help-rejecting complaining
help-seeking behavior
"he-man" (fentanyl)
hemangioma of the brain
hematophobia
hemianopsia
    bitemporal
    homonymous
hemiballismic movements
hemic disorder, psychogenic
hemifacial spasm
hemifield of vision
hemilaryngectomy
hemiparesis
hemiparesthetic migraine headache
hemiplegia, hysterical
hemiplegic idiocy
hemiplegic migraine headache
hemisensory loss
hemispheral dysfunction
hemisphere
    cerebral
    left
    right
hemisphere dominance
    left
    left/right
    right
hemispheric reliance
hemispherical dysfunction
hemochromatosis
hemophobia
hemorrhage
    extradural
    intracerebral
    subarachnoid
    subdural

"hemp" (cannabis)
Henderson-Moriarty ESL/Literacy
    Placement Test
Hendler Test for Chronic Pain
    (HTCP)
Henmon-Nelson Ability Test,
    Canadian Edition
Henmon-Nelson Tests of Mental
    Ability, The
"henpicking" (re: crack acquisition)
"Henry" (heroin)
"Henry VIII" (cocaine)
hepatic conditions, dementia due to
hepatic encephalopathy (HE), delirium
    due to
hepatic encephalopathy tremor
hepatic function
hepatitis, toxic
hepatolenticular degeneration,
    dementia in
hepatorenal syndrome
"her" (cocaine)
"Herb" (cannabis)
"herba" (cannabis)
"Herb and Al" (cannabis and alcohol)
herd instinct
here-and-now approach
hereditary deficiency
hereditary hearing loss
heredity, environment and (E&H)
heredofamilial tremor
Hereford Parental Attitude [survey]
    (HPA)
hermaphrodite
hermaphroditism
    bilateral
    false
    transverse
    true
    unilateral
"herms" (phencyclidine)
"hero" (heroin)

heroin (street names)
AIP
antifreeze
Aries
atom bomb
Aunt Hazel
bad seed
ballot
beast, the
Belushi
big bag
big H
big Harry
black pearl
black stuff
black tar
blanco
bonita
bozo
brick gum
brown
brown crystal
brown rhine
brown sugar
bundle
butu
capital H
caps
carga
carne
Charley
chasing the dragon
chicle
chieva
China cat
China white
Chinese red
chip
cotics
cotton brothers
courage pills
crap/crop

heroin *(cont.)*
cura
cut-deck
dead on arrival
deuce
dirt
dog food
dogie
doogie/doojee/dugie
dooley
dreck
duji
dynamite
dyno
dyno-pure
eightball
eighth
el diablito
el diablo
estuffa
ferry dust
flamethrower
flea powder
Florida snow
foo foo stuff
foolish powder
Frisco special
Frisco speedball
gag
galloping horse
gamot
gato
George smack
girl
glancines
golden girl
golpe
goma
good and plenty
good H
gravy
H

heroin *(cont.)*
hache
hairy
H & C
hard candy
hard stuff
Harry
Hazel
H Caps
heaven dust
Helen
hell dust
Henry
hero
heroina
herone
hero of the underworld
hessle
him
hombre
hong-yen
horning
horse
hot dope
HRN
Isda
jee gee
jive
jive doo jee
jojee
Jones
joy flakes
joy powder
junk
kabayo
Karachi
LBJ
lemonade
little bomb
Matsakow
mayo
Mexican brown

heroin *(cont.)*
  Mexican horse
  Mexican mud
  Mojo
  moonrock
  Morotgara
  mortal combat
  mud
  muzzle
  nanoo
  New Jack Swing
  nice and easy
  nickel bag
  nickel deck
  noise
  nose
  nose drops
  number 1
  number 3
  number 4
  number 8
  ogoy
  oil
  Old Steve
  pack
  Pangonadalot
  parachute
  Peg
  Perfect High
  P-funk
  poison
  polvo
  poppy
  powder
  pulborn
  pure
  quill
  racehorse charlie
  ragweed
  Rambo
  rane
  ready rock

heroin *(cont.)*
  red chicken
  red eagle
  reindeer dust
  Rhine
  sack
  salt
  scag
  scat
  scate
  Scott
  shmeck/schmeek
  skag
  skid
  sleeper
  slime
  smack
  smoke
  smoking gun
  snow
  snowball
  speedball
  spider blue
  stuff
  sugar
  Sweet Jesus
  sweet stuff
  tar
  taste
  tecate
  thing
  T.N.T.
  Tootsie Roll
  whack
  white boy
  white girl
  white junk
  white lady
  white nurse
  whiz bang
  wings
  witch
  witch hazel

"heroina" (heroin)
heroin addiction
Heroin Antagonist and Learning
    Therapy (HALT)
"hero of the underworld" (heroin)
"herone" (heroin)
herpes simplex virus meningitis
herpes zoster meningitis
herpetophobia
hertz (Hz)
Hertz positive spike-waves
Heschl gyri
hesitation phenomena
"hessle" (heroin)
Hess School Readiness Scale (HSRS)
Heston Personality Index (HPI)
heterocyclic antidepressant
heteroerotism
heterogeneity, neurophysiological
heterogeneous group
heterogeneous word
heteronomous psychotherapy
heterophasia
heterophemy
Heterosexual Attitudes Toward
    Homosexuality [scale] (HATH)
heterosexuality
heterosexual marriage
heterosexual orientation
heterosexual pedophilia
heterosuggestion
heterotopy
heterotrimeric G proteins
heterozygous
heuristic
HEW (Department of Health,
    Education and Welfare)
hexing, illness ascribed to
HF (high frequency)
HF audiometry
HF average full-on gain
HF average SSPL output

HF deafness
HFD (Human Figure Drawing)
HFF (high filter frequency)
HGSHS (Harvard Group Scale of
    Hypnotic Susceptibility)
hiccough, psychogenic
HICROS (high frequency CROS)
hidden meaning
hiding behavior, cunning and
HIE (hypoxic-ischemic encepha-
    lopathy)
hierarchical functioning
hierarchical regression analysis
hierarchical scale of ADLs
hierarchical structure
hierarchy
    response
    social
hieromania
hierophobia
"high"
    feeling
    get (re: drug intoxication)
high adaptive level
high affectivity ratio
high-amplitude sucking technique
    (HAS)
high anxiety (HA)
"highbeams" (re: crack use)
high-dose drug
high-dose use of substance
high-energy level
higher cerebral dysfunction (HCD)
higher cortical dysfunction
higher integrative language processing
higher level cognitive function
higher level function
high-filter frequency (HFF)
high frequency (HF)
high-frequency audiometry
high-frequency average full-on gain
high-frequency CROS (HICROS)

high-frequency deafness
high-frequency of drug use
high-grade defect
high impulsiveness
    high anxiety (HIHA)
    low anxiety (HILA)
high-level perceptual disturbance
high-pass filter
high-pitched cry
high potential for painful consequences
high-risk activity
high-risk behavior
high risk for suicide
high-risk group
high-risk variables
High School Career-Course Planner
    (HSCCP)
High School Personality Questionnaire
    (HSPQ)
high standards of performance, self-
    imposed
high-stimulus speech
high strung
high tolerance potential
high value
high vowel
HIHA (high impulsiveness, high
    anxiety)
"hikori" (mescaline)
"hikuli" (mescaline)
HILA (high impulsiveness, low
    anxiety)
Hill Interaction Matrix (HIM)
Hilson Adolescent Profile
Hilson Personnel Profile/Success
    Quotient (HPP/SQ)
"him" (heroin)
HIM (Hill Interaction Matrix)
"Hinkley" (phencyclidine)
HIP (Hypnotic Induction Profile)
"hippie crack" (inhalant)
hippocampal amnesia

hippocampal amnesic
hippocampal epilepsy
hippocampus
hippomania
hippophobia
"hiroppon" (methamphetamine
    hydrochloride)
Hirschsprung disease
HIS (Haptic Intelligence Scale)
Hiskey-Nebraska Test of Learning
    Aptitude (HNTLA)
HISMS (How-I-See-Myself Scale)
Hispanic English
histamine headache
histidine
histogram
history
    cyclic
    depression
    detailed
    drinking
    educational
    family
    known
    life
    lifetime
    marital (MH)
    medical
    military
    neuro-ophthalmologic
    occupational (OH)
    pain
    past (PH)
    personal (PH)
    premorbid
    previous
    prior
    psychiatric
    psychosexual
    school
    seizure
    sexual

history *(cont.)*
   social (SH, S.H.)
   suicide attempt
history and physical (H&P) exam
history of (H/O)
histrionic character
histrionic personality disorder
   (hysterical personality)
histrionic presentation
histrionic situation
histrionism
HIT (Holtzman Inkblot Technique)
"hit" (cannabis cigarette; crack)
"hit and run" effect
"hit of acid"
"hit the hay" (re: cannabis use)
"hit the main line" (re: drug injection)
"hit the needle" (re: drug injection)
hitting one's own body, nonfunctional
   and repetitive
HIV (human immunodeficiency virus)
   HIV-based dementia
   HIV disease
HL (hearing level)
HMT (Hodkinson Mental Test)
HNTLA (Hiskey-Nebraska Test of
   Learning Aptitude)
H/O (history of)
hoarseness
   dry
   rough
   wet
hoboes, hospital (Munchausen
   syndrome)
"hocus" (cannabis; opium)
Hodkinson Mental Test (HMT)
hodomania
hodophobia
"hog" (phencyclidine)
Hogan Personality Inventory
Hogan Personnel Selection Series

hole, bore
holiday, drug
holism
holistic medicine
holistic psychology
holophrastic utterances
Holtzman Inkblot Technique (HIT)
"hombre" (heroin)
"hombrecitos" (psilocybin)
home assessment
home environment, disturbed
Home Environment Questionnaire
home evaluation
home language
homeless
homemade marijuana
homemaking responsibilities
Home Observation for Measurement
   of the Environment
homeostasis
homeostatic balance
Home Screening Questionnaire
home setting
homichlophobia
homicidal behavior
homicidal ideation
homicidal intent
homicidal plan
homicidal preoccupation
homicidal rumination
homicidomania
homilophobia
homocysinuria
homoerotic
homoeroticism
homoerotism
homogeneous scintillating scotoma
homogeneous word
homograph
homonym
homonymy, analysis of
homophenes

homophobe
homophobia
homophone
homorganic
homosexual activity
homosexual, closet
homosexual complex
homosexual conflict disorder
homosexuality
  ego-dystonic
  female
  latent
  male
  overt
  pedophilic
  unconscious
homosexual marriage
homosexual neurosis
homosexual orientation
homosexual panic, acute
homosexual pedophilia
homovanillic acid (HVA), plasma
"honey" (re: currency)
"honey blunts" (cannabis cigars sealed
  with honey)
"honey oil" (inhalant; ketamine)
"honeymoon" (re: drug use)
"hong-yen" (heroin in pill form)
honorable discharge
"hooch" (cannabis)
Hood masking technique
HOOI (Hall Occupational Orientation
  Inventory)
"hooked" (addicted)
Hooper Visual Organization Test (VOT)
"hooter" (cannabis; cocaine)
"hop/hops" (opium)
hopelessness, feelings of
Hopkins Symptom Checklist-90 Total
  Score (HSCL-90 T)
"hopped up" (re: drug influence)
horizontal canal

horizontal jut
horizontal nystagmus
horizontal plane
hormephobia
hormonal level
hormonal self-treatment
hormonal sex-reassignment
hormone ingestion
"horn" (re: cocaine or crack use)
Horney, Karen (1883-1952)
"horning" (heroin)
horrific impulses
"horse" (heroin)
"horse heads" (amphetamine)
"horse tracks" (phencyclidine)
"horse tranquilizer" (phencyclidine)
hospital
  day
  mental
  night
  open
  private psychiatric
  psychiatric
  state mental (SMH)
  teaching
  weekend
hospital addiction syndrome
  (Munchausen syndrome)
Hospital and Community Psychiatry
Hospital Anxiety and Depression
  Scale
hospital-based psychiatry
hospital-based study
hospital consultation/liaison service
hospital hoboes (Munchausen syndrome)
hospitalism
hospitalization
  involuntary
  need for
  partial
  voluntary

hospital-patient relations
hospital-physician relations
hospital regulations, noncompliance
    with
hospital routine
hospital unit, locked
hostage status
host culture
hostile aggressiveness
hostile behavior
hostile identity
hostile response
Hostility and Direction of Hostility
    (HDH)
Hostility and Direction of Hostility
    Questionnaire (HDHQ)
hostility, voice
"hotcakes" (crack)
"hot dope" (heroin)
"hot heroin" (poisoned heroin given
    to a police informant)
"hot ice" (smokable methampheta-
    mine)
"hot load/hot shot" (re: drug injec-
    tion)
"hot stick" (cannabis cigarette)
hour (h., hr.)
"house fee" (re: crack use)
household, dual-earner
household duties, neglect of
household responsibilities
"house piece" (re: crack use)
house-tree-person test (HTP, H-T-P)
house-tree test (HT, H-T)
housing problem
Houston Test for Language Develop-
    ment
"How do you like me now?" (crack)
Howell Prekindergarten Screening
    Test
How-I-See-Myself Scale (HISMS)
"hows" (morphine)

HP (hyperphoria)
HPA (Hereford Parental Attitude)
    (survey)
HPA (hypothalamic-pituitary-adrenal)
    axis
HPD (hearing protection device)
HPI (Heston Personality Index)
HPNT (The Hundred Pictures Naming
    Test)
HPP/SQ (Hilson Personnel Profile/
    Success Quotient)
hr. (hour)
"HRN" (heroin)
HRNES (Halstead-Russell Neuro-
    psychological Evaluation System)
HRNTB (Halstead-Reitan Neuro-
    psychologic Test Battery)
h.s. (hour of sleep; bedtime)
HSCCP (High School Career-Course
    Planner)
HSCL-90 T (Hopkins Symptom
    Checklist-90 Total Score)
HSPQ (High School Personality
    Questionnaire)
HSRS (Hess School Readiness Scale)
HT (Hand Test)
HT (house-tree) test
HTCP (Hendler Test for Chronic Pain)
HTL (hearing threshold level)
HTP, H-T-P (house-tree-person) test
"Hubba, I am back" (crack)
"hubba pigeon" (re: crack user)
"hubbas" (crack)
"huff" or "huffer" (inhalant)
huffing
"hulling" (re: stealing drugs)
human foibles, common
human growth factor (HGF)
Human Information Processing Survey
human movement responses
humanistic psychology
human-pet bonding

humiliation, fear of
hum noise, sixty-cycle
humorless
hunches, tendency to play
Hundred Pictures Naming Test
  (HPNT)
hunger drive
"hunter" (cocaine)
Huntington chorea (HC)
Hunt syndrome
husband-to-wife aggression
"hustle" (re: drug dealing)
Hutchins Behavior Inventory (HBI)
Hutchinson teeth
HVA (homovanillic acid)
HVA levels in schizophrenia, plasma
HVS (hyperventilation syndrome)
hx (history)
hyalophobia
hyaluronidase inhibitor, physiological
  (PHI)
"hyatari" (mescaline)
hydantoin
hydrargyromania
hydrocarbon (inhalation) dependence
hydrocephalic idiocy
hydrocephalus
  communicating
  congenital
  normal pressure (NPH)
  obstructive
hydrodipsomania
hydromania
hydrophobia
hydrophobophobia
hydrops
  endolymphatic
  labyrinthine
  vestibular
hygiene
  deterioration in
  impaired personal

hygiene *(cont.)*
  inadequate sleep
  lack of minimal
  lapses in
  mental
  minimal personal
  personal
  sleep
hygrophobia
hylephobia
hylomania
hylophobia
Hymovich Chronicity Impact and
  Coping Instrument (CICI)
hyoglossal (hyoglossus) muscle
hyoid bone
HYP, Hyp (hypnosis)
hypacusic
hypacusis
"hype" (heroin addict)
hypegiaphobia
hypengyophobia
hyperacousis
hyperactive behavior
hyperactive child syndrome
hyperactive-impulsive attention-
  deficit/hyperactivity disorder
hyperactive-impulsive combined
  behavior
hyperactive sexual desire
hyperactivity, autonomic
hyperactivity disorder, attention-deficit
  (ADHD)
hyperactivity-impulsivity
hyperactivity indices
hyperactivity signs, autonomic
hyperacusis
hyperadrenocorticism
hyperalert
hyperalgesia
hyperamnesia

hyperarousal, autonomic
hyperbole (figure of speech)
hypercalcemia
hypercarbia
hyperdefensive attitude
hyperdopaminergic state
hyperemotional
hyperesthenia
hyperesthesia, laryngeal
hyperexcitability
hypergnosis
hypergraphia
hyperhedonia
hyperhedonism
hyperhidrosis
hyperintensity, white matter
hyperirritability
hyperkalemia
hyperkeratosis
hyperkinesia of the false folds
hyperkinesis index
hyperkinesis sign, Claude
hyperkinetic conduct disorder
hyperkinetic conversion reaction
hyperkinetic disturbance
hyperkinetic dysarthria
hyperkinetic dysphonia
hyperkinetic reaction
hyperkinetic speech
hyperkinetic syndrome of childhood
hyperlexia
hypermania
hypermimia
hypermnesia
hypermnesic
hypernatremia
hypernoia
hyperorexia
hyperphagia
hyperphoria (HP)
hyperphrenia
hyperplasia, congenital adrenal

hyperplastic laryngitis
hyperpragia
hyperpragic
hyperpraxia
hyperpyrexia
hyperquantivalent idea
hyperreflexia
    autonomic
    generalized
hyperreligiosity
hyperresponsible worries
hyperrexia
hyperrhinolalia voice disorder
hyperrhinophonia voice disorder
hypersensibility
hypersensitive
hypersensitivity
hypersensitization
hypersexual complex
hypersexuality
hypersomnia
hypersomnolence
hypersomnolent
hypertensive crisis
hypertensive encephalopathy
hyperthermia, malignant
hyperthymia
hyperthymic personality disorder
hyperthymism
hypertonia
hypertonic tongue
hypertrophic pyloric stenosis,
    congenital
hyperventilate
hyperventilation
    autonomic
    central neurogenic
    psychogenic
hyperventilation syndrome (HVS)
hypervigilance
hypervigilant
hypesthesia

"hype stick"
hyphedonia
hypnagogic hallucination
hypnagogic hallucination imagery
hypnagogic state
hypnagogue
hypnalgia
hypnic
hypno. (hypnosis, hypnotism, hypno-
    tist)
hypnoanalysis
hypnoanesthesia
hypnocinematograph
hypnodrama
hypnogenetic
hypnogenic
hypnogenous
hypnoidal
hypnoid state
hypnolepsy
hypnology
hypnomania
hypnopedia
hypnophobia
hypnopompic hallucination
hypnopompic image
hypnopompic state
hypnosis (HYP, Hyp, hypno.)
    diagnostic use of
    direct suggestion under (DSUH)
    lethargic
    major
    minor
    suggestion
    symptom relief through
hypnosophy
hypnot. (hypnotic, hypnotism)
hypnotherapy
hypnotic (hypnot.)
hypnotic abreaction
hypnotic abuse
hypnotic-dependent patient

hypnotic drug abuse; dependence
hypnotic-induced anxiety
Hypnotic Induction Profile (HIP)
hypnotic interview
hypnotic intoxication delirium
hypnotic psychotherapy
hypnotic-related disorder
hypnotic relaxation technique training
hypnotic state
hypnotic-type withdrawal
hypnotic use disorder
hypnotic withdrawal delirium
hypnotic withdrawal symptom,
    sedative
hypnotism (hypno., hypnot.)
hypnotist (hypno.)
hypnotizability
hypnotization
hypnotize
hypoactive sexual desire disorder
    acquired-type
    generalized-type
    lifelong-type
    situational-type
hypoacusis
hypocalcemia
hypochondria
hypochondriac
hypochondriacal disorder, psychogenic
hypochondriacal melancholia
hypochondriacal neurosis
hypochondriacal psychoneurosis
hypochondriacal psychoneurotic
    reaction
hypochondriacal reaction
hypochondriacal symptoms
hypochondriasis
hypoesthesia
hypoesthetic
hypofunction, testicular
hypoglossal nerve (cranial nerve XII)
hypoglottis

hypoglycemia
hypoglycemic delirium
hypogonadism
hypokalemia
hypokinesia
hypokinesis
hypokinetic dysarthria
hypokinetic speech
hypologia
hypomania
hypomaniac
hypomanic disorder
hypomanic-like episode
hypomanic manic-depressive reaction
hypomanic personality, chronic
hypomanic psychosis
hypomanic reaction
hypomanic tendencies
hypomanic-type manic-depressive
    psychosis
hypomelancholia
hypometabolism
    frontotemporal
    striatal
hypomnesis
hyponatremia
hyponoia
hypopharynx
hypophonia
hypophonic aphasia
hypophrasia
hypophrenia
hypophrenic
hypoplasia
    lingual
    mandibular
hypoprosody
hyposensitive
hyposensitivity
hyposensitization
hyposexuality
hyposomnia

hypotaxia
hypotension, orthostatic
hypothalamic-pituitary-adrenal (HPA)
    axis
hypothermia
hypothesis
    biogenic amine
    dopamine
    falsifiable
    null
hypothesize
hypothymic personality disorder
hypothymism
hypotonic cerebral palsy (CP)
hypoventilation syndrome, central
    alveolar
hypoxia, toxic
hypoxic-ischemic encephalopathy
    (HIE)
hypoxyphilia
hypsiphobia
hypsophobia
HYS, hys. (hysteria, hysterical)
hysteria (HYS, hys.)
    anxiety
    canine
    Charcot grand
    conversion
    dissociative
    epidemic
    fixation
    major
    minor
    studies on
hysteria psychoneurosis
    conversion
    dissociative
hysteria psychosis
hysterical (HYS, hys.)
hysterical amnesia
hysterical anesthesia
hysterical aphonia

hysterical astasia-abasia
hysterical ataxia
hysterical aura
hysterical blindness
hysterical conversion reaction (HCR)
hysterical convulsion
hysterical deafness
hysterical delirium
hysterical depression
hysterical disorder, psychogenic
hysterical epilepsy
hysterical fugue state
hysterical gait
hysterical hemiplegia
hysterical insanity
hysterical mania
hysterical movement disorder
hysterical mutism
hysterical neurosis
    conversion-type
    dissociative-type
hysterical overbreathing, voluntary
hysterical personality
hysterical pregnancy
hysterical pseudodementia

hysterical psychomotor disorder
hysterical psychoneurotic reaction
    conversion-type
    dissociative-type
hysterical psychosis
hysterical reaction, dissociative
hysterical seizure
hysterical stuttering
hysterical trance
hysterical tremor
hysterical visual loss
hysteric aphonia
hysteric coma-like state
hystericism
hysteric lethargy
hysterics
hystericus, globus
hysteriform
hysteroepilepsy
hysteroid convulsion
hysteroid defenses
hysteroid features
hysteroid personality
hysteromania
Hz (Hertz or cycles per second)

I, i

I (iodine)
IA (inactive alcoholic)
IAAT (Iowa Algebra Aptitude Test, Fourth Edition)
"I am back" (crack)
iambic stress
IAS (Integrated Assessment System)
IASP (International Association for the Study of Pain)
iatrogenesis
iatrogenic addiction
iatrogenic induction
iatrogenic seizure
iatrophobia
IBS (Interpersonal Behavior Study)
IBT (inkblot test)
IC (inspiratory capacity)
ICA (Infancy, Childhood and Adolescence)
ICD-9-CM (*International Classification of Diseases*, 9th ed., *Clinical Modification*)
ICD-10 system
ICE (Individual Career Exploration)
"ice" (cocaine; methamphetamine hydrochloride; methylenedioxymethamphetamine and phencyclidine; smokeable amphetamine)

"ice cream habit" (re: occasional drug use)
"ice cube" (crack)
ICET (48-Item Counseling Evaluation Test)
ichthyomania
ichthyophobia
"icing" (cocaine)
iconic memory
iconomania
icons
ICPS (Interpersonal Cognitive Problem-Solving)
ICRT (Individualized Criterion Referenced Testing)
ICRTM (Individualized Criterion Referenced Testing Mathematics)
ICRTR (Individualized Criterion Referenced Test Reading)
ICSD (*International Classification of Sleep Disorders: Diagnostic and Coding Manual*)
ICT (insulin coma therapy)
ictal amnesia
ictal amnesic
ictal automatism
ictal confusional seizure

ictal depression phase of seizure, past
ictal period
id
idea (pl. ideas)
  autochthonous
  compulsive
  disconnected
  dominant
  fixed
  flight of (FOI)
  flow of
  hyperquantivalent
  imperative
  intruding
  intrusive distressing
  morbid
  obsessional
  overvalued
  permanent dominant
  persistent
  persistent inappropriate
  persistent intrusive
  poverty of
  recurring
  referential
  repetitive
  separation of feelings from
  strongly held
  unreasonable
  unwarranted
ideal, ego
idealization
idealized value
IDEA Oral Language Proficiency
  Test II
IDEAS (Interest Determination,
  Exploration and Assessment
  System), Enhanced Version
ideas of reference, transient
ideation
  AWOL (absent without leave)
  elopement

ideation *(cont.)*
  homicidal
  paranoid
  persecution
  recurrent suicidal
  stress-related paranoid
  suicidal
  suspicious
  transient
ideational apraxia
ideational shield
ideational style of coping
ideatory apraxia
idée fixe
identical twins
identifiable pattern of sleep and wakefulness
identifiable stress
identifiable stressor
identification
  cosmic
  cross-gender
  deep-trance
  gender
  healthy
  letter-word
  projective
  social
identification audiometry
identification with the aggressor
identifying with aggression
identity (pl. identities)
  adolescent sexual
  alteration in
  alternate
  controlling
  core gender
  cultural
  ego
  female-to-male transgender
  former
  gender

identity *(cont.)*
  hostile
  male-to-female transgender
  masculine
  multiple distinct
  new
  particular
  personal
  place
  primary
  "protector"
  sense of
  sense of personal
identity confusion
identity crisis, psychosexual
identity disorder
  dissociative
  gender (GID)
  psychosexual
  sexual
  sexual and gender
identity disorder of adolescence
identity disorder of childhood
identity disturbance
identity problem
  adolescent
  gender
identity states
ideodynamism
ideogenetic
ideogenous
ideoglandular
ideogram
ideographs
ideokinetic apraxia
ideology
ideometabolic
ideometabolism
ideomotion
ideomotor aphasia
ideomotor apraxia
ideomuscular

ideo-obsessional constitution
ideophobia
ideoplastia
ideovascular
idiocy
  amaurotic
  athetosic
  Aztec
  Bielschowsky
  cretinoid
  developmental
  diplegic
  eclamptic
  epileptic
  erethistic
  family
  genetous
  hemiplegic
  hydrocephalic
  infantile
  intrasocial
  juvenile
  Kalmuk
  microcephalic
  mongolian
  moral
  paralytic
  paraplegic
  plagiocephalic
  profound
  scaphocephalic
  sensorial
  spastic amaurotic axonal
  torpid
  traumatic
  Vogt-Spielmeyer
  xerodermic
idioglossia
idioglottic
idiographic
idiohypnotism
idio-imbecile

idiolalia
idiolect
idiologism
idiom (figure of speech)
idioneurosis
idiopathic dystonias
idiopathic encephalopathy
idiopathic epilepsy
idiopathic insomnia
idiopathic language retardation
idiophrenic insanity
idiophrenic psychosis
idiopsychologic
idiosyncrasy
idiosyncratic alcohol intoxication
idiosyncratic material, evidence of
    intrusion of
idiosyncratic meaning
idiosyncratic processes
idiosyncratic reaction
idiosyncratic reasoning
idiosyncratic thinking
idiot
    erethistic
    mongolian
    oxycephalic
    pithecoid
    profound
    superficial
    torpid
"idiot pills" (barbiturate)
idiot-prodigy
idiotropic
idiot-savant
idolomania
IDT (Interdisciplinary Team)
IER (Institute of Educational Research
    [intelligence] test
I-E Scale (internal versus external
    scale)
IFA (International Fluency Associa-
    tion)

IFI (Institutional Functioning
    Inventory)
IFROS (ipsilateral frontal routing of
    signals)
IGI (Institutional Goals Inventory)
IIP (Intra- and Interpersonal [Relations
    Scale])
ILA-II (Inventory of Language
    Abilities II)
[123]I-labeled cocaine analog
    ([123]beta-CIT)
ILEAD (Instructional Leadership
    Evaluation and Development
    Program)
ileus, paralytic
iliocostal muscle of thorax
ill
    chronically mentally (CMI)
    commitment of mentally
ill-at-ease, mentally
illegal drug purchases
illegitimacy
illegitimate child
illicit drug
illicit lover
illicit psychoactive substance
Illinois Children's Language Assess-
    ment Test
Illinois Test of Psycholinguistic
    Abilities (ITPA)
illness (pl. illnesses)
    emotional
    factitious
    folk
    iatrogenic
    life-threatening
    manic-depressive
    mental (MI)
    no mental (NMI)
    preexisting
    present (PI)
    progressive dementing

illness *(cont.)*
  psychiatric
  psychosomatic
  psychotic
  usual childhood (UCI)
illness ascribed to hexing
Illness Behavior Questionnaire
illness during pregnancy, psychiatric
illness phase
illogical communication
illogical reasoning
illogical thinking
illuminism
illusion (pl. illusions)
  bodily
  optic
  fleeting
  recurrent
  transient auditory
  transient tactile
  transient visual
illusionary misconceptions
ILSA (Interpersonal Language Skills
  and Assessment)
IM or I.M. (intramuscular)
image
  body
  distorted body
  disturbed body
  eidetic
  hypnagogic
  hypnagogic hallucination
  hypnopompic
  memory
  mental
  motor
  negative body
  obsessional mental
  peripheral field
  persistence of visual
  persistent inappropriate
  persistent intrusive

image *(cont.)*
  splitting of
  tactile
  trailing
  transient
image control
image-distorting level
image distortion, body
image intensification
image intensifier
image of others, splitting of
imagery
  eidetic
  guided affective (GAI)
  paraphiliac
  visual (VI)
Imagery and Disease (IMAGE-CA;
  IMAGE-DB; IMAGE-SP)
imaginal processes
imaginary language
imaginary playmate
imaginative play
imagined abandonment
imagined defect
imagined loss
imaging
  functional brain
  structural brain
imaging studies, brain
imago
I marker (intentional marker)
imbalance
  biochemical
  central language
  developmental
  electrolyte
  orofacial muscle
imbecile
imbecility
  moral
  old age
  phenylpyruvic
  senile

imbibe
IMI (Impact Message Inventory),
   Research Edition
imitation
   elicited
   spontaneous
imitative behavior
imitative movement, repetitive
imitative word repetition, senseless
immature personality
immaturity
   perceptual
   social
immaturity reaction
   aggressive
   emotional instability
immediate anxiety
immediate echolalia
immediate environment
immediate gratification
immediate memory
immediate memory test
immediate sentence constituents
immediately (STAT, stat)
immigrant status
immittance measurement test, acoustic
immobility
   motor
   motoric
immobilized
immune disorders, dementia due to
immune function, impaired
immune functioning, potential impairment of
immune mechanism
immunity, stress
impacted cerumen
impacted grief
Impact Message Inventory, Research
   Edition (IMI)
Impact of Event Scale
impact, potential

impaired
   communicatively
   emotionally
   functionally
   severely mentally (SMI)
   speech and language (SLI)
impaired affect modulation
impaired arousal, sexual dysfunction
   with
impaired communication ability
impaired function
impaired insight
impaired judgment
impaired language
impaired memory
impaired orientation
impaired performance
impaired relationships
impaired social functioning
   anxiety-induced
   frustration-induced
impaired speech
impaired thinking ability
impairment
   aphasic
   cerebral
   cognitive
   degree of
   disproportionate
   emotional
   focal neurological
   functional
   gaze
   generalized intellectual
   graphic
   hearing
   intellectual
   language
   marked
   measurable
   memory
   mental

impairment *(cont.)*
  motor
  neurologic
  neuropsychological
  objective symptoms of
  occupational
  organic
  perceptual-motor
  perceptual-motor abilities
  permanent residual
  physical
  reading comprehension
  residual
  reversible memory
  school functioning
  sensory
  significant
  social functioning
  speech
  subjective symptoms of
  visual
  visual-motor
impairment criterion
impasse, therapeutic
impedance
  acoustic
  static acoustic
impedance matching
impedance measures
impediment, speech
impel
impelled
impending death
impending decompensation
impending doom, sense of
imperative idea
imperative mood
imperative sentence
imperception, auditory
imperfections revealed, fear of
impersistence, motor
impetus

implant, cochlear
implication, semantic
implications, management
implicit language
implicit memory
implicit stuttering
implied criticism
implosion (flooding)
implosive consonant formation
implosive therapy
impose
imposition of legal sanctions
imposition of social sanctions
impostors
impotence
  , erectile
  sexual
impoverished early environment
impoverished fantasy life
impoverished speech
impoverished thoughts
impoverishment in thinking
impoverishment, personality
impractical
impression
  erroneous
  good (Gi)
impressionable/impressionability
impressionistic phonetics
impressionistic speech, excessively
impressive aphasia
imprinting, filial
Improving Writing, Thinking, and
  Reading Skills test
improvisation
IMPS (Inpatient Multidimensional
  Psychiatric Scale)
impulse (pl. impulses)
  aggressive
  base
  forbidden
  horrific

impulse *(cont.)*
  irresistible
  morbid
  obsessional
  persistent inappropriate
  persistent intrusive
  repressed
impulse control
  impaired
  poor
impulse-control disorder
impulse-control interface disorder
impulse-control problems
impulse disorder
impulse regulation, lack of
impulse test, irresistible
impulsion
impulsive activity
impulsive behavior
impulsive/compulsive psychopathology
impulsive dyscontrol
impulsive insanity
impulsiveness
impulsive neurosis
Impulsive Nonconformity Scale
impulsive petit mal epilepsy
impulsive tendencies
impulsivity
  lack of
  self-damaging
  tendency toward
"in" (re: drug suppliers)
inability to cope
inability to experience pleasure
inability to function
inability to sleep
inability to take criticism
inaccuracy
  general oral
  oral
inactive alcoholic (IA)
inadequacy, feelings of

inadequate discipline
inadequate information
inadequate personality
inadequate personality disorder
inadequate rapport
inadequate school environment
inadequate sleep hygiene
inanimate
inanition
inappropriate affect
inappropriate attitude
inappropriate behavior
inappropriate circumstances
inappropriate compensatory behavior
inappropriate dependent care
inappropriate ideas, persistent
inappropriate images, persistent
inappropriate impulses, persistent
inappropriate laughter
inappropriateness
inappropriate passage of feces, repeated
inappropriate posture
inappropriate quality of obsessions
inappropriate sexual behavior
inappropriate social relatedness, developmentally
inappropriate thoughts, persistent
inappropriate urges, persistent
inappropriate voiding of urine, repeated
inappropriate words
  sexual
  social
inarticulate
inattention, selective
inattention to the environment
inattentive behavior
inattentive-type attention-deficit/hyperactivity disorder, predominantly
"in-betweens" (amphetamine; barbiturate; lysergic acid diethylamide)

inborn errors of metabolism
"Inca message" (cocaine)
incapacitate
incapacitated
incapacitating fear
incapacitating injury
incarceration
incentive
    aversive
    positive
incentive motivation
incessant speech
incest
incestual relationship
incestuous
incidence
incident wave
incidental learning
incipient psychosis
incipient schizophrenia
incipient schizophrenic psychosis
incipient stuttering
incisive foramen
incisiveness, feelings of
incisor teeth
    central
    lateral
incoherence
incoherent behavior
incoherent patient
incoherent speech
incompatibility
incompatible behavior
incompetence
    ejaculatory
    velopharyngeal
incompetency, certificate of
incompetent
incomplete alexia
incomplete cleft palate
incomplete phrases
incomplete recruitment

Incomplete Sentences Survey
Incomplete Sentences Task
incomprehensible speech
incomprehensible thought
incongruent
incongruous affect
inconsistent contact with reality
inconsistent discipline
inconsistent manner
inconsistent parental discipline
inconsistent recall
incontinence
    affective
    emotional
    fecal
    urinary
incontrovertible evidence (proof)
incoordination
incorporation
incurable problem drinker (IPD)
incus
indecision
indecisiveness
indefinite vowel
independence, physical
independent clause
independent functioning
independent group (experimental study
    designs)
independent living, capacity for
Independent Living Behavior
    Checklist
independent variable
in-depth analysis
indeterminate sex
indeterminate sleep
index (pl. indices) (see also *test*)
    ADL (activities of daily living)
    alpha
    alphabetical
    ambulation
    anxiety (AI)

index *(cont.)*
  articulation
  Barthel ADL
  beta
  body mass (BMI)
  delta
  hyperactivity
  hyperkinesis
  maturation
  multi-item
  physiological sleepiness
  schizophrenia
  shift referential
  spouse abuse
  switch referential
  tabular
  theta
  total response (TRI)
Index of Spouse Abuse
Index of Well-Being (IWB)
index/position, self
"Indian boy" (cannabis)
"Indian hay" (cannabis)
Indian hemp dependence
"Indica" (cannabis)
indicative mood
indicator (pl. indicators) (see *test*),
  risk
indices (see *index*)
indictment
indifference
  belle (also, la belle indifférence)
  sexual
indifferent to surroundings
indigenous worker
indirect laryngoscopy
indirect motor system
indirect object
indirect self-destructive behavior
  (ISDB)
indiscretion, sexual
indiscriminate sexual encounters

indistinct speech
indistinguishable
individual
  age-matched
  androgynous
  insightless
individual care
Individual Career Exploration (ICE)
individual counselor
individuality
Individualized Criterion Referenced
  Testing (ICRT)
Individualized Criterion Referenced
  Testing Mathematics (ICRTM)
Individualized Criterion Referenced
  Test Reading (ICRTR)
Individual Phonics Criterion Test
individual psychology
individual psychotherapy
individual responsibility
individual skill
individual therapy (IT)
individuation problem
"Indo" (cannabis)
indoctrination while captive
Indoklon therapy
indolamine
indole
"Indonesian bud" (cannabis; opium)
induced lethargy
induced paranoid disorder
induced psychosis
induced psychotic disorder
inductance
induction
  iatrogenic
  negative mood
induction coil
induction loop
inductive reactance
inductor
industrial audiometry

industrial deafness
industrial psychiatry
industrial psychology
industrialized culture
indwelling low pressure voice
  prosthesis
inebriation
inebriety
ineffability
ineffective anger
ineffective decision making
ineffectiveness, feelings of
ineffectual parent
inept
inertial bone conduction
inevitability, ejaculatory
infancy and early childhood disturbances in feeding and eating
Infancy, Childhood and Adolescence
  (ICA)
infant behavior
infantile affect
infantile amnesia
infantile aphasia
infantile autism
infantile behavior
infantile convulsion
infantile dynamics
infantile idiocy
infantile perseveration
infantile psychosis, symbiotic
infantile speech
infantile sexuality
infantile swallowing
infantilism
  regressive
  sexual
infantilized
Infant Reading Tests
Infant/Toddler Environment Rating
  Scale (ITERS)
infarct dementia, repeated

infarct, lacunar
infection-exhaustion psychosis
infection-type organic psychosis
  brain
  intracranial
infective psychosis
  acute
  subacute
inference (pl. inferences), statistical
inferential behavioral monitoring
  distortion of
  exaggeration of
inferential perception
  distortion of
  exaggeration of
inferential thinking
  distortion of
  exaggeration of
inferior constrictor muscle of pharynx
inferior frontal sulcus
inferiority complex
inferiority, constitutional psychopathia
  (CPI)
inferiority feelings, premorbid (PIF)
inferiority to others, feelings of
inferior laryngotomy
inferior longitudinal muscle of tongue
inferior maxillary bone
inferior meatus, nasi
inferior nasal concha
inferior sibling lifestyle
inferior temporal sulcus
Inferred Self-Concept Scale
infibulation (pinning and piercing)
infidelity
  delusion of
  marital
infinitive (parts of speech)
infixation
infix morpheme
inflammatory croup

inflated identity
inflated knowledge
inflated power
inflated worth
inflection, speech
inflectional endings
inflectional morpheme
inflexibility, enduring pattern of
inflexible attitude
inflexible pattern
influential
informal contract
informal method
Informal Reading Comprehension
  Placement Test
informal retention
informant
information center, drug (DIC)
information log, drug (DIL)
information processing, disturbance in
  speed of
information processing speed
information subtest
information test
  fund of
  recall of
information theory
informed consent
infradian rhythms
infraglottic
infrahyoid extrinsic muscles
infrahyoid muscles
infrasonic frequency
infraversion of teeth
ingestion, caustic
ingratiating behavior
inhalant (street names)
  air blast
  amyl nitrate
  bullet bolt
  butyl nitrate
  heart-on

inhalant *(cont.)*
  hippie crack
  honey oil
  huff
  isobutyl nitrate
  kick
  nitrate
  Oz
  poor man's pot
  pulmonary absorption of
  satan's secret
  sniff
  spray
  toilet water
inhalant abuse
inhalant dependence
inhalant intoxication delirium
inhalant-related disorder
inhalant use disorder
inhalational anesthetics, halogenated
inhalation (forced) muscles
inhalation (quiet) muscles
inhalation method of esophageal
  speech
inhalation of drug
inhaling intoxicating vapors, method
  of
inheritance, polygenic
inherited abnormality
inherited disease
inherited progressive degenerative
  disease
inhibit
inhibited female orgasm
inhibited grieving
inhibited male orgasm
inhibited mania
inhibited sexual desire
inhibited sexual excitement
inhibited-type reactive attachment
  disorder

inhibition
  academic
  emotional
  proactive (PI)
  reactive
  reciprocal
  retroactive (RI)
  work
inhibition and desensitization,
  reciprocal
inhibition factor, feedback (FIF)
inhibitions level, mental
inhibitive
inhibitor
  MAO (monoamine oxidase)
  physiological hyaluronidase (PHI)
  selective serotonin reuptake
  serotonin reuptake
inhibitory obsession
inhibitory tone
inhospitability
inhospitable
initial consonant, deletion of
initial consonant position
initial dominant, bystander dominates
  (BDID)
initial insomnia
initial interview
initial lag
initial masking
initial phase of insomnia
initial string
initial teaching alphabet
initiating and maintaining sleep,
  disorder of (DIMS)
initiating insomnia
initiation of goal-directed behavior
initiative, lack of
injectable steroid
injection drug users
injection method, cross-consonant
injection method of esophageal speech

injury
  brain
  potential for
  self-induced
  self-inflicted bodily
  toxic
  traumatic
  traumatic brain (TBI)
injustice gathering
inkblot test (IBT)
innate drive
innateness theory
  language
  speech
inner barrenness
inner battery clusters
inner child issues
inner-directed person
inner ear
inner experience
inner language
inner life
inner self helper
inner speech
inner tension
innervation apraxia
innervation, patterns of motor
Inpatient Multidimensional Psychiatric
  Scale (IMPS)
inpatient patient populations
in-phase wave
input, acoustic
Input Receptive Language Processing
INQ (Inquiry Mode Questionnaire: A
  Measure of How You Think and
  Make Decisions)
inquiry forensic psychiatry, Clunis
Inquiry Mode Questionnaire (INQ): A
  Measure of How You Think and
  Make Decisions
insane

insanity
  adolescent
  affective
  alcoholic
  alternating
  basedowian
  choreic
  circular
  climacteric
  communicated
  compulsive
  confusional
  criminal
  cyclic
  degenerative
  delusional
  double
  doubting
  dread of
  drug
  hysterical
  idiophrenic
  impulsive
  intermittent
  manic-depressive
  moral
  partial
  periodic
  religious
  senile
  simultaneous
  toxic
insanity defense
insanoid
insatiable
insecticide, organophosphate
insect infestation, sensation of
insecurity, social
insensible
insensitive
insensitivity syndrome, androgen
insertion loss

insertion, thought
insidious onset
insight
  emotional
  impaired
  intellectual
  lack of
  myopic
  poor
insightless individuals
insightless tendency
insight-oriented psychotherapy
insight therapy
insincerity
insomnia
  alcohol-related
  bouts of
  chronic
  cocaine-produced
  drug-dependent
  drug-related
  idiopathic
  initial
  initiating
  maintenance
  middle
  mild
  nonorganic origin
  persistent
  primary
  psychophysiological
  significant
  situational
  sleep disorder
  sleep-onset
  terminal
  transient
  withdrawal
insomnia-type caffeine-induced sleep
  disorder
insomnia-type sleep disorder due to
  GMC (general medical condition)

insomnia-type substance-induced sleep
   disorder
insomniac
insomnic
inspiration
inspiratory capacity (IC)
inspiratory reserve volume (IRV)
inspiratory voice
instability
   affective
   emotional
   family
   job
   marital
instability in interpersonal relationships, pattern of
installation
instantaneous power
"instant zen" (lysergic acid diethylamide)
instinct
   aggressive
   death
   ego
   herd
   life
   mother
   sexual
   social
instinctive
instinctual drives, repressed
Institute for Personality and Ability
   Testing (IPAT)
Institute of Educational Research
   (intelligence) Test (IER test)
Institute of Personality Assessment
   and Research (IPAR)
institution
   marriage
   religious
   treatment
institutional environments

Institutional Functioning Inventory
   (IFI)
Institutional Goals Inventory (IGI)
institutionalized
Instructional Environment Scale, The
   (TIES)
Instructional Leadership Evaluation
   and Development Program
   (ILEAD)
Instructional Leadership Inventory
instructional objective
instrumental ADL measurement
instrumental affair
instrumental case (parts of speech)
instrumental conditioning
instrumental support
instrumental tasks
Instrument Timbre Preference Test
insufficiency
   basilar
   corticoadrenal
   mental
   palatal
   role
   velar
   velopharyngeal
   vertebrobasilar
insufficient nocturnal sleep
insufficient stimulation
insulin coma therapy (ICT)
insulin treatment, subcoma
insult
   CNS (central nervous system)
   nutritional
intact motor function
intact reflexes
intact sensory function
intake worker
intangible benefits of the "sick" role
integrate
Integrated Assessment System (IAS)

Integrated Literature and Language
 Arts Portfolio Program
integrating auditory information with
 motor activity, disturbance in
integrating responses/anchors
integrating tactile information with
 motor activity
integration
 binaural
 competing messages
 ego
 personality
 social
 visual-motor
integrative aspect
integrative language
integrative language processing,
 higher
integrative learning
integrity
integrity of brain function
integrity test, organic [Tien] (OIT)
integumentary system
intellect, structure of (SI)
intellectual ability, impaired
intellectual aphasia
intellectual aura
intellectual capacity
intellectual deterioration
intellectual development
intellectual faculties
intellectual function, discrepant
intellectual functioning
 borderline
 current level of
 discrepant
 general
 generalized
 subaverage
intellectual insight
intellectualization
intellectual resources

intellectual skill
intellectually sharp
intelligence
 above-average
 abstract
 low
 measured
 mechanical
 psychomotor
 social
 superior
intelligence period, sensorimotor
intelligence quotient (IQ)
intelligence scale (see *test*)
intelligence test (see *test*)
intelligibility, speech
intelligibility test (see *test*)
intelligibility threshold
intelligible threshold
intemperance
intense affect
intense autonomic arousal
intense episodic dysphoria
intense intoxication
intense psychological distress
intense relationship
intense sexual behavior
intense sexual fantasies
intense sexual urges
intense wish
intensification, image
intensified action
intensifier, image
intensity, sound
intensive habit pattern
intensive psychotherapy
intensive treatment unit (ITU)
intent
 homicidal
 suicidal
intentional fire setting
intentionally produced symptoms

intentional marker (I marker)
intentional production of symptoms
intentional stereotyped movements
intentional tremor
intention semantics
intention to deceive
intention tremor
interaction
  accelerated
  affective
  communicative
  complementarity of
  drug (DI)
  impaired social
  impairment in reciprocal social
  interpersonal
  occupational
  peer
  sexual
  social
interactional group psychotherapy,
  structured
interactional psychosis, childhood
interactional situation, peer
interaction with the legal system
interactive phenomenon
intercalation
interconsonantal vowel
intercostal muscle
  internal
  external
intercourse
  anal
  sexual
intercurrent anxiety
interdental sound
interdepartmental relations
Interdisciplinary Team (IDT)
interepisode functioning
interepisode recovery, full
interepisode residual symptoms of
  schizophrenia

interest
  cross-gender
  decreased
  loss of
  low sexual
  range of
  stereotyped
interest blank (see *test)*
Interest Check List
interest inventory (see *test)*
interest scale (see *test)*
interest schedule (see *test)*
interest survey (see *test)*
interface
  acoustic
  emotion-cognition
interface disorder
  adjustment
  dissociative
  factitious
  impulse-control
  noise (NIL)
  psychiatric system
  somatoform
  speech (SIL)
interference modification
interference, semantic
intergenerational relations
interhemispheric asymmetry
interictal behavior
interictal period
interinstitutional relations
interior turbinated bone
interiorized stuttering
interjection (parts of speech)
interleaved learning
Intermediate Booklet Category Test
Intermediate Personality Questionnaire
  (IPQ)
intermediate string
intermediate structure
intermission

intermittent aphonia
intermittent explosive behavior
intermittent explosive disorder
intermittent explosive disturbance
intermittent insanity
intermittent melancholia
intermittent pain
intermittent wakefulness
intermixed
internal acoustic meatus
internal auditory canal
internal auditory meatus
internal conflict
internal drive
internal-external control
internal, fixed (FI)
internal intercostal muscle
internalize
internalizing style of conflict resolution
internal juncture
internal speech
internal stimulus
internal stressor
internal stuttering
internal versus external scale
(I-E Scale)
internal world of belief
internal world of expectation
internal world of fantasy
internal world of perception
International Association for the Study of Pain (IASP)
International Classification of Diseases, 9th ed., *Clinical Modification (ICD-9-CM)*
International Classification of Sleep Disorders (ICSD): Diagnostic and Coding Manual
International Fluency Association (IFA)

International Organization for Standardization (ISO)
International Phonetic Alphabet (IPA)
International Phonetic Association
International Primary Factors (test battery) (IPF)
International Society for the Study of Dissociation
International Society for Traumatic Stress Studies
International Standard Manual Alphabet
Iternational Stuttering Association (ISA)
International Test for Aphasia
International Version of the Mental Status Questionnaire
Internet addiction
internship
interoceptive awareness, lack of
interoceptor
interpersonal behavior
Interpersonal Behavior Study (IBS)
Interpersonal Cognitive Problem-Solving (ICPS)
interpersonal conflict
interpersonal control, pattern of
interpersonal dependency
interpersonal difficulty
interpersonal distrust
interpersonal dysfunction
interpersonal effectiveness skills
interpersonal exploitation
interpersonal function
interpersonal functioning
interpersonal interaction
Interpersonal Language Skills Assessment (ILSA), Final Edition
interpersonal loss
interpersonal networks
Interpersonal Perception Scale (IPS)
interpersonal personality traits

interpersonal psychotherapy (IPT)
interpersonal rapport, poor
Interpersonal Reaction Test (IPRT)
interpersonal rejection
    pathological sensitivity to perceived
    perceived
interpersonal relations
interpersonal relationships, disturbed
    (DIR)
interpersonal research orientation
interpersonal responsibilities
interpersonal roles
interpersonal skills
interpersonal spacing (communication
    pattern)
interpersonal strain
interpersonal style, dramatic
Interpersonal Style Inventory
interpersonal withdrawal
Inter-Person Perception Test (IPPT)
"interplanetary mission" (re: crack
    acquisition)
interpretation
    abstract
    differences in
    dream
    personalized
    psychoanalytic
interpretation and treatment, psycho-
    dynamic
interpretation of a perceptual distur-
    bance, delusional
Interpretation of Dreams, The
interpretation of events
interpretation of test results
interpretation test
interpreter role
interprofessional relations
interpsychic relationship
interracial marriage
interrogative sentence
interrupted tracing (I tracing)

interrupter device
interruption of thought
interruptions
    evidence of
    repeated REM-sleep
    speech
interruptus, coitus
intersecting pentagons test, copy
intersensory transfer
intersex
    female
    male
intersex condition
    congenital
    physical
intersexual
intersexuality
interstitial word
interval reinforcement schedule
    fixed
    variable
intervening validity
intervening variable
intervention
    associated
    barriers to
    cognitive-behavioral
    crisis
    evolutionary
    generative
    outpatient
    paradoxical
    pharmacotherapeutic
    psychopharmaceutical
    psychosocial
    remedial
    "stop, look, and listen"
interventions for mental disorders
interview
    Amytal
    barbiturate-facilitated
    clinical

interview *(cont.)*
  hypnotic
  initial
  open-ended
  psychological
  semistructured diagnostic
interviewer
  biased
  unbiased
Interviewer's Guide to the Structured
  Clinical Interview for DSM-IV
  Dissociative Disorders (SCID-D),
  Revised
intervocalic consonant position
intestinal disorder, psychogenic
in-the-ear (ITE) hearing aid
Intimacy Potential Quotient (IPQ)
intimate feelings
intimidating behavior
intimidating others
intolerable
intolerance
  drug
  food
intonation contour
intoxicated, driving while (DWI)
intoxicating vapors, method of inhaling
intoxication
  acute
  alcohol
  alcohol idiosyncratic
  amphetamine
  anticonvulsant
  anxiolytic
  caffeine
  cannabis
  carbon dioxide
  carbon monoxide
  characteristic durations of
  chronic
  cocaine

intoxication *(cont.)*
  glutethimide
  hallucinogen
  hallucinogenic
  hangover effects
  hypnotic
  inhalant
  intense
  manganese
  narcotic chemical
  nicotine
  opioid
  pathological drug
  phencyclidine
  physiological
  sedative
  severe
  signs of alcohol
  substance
  water
intoxication criteria, equivalent
intoxication delirium
  alcohol
  amphetamine
  anxiolytic
  cannabis
  cocaine
  hallucinogen
  hypnotic
  inhalant
  opioid
  phencyclidine
  sedative
  substance
intoxication syndrome
intoxication-type organic psychosis
  alcohol
  drug
Intra- and Interpersonal [Relations
  Scale] (IIP)
intra-aural attenuation
intra-aural reflex

intracerebral hemorrhage
intracorporeal pharmacological testing
intracranial infection organic
    psychosis
intractable pain
intrafamilial conflict
intrafamilial relationships
intramedullary canal
intramuscular (IM or I.M.)
intranasal drug
intraneuronal argentophilic Pick
    inclusion bodies
intransitive verb
intraoral pressure
intrapleural pressure
intrapsychical function
intrapsychic ataxia
intrapsychic conflict
intrapsychic distress
intrapsychic personality traits
intrapulmonic pressure
intrasocial idiocy
intra-subtest variability
intratest scatter
intrathoracic pressure
intravenous (IV or I.V.)
intravenous drug
Intrex Questionnaires
intriguing manner
intrinsic muscles of larynx
intrinsic muscles of tongue
introject
introjection
intropunitive view
introspection
introspective and ruminative
introtensive personality style
introtensive style
introversion, social (SI)
introversive problem-solving style
introversive tendencies
introvert

introverted disorder of adolescence
introverted disorder of childhood
introverted personality
introverted schizoid personality
introverted schizothymia
Introvertive Anhedonia Scale
intruding idea
intrusion, ego-dystonic
intrusion of idiosyncratic material,
    evidence of
intrusion of private material, evidence
    of
intrusive distressing idea
intrusive ideas, persistent
intrusive images, persistent
intrusive impulses, persistent
intrusive quality of obsessions
intrusive recollection
intrusive thoughts, persistent
intrusive urges, persistent
intubation
invalidating environment
invariable behavior
invasion, aggressive
invasive operation
inventory (pl. inventories) (see also
    test)
    academic
    acute panic
    adaptive behavior
    adjustment
    adolescent
    adult personal data
    alcohol use
    anxiety status
    aptitude
    attitude
    behavior
    career
    child abuse
    child care
    child development

inventory *(cont.)*
  clinical
  coping
  counseling
  cultural
  depression
  diagnostic
  eating disorder
  employment
  environmental
  interest
  language
  leadership
  learning
  management
  motivational
  occupational
  parent
  perception
  personality
  picture
  psychological
  reading
  relationship
  risk
  satisfaction
  screening
  self-report personalities
  self-report psychological
  skill
  social stress and functionability
  stress
  suicide
  teacher
  values
  vocational
Inventory for Client and Agency Planning
Inventory for Counseling and Development
Inventory of Individually Perceived Group Cohesiveness

Inventory of Language Abilities and Inventory of Language Abilities II (ILA, ILA-II)
inventory of loss
Inventory of Peer Influence on Eating Concerns
Inventory of Perceptual Skills (IPS)
Inventory of Psychosocial Development (IPD)
inverse feedback
inverse-square law
inversion
invert
investigation, principal
in vivo benzodiazepine receptor binding
in vivo magnetic resonance spectroscopy in psychiatric brain disorders
involuntary commitment
involuntary hospitalization
involuntary motion
involuntary movement
involuntary movement disorder, abnormal (AIMD)
involuntary movement scale, abnormal (AIMS)
involuntary pauses in speech
involuntary retention
involuntary speech elements
involuntary state of trance
involuntary twitch/twitching
involuntary whispering
involuntomotor
involution
involutional depression
involutional melancholia
involutional paranoid state
involutional paraphrenia
involutional psychosis
  affective
  depressive
  paranoid

involutional reaction
  melancholic
  paranoid
  psychotic
Inwald Personality Inventory (IPI),
  Revised
iodine (I)
iodine-123-labeled cocaine analog
  (^{123}beta-CIT)
iodine-123-labeled iomazenil
  (^{123}I iomazenil)
ion
  negative
  positive
iophobia
Iowa Algebra Aptitude Test, Fourth
  Edition (IAAT)
Iowa Conners Rating Scale
Iowa Pressure Articulation Test
  (IPAT)
Iowa's Severity Rating Scales for
  Speech and Language Impairments
Iowa Tests of Basic Skills, Forms G
  and H
Iowa Tests of Educational Develop-
  ment, Forms X-8 and Y-8
IPA (International Phonetic Alphabet)
IPAT (Iowa Pressure Articulation
  Test)
IPAT Anxiety Scale
IPAT Depression Scale
IPD (incurable problem drinker)
IPD (Inventory of Psychosocial
  Development)
IPF (International Primary Factors
  [test battery])
IPI (Inwald Personality Inventory
  [Revised])
I.P.I. Aptitude-Intelligence Test Series
IPPT (Inter-Person Perception Test)
IPQ (Intermediate Personality
  Questionnaire)

IPQ (Intimacy Potential Quotient)
IPRT (Interpersonal Reaction Test)
IPS (Interpersonal Perception Scale)
IPS (Inventory of Perceptual Skills)
ipsilateral cerebellar ataxia
ipsilateral frontal routing of signals
  (IFROS)
ipsilateral headache
ipsilateral loss
ipsilateral palsy
ipsilateral routing of signals (IROS)
IPT (interpersonal psychotherapy)
IQ (Intelligence Quotient) score
  full-scale
  performance
  verbal
irascible
irascibility
irate
IRI (Burns/Roe Informal Reading
  Inventory: Preprimer to Twelfth
  Grade, Third Edition)
Irish Study of High-Density
  Schizophrenia Families
irony (figure of speech)
IROS (ipsilateral routing of signals)
irradiation-induced mental deterioration
irrational behavior
irrational fear
irrationality
irreconcilable
irregular movement
irregular sleep patterns
irregular sleep-wake pattern
irrelevancy
irrelevant speech
irrelevant stimuli, screen out
irresistible impulse
irresistible impulse test
irresponsibility, consistent
irresponsible work behavior

irreverent communication
irreversible coma
irritability
    electric
    feelings of
    marked
    myotatic
irritable mood, prominent
irritation
IRT (item response theory)
IRV (inspiratory reserve volume)
ISA (International Stuttering Association)
ischemia-type organic psychosis, cerebrovascular
ischemic attack, transient (TIA)
"Isda" (heroin)
ISDB (indirect self-destructive behavior)
island of control
ISO (International Organization for Standardization)
isobutyl nitrate inhalant
isobutyl nitrite (street names)
    aroma of men
    hardware
    quicksilver
    rush snappers
    thrust
    whiteout
isochronal
isogloss
isoglosses, bundle of
isolated, emotionally
isolated explosive disorder
isolated explosive disturbance

isolated phobia
isolate, social (noun)
isolation aphasia
isolation of affect
isolation, social
isolation syndrome
isolative behavior
isophilic
isopterophobia
isotope cisternography
"issues" (crack)
issues
    inner child
    preexisting underlying emotional
    to process
    reality
"I" statements
Is This Autism? A Checklist of Behaviors and Skills for Children Showing Autistic Features
isthmus of fauces
IT (individual therapy)
Italomania
"itchlike" sensation of the scalp
item response theory (IRT)
ITERS (Infant/Toddler Environment Rating Scale)
I-Thou
ITPA (Illinois Test of Psycholinguistic Abilities)
I tracing (interrupted tracing)
ITSC (It Scale for Children)
It Scale for Children (ITSC)
ITU (intensive treatment unit)
IV or I.V. (intravenous)
IWB (Index of Well-Being)

J, j

"J" (cannabis cigarette)
J (joule)
jabbing pain
"jab/job" (re: drug injection)
"jack" (re: to steal drugs)
"jackpot" (fentanyl)
Jackson epilepsy
Jackson Evaluation System
jacksonian convulsion
jacksonian epilepsy
jacksonian seizure
Jackson Personality Inventory (JPI)
Jackson syndrome
Jackson Vocational Interest Survey
    (JVIS)
"jack-up" (re: drug injection)
jactitation
"jag" (re: drug influence)
Jakob-Creutzfeldt disease, dementia in
Jakob-Creutzfeldt disease organic
    psychosis
"jam" (amphetamine; cocaine)
"jam cecil" (amphetamine)
jamais vu
jamais vu aura
James Language Dominance Test
"Jane" (cannabis)

Janet disease
Janet, Pierre (1859-1947)
Jansky Screening Index (JSI)
Japanophobia
jargon agraphia
jargon aphasia
jargon paraphasia, extended
JAS (Jenkins Activity Survey)
JAS (Job Attitude Scale)
jaw-closing muscle reflexes
jaw dysfunction stuttering
"jay" (cannabis cigarette)
"jay smoke" (cannabis)
JBC (Jesness Behavior Checklist)
JCAHO (Joint Commission on
    Accreditation of Healthcare
    Organizations)
JDI (Job Descriptive Index)
jealous-type delusions
jealous-type schizophrenia
jealousy
    alcoholic
    delusion of
    delusional
    morbid
    sibling
"jee gee" (heroin)

"Jefferson Airplane" (re: cannabis
equipment)
"jellies" (barbiturate; temazepam)
"jelly" (cocaine)
"jelly baby" (amphetamine)
"jelly beans" (amphetamine sulfate;
crack)
Jenkins Activity Survey (JAS)
Jenkins Non-Verbal Test
JEPI (Junior Eysenck Personality
Inventory)
jerking movement
Jesness Behavior Checklist (JBC)
Jesness Inventory (JI)
"jet" (ketamine)
"jet fuel" (phencyclidine)
jet lag
jet lag-type dyssomnia
Jette Functional Status Index
Jevs Work Sample Battery
Jewett wave
Jezebel
JI (Jesness Inventory)
"Jim Jones" (cannabis laced with
cocaine and phencyclidine)
JIRI (Johnston Informal Reading
Inventory)
jitter, frequency
jittery
"jive" (cannabis; heroin)
"jive doo jee" (heroin)
"jive stick" (cannabis)
JKST (Johnson-Kenney Screening
Test)
JLO (Judgment of Line Orientation)
JND (just noticeable difference)
Job Attitude Scale (JAS)
Job Descriptive Index (JDI)
job-related hearing loss
job satisfaction
Job Seeking Skills Assessment
Jocasta complex

jock
"Johnson" (crack)
Johnson-Kenney Screening Test (JKST)
Johnston Informal Reading Inventory
(JIRI)
joint
cricoarytenoid
temporomandibular (TMJ)
"joint" (cannabis)
Joint Commission on Accreditation of
Healthcare Organizations (JCAHO)
Joint Commission on Mental Health of
Children
Joint Commission on Mental Illness and
Health
joint custody
joint disorder, psychogenic
joint syndrome, temporomandibular
"jojee" (heroin)
"jolly bean" (amphetamine)
"jolly green" (cannabis)
"jolly pop" (re: heroin user)
"jolt" (re: drug injection; drug reaction)
JOMACI (judgment, orientation,
memory, abstraction, and calculation
intact)
Jonah words
"Jones" (heroin)
Jones, Ernest (1879-1958)
"Jonesing" (re: needing drugs)
Jordan Left-Right Reversal Test
Joseph Pre-School and Primary Self-
Concept Screening Test
joule (J)
journaling exercise
"joy flakes" (heroin)
"joy juice" (barbiturate)
"joy plant" (opium)
"joy pop" (re: drug injection)
"joy popping" (re: drug use)
"joy powder" (cocaine; heroin)
"joy smoke" (cannabis)

"joy stick" (cannabis cigarette)
JPI (Jackson Personality Inventory)
JSI (Jansky Screening Index)
"Juan Valdez" (cannabis)
"Juanita" (cannabis)
Judaeophobia
Judeophobia
judgment
    clinical
    diagnostic
    faulty
    impaired
    lack of
    negative
    poor
    social
    value
judgment and insight
Judgment of Line Orientation (JLO)
Judgment of Occupational Behavior-
    Orientation
judgment, orientation, memory,
    abstraction, and calculation intact
    (JOMACI)
judgment score, practical social
Judophobia
"juggle" (re: drug dealing)
"juggler" (re: drug dealer)
"jugs" (amphetamine)
"juice" (steroids, phencyclidine)
"juice joint" (cannabis cigarette
    sprinkled with crack)

"ju-ju" (cannabis cigarette)
"jum" (re: crack container)
jumbling of teeth
"jumbos" (re: crack containers)
jumpy
junction, pharyngoesophageal (PE)
junctural feature
juncture
    closed
    internal
    open
    plus
    terminal
Jung, Carl Gustav (1875-1961)
jungian psychoanalysis
jungian theory
Jung method
Junior Eysenck Personality Inventory
    (JEPI)
"junk" (heroin)
"junkie" (drug addict)
justifiable reaction
just noticeable difference (JND)
juvenile delinquent
juvenile fire setting
juvenile idiocy
juvenile neurotic delinquency
juvenile papillomatosis
JVIS (Jackson Vocational Interest
    Survey)

K, k

"K" (phencyclidine)
KAB (knowledge, attitude, behavior)
"kabayo" (heroin)
KABC (Kaufman Assessment Battery
　for Children)
"Kabuki" (re: crack equipment)
Kahn Intelligence Tests (KIT)
Kahn Test of Symbol Arrangement
　(KTSA)
kainomania
kainophobia
KAIT (Kaufman Adolescent and Adult
　Intelligence Test)
kakorrhaphiophobia
"Kaksonjae" (smokable methampheta-
　mine)
"Kali" (cannabis)
Kalmuk idiocy
"kangaroo" (crack)
Kanner syndrome
kappa opiate receptors
kappa receptors
"kaps" (phencyclidine)
"Karachi" (heroin)
KAS (Katz Adjustment Scales)
Kasanin-Hanfmann Concept Formation
　Test

KAST (Kindergarten Auditory
　Screening Test)
katagelophobia
kathisomania
kathisophobia
Katz Adjustment Scales (KAS)
Katz ADL Index
Kaufman Adolescent and Adult
　Intelligence Test (KAIT)
Kaufman Assessment Battery for
　Children (KABC)
Kaufman Brief Intelligence Test
　(K-BIT)
Kaufman Development Scale
Kaufman Infant and Preschool Scale
Kaufman Survey of Early Academic
　and Language Skills (K-SEALS)
Kaufman Test of Education Achieve-
　ment
"kaya" (cannabis)
K-BIT (Kaufman Brief Intelligence
　Test)
"K-blast" (phencyclidine)
kc (kilocycle)
KCI (Kolbe Conative Index)
K-complex
K-corrected raw score

Keegan Type Indicator
Keirsey Temperament Sorter
Kendrick Cognitive Tests for the
  Elderly
Kenny ADL Index
Kenny Self-Care Evaluation
Kenny Self-Care Questionnaire
kenophobia
Kent Infant Development Scale
"Kentucky blue" (cannabis)
keraunophobia
Kerby Learning Modality Test,
  Revised
kernel sentence
ketamine (street names)
  cat valium
  green
  honey oil
  jet
  purple
  special "K"
  special la coke
  super acid
  super C
keyed up, feeling
Key, Fitzgerald
KeyMath Revised: A Diagnostic Inventory of Essential Mathematics
key word method
KFD (Kinetic Family Drawings)
"KGB" (killer green bud) (cannabis)
"khat" (narcotic)
Khatena-Torrance Creative Perception
  Inventory
"K-hole" (ketamine-induced confusion)
K-hole (effect of "Special K")
"Kibbles & Bits" (small crumbs of
  crack)
"kick" (inhalant; re: drug withdrawal)
"kick stick" (cannabis cigarette)
"kiddie dope" (prescription drugs)

kidnapping
"kif" (cannabis)
killer
  serial
  serial sexual
"killer" (cannabis; phencyclidine)
killer cults
"killer weed" (cannabis; phencyclidine)
"kilo" (2.2 pounds)
kilocycle (kc)
"kilter" (cannabis)
"kind" (cannabis)
Kindergarten Auditory Screening Test
  (KAST)
Kindergarten Language Screening Test
  (KLST)
Kindergarten Readiness Test (KRT)
kinesic gestures
kinesics
kinesigenic ataxia
kinesiology
kinesis
kinesomania
kinesthesia
kinesthesis
kinesthetic analysis
kinesthetic aura
kinesthetic cue
kinesthetic feedback
kinesthetic hallucination
kinesthetic method
kinesthetic perception, tactile
kinesthetic sense
kinesthetic technique
kinetic analysis
kinetic energy
Kinetic Family Drawings (KFD)
kinetics
kinetic tremor
"king ivory" (fentanyl)
"King Kong pills" (barbiturate)
"king's habit" (cocaine)

kinky hair disease
Kirkbridge, Thomas S. (1809-1883)
KIT (Kahn Intelligence Tests)
"kit" (re: drug injection paraphernalia)
"KJ" (phencyclidine)
"Kleenex" (methylenedioxymethamphetamine)
Klein's death wish
Kleine-Levin syndrome
Klein, Melanie (1882-1960)
Klein suffocation alarm theory
kleptolagnia
kleptomania
kleptophobia
Klinefelter syndrome
"Klingons" (crack addicts)
klismaphilia
KLST (Kindergarten Language Screening Test)
Klüver-Bucy syndrome
knowledge, attitude, behavior (KAB)
knowledge, linguistic
Knowledge of Occupations Test (KOT)
Knox's Cube Test
Kohs Block Design
KOIS (Kuder Occupational Interest Survey)
Kojevnikoff epilepsy
"Kokomo" (crack)
Kolbe Conative Index (KCI)
"koller joints" (phencyclidine)
koniophobia
"kools" (phencyclidine)
kopophobia
Koppitz Scoring System for Organicity
koro (culture-specific syndrome)
Korsakoff amnesia
Korsakoff amnesic

Korsakoff disease
Korsakoff psychosis
alcoholic
nonalcoholic
Korsakoff syndrome
Koshevnikoff (see *Kojevnikoff*)
Koshevnikoff epilepsy
KOT (Knowledge of Occupations Test)
KPR-V (Kuder Preference Record-Vocational)
Krabbe's disease
Kraepelin, Emil (1865-1926)
kraepelinian view of psychosis
Kretschmer, Ernest (1888-1964)
Kretschmer types
KRT (Kindergarten Readiness Test)
"Kryptonite" (crack)
"krystal" (phencyclidine)
"krystal joint" (phencyclidine)
K-SEALS (Kaufman Survey of Early Academic and Language Skills)
KTSA (Kahn Test of Symbol Arrangement)
Kuder General Interest Survey, Form E
Kuder Occupational Interest Survey (KOIS)
Kuder Preference Record-Vocational (KPR-V)
Kufs disease
"Kumba" (cannabis)
Kuru
Kussmaul aphasia
"KW" (phencyclidine)
Kwell bath
kymogram
kymograph
kynophobia

L, l

"L" (lysergic acid diethylamide; LSD)
LA (long-acting; low anxiety)
lab (laboratory)
LAB (Leisure Activities Blank)
labeling
la belle indifférence
labial cleft
labile affect
labile emotionality
labile mood
labile personality disorder
labile range of affect
labile-type personality disorder
lability
   affective
   emotional
   mood
labiodental area consonant placement
labioglossolaryngeal paralysis
labioglossopharyngeal paralysis
labioversion
labioversion of teeth
labored speech
labyrinth
   bony
   membranous
   osseous

labyrinthine aplasia
labyrinthine deafness
labyrinthine disorder, acute
labyrinthine hydrops
labyrinthine vertigo
"lace" (cocaine and cannabis)
lacrimal bone
lacrimal skull bone
LACT (Lindamood Auditory
   Conceptualization Test)
lacunaire, etat (multiple small strokes)
lacunar amnesia
lacunar dementia
lacunar infarct
lacunar state
lacunar stroke
lacunar syndrome
LAD (language acquisition device)
ladder, abstraction
"lady" (cocaine)
"lady caine" (cocaine)
"lady snow" (cocaine)
lag
   initial
   jet
   maturational
   terminal

"L.A. glass" (smokable methamphetamine)
"L.A. ice" (smokable methamphetamine)
laissez-faire (leadership pattern)
"lakbay diva" (cannabis)
laliophobia
lalling
lalochezia
lalognosis
lalomania
laloneurosis
lalopathology
lalopathy
lalophobia
lalorrhea
lambdacism
Lambeth Disability Screening
    Questionnaire
"Lamborghini" (re: crack equipment)
laminograph
Landau-Kleffner syndrome (acquired
    epileptic aphasia)
Langat viral encephalitis
language
    American Indian Sign (Amerind)
    American Sign (ASL) (Ameslan)
    automatic
    body
    common
    confused
    daughter
    delayed
    deviant
    dominant
    egocentric
    emergent
    emotive
    executive
    expressive
    female
    first

language *(cont.)*
    gesture
    home
    imaginary
    impaired
    implicit
    inner
    integrative
    native
    negotiating
    nonspecific
    nonstandard
    oral
    organ
    parent
    pattern of
    primary
    receptive
    reduced body
    school
    sign
    source
    standard
    subcultural
    substandard
    syntaxic
    target
    true
    twin
    unknown
    vulgar
    written
language abilities
language acquisition device (LAD)
language and communication
    distortion of
    exaggeration of
language area
language areas of brain, mapping of
language arts
language barrier
language boundary

language change
language center
language comprehension and production
language content
language deficit, central
language development
  expressive
  receptive
  slow rate of
language development disorder, expressive
language difference
language difficulties
language disabilities
language disorder
  central (CLD)
  expressive
  mixed receptive-expressive
  receptive
  schizophrenic speech and
  speech and
language disorder in dementia
language disorders in psychiatry, speech and
language disturbance
language dysfunction
language empiricist theory
language faculty
language form
language formulation
language function
language imbalance
language impairment
language innateness theory
language in schizophrenia
  distorted
  exaggerated
language innateness theory
language-learning environment
language learning theory
Language Modalities Test for Aphasia

language of lying
language problem
  expressive
  receptive
language processing
  higher integrative
  input receptive
language-processing quotient, receptive
Language Processing Test
language purists
language quotient
  adolescent
  expressive
  grammar
  listening
  reading
  spoken
  verbal
  vocabulary
  written
language retardation, idiopathic
Language Sampling, Analysis, and Training
language scale (see *test*)
language screening (see *test*)
language skills learning retardation
language spoken at home (communication pattern)
language spoken outside home (communication pattern)
language structure
Language-Structured Auditory Retention Span (LARS)
language syndrome, confused (CLS)
language tests and procedures
language theory, biolinguistic
language therapist
language universals
language use
lapse of awareness
lapses in hygiene

LARS (Language-Structured Auditory
    Retention Span)
larval epilepsy
laryngeal anesthesia
laryngeal anomaly
laryngeal atresia
laryngeal cancer
laryngeal dysarthria
laryngeal dyskinesia
laryngeal epilepsy
laryngeal fissure
laryngeal hyperesthesia
laryngeal motor paralysis
laryngeal oscillation
laryngeal paralysis, bilateral
laryngeal paresthesia
laryngeal-pharyngeal spasm
laryngeal prominence
laryngeal psychophysiologic reaction
laryngeal reflex
laryngeal respiration
laryngeal sensory paralysis
laryngeal stuttering
laryngeal tension
laryngeal trauma
laryngeal web
laryngectomy
    anterior partial
    frontolateral
    subtotal
    total
larynges (see *larynx*)
laryngismus
laryngitic
laryngitis
    acute
    chronic
    chronic subglottic
    croupous
    hyperplastic
    membranous
    spasmodic
    stridulous

laryngocele
laryngograph
laryngology
laryngomalacia
laryngoparalysis
laryngopathy
laryngophantom
laryngopharyngeal
laryngopharyngectomy
laryngopharyngitis
laryngopharynx
laryngophony
laryngophthisis
laryngoplasty
laryngoplegia
laryngoptosis
laryngorhinology
laryngoscope
laryngoscopy
    direct
    indirect
    suspension
laryngospasm
laryngostenosis
laryngostomy
laryngostroboscope
laryngotome
laryngotomy
    inferior
    median
    superior
laryngotracheal
laryngotracheitis
laryngotracheobronchitis
laryngotracheotomy
laryngoxerosis
larynx (pl. larynges)
    blunt trauma to
    cysts of
    electrical artificial
    electronic artificial
    malignant neoplasm of

larynx *(cont.)*
  pneumatic artificial
  reed artificial
  ventricular
larynx muscles
  extrinsic
  intrinsic
"las mujercitas" (psilocybin)
Lasègue disease
Lasègue sign
LAS-O (Language Assessment
  Scales–Oral)
"lason sa daga" (lysergic acid diethylamide)
LASS (Linguistic Analysis of Speech
  Samples)
LASSI (Learning and Study Strategies
  Inventory)
latah (culture-specific syndrome)
late adolescence
late-age trauma and posttraumatic
  stress disorder
late life
late-life migraine headache
late luteal phase dysphoric disorder
late luteal phase of menstrual cycle
late onset of schizophrenia
late paraphrenia
late speech development
late traumatic epilepsy
latency
  mean sleep
  prolonged sleep
  reduced rapid eye movement
  reflex
  short sleep
  short REM
  sleep
latency period
latency period psychosexual development
latency phase

latency responses
  long
  middle
latent class analysis
latent content
latent epilepsy
latent homosexuality
latent learning
latent meaning
latent response
latent schizophrenia
latent schizophrenic reaction
lateral adenoidectomy
lateral canal
lateral consonant formation
  dark
  light
lateral cricoarytenoid muscle
lateral dominance
lateral gaze palsy
lateral incisor teeth
laterality
  crossed
  mixed
Laterality Preference Schedule
laterality theory of stuttering
lateralization, cortical
lateralized dysfunction
lateralizing abnormalities
lateral lisp
lateral occipital sulcus
lateral sulcus
lateral trim of adenoid
"Latin lettuce" (cannabis)
latissimus dorsi muscle
"laugh and scratch" (re: drug injection)
"laughing gas" (nitrous oxide)
"laughing grass" (cannabis)
"laughing weed" (cannabis)
law
  Bernoulli
  Fourier

law *(cont.)*
  inverse-square
  Ohm
  Semon
  Semon-Rosenbach
  talion (or talion principle)
LAW R/W (Language Assessment Scales, Reading and Writing)
lawful behavior
laws of cause and effect
laxative abuse
"laxative habit" abuse
lax consonant
lax phoneme
lax toilet training
lax vowel
"lay back" (barbiturate)
"lay-out" (re: drug equipment)
LBAII (Leader Behavior Analysis II)
LBDQ (Leader Behavior Description Questionnaire)
"LBJ" (heroin; lysergic acid diethylamide; phencyclidine)
LCT (Listening Comprehension Test)
LCU (life change units)
LD (learning disabled)
LD (lithium discontinuation)
LDES (Learning Disability Evaluation Scale)
L-dopa, on-off effect of
leaden paralysis
Leader Behavior Analysis II (LBAII)
Leader Behavior Description Questionnaire (LBDQ)
leaderless group discussion (LGD)
leader role
Leadership Ability Evaluation
leadership behavior
Leadership Evaluation and Development Scale (LEADS)
Leadership Opinion Questionnaire (LOQ)

leadership pattern
  authoritarian
  democratic
  laissez-faire
  power struggle
leadership potential
Leadership Practices Inventory (LPI)
leadership role
Leadership Skills Inventory
leader, team (TL)
leading
"lead-pipe" rigidity
lead poisoning
lead system
LEADS (Leadership Evaluation and Development Scale)
"leaf" (cannabis; cocaine)
"leaky bolla" (phencyclidine)
"leaky leak" (phencyclidine)
"leapers" (amphetamine)
"leaping" (re: drug influence)
Lear complex
learned drive
learned dysfunctional behavior
learned helplessness
learning
  associate
  association
  avoidance
  critical period of
  discrimination
  escape
  incidental
  integrative
  interleaved
  latent
  maze
  operant
  paired associate
  passive
  probability
  problem-based

learning *(cont.)*
  reversal
  rote
  serial
  serial list
  verbal
learning ability
  impaired
  general (G)
Learning and Study Strategies Inventory (LASSI)
learning aptitude
learning aptitude test
learning cues
learning defect
learning development disorder
learning difficulties
learning disability
Learning Disability Evaluation Scale (LDES)
Learning Disability Rating Procedure
learning disabled (LD)
  emotionally disturbed (ED/LD)
  psychogenic
learning disorder
Learning Efficiency Test-II (LET-II)
learning information
Learning Inventory of Kindergarten Experiences (LIKE)
learning new information
learning problems, developmental (DLP)
learning retardation
  arithmetical
  language
  reading
Learning Style Profile (LSP)
Learning Styles Inventory
learning test (see *test*)
learning theory
  language
  social

learning theory of stuttering
Least Preferred Coworker Score
leather restraints
Leatherman Leadership Questionnaire (LLQ)
leave
  absent without (AWOL)
  unauthorized (UL)
leaving parental control problem
"Lebanese red" (cannabis)
LEC (Life Experiences Checklist)
Leeds Scales for the Self-Assessment of Anxiety and Depression
left bundle branch block
left hemisphere dominance
left-out sibling profile
left/right hemisphere dominance
legal action
legal aspects of assaultive client care
legal aspects of dementia
legal contract
legal counselor
legal psychiatry
legal responsibilities
legal sanctions
"legal speed" (over-the-counter asthma drug)
legal system
leisure activities
Leisure Activities Blank (LAB)
leisure awareness
Leisure Diagnostic Battery, The
leisure skills
Leiter Adult Intelligence Scale
Leiter International Performance Scale
Leiter Recidivism Scale
"lemon 714" (phencyclidine)
"lemonade" (heroin; poor quality drugs)
Lengthened-Off-Time (LOT)
length, mean sentence (MSL)
length of response

length of stay (LOS)
length of utterance
lenis consonant
lenis phoneme
Lennon-Gastaut (petit mal variant)
   seizure
"lens" (lysergic acid diethylamide)
lenticular aphasia
lepraphobia
lesbian
lesbianism
Lesch-Nyhan syndrome
lesion
   brain
   brain stem
   callosal
   cerebral
   keratotic
LET-II (Learning Efficiency Test-II)
lethal catatonia
"lethal weapon" (phencyclidine)
lethargic patient
lethargy
   hysteric
   induced
letheomania
lethica, aphasia
lethologica
"Let's Talk" Inventory for Adolescents
letter cancellation test
letter dysgnosia, visual
letter reversal
letter symbols
letter-word identification
"lettuce" (re: currency)
"lettuce opium" (narcotic)
leukodystrophy, metachromatic
leukoencephalopathy, progressive
   multifocal
level (pl. levels)
   action
   activity

level *(cont.)*
   alcohol
   alertness
   anxiety
   aspiration
   automatic phrase
   blood
   blood alcohol
   cognitive impairment
   cohesiveness
   conflict
   current defense
   defense
   defensive dysregulation
   demarcation in sensory testing
   denervation
   desire
   difficulty
   disability
   disavowal
   discomfort
   drug
   effort
   engagement
   functioning
   GGT
   hearing (LH)
   hearing threshold (HTL)
   high adaptive
   high energy
   hormonal
   image-distorting
   intellectual functioning
   intoxication
   loudness
   low educational
   mental inhibition
   noise interference (NIL)
   occupational functioning
   operant
   overall sound
   peak and trough
   perceived noise (PNdB)

level *(cont.)*
  predominant defense
  psychopathology
  reference zero
  resistance
  saturation sound pressure (SSPL)
  sensation (SL)
  sensory
  sensory loss
  serotonin
  serum calcium
  significance
  social functioning
  society
  sound
  speech interference (SIL)
  tolerance
  toxic
  uncomfortable loudness (UCL)
  zero hearing
leveling, dialect
level of consciousness
  altered
  change in
Level of Psychosocial Stress (Axis IV)
level tone
Levine-Pilowsky Depression Questionnaire
levophobia
Lewin, Kurt (1890-1946)
Lewy body disease
Lewy body variant of Alzheimer
  disease
lexical agraphia
lexical ambiguity
lexical categories
lexical concepts
lexical gap
lexical measuring
lexical memory
lexical morpheme
lexical paraphrases

lexical word
lexicography
lexicon
Leyton Obsessive Inventory (LOI)
LF (low frequency)
LFF (low filter frequency)
LGD (leaderless group discussion)
liaison
liar, pathological
"lib" (Librium)
libidinal energy
libidinous
libido
  bisexual
  diminished
  ego
  normal (NL)
  object
libido theory
licensed psychologist
Licensed Vocational Nurse (LVN)
licensing board
Lichtheim aphasia
"licorice" (tincture of opium)
"lid" (1 ounce of cannabis)
"lid poppers" (amphetamine)
lid tic, transient disorder of childhood
lie detection
lie, living a
Liepmann apraxia
life
  adult
  enjoyment of
  everyday
  family
  impoverished fantasy
  inner
  late
  later in
  loss of
  ordinary demands of
  satisfaction with

life *(cont.)*
  sexual
  sheltered
  the time of your
  vegetative
  viscissitudes of
life activity, major
life change
  affectional
  biophysical
  major
  socioeconomic
life change events
life change units (LCU)
life circumstance problem
life circumstances
  altered
  difficult
life-cycle adjustment
life-cycle change
life-cycle transition
life difficulties
Life Event Scale Adolescents
Life Event Scale Children
Life Experiences Checklist (LEC)
life experience, stressful
life history
life instinct
Life Interpersonal History Enquiry
  (LIPHE)
life lie
lifelong sexual dysfunction
lifelong-type dyspareunia
lifelong-type female orgasmic disorder
lifelong-type female sexual arousal
  disorder
lifelong-type hypoactive sexual desire
  disorder
lifelong-type male erectile disorder
lifelong-type male orgasmic disorder
lifelong-type sexual aversion disorder
lifelong-type vaginismus

Life Satisfaction Index (LSI)
Life Skills, Forms 1 & 2
Life Skills Program
life span
life stress
life's stressors
lifestyle
  inferior sibling
  sedentary
Life Styles Inventory (LSI)
life-threatening disease
life-threatening illness
life-threatening medical condition
lifetime history
lift, palatal
Lifwynn Foundation
ligand, free
ligand-gated receptor
light, cone of
light drinking
lighter fluid (sniffing) dependence
light lateral consonant formation
"lightning" (amphetamine)
"light stuff" (cannabis)
light therapy
light therapy-induced mood disorder
light touch sensation
light treatment for winter depression
light voice
light vowel
likability, peer
likable or likeable
LIKE (Learning Inventory of Kindergarten Experiences)
lilliputian hallucination
"lilly" (amobarbital)
"Lima" (cannabis)
limb (pl. limbs)
  abnormal positioning of distal
  phantom
limb disorder
limbic dysregulation

limbic forebrain
limbic system disorders
"lime acid" (lysergic acid diethylamide)
limen, difference (DL)
limitations, functional (emotional problems)
limited activity
limited diet
limited-range audiometry
limited speech
limited support
limited-symptom attacks
limited to pain
limiter, noise
limit-setting for adolescents
limit-testing behavior
limits
    to follow
    to press
    within normal (WNL)
limnophobia
Limon Self-Image Assessment
Lincoln-Oseretsky Motor Development Scale
Lincoln-Oseretsky Motor Performance Test (LOMPT)
Lindamood Auditory Conceptualization Test (LACT)
"line" (cocaine)
linear thought processes
lingua-alveolar area
lingua-alveolar area consonant placement
linguadental area consonant placement
lingua franca
lingual airway dysfunction
lingual frenum
lingual hypoplasia
lingual lisp
lingual paralysis
lingual raphe

lingual sulcus
    medial
    median
linguist
Linguistic Analysis of Speech Samples (LASS)
linguistic aspects
Linguistic Awareness in Reading Readiness
linguistic borrowing
linguistic competence
linguistic deficit
linguistic determinism
linguistic disorganization
linguistic disorganization in schizophrenia
linguistic knowledge
linguistic mechanisms
linguistic performance
linguistic phonetics
linguistic relativity
linguistic retention
linguistics
    comparative
    contrastive
    descriptive
    diachronic
    sign
    structural
    synchronic
    theoretical
linguistic savant
linguistic set of disturbances
linguistic skills, impaired
linguistic stimulation
linguistic universals theory
linguistic variation
linguodental area
linguoversion of teeth
linkage study, genetic
link, causal

linking verb
linonophobia
lip
  bilateral cleft
  median cleft
  unilateral cleft
lip dysfunction stuttering
LIPHE (Life Interpersonal History Enquiry)
lipidosis, cerebral
lipoid metabolism
lipreading
lipreading aural rehabilitation
lip rounded vowel
lip rounding
lip smacking
lip tremor
"Lipton tea" (poor quality drugs)
liquid consonant formation
liquid, gliding of
liquid sounds
lisp
  dental
  frontal
  lateral
  lingual
  nasal
  occluded
  protrusion
  strident
lisping
list (see *test*)
Lista de Destrezas en Desarrollo (La Lista)
listening
  dichotic
  diotic
  selective
  visual
Listening Comprehension Test (LCT)
listening language quotient
listening tasks, dichotic

list learning, serial
listless
listlessness
literacy, visual
literal agraphia
literal meaning
literal paraphasia
lithium
  cellular effects of
  clinical action of
  therapeutic action of
  toxic action of
lithium action on first messengers
lithium action on membranes
lithium action on second messengers
lithium discontinuation (LD)
lithium-induced postural tremor
lithium therapy
lithium toxicity
lithium tremor
  nontoxic
  toxic
litigious paranoia
litotes (figure of speech)
"little bomb" (amphetamine; barbiturate; heroin)
"little ones" (phencyclidine)
little sense of other people's boundaries
"little smoke" (cannabis; psilocybin/psilocin)
"lit up" (re: drug influence)
"live ones" (phencyclidine)
liver-disease-type organic psychosis, alcoholic
liver function tests
live voice audiometry
living
  activities of daily (ADL)
  daily
  group
  independent

living *(cont.)*
  normal activities of daily
  simulated activities of daily (SADL)
  standard of
living a lie
living in a crime-ridden neighborhood
living in a dream world
living in the opposite sex role
living skills, activities of daily (ADLS)
"L.L." (cannabis)
"llesca" (cannabis)
LLQ (Leatherman Leadership Questionnaire)
LNNB (Luria-Nebraska Neuropsychological Battery)
LOA (loosening of associations)
"load" (25 bags of heroin)
"loaded" (re: drug influence)
"loaf" (cannabis)
loan word
loathsome
lobe
  frontal
  occipital
  parietal
  temporal
lobe dysfunction
  contralateral parietal
  frontal
  parietal
"lobo" (cannabis)
lobotomy
  frontal
  prefrontal
lobotomy syndrome
loc (level of consciousness)
LOC (Locus of Control)
LOC-C (Locus of Control-Chance)
LOC-E (Locus of Control-External)
LOC-I (Locus of Control-Internal)
LOC-PO (Locus of Control-Powerful Others)

local convulsion
localization
  auditory
  cerebral
  sound
localized amnesia
localized epilepsy
localized weakness
locative case (parts of speech)
locked hospital unit
locked in state
locked seclusion
"locker room" (butyl nitrite)
locomotion
locomotor ataxia
"locoweed" (cannabis)
locus
locus ceruleus neurons
Locus of Control (LOC)
Locus of Control-Chance (LOC-C)
Locus of Control-External (LOC-E)
Locus of Control-Internal (LOC-I)
Locus of Control-Powerful Others
  (LOC-PO)
locutions
Loevinger's Washington University
  Sentence Completion Test
loft register
"log" (cannabis cigarette; phencyclidine)
logagnosia
logagraphia
logamnesia
logaphasia
logasthenia
log, drug information (DIL)
logic
  perverted
  trance
logical memory test
logical operations
logoclonia

logographic
logokophosis
logomania
logoneurosis
logophobia
"Logor" (lysergic acid diethylamide)
logorrhea
logospasm
logotherapy
LOI (Leyton Obsessive Inventory)
Lollipop Test: A Diagnostic Screening
    Test of School Readiness
Lombard Test
LOMPT (Lincoln-Oseretsky Motor
    Performance Test)
London Psychogeriatric Scale (LPS)
loneliness
    deep-seated
    fear of
    feelings of
loner, psychological
long-acting drug (LA)
long-half-life anxiolytic substances
longitudinal cerebral fissure
longitudinal evaluation
longitudinal (experimental study
    designs)
Longitudinal Interval Follow-Up
    Evaluation
longitudinal mental status examination
longitudinal muscle of tongue
    inferior
    superior
longitudinal observation
longitudinal raphe, median
longitudinal wave
long latency responses
long sleepers
long spinal white matter
long-suffering
long-term chase (gambling)
long-term data

long-term effect
long-term goals
long-term heavy use
long-term memory
long-term mortality rate
long-term outcome
long-term pattern
long-term patterns of functioning
long-term therapy
long vowel
Look and Say Articulation Test
loop, calibrated
loop-induction auditory trainer
loose associations
loose boundaries
loosening of associations
LOQ (Leadership Opinion Question-
    naire)
loquacity
"lords" (hydromorphine)
Lorge-Thorndike Cognitive Abilities
    Test
Lorge-Thorndike Intelligence Test
LOS (length of stay)
losing control
losing one's mind
losing time
loss
    appetite
    approval
    autonomy
    axon
    bilateral muscle
    central sensory
    "chasing" one's
    complete visual
    conductive hearing
    cortical sensory
    dense sensory
    dissociated sensory
    excessive semen
    extreme hearing

loss *(cont.)*
  functional
  hearing
  hemisensory
  hysterical visual
  imagined
  insertion
  interpersonal
  inventory of
  ipsilateral
  job
  major
  mechanical functional
  memory
  monocular visual
  motor
  nerve
  neuronal
  parental
  past
  perceptive hearing
  peripheral sensory
  real
  recent
  sensory
  significant
  sleep
  stocking-glove sensory
  unresolved
  visual
  weight
loss discrimination
loss of:
  belief
  biographical memory
  bladder control
  body control
  bowel control
  breadwinner
  consciousness
  desire
  ego boundaries

loss of *(cont.)*
  energy
  erectile functioning
  experience
  faith
  freedom
  language (global)
  life
  memory
    amnesia
    anterograde
    retrograde
  motivation
  orientation
  pain sensation
  pleasure
  previously stabilizing social
    situations
  sensation
  sensory modalities
  sexual desire
  significant supporting persons
  speech
  spontaneity
  support
  touch
  touch sensation
  vision
  zest
lost in thought
lost performative
LOT (Lengthened-Off-Time)
LOTE Reading and Listening Tests
loudness balance
  alternate binaural (ABLB)
  alternate monaural (AMLB)
loudness contours, equal
loudness level
loudness perception
loudness range
loudness unit
loud snoring

loudspeaker
loud speech
Lou Gehrig's disease (ALS; amyotrophic lateral sclerosis)
Louisville Behavior Checklist
"loused" (re: drug injection)
"love" (crack)
"love affair" (cocaine)
"love boat" (cannabis; phencyclidine)
"love drug" (barbiturate; methylenedioxymethamphetamine)
"lovelies" (cannabis laced with phencyclidine)
"lovely" (phencyclidine)
love object
"love pearls" (alpha-ethyltryptamine)
"love pills" (alpha-ethyltryptamine)
lover, illicit
love, transference
"love trip" (methylenedioxymethamphetamine and mescaline)
"love weed" (cannabis)
loving feelings
low-activity situation
low anxiety (LA)
low back disorder, psychogenic
low-complexity movements
low delirium
"low" desire
low educational level
low energy
low fence
low filter frequency (LFF)
low frequency (LF)
low frequency of drug use
low intelligence
low self-confidence
low self-esteem as cause for impaired social functioning
low self-worth, feelings of
low sensory environment
low-set ears

low sexual desire
low sexual interest
low stimulation environment
low-stimulation situation
low tolerance potential
low tone deafness
low-tyramine diet
low vowel
LP (lumbar puncture)
LPI (Leadership Practices Inventory)
LPT (Language Proficiency Test)
LSD (lysergic acid diethylamide)
LSD-type perceptions
LSES (Salamon-Conte Life Satisfaction in the Elderly Scale)
LSI (Life Satisfaction Index)
LSI (Life Styles Inventory)
LSP (Learning Style Profile)
LSV2 (Vocational Learning Styles)
"lubage" (cannabis)
"Lucy in the sky with diamonds" (LSD)
"luding out" (barbiturate)
"luds" (barbiturate)
lumbar iliocostal muscle
"lump in the throat"
lung capacity, total
lung volume
Luria-Nebraska Neuropsychological Battery
Luria's Neuropsychological Investigation
luteal phase
lying, repetitive
lysergic acid diethylamide (LSD) (street names)
    A
    animal
    backbreakers
    barrels
    battery acid
    beast

lysergic acid diethylamide *(cont.)*

  big D
  black star
  black sunshine
  black tabs
  blotter
  blotter acid
  blotter cube
  blue acid
  blue barrels
  blue chairs
  blue cheers
  blue mist
  blue moons
  blue vials
  brown bombers
  brown dots
  California sunshine
  cap
  chief
  chocolate chips
  coffee
  conductor
  contact lens
  crackers
  crystal tea
  cube
  cupcakes
  D
  deeda
  domes
  dots
  double dome
  Electric Kool Aid
  fields
  flash
  flat blues
  Frisco special
  Frisco speedball
  ghost
  golden dragon
  goofy's

lysergic acid diethylamide *(cont.)*

  grape parfait
  green double domes
  green single domes
  green wedge
  grey shields
  hats
  Hawaiian sunshine
  hawk
  haze
  headlights
  inbetweens
  instant zen
  L
  lason sa daga
  LBJ
  lens
  lime acid
  Logor
  Lucy in the sky with diamonds
  mellow yellow
  Mighty Quinn
  mind detergent
  one way
  optical illusions
  orange barrels
  orange cubes
  orange haze
  orange micro
  orange wedges
  outerlimits
  Owsley
  Owsley's acid
  pane
  paper acid
  peace
  peace tablets
  pearly gates
  pellets
  pink blotters
  Pink Panther
  pink robots

lysergic acid diethylamide *(cont.)*
- pink witches
- potato
- pure love
- purple barrels
- purple flats
- purple haze
- purple hearts
- purple ozoline
- recycle
- royal blues
- Russian sickles
- sacrament
- sandoz
- sheet rocking
- smears
- sugar
- sugar lumps

lysergic acid diethylamide *(cont.)*
- sunshine
- tabs
- tail lights
- ticket
- trip
- twenty-five
- vodka acid
- wedding bells
- wedge
- white dust
- white Owsley's
- window glass
- yellow
- yellow dimples
- yellow sunshine
- zen
- zig zag man

M, m

"M" (cannabis, morphine)
M (manual dexterity)
MA (mental age)
M/A (mood and/or affect)
MAACL (Multiple Affect Adjective Check List)
MAB (management of assaultive behavior)
MAC (Minimum Auditory Capabilities) Test
MacAndrew Addiction Scale (MAS)
machiavellianism
"machinery" (cannabis)
"macho" manner
Machover Draw-A-Person (MDAP) test
MACI (Millon Adolescent Clinical Inventory)
MacKenzie syndrome
Macmillan Graded Word Reading Test
"Macon" (cannabis)
"maconha" (cannabis)
macrocephaly
macrocheilia
macroglossia
macrognathia
macromania
macropsia

macrostomia
"mad dog" (phencyclidine)
"madman" (phencyclidine)
madness
MADRS (Montgomery and Asberg Depression Rating Scale)
MAE (Multilingual Aphasia Examination)
MAF (minimum audible field)
Maferr Inventory of Masculine Values (MIMV)
Magenblase syndrome
"magic" (phencyclidine; psilocin/psilocybin)
"magic dust" (phencyclidine)
"magic mushroom" (psilocybin/psilocin)
"magic smoke" (cannabis)
magnetic apraxia
magnetic resonance imaging (MRI)
magnetic resonance spectroscopy (MRS)
magnetoencephalogram
MAGS (Multidimensional Assessment of Gains in School)
MAI (Marriage Adjustment Inventory)
MAI (Morbid Anxiety Inventory)
maieusiophobia

313

MAII (Milwaukee Academic Interest
   Inventory)
"main line" (re: drug injection)
"mainliner" (re: drug injection)
"mainlining" (re: cocaine)
mainstreaming
maintaining sleep
   difficulty
   disorder of initiating and (DIMS)
maintenance
   drug
   methadone
maintenance dose
maintenance insomnia
maintenance of pain
maintenance treatment
main verb
major affective disorder
major attachment figures
major depression
major depressive affective psychosis
   recurrent episode
   single episode
major depressive disorder (MDD)
   recurrent episode
   single episode
major depressive episode (MDE)
major epilepsy (grand mal)
major hysteria
major image-distorting level
major impairment of functioning
majority society
major life activity
major mental disorder
major mood disorder
major motor aphasia
major motor seizure
major role obligations
major role therapy (MRT)
major tranquilizer
make amends symbolically
Make-A-Picture-Story (MAPS)

make-believe play
"make up" (re: drugs acquisition)
makeup application
mal
   grand
   haut
   petit
malabsorption, disaccharide
maladaptive behavior
maladaptive behavioral changes
maladaptive feelings
maladaptive gambling behavior
maladaptive health behavior
maladaptive pattern
maladaptive pattern of substance use
maladaptive personality
maladaptive personality traits
maladaptive psychological changes
maladaptive reaction to a stressor
maladaptive response
maladaptive way
malady
malar bones
malar skull bones
male dyspareunia
male erectile arousal disorder
   acquired-type
   generalized-type
   lifelong-type
   situational-type
male erectile disorder due to combined factors
male erectile disorder due to psychological factors
male erectile dysfunction
Male Impotence Test (MIT)
maleness
male orgasmic disorder
   acquired-type
   generalized-type
   lifelong-type
   situational-type

male orgasmic disorder due to
combined factors
male orgasmic disorder due to
psychological factors
male orgasm, inhibited
male-to-female transgender identity
malevolent distrust
malignant brain neoplasm
malignant hyperthermia
malignant syndrome
malinger
malingerer
malingering
malingering disorder
mallet, anger
malleus, handle of
malocclusion, teeth
malpositions, teeth
maltreatment and PTSD (posttraumatic
stress disorder)
maltreatment of children
"mama coca" (cocaine)
management
behavioral
case
clinical
contingency
crisis
pain
pharmacological
psychological
stress
time
Management Appraisal Survey (MAS)
management by medication
Management Development Profile
management implications
Management Inventory on Leadership,
Motivation and Decision- Making
(MILMD)
management of assaultive behavior
(MAB)

Management Philosophies Scale
(MPS)
Management Position Analysis Test
Management Readiness Profile
Management Styles Inventory
Managerial Style Questionnaire
(MSQ)
Manager Profile Record
Manager Style Appraisal
Mandel Social Adjustment Scale
(MSAS)
mandible, alveolar border of
mandible skull bone
mandibular hypoplasia
mandibular movement
mandibular restriction
mandibulofacial dysostosis
"M&M" (barbiturate)
maneuver, body concept-exploration
manganese intoxication
"Manhattan silver" (cannabis)
mania (pl. manias)
ablutomania
abulomania
acromania
acute
agoramania
agyiomania
aidoiomania
ailuromania
akinetic
alcohol
alcoholic
alcoholomania
amaxomania
amenomania
Americamania
andromania
Anglomania
anthomania
aphrodisiomania
apimania

mania *(cont.)*
arithmomania
automania
autophonomania
ballistomania
Bell
bibliokleptomania
bibliomania
bruxomania
cacodemonomania
callomania
cheromania
Chinamania
chionomania
choreomania
chrematomania
chronic
clinomania
compulsive
coprolalomania
cremnomania
cresomania
cynomania
dancing
Dantomania
delirious
demomania
demonomania
dinomania
dipsomania
doramania
doubting
drapetomania
dromomania
ecdemiomania
ecomania
edeomania
egomania
eleuthromania
empleomania
enomania
entheomania

mania *(cont.)*
entomomania
epileptic
eremiomania
ergasiomania
ergomania
eroticomania
erotographomania
erotomania
erythromania
etheromania
florimania
Francomania
Gallomania
gamomania
gephyromania
Germanomania
graphomania
Grecomania
gymnomania
gynecomania
hallucinatory
hamartomania
hedonomania
heliomania
hieromania
hippomania
hodomania
homicidomania
hydrargyromania
hydrodipsomania
hydromania
hylomania
hypermania
hypnomania
hypomania
hysterical
hysteromania
ichthyomania
iconomania
idolomania
inhibited

mania *(cont.)*
Italomania
kainomania
kathisomania
kinesomania
kleptomania
lalomania
letheomania
logomania
lycomania
lypemania
macromania
megalomania
melomania
mentulomania
mesmeromania
methomania
metromania
micromania
monomania
morphinomania
musicomania
musomania
mythomania
narcomania
narcosomania
necromania
noctimania
nosomania
nostomania
nudomania
nymphomania
ochlomania
oestromania
oikomania
oinomania
oligomania
oniomania
onomatomania
onychotillomania
ophidiomania
opiomania

mania *(cont.)*
opsomania
orchidomania
orinthomania
paramania
parousiamania
pathomania
peotillomania
peracute
periodical
phagomania
phaneromania
pharmacomania
philopatridomania
phonomania
photomania
phronemomania
phthiriomania
plutomania
politicomania
poriomania
pornographomania
potomania
pseudomania
puerperal
pyromania
Ray
reasoning
recurrent episode
religious
Russomania
satyromania
scribblemania
scribomania
senile
siderodromomania
single episode
sitomania
sophomania
squandermania
stupor
submania

mania *(cont.)*
  symmetromania
  Teutonomania
  thalassomania
  thanatomania
  theomania
  theotromania
  timbromania
  tomomania
  transitory
  trichomania
  trichorrhexomania
  trichotillomania
  tristimania
  tromomania
  Turkomania
  typomania
  unproductive
  uteromania
  verbomania
  xenomania
  zoomania
mania à potu (delirium tremens)
maniac
maniacal
Mania "9" Scale
maniaphobia
mania rating scale (MRS)
manic affective psychosis
  atypical
  recurrent episode
  single episode
manic atypical psychosis
manic bipolar disorder
manic delirium
  acute
  recurrent episode
  single episode
manic depression
manic-depressive affective psychosis
manic-depressive disorder
manic-depressive illness

manic-depressive insanity
manic-depressive-like episodes
manic-depressive psychosis
  alternating
  atypical manic-type
  circular
  depressive
  hypomanic
  mixed
  perplexed
  stuporous
manic-depressive reaction
  depressed
  hypomanic
manic-depressive syndrome
manic disorder
manic episode
manic excitement
  recurrent episode
  single episode
manic features
manicky
manic-like episodes
manic phase
manic psychosis
manic reaction
manic speech
manic symptoms
manifest content
manifestation
  behavioral
  neurotic
  psychophysiologic
  psychotic
manifestation of behavioral dysfunction
manifestation of biological dysfunction
manifestation of pain
manifestation of pathology
manifestation of psychological dysfunction
manifested disability

manipulation
  digital
  emotional
manipulative behavior
manipulative behavior for material
  gratification
manipulative behavior to attain power
manipulative behavior to gain profit
manipulative pseudohallucination
manipulatory tasks
manliness
man-machine systems
man-made disasters
manner (pl. manners)
  deterioration of
  devious
  guarded
  inconsistent
  intriguing
  "macho"
  patronizing
  secretive
  superior
  sustained
  unkempt
  unusual
manner and dress
mannerisms
  feminine
  speech
manner of articulation
manometer, oral
manometric flame
manual communication
manual dexterity (M)
manual stimulation
manual volume control
manubrium (pl. manubria)
manufacturing amphetamines
MAO (monoamine oxidase)
MAO inhibitor
MAOI (monoamine oxidase inhibitor)

MAOI-meperidine
MAOI-serotonergic agents
MAOI-tricyclides
map (mapping)
  apraxia
  behavioral
  brain
  brain electrical activity (BEAM)
  cognitive
  cortical function
  language areas of brain
  reality
  topographic
MAP (minimum audible pressure)
MAP (Musical Aptitude Profile)
MAPE (Multidimensional Assessment
  of Philosophy of Education)
MAPS (Make-A-Picture-Story)
marathon, Gestalt therapy
marathon group psychotherapy
"marathons" (amphetamine)
Marfan syndrome
marginal function
marginal member of society
marginal thinking
"Mari" (marijuana cigarette)
mariguana (see *marijuana*)
marihuana (see *marijuana*)
marijuana (MJ) (see also *cannabis*)
  Colombian
  Hawaiian
  homegrown
  Mexican
  sinsemillan
  Thai
marijuana extract
marijuana smoking
Marital Attitudes Evaluation (MATE)
Marital Communication Scale
marital conflict
marital counseling
marital counselor

marital discord
marital disruption
marital dissatisfaction
marital history (MH)
marital infidelity
marital instability
Marital Satisfaction Inventory
marital stability
marital status
marital therapy
marker
  genetic
  I (intentional marker)
  sign
markers of heavy drinking
marking, analog
Marlow-Crowne (Social Desirability)
  Scale (MCS)
marriage (pl. marriages)
  arranged
  consanguineous
  heterosexual
  homosexual
  institution of
  interracial
  nonconsanguineous
  open-end (OEM)
  related by
  same-sex
  troubled
Marriage Adjustment Inventory (MAI)
Marriage and Family Attitude Survey
marriage counselor
marriage problem
marriage therapy
MARS (Mathematics Anxiety Rating
  Scale)
MARS-A (Mathematics Anxiety
  Rating Scale, Adolescents)
"marshmallow reds" (barbiturate)
martialis, psychopathia
Martinez Assessment of the Basic
  Skills

Martin S-D (suicide-depression)
  Inventory (MSDI)
martyr complex
"Mary" (cannabis)
"Mary and Johnny" (cannabis)
"Mary Ann" (cannabis)
"Mary Jane" (cannabis)
"Mary Jonas" (cannabis)
Maryland Parent Attitude Survey
"Mary Warner" (cannabis)
"Mary Weaver" (cannabis)
MAS (MacAndrew's Addiction Scale)
MAS (Management Appraisal Survey)
MAS (Manifest Anxiety Scale)
MAS (Maternal Attitude Scale)
MAS (Memory Assessment Scales)
masculine identity
masculine protest
Masculinity-femininity "5" Scale
masculinization
"Maserati" (re: crack equipment)
masked depression
mask (of parkinsonism) facies
masking
  backward
  central
  effective
  forward
  frequency
  initial
  maximum
  perceptual
  peripheral
  upward
masking efficiency
masking technique
  Hood
  plateau
  sensorineural acuity level
  shadowing
  threshold shift
masklike facies

Maslach Burnout Inventory (MBI),
Second Edition
masochism
sadism and (S&M)
sexual
masochist
masochistic personality
masochistic ritual
masochistic sexual activity
masochistic sexual behavior
masochistic sexual fantasy
masochistic sexual urges
mass behavior
MAST (Michigan Alcoholism Screening Test)
Master of Science in Nursing (MSN)
Master of Social Work (MSW)
Masters and Johnson
mastery motive
mastication
mastigophobia
mastoid, artificial
mastoidectomy
modified
radical
mastoid process
masturbation, compulsive
masturbatory activity
MAT (Manipulative Aptitude Test)
MAT (Metropolitan Achievement
Tests)
MAT (Miller Analogies Test)
MAT (Motivation Analysis Test)
MAT (Music Achievement Tests 1, 2,
3, and 4)
MAT7 (Metropolitan Achievement
Tests, Seventh Edition)
"matchbox" (1/4 ounce of cannabis;
6 cannabis cigarettes)
matched groups
Matching Familiar Figures Test
(MFFT)

matching, impedance
match, perceptual-motor
mate (verb and noun)
mate, age
MATE (Marital Attitudes Evaluation)
material
current
genetic
material aspects of the body
material gratification
materialistic
Maternal Attitude Scale (MAS)
maternal behavior
maternal deprivation
Math Achievement
mathematical ability
mathematical skills
mathematical symbols
Mathematics Anxiety Rating Scale
(MARS)
Mathematics Anxiety Rating Scale
Adolescents (MARS-A)
mathematics disorder
matrix (pl. matrixes or matrices)
Matrix Analogies Test
matrix sentence
"Matsakow" (heroin)
matter
central gray
cortical gray
dorsal gray
gray (of CNS)
long spinal white
midbrain
periventricular white
subcortical white
white (of CNS)
maturational lag
maturation index
maturation, rate of
maturity fears
maturity rating

maturity scale (see *test*)
Maudsley Obsessional Compulsive
Inventory (MOCI)
Maudsley Personality Inventory
"Maui wauie" (cannabis)
"Max" (gamma hydroxybutyrate and
amphetamines)
Maxfield-Buchholz Social Maturity
Scale for Blind Preschool
Children
maxibolin (oral steroid)
maxilla, alveolar process of
maxillary bone
inferior
superior
maximal contrasts
maximal effect
maximal electroshock (MES)
maximal electroshock seizures (MES)
maximum acoustic output
maximum amplitude
maximum duration of phonation
maximum duration of sustained blowing
maximum frequency range
maximum masking
maximum power output (MPO)
maximum security unit
Mayer reflex
"mayo" (cocaine; heroin)
maze learning
Mazes, Foster
maze test
MBD (minimal brain dysfunction)
syndrome
MBHI (Millon Behavioral Health
Inventory)
MBI (Maslach Burnout Inventory)
MBSP (Monitoring Basic Skills
Progress)
MBTI (Myers-Briggs Type Indicator)

McCarthy Scales of Children's
Abilities (MSCA)
McCarthy Screening Test
MCDI (Minnesota Child Development
Inventory)
McGill Pain Questionnaire
MCLR (most comfortable loudness
range)
McMaster Health Index Questionnaire
MCMI (Millon Clinical Multiaxial
Inventory)
MCMI-II (Millon Clinical Multiaxial
Inventory II)
MCPS (Missouri Children's Picture
Series)
MCRE (The Mother-Child Relation-
ship Evaluation)
MCS (Marlow-Crowne [Social Desir-
ability] Scale)
MD (mental deficiencies)
MD (mentally deficient)
MDA (methylene dioxyamphetamine)
MDAP (Machover Draw-A-Person)
MDB (Mental Deterioration Battery)
MDD (major depressive disorder)
MDDA (Minnesota Differential Diag-
nosis of Aphasia)
MDE (major depressive episode)
MDI (Multiscore Depression Inven-
tory)
MDM or MDMA (amphetamine/
methamphetamine; methylene-
dioxymethamphetamine)
MDQ (Menstrual Distress Question-
naire)
MDSO (mentally disordered sex
offender)
meals
after (p.c.)
before (a.c.)
mean deviation

"mean green" (phencyclidine)
mean half-life (of a pharmaceutical)
meaning
  double
  figurative
  grammatical
  hidden
  idiosyncratic
  latent
  literal
  symbolic
  transferred
meaningful, psychologically
meaningful relationship
meaningless
meaning reframing
mean length of response (MLR)
mean length of utterance (MLU)
mean peak frequency
mean relational utterance (MRU)
mean sentence length (MSL)
mean sleep latency
MEAP (Multiphasic Environmental
  Assessment Procedure)
measurable impairment
measure (see *test*)
measured capacity
measured intelligence
measurement (pl. measurements) (see
  also *test*)
  auditory function
  core body temperature
  EEG activity
  global (of disability)
  instrumental ADL
  physiological
  reproductive hormonal
  speech production
Measurement of Language Development
measures of disability
Measures of Musical Abilities

Measures of Psychosocial Development (MPD)
measuring, lexical
MEAT (Minnesota Engineering
  Analogies Test)
meatus (pl. meatus)
  acoustic
  acusticus externus
  acusticus internus
  external acoustic
  external auditory
  internal acoustic
  internal auditory
  nasi inferior
  nasi medius
  nasi superior
  nasopharyngeus
mechanical functional loss
mechanical intelligence
Mechanical Technology (NOCTI
  Teacher Occupational Competency
  Test)
mechanics, body
mechanism
  airstream
  association
  balance
  coping
  defense
  direct causative pathophysiological
  ego-defense
  immune
  linguistic
  mental
  neutralizing
  pathophysiological
  physiologic
  sex arousal (SAM)
  shared
  sleep
  specific pathophysiological
  speech
  triggering

mechanophobia
medial consonant position
medial nasal concha
medial turbinate bone
median age
median cleft lip
median laryngotomy
median lingual sulcus
median longitudinal raphe
median sagittal plane
mediated function
mediated response
mediation, verbal
Medicaid
medical ethics
medical etiology
medical futility
medical history
medically related position
medical/neurological disorder
Medical Outcomes Study Short
   Form-36
medical/psychiatric sleep disorder
medical psychology
medical services
medical sociology
medical stress
medical taper schedule
Medicare
medication (descriptive terms)
   adverse effects of
   agonist
   antagonist
   beta-adrenergic
   cheeking
   management by
   NSAID
   overuse of
   psychoactive
medication (drugs) (for *illicit drugs*,
   see *dependence*; *drugs, street*)
   abecarnil
   acarbose

medication *(cont.)*
   acepromazine
   acetaminophen
   acetazolamide
   acetophenazine maleate
   acetylcarbromal
   acetylsalicylic acid
   Aches-N-Pain
   Acutrim
   Adapin (doxepin)
   ADH (antidiuretic hormone)
   adinazolam
   Advil
   Akineton (biperiden)
   Alcar
   Aldactone
   Aleve
   alpidem
   alprazolam
   aluminum glycinate
   aluminum hydroxide
   Alurate
   amantadine hydrochloride
   Amaphen
   amineptine
   Amitril
   amitriptyline hydrochloride
   amobarbital sodium
   amoxapine
   amperozide
   amphetamine sulfate
   amylobarbitone
   Amytal Sodium
   Anacin; Anacin-3
   Anafranil
   Anaprox
   Anoquan
   Antabuse (disulfiram)
   antidiuretic hormone (ADH)
   Antivert (meclizine)
   Anxanil
   APF (Arthritis Pain Formula)
   aprobarbital

medication *(cont.)*
Arcet
Aricept
Artane (trihexyphenidyl HCl)
Arthritis Pain Formula
Arthropan
Ascriptin
Ascriptin A/D
Asendin (amoxapine)
aspirin
Atarax (hydroxyzine HCl)
Atarax 100
Atenolol (timolol)
Athymil
Ativan
Atozine
atropine sulfate
Aventyl
Axotal
baclofen
Bancap HC
B & O (or B and O)
Banthine (methantheline bromide)
barbital
Barbita
barbitone
Bayer Aspirin
belladonna
Bellergal-S
Bel-Phen-Ergot S
Benadryl
benperidol
Bentyl (dicyclomine HCl)
Benzedrine
benzodiazepine
benzphetamine hydrochloride
benztropine mesylate
Betachron E-R
bethanechol chloride
biperiden HCl
Biphetamine
boldenone

medication *(cont.)*
Bontril
bretazenil
brofaromine
bromine
bromocriptine mesylate
brompheniramine
Bucet
Bufferin
Buprenex
buprenorphine hydrochloride
bupropion
BuSpar (buspirone HCl)
buspirone hydrochloride
buspirone transdermal patch
butabarbital
butabarbitone
butalbital
butaperazine
butriptyline
Buticaps
Butisol Sodium
butorphanol tartrate
Cafatine
Cafergot
Cafergot P-B
Cafetrate
caffeine
calcium gluconate
Cama
cannabis
Capital with codeine
carbamazepine
Carbatrol
carbidopa
carbromal
carisoprodol
carphenazine
Catapres
Catatrol
cefadroxil
Celontin

medication *(cont.)*
Centrax
Cerebyx
Children's Advil
Children's Motrin
chloral hydrate
chlordiazepoxide hydrochloride
chlormezanone
Chlorpazine
chlorphenesin carbamate
chlorpromazine hydrochloride
chlorprothixene
chlorzoxazone
Choledyl
choline salicylate
Cibalith-S
cinnamedrine hydrochloride
citalopram
citicoline sodium
clindamycin
clobazam
clomipramine hydrochloride
clonazepam
clonidine
clorazepate dipotassium
clorgyline
clozapine
Clozaril (clozapine)
codeine phosphate
codeine sulfate
Cogentin (benztropine mesylate)
Co-Gesic
Cognex
Compazine (prochlorperazine
    maleate)
Consonar
Cope
Cognex
cyclobenzaprine hydrochloride
cycloserine
cycrimine
Cylert (pemoline)

medication *(cont.)*
cyprolidol
cyproheptadine
cyproterone acetate
Dalmane (flurazepam HCl)
Dantrium (dantrolene sodium)
dantrolene sodium
Darvocet-N
Darvon
Darvon Compound
Darvon-N
Darvon with ASA
Datril
Dazamide
delta-9-tetrahydrocannabinol
Demerol
Depakene
Depakote
Depo-Provera (medroxyproges-
    terone acetate)
Deprol
desipramine hydrochloride
Desoxyn
Desyrel (trazodone HCl)
Dexatrim
Dexedrine
dexfenfluramine hydrochloride
dextroamphetamine sulfate
dextromethorphan
D.H.E. 45
DHT
Diamox
diazepam
dibenzodiazepine
dibenzoxazepine
dichloralphenazone
dicyclomine
Didrex (benzphetamine HCl)
dihydrotachysterol
diethylpropion hydrochloride
diflunisal
dihydrocodeine bitartrate

medication *(cont.)*
dihydroergotamine mesylate
dihydroindolone
Dilantin (phenytoin)
Dilantin Infatab
Dilaudid
Dilaudid-HP
Dilone
Dimensyn
Dimetane (brompheniramine
maleate)
diphenylbutylpiperidine
dimethyltryptamine (DMT)
diphenhydramine citrate
diphenhydramine hydrochloride
Diphenylan Sodium
disopyramide
disulfiram
divalproex sodium
DMT (dimethyltryptamine)
Dolobid
Dolophine
donepezil
Dopar
Doral (quazepam)
Dorcol
Doriden
Doriglute
Dormalin
dothiepin hydrochloride
doxepin hydrochloride
doxylamine
droperidol
Durrax
Dyazide
Easprin
Ecotrin
Effexor
Elavil (amitriptyline HCl)
Eldepryl (selegiline HCl)
Emitrip
Empirin

medication *(cont.)*
Empirin with codeine
Empracet with codeine
enciprazine
encyprate
Endep (amitriptyline HCl)
Endolor
Enovil
ephedrine sulfate
Epitol
Equagesic
Equanil
Ercaf
ergoloid mesylate
Ergomar
Ergostat
ergotamine tartrate
Esgic
Esgic-Plus
Eskalith
Eskalith CR
estazolam
ethchlorvynol
ethinamate
ethopropazine hydrochloride
ethosuximide
ethotoin
etoperidone
Etrafon-A
Etrafon-Forte
etryptamine
E-Vista
Excedrin
Excedrin P.M.
Ex-Lax
Excedrin IB
Excegran
Fastin
felbamate
Felbatol
Femcet
fenfluramine hydrochloride

medication *(cont.)*
  fenoprofen calcium
  fentanyl citrate
  Fioricet
  Fiorgen PF
  Fiorinal
  Fiorinal with codeine
  Flexeril
  flumazenil
  fluoxetine hydrochloride
  flupenthixol
  fluphenazine decanoate
  fluphenazine enanthate
  fluphenazine hydrochloride
  flurazepam hydrochloride
  fluvoxamine
  fosphenytoin
  Frisium
  gabapentin
  Gemnisyn
  Gemonil
  Genpril
  Gen-XENE
  gepirone
  Gerimal
  glutethimide
  guaifenesin
  Habitrol Patch
  halazepam
  Halcion (triazolam)
  Haldol Decanoate
  haloperidol
  Halperon
  Haltran
  heptachlor
  heroin
  H.P. Acthar Gel
  Hydergine LC
  hydrocodone bitartrate
  Hydro-Ergoloid
  Hydroloid-G
  hydromorphone hydrochloride

medication *(cont.)*
  hydroxyzine hydrochloride
  hydroxyzine pamoate
  Hy-Pam
  Hy-Phen
  Hytakerol
  Hyzine-50
  Ibuprin
  Ibuprohm
  ibuprofen
  Ibu-Tab
  idazoxan
  imipramine hydrochloride
  imipramine pamoate
  Imitrex
  Inapsine
  Inderal
  Inderal LA
  iodine-123 iomazenil (^{123}I)
  iodine-123-labeled cocaine analog
    (^{123}I beta-CIT)
  Ionamin
  ipecac
  iprindole
  iproniazid
  ipsapirone
  isocarboxazid
  Isocet
  Isollyl Improved
  isometheptene mucate
  Janimine Oral
  Kadian
  Kalcinate
  Kemadrin
  Ketalar
  ketamine
  ketoprofen
  Klonopin
  Lamictal
  lamotrigine
  Lanorinal
  Largon

medication *(cont.)*
Larodopa
laroxyl
levacecarnine
levodopa
Levo-Dromoran
Levoprome
levorphanol tartrate
Libritabs
Librium
lidocaine
Limbitrol
Limbitrol DS
Lioresal
Lipoxide
Liquiprin
Lithane
lithium carbonate
lithium citrate
Lithobid
Lithonate
Lithotabs
Lopressor
lorazepam
Lotusate
loxapine hydrochloride
loxapine succinate
Loxitane
Loxitane C
Loxitane IM
Ludiomil (maprotiline)
Lupron (leuprolide acetate)
Luvox
Magan
magnesium carbonate
magnesium hydroxide
magnesium oxide
magnesium salicylate
magnesium sulfate
Maolate
maprotiline hydrochloride
Margesic

medication *(cont.)*
Marnal
Marplan
Marsilid
Mazanor
mazindol
mebanazine
Mebaral
meclizine
meclofenamate sodium
Meclomen
medazepam
Medigesic
Medihaler Ergotamine
Medipren
medroxyprogesterone acetate
mefenamic acid
Mellaril
Mellaril-S
Menadol
Mentane
Mepergan
Mepergan Fortis
meperidine hydrochloride
mephenytoin
mephobarbital
Mephyton (methadone)
meprobamate
Meprospan
mertazepine
Mesantoin
mesoridazine besylate
Mestinon
metaproterenol
metaxalone
methadone
methadone hydrochloride
methamphetamine hydrochloride
methandrostenolone
methapyrilene
methaqualone
metharbital

medication *(cont.)*
  Methedrine
  methenolone
  methocarbamol
  methotrimeprazine
  methsuximide
  methylmorphine
  methylphenidate hydrochloride
  methyprylon
  methysergide maleate
  metoprolol
  mianserin
  Micrainin
  midazolam hydrochloride
  Midol
  Midol IB
  Midol PMS
  Midol 200
  Midrin
  Millazine
  Milontin
  Miltown
  Miltown-600
  Mirapex
  mirtazepine
  Mitran
  Moban (molindone HCl)
  moclobemide
  Mogadon
  molindone hydrochloride
  Momentum
  monoamine oxidase inhibitor
    (MAOI)
  moperone
  morphine
  morphine sulfate (MS)
  Motrin IB
  MS Contin
  Mucomyst
  Mysoline
  nafcillin
  nalbuphine hydrochloride

medication *(cont.)*
  Nalfon
  nalmefene hydrochloride
  naloxone hydrochloride
  naltrexone hydrochloride
  Naprosyn
  naproxen sodium
  Narcan
  Nardil (phenelzine sulfate)
  Navane (thiothixene)
  nefazodone hydrochloride
  Nembutal (pentobarbital)
  Nembutal Sodium
  Neucalm
  Neuramate
  Neurontin
  neuroleptic
  nialamide
  Nicoderm
  Nicoderm CQ
  Nicoderm HP
  Nicorette DS Gum
  Nicotrol Patch
  nicotine polacrilex
  Nicotrol
  Nicotrol NS
  nimodipine
  nitrazepam
  Noctec
  Noludar
  norepinephrine
  Norflex
  Norgesic
  Norgesic Forte
  Norpace
  Norpramin (desipramine HCl)
  nortriptyline hydrochloride
  Nubain
  Numorphan
  Nuprin
  olanzapine
  opium

medication *(cont.)*
Oramorph SR
Orap (pimozide)
Ormazine
orphenadrine citrate
Orudis
Oruvail
oxandrolone
oxazepam
oxiracetam
oxtriphylline
oxycodone hydrochloride
oxycodone terephthalate
oxymorphone hydrochloride
oxypertine
Pabalate
Pabalate-SF
pamabrom
Pamelor (nortriptyline)
Panadol
Paradione
Paraflex
Parafon
Parafon Forte
Paral
paraldehyde
paramethadione
Parlodel (bromocriptine mesylate)
Parnate (tranylcypromine sulfate)
paroxetine
Parsidol (ethopropazine HCl)
Paxarel
Paxil
Paxipam
PBZ (pyribenzamine)
Peganone
pemoline
pentazocine hydrochloride
pentazocine lactate
pentobarbitone
pentobarbital sodium
Pentothal

medication *(cont.)*
Percocet
Percodan
Percodan-Demi
Percogesic
pericyazine
Permitil (fluphenazine HCl)
Permitil Oral
perphenazine
Pertofrane (desipramine HCl)
phenacemide
phenaglycodol
Phenaphen
Phenaphen with codeine
phencyclidine
phendimetrazine tartrate
phenelzine sulfate
Phenerbel-S
pheniprazine
pheniramine
phenmetrazine hydrochloride
phenobarbital sodium
phenobarbitone
phenothiazine
phensuximide
phentermine hydrochloride
phentermine resin
Phenurone
phenylalanine
phenylpropanolamine hydro-
    chloride
phenylephrine
phenyltoloxamine citrate
phenytoin sodium
Phrenilin
Phrenilin Forte
physostigmine
pimozide
piperacetazine
piribedil
Placidyl
Plegicil

medication *(cont.)*
Plegine
Pondimin (fenfluramine)
Ponstel
potassium salicylate
pramipexole
prazepam
Precose
Prelu-2
Preludin
primidone
procainamide
procaine
prochlorperazine maleate
procyclidine hydrochloride
Prolixin (fluphenazine HCl)
Prolixin Decanoate
Prolixin Enanthate
promazine hydrochloride
promethazine hydrochloride
Pronestyl
propiomazine hydrochloride
propoxyphene hydrochloride
propoxyphene napsylate
propranolol hydrochloride
ProStep Patch
Prothiaden
prothipendyl
protriptyline hydrochloride
Prozac (fluoxetine)
Prozine-50
pseudoephedrine
pyridostigmine bromide
pyrilamine maleate
Quaalude
quazepam
quetiapine
Quide
Quiess
quinalbarbitone
Quinamm
quinine ascorbate

medication *(cont.)*
quinine sulfate
raclopride
ranitidine
Raudixin
Rauverid
rauwolfia serpentina
Redux
Regonol Injection
Remeron
Reminyl
remoxipride
Repan
Reposans-10
reserpine
Restoril (temazepam)
Revex
ReVia
Rezine
Risperdal
risperidone
Ritalin
Ritalin-SR
ritanserin
RMS
Robaxin
Robaxisal
Roxanol
Roxiam
Rufen
sabeluzole
Sabril
Saleto-200
Saleto-400
salicylamide
Sanorex
Sansert
saroten
scopolamine
secobarbital sodium
Seconal Sodium
Sedabamate

medication *(cont.)*
Sedapap-10
Seldane (terfenadine)
selective serotonin reuptake
  inhibitor
selegiline HCl
Serax (oxazepam)
Serentil
Serlect
Seromycin (cycloserine)
Seroquel
serotonin metabolite 5-HIAA
  (5-hydroxyindoleacetic acid)
sertindole
sertraline HCl
Serzone
Sinemet
Sinequan (doxepin HCl)
Sintoclar
Skelaxin
sodium aminobenzoate
sodium amytal
sodium butabarbital
sodium lactate
sodium salicylate
sodium thiosalicylate
sodium valproate
Solfoton
Soma
Soma Compound
Soma Compound with codeine
Sonazine
Sopor
Sparine
spiperone
spironolactone
SSRI (selective serotonin reuptake
  inhibitor)
Stadol
Stelazine (trifluoperazine HCl)
St. Joseph Aspirin
strychnine

medication *(cont.)*
Sublimaze
sulpiride
sumatriptan succinate
Suprazine
suprofen
Suprol
Surmontil (trimipramine maleate)
Symmetrel (amantidine HCl)
Synalgos
Synalgos-DC
synthetic delta-9-THC
tacrine HCl
Talacen
talbutal
Talwin (pentazocine lactate)
Talwin Compound
Talwin NX
Taractan
tefludazine
Tegretol (carbamazepine)
temazepam
Tempra
Tencet
Tencon
Tenuate (diethylpropion HCl)
Tenuate Dospan
Tepanil
terbutaline
terfenadine
tetrabenazine
tetrahydroaminoacridine
THC
thiamine
thiazesim
thiocyclidine
thiopental sodium
thioridazine hydrochloride
thiothixene
Thorazine (chlorpromazine)
Thor-Prom
tianeptine

medication *(cont.)*
Tigan
Tindal
timolol
Tipramine
tizanidine hydrochloride
tocainide
Tofranil (imipramine)
Tofranil-PM
tolamolol
Topimax
topiramate
tramadol
Trancopal
Tranmep
Tranxene (clorazepate dipotassium)
Tranxene-SD
tranylcypromine sulfate
trazodone hydrochloride
Trendar
Trexan
Triad
Trialodine
triamterene
Triaprin
Triavil
triazolam
Tridione
trifluoperazine hydrochloride
trifluperidol
triflupromazine hydrochloride
Trihexy-2
Trihexy-5
trihexyphenidyl hydrochloride
Trilafon (perphenazine)
trimethadione
trimethobenzamide
trimethoxyamphetamine
trimipramine maleate
Trimstat
tripelennamine
Trofan

medication *(cont.)*
Trofan-DS
tryptophan
tryptizol hydrochloride
Tuinal
Two-Dyne
Tycolet
Tylenol
Tylenol Allergy Sinus
Tylenol Allergy Sinus NightTime
Tylenol Cold
Tylenol with codeine
Tylox
Ultram
Uni-Pro
Valium
Valmid
valproate sodium
valproic acid
Valrelease
Vamate
Vanquish
vasopressin
velnacrine maleate
venlafaxine hydrochloride
Versed
Vesprin
Viagra
Vicodin
vigabatrin
viloxazine hydrochloride
Vistacon
Vistaject-25
Vistaject-50
Vistaquel 50
Vistaril (hydroxyzine pamoate)
Vistazine 50
Vivactil (protriptyline HCl)
Wellbutrin (bupropion HCl)
Wellbutrin SR
Wigraine
Wolfina

medication *(cont.)*
  Wygesic
  Xanax (alprazolam)
  Xanax SR
  Xanax XR
  Xylocaine
  Xylocaine hydrochloride
  Xylocaine MPF
  Xylocaine Viscous
  Yocon (yohimbine HCl)
  yohimbine HCl
  Zanaflex
  Zantac (ranitidine)
  Zarontin
  Zaxopam
  Zetran
  Zoloft
  zolpidem
  Zonalon topical cream
  zonisamide
  Zorprin
  Zydone
  Zyprex
medication-induced movement
  disorder
medication-induced movements
medication-induced postural tremor
medication side effect
medication trial
medicinals, abuse of patent
medicine
  behavioral
  concepts in
  family
  history of
meditate, meditation
medulla oblongata
medullary canal
Meeting Street School Screening Test
  (MSSST)
"Meg," "Megg," "Meggie" (cannabis
  cigarette)

megalomania
megalomanic
megalophobia
megavitamin therapy
Mega Test, The
mel (tone pitch unit)
melancholia
  acute
  affective
  agitated
  chronic
  climacteric
  convulsive
  hypochondriacal
  intermittent
  involutional
  menopausal
  panphobic
  paretic
  puberty
  puerperal
  reactive
  recurrent
  senile
  sexual
  stuporous
  suicidal
melancholia agitata
melancholia attonita
melancholia hypochondriaca
melancholia religiosa
melancholia simplex
melancholia stuporosa
melancholia with delirium
melancholic features
melancholic involutional reaction
melancholy
melatonin
melissophobia
"mellow yellow" (lysergic acid
  diethylamide)
melomania

membrane (pl. membranes)
  basilar
  drum
  mucous
  Reissner's
  vestibular
membrane ion channel
membranous labyrinth
membranous laryngitis
memory (pl. memories)
  affect
  amnesia loss of
  anterograde
  anterograde loss of
  auditory
  behavioral
  biographical
  body
  childhood trauma
  delayed
  distributed
  disturbance in
  echoic
  eye
  explicit
  false
  figural
  gaps in
  iconic
  immediate
  impaired
  implicit
  lack of
  lexical
  long-term
  loss of
  poor
  recent
  recognition
  recurrence of a
  recursive autoassociative
  remote

memory (cont.)
  retrograde loss of
  retrospective gaps in
  rote
  screen
  selective
  semantic
  senile
  sequential
  short-term (STM)
  somatic
  state dependent
  subconscious
  traumatic
  verbal
  visual
  visual-spatial
memory ability
memory amplification
Memory Assessment Scales (MAS)
memory bias
memory deficit
memory difficulties
memory distortion
memory disturbance
memory encoding
Memory-for-Designs test (MFD)
memory for digits test
memory gaps
memory image
memory impairment
  reversible
  severe
memory intact for remote, recent, and
  immediate events
memory loss
memory passages
memory problems
memory questionnaire
memory quotient (MQ)
memory recall
memory retention

memory scale (see *test*)
memory score (see *test*)
memory skills
memory test
memory traces
Memphis Educational Model Providing Handicapped Infant Services (MEMPHIS)
menarche
mendacity
Meniere disease
meningitis
  bacterial
  cryptococcal
  herpes simplex virus
  herpes zoster
  syphilitic
  viral
meningitophobia
meningoencephalitis viral encephalitis
meniscus (pl. menisci)
menopausal melancholia
menopausal paranoid psychosis
menopausal paranoid reaction
menopausal paranoid state
menopausal paraphrenia
menopausal psychosis
menopause, male
menopause neurosis
menses, irregular
mens rea
menstrual disorder
Menstrual Distress Questionnaire (MDQ)
menstruation, psychogenic painful
mental abuse
mental aberration
mental activity
mental age (MA)
mental agitation
mental agraphia
mental capacity

mental changes
mental competency
mental condition
mental confusion
mental control
"mental defect"
mental deficiencies (MD)
mental deficit
mental depression
mental derangement
mental deterioration
Mental Deterioration Battery (MBD)
mental disability
mental disorder
  anxiety-related
  biology of major
  co-occurring
  delirium-related
  dementia-related
  depression-related
  drug-induced
  neurotic
  non-substance-induced
  organic
  preexisting
  presenile
  psychoneurotic
  psychotic
  primary
  substance-induced
mental disorder affecting GMC
mental disturbance in children
mental excitement
mental exhaustion
mental faculty
mental fatigue
mental health
Mental Health Association
mental health clinic (MHC)
mental hospital
mental health resource
mental health services

mental hygiene
mental illness (MI)
mental image
mental impairment
mental inhibitions level
mental insufficiency
mentality
mentally competent
mentally deficient (MD)
mentally deranged
mentally disordered offenders
mentally disordered sex offender
　(MDSO)
mentally handicapped
mentally ill
mentally impaired
mentally obtunded
mentally retarded
mental mechanism
mental obtundation
mental processes
mental retardation
　mild
　moderate
　profound
　severe
mental scotoma
mental state
mental status
　altered
　disordered
mental status changes
mental status examination (MSE)
Mental Status Examination Record
　(MSER)
mental status schedule (MSS)
mental subnormality disorder
mental syndrome
mental upset
mentation
　change in
　normal

mentation rate
mentis, abalienatio
mentulomania
MEP (multimodality-evoked potential)
　brain test
meperidine, analog of
meperidine dependence
"merchandise" (re: drugs)
mercurial behavior
mercyism
merinthophobia
"merk" (cocaine)
Mertens Visual Perception Test
　(MVPT)
MES (maximal electroshock)
"mesc" (mescaline)
"mescal" (mescaline)
mescaline (street names)
　bad seed
　barf tea
　beans
　big chief
　blue caps
　britton
　buttons
　cactus
　chief
　half moon
　hikori
　hikuli
　hyatari
　mescal
　mesc
　mese
　mezc
　moon
　nubs
　peyote
　seni
　topi
　tops
"mese" (mescaline)

mesioclusion of teeth
mesioversion of teeth
mesmerism
mesmeromania
message (pl. messages)
    covert
    dichotic
    overt
    peer
message integration
messengers
    chemical
    lithium's action on first
    lithium's action on second
"messorole" (cannabis)
MET (Minimum Essentials Test)
metabolic abnormalities
metabolic acidosis
metabolic alkalosis
metabolic amyloidosis
metabolic coma
metabolic condition
metabolic derangements
metabolic disturbance
metabolic rate
metabolic tremor
metabolic-type organic psychosis
    acute
    cerebral glucose
    subacute
metabolic volume depletion
metabolism
    brain
    dopamine
    inborn errors of
    lipoid
    mineral
    myelin
    neuronal
    plasma protein
    porphyrin
    purine
    pyrimidine

metachromatic leukodystrophy
metalanguage
metalinguistics
metallophobia
metal screen, heavy
meta-model
meta-outcome
meta-person
Metaphon
metaphor (figure of speech)
metaphorical speech
metaphrenia
metapsyche
metapsychiatry
metapsychics
metapsychology
metathesis
meteorophobia
meter
    biofeedback
    vibration
    volume unit (VU meter)
"meth" (methamphetamine hydro-
    chloride)
methadone (street names)
    amidone
    fizzies
methadone maintenance treatment
methamphetamine (street names)
    batu
    bombit
    chalk
    crank
    croak
    crink
    cris
    Cristina
    Cristy
    crystal
    crystal meth
    domes
    fire
    hiroppon

methamphetamine *(cont.)*
  hot ice
  ice
  Kaksonjae
  L.A. glass
  L.A. ice
  meth
  methylphenidate
  quill
  shabu
  speed
  super ice
  water
  white cross
  X
  yellow bam
methamphetamine abuse
methamphetamine/amphetamine
methaqualone (street names)
  ludes
  sopors
methaqualone compound
methatriol (injectable steroid)
methcathinone (street names)
  bathtub speed
  the C
  cat
  ephedrone
  gaggers
  go-fast
  goob
  slick superspeed
  sniff
  star
  stat
  tweeker
  wild cat
"meth head" (re: methamphetamine
  user)
"meth monster" (re: methamphetamine user)

method
  acoupedic
  acoustic
  administration
  analytic
  artificial
  ascertainment
  assessment
  aural rehabilitation
  bisensory
  breathing
  chewing
  combined
  consonant-injection
  cross-consonant injection
  defining criteria
  formal
  Freud cathartic
  informal
  inhalation
  inhaling intoxicating vapors
  injection
  Jung
  key word
  kinesthetic
  manual
  monitoring
  nonpurging
  numerical cipher
  optimal
  oral-aural
  pavlovian
  plateau
  plosive-injection
  poor
  preferred
  purging
  rehabilitation
  retrieval
  review
  Rochester

method *(cont.)*
  shadowing
  sniff
  synthetic
  verbotonal
  visual
  weight loss
method factors
method of esophageal speech
  breathing
  inhalation
  injection
  sniff
  suction
  swallow
method sine wave
method threshold shift
methomania
methoxyhydroxyphenylglycol level
  (in bipolar disorders)
methyl acceptor
methyl alcohol addiction
methylated spirit addiction
methyldimethoxyamphetamine (DOM)
methylene chloride
methylenedioxyamphetamine (MDA)
methylenedioxymethamphetamine
  (street names)
  decadence
  doctor
  domex
  ecstasy
  essence
  ice
  Kleenex
  love drug
  love trip
  MDM
  MDMA
  rolling
  running
  speed for lovers

methylenedioxymethamphetamine *(cont.)*
  X
  X-ing
  XTC
methylphenidate challenge test
methyltestosterone (oral steroid)
methylxanthine-induced postural
  tremor
metonymy (figure of speech)
Metrazol shock therapy or treatment
metromania
Metropolitan Achievement Tests,
  Seventh Edition (MAT7)
Metropolitan Language Instructional
  Test
Metropolitan Readiness Tests, Fifth
  Edition (MRT)
"Mexican brown" (cannabis; heroin)
"Mexican horse" (heroin)
Mexican marijuana
"Mexican mud" (heroin)
"Mexican mushroom" (psilocybin/
  psilocin)
"Mexican red" (cannabis)
"Mexican reds" (barbiturate)
Meyer, Adolf (1866-1950)
Meyer-Kendall Assessment Survey
  (MKAS)
"mezc" (mescaline)
MFD (Memory-for-Designs) test
MFFT (Matching Familiar Figures
  Test)
MH (marital history)
MHAQ (Modified Health Assessment
  Questionnaire)
MHC (mental health clinic)
MHPA (Minnesota-Hartford
  Personality Assay)
MI (mental illness)
MI (mentally impaired)
miasma
Michigan Alcoholism Screening Test
  (MAST)

Michigan Alcohol Screening Test
Michigan English Language
  Assessment Battery
Michigan Picture Inventory
Michigan Picture Stories
Michigan Picture Test Revised
Michigan Screening Profile of
  Parenting
"Mickey" or "Mickey Finn" (barbiturate)
microbiophobia
microcephalic idiocy
microcephalus
microcephaly
microcheilia
"microdot" (lysergic acid diethylamide)
microglossia
micrognathia
micromania
microphobia
microphone
  directional
  nondirectional
  omnidirectional
  probe tube
microphone measurements
microphonia, cochlear
microphonics
micropsia
microscopic examination
microstomia
microtia
MICS (Mother/Infant Communication
  Screening)
micturition disorder
midbrain deafness
midbrain dysfunction
middle constrictor muscle of pharynx
midlife crisis
"midnight oil" (opium)
mid vowel

"Mighty Joe Young" (barbiturate)
"mighty mezz" (cannabis cigarette)
"Mighty Quinn" (lysergic acid
  diethylamide)
migraine (migraine headache)
  acute confusional
  aphasic
  basilar
  bilateral
  circumstantial
  classical
  cluster
  common
  complicated
  confusional
  familial
  hemiparesthetic
  hemiplegic
  late-life
  ocular
  paroxysmal
  recurrent
  seasonal
  tension
  unilateral
  vestibular
migraine aura
migrainous syndrome
migration, cultural adjustment following
Miles ABC Test of Ocular Dominance
milestones, developmental
milieu
  structured
  therapeutic
milieu therapy
military combat
Military Environment Inventory
military history
military neurosis
military psychiatry

military psychology
Miller Analogies Test (MAT)
Miller Assessment for Preschoolers
Miller-Yoder Language Comprehension Test (Clinical Edition)
Mill Hill Vocabulary Scale
Millon Adolescent Clinical Inventory (MACI)
Millon Adolescent Personality Inventory
Millon Behavioral Health Inventory II (MBHI-II)
Millon Clinical Multiaxial Inventory (MCMI)
MILMD (Management Inventory on Leadership, Motivation and Decision-Making)
Milton-model
Milwaukee Academic Interest Inventory (MAII)
mimetic addiction
mimetic convulsion
mimetic speech
mimic convulsion
mimicked
mimic speech
MIMV (Maferr Inventory of Masculine Values)
mind/body dualism
mind control
"mind detergent" (lysergic acid diethylamide)
mindedness, psychological
mind going blank
mind reading
mind pain
mind powers
mind, state of
mineral metabolism
"minibennie" (amphetamine)
MINICROS (contralateral routing of signals)

Mini Inventory of Right Brain Injury (MIRBI)
minimal brain dysfunction (MBD)
minimal role
Mini-Mental State Examination
minimization of emotional detail
minimum acceptable skill
minimum audible field (MAF)
minimum audible pressure (MAP)
Minimum Auditory Capabilities (MAC) Test
Minimum Essentials Test (MET)
minimum self-support
Minnesota Child Developmental Inventory (MCDI)
Minnesota Clerical Assessment Battery
Minnesota Clerical Test
Minnesota Differential Diagnosis of Aphasia (MDDA)
Minnesota Engineering Analogies Test (MEAT)
Minnesota-Hartford Personality Assay (MHPA)
Minnesota Importance Questionnaire
Minnesota Infant Development Inventory
Minnesota Job Description Questionnaire (MJDQ)
Minnesota Manual Dexterity Test
Minnesota Multiphasic Personality Inventory (MMPI)
Minnesota Multiphasic Personality Inventory, Adolescent (MMPI-A)
Minnesota Multiphasic Personality Inventory, Second Edition (MMPI-2)
Minnesota Percepto-Diagnostic Test (MPDT)
Minnesota Preschool Scales
Minnesota Rate of Manipulation Tests
Minnesota Satisfaction Questionnaire (MSQ)

Minnesota Satisfaction Scales (MSS)
Minnesota Scholastic Aptitude Test
(MSAT)
Minnesota Spatial Relations Test
(MSRT)
Minnesota Teacher Attitude Inventory
(MTAI)
Minnesota Test for Differential
Diagnosis of Aphasia
Minnesota Test of Aphasia
Minnesota Vocational Interest
Inventory (MVII)
minor, emancipated
minor epilepsy (petit mal)
minor hysteria
minor image-distorting level
minor stimuli
minor tranquilizer
"mint leaf" (phencyclidine)
"mint weed" (phencyclidine)
Minutes of the Vienna Psychoanalytic
Society
"mira" (opium)
MIRBI (Mini Inventory of Right
Brain Injury)
mirror focus
mirroring, cross-over
mirror speech
misaction
misanthropy
misattribute
misattribution
mischievous behavior
miscommunication
misconceptions, illusionary
misdemeanor
misinterpretation
Miskimins Self-Goal-Other Discrepancy Scale
misogamy
misogyny
misophobia

misperception, sleep state
misplaced objects test
mispronunciation
misrepresentation
"Miss Emma" (morphine)
"missile basing" (crack liquid and
phencyclidine)
"mission" (re: crack acquisition)
Missouri Children's Picture Series
(MCPS)
Missouri Kindergarten Inventory of
Developmental Skills
Missouri Occupational Card Sort
misstatement
"mist" (crack smoke; phencyclidine)
"mister blue" (morphine)
mistreatment
mistrustful
MIT (Male Impotence Test)
MIT (Motor Impersistence Test)
Mitchell, S. Weir (1830-1914)
mitigated echolalia
mixed anxiety and depressed mood
mixed anxiety/depressed mood
mixed aphasia
mixed bipolar disorder
mixed cerebral dominance
mixed compulsive psychasthenia
mixed conduct/emotional adjustment
reaction
mixed conduct/emotional disturbance
mixed deafness
mixed disturbance stress reaction
mixed drug abuse
mixed episode
mixed features
mixed hearing loss
mixed laterality
mixed-mood state
mixed nasality
mixed nasality voice disorder
mixed neurosis

mixed paralytic conversion reaction
mixed paranoid/affective organic
    psychosis
mixed presentation
mixed psychoneurotic disorder
mixed psychopathic personality
mixed receptive-expressive language
    disorder
mixed schizophrenia
mixed schizophrenic/affective
    psychosis
mixed sedative
mixed sleep apnea
mixed symptom picture with percep-
    tual disturbances
mixed-type delusions
mixed-type epilepsy
mixed-type manic-depressive
    psychosis
mixed-type of symptom
mixed-type schizophrenia
mixoscopia
mixture approach
MJ (marijuana; cannabis)
MJDQ (Minnesota Job Description
    Questionnaire)
MKAS (Meyer-Kendall Assessment
    Survey)
MLB (Monaural Loudness Balance)
    Test
MLQ (Multifactor Leadership
    Questionnaire)
MLR (mean length of response)
MLU (mean length of utterance)
MMPI (Minnesota Multiphasic
    Personality Inventory)
MMPI-A (Minnesota Multiphasic
    Personality Inventory, Adolescent)
MMPI Code Type
MMPI-2 (Minnesota Multiphasic
    Personality Inventory, Second
    Edition)

MMTIC (Murphy-Meisgeier Type
    Indicator for Children)
MMY (Mental Measurements Year-
    book)
M'Naghten rule
mnemenic
mnemic
mnemonics
"M.O." (cannabis)
Mo (mother)
mobility disability
mobilization, stapes
Mobius syndrome
MOCI (Maudsley Obsessional Com-
    pulsive Inventory)
modal auxiliary verb
modal frequency
modality (pl. modalities)
    auditory sensory
    gustatory sensory
    olfactory sensory
    sensory
    tactile sensory
    therapeutic
    visual sensory
modal operators
modal tone
modal verb
"modams" (cannabis)
model
    biopsychosocial
    categorical
    dimensional
    ego
    psychological
modeled (not mottled) behavior
modeling procedures for anxiety
    disorders in children
model of schizophrenia
Modern Language Aptitude Test
Modern Occupational Skills Test
    (MOST)

mode, vocal
modification
  active
  behavior (B-mod)
  carbonyl
  interference
Modified Health Assessment Questionnaire (MHAQ)
modified mastoidectomy
modified self-report measure of social adjustment measure
Modified Vygotsky Concept Formation Test
Modified Word Learning Test (MWLT)
modifier
  nonrestrictive
  restrictive
modulated affect
modulation
  amplitude (AM)
  emotion
  impaired affect
mogilalia
"mohasky" (cannabis)
MOJAC (mood, orientation, judgment, affect, content)
"Mojo" (cocaine; heroin)
molar
  first deciduous
  second deciduous
molar teeth
molds, ear
molecular neurobiology
molestation, child
molysmophobia
moment, product
monaural hearing aid
Monaural Loudness Balance (MLB) Test
Monday morning headache
Mondini deafness

monetary value
mongolian
mongolian idiocy
mongolian idiot
mongolism, translocation
mongoloid
monitoring
  baseline
  behavioral
  method of
monitoring audiometry
Monitoring Basic Skills Progress (MBSP)
"monkey" (cocaine-laced cigarette; drug dependency)
"monkey dust" (phencyclidine)
"monkey tranquilizer" (phencyclidine)
monoamine oxidase (MAO)
monoamine oxidase inhibitor (MAOI)
monoamine oxidase inhibitor-serotonergic agent
monoamine oxidase inhibitor tricyclic agent
monocular visual loss
monocyclic antidepressant
monogamous relationship
monogynous
monogyny
monologue, collective
monomania
monomoria
monomorphemic
mononoea
monopathophobia
monophasia
monophasic
monophobia
monophthong
monoplegia
monoplegic disorder
monopolar depression
monopolization (communication pattern)

"monos" (cocaine-laced cigarette)
monosyllabic processes
monosyllabic speech
monosyllabic word
Monotic Word Memory Test
  (MWMT)
monotone speech
monozygotic twins
"monte" (cannabis)
Montgomery and Asberg Depression
  Rating Scale (MADRS)
month-of-year test
"mooca/moocah" (cannabis)
mood
  abnormal
  anxious
  cranky
  dejected
  depressed
  dysphoric
  elevated
  erratic
  euphoric
  expansive
  euthymic
  imperative
  indicative
  irritable
  labile
  lowered
  nondepressed
  prominent irritable
  sad
  subjunctive
mood-altering substance
mood and/or affect (M/A)
mood-balance
mood changes
mood congruent
mood-congruent delusion
mood-congruent hallucination
mood-congruent psychotic features

mood disorder
  alpha-methyldopa-induced
  amitriptyline-induced
  amphetamine-induced
  cocaine-induced
  electroconvulsive therapy-induced
  gender differences in
  light therapy-induced
  major
  seasonal
  substance-induced
  unknown substance-induced
mood disturbance
mood-elevating drug
mood episode
mood-incongruent delusion
mood-incongruent hallucination
mood-incongruent psychotic features
mood induction
mood lability
mood, orientation, judgment, affect,
  content (MOJAC)
mood shifts
mood swings
mood symptomatology
mood symptoms
"moon" (mescaline)
Mooney Problem Check List (MPCL)
Moonies
"moonrock" (crack and heroin)
"mooster" (cannabis)
"moota/mutah" (cannabis)
"mooters" (cannabis cigarette)
"mootie" (cannabis)
"mootos" (cannabis)
"mor a grifa" (cannabis)
moral (pl. morals)
moral ataxia
moral behavior
moral deficiency personality disorder
moral development
morale

moral idiocy
moral imbecility
moral insanity
moral oligophrenia
moral outrage
moral treatment
moral values
Morbid Anxiety Inventory (MAI)
morbid doubt
morbid idea
morbid impulse
morbidity
morbid jealousy
morbid responses
morbid rumination
"more" (phencyclidine)
mores, sexual
"morf" (morphine)
moria
moribund state
Morita therapy
morning drinking
morning glory seeds (street names)
  flower power
  heavenly blue
  pearly gates
morning headache
"morning wake-up" (re: crack use)
moron
moronity
Moro reflex
"Morotgara" (heroin)
morpheme
  bound
  circumfix
  derivational
  free
  grammatical
  infix
  inflectional
  lexical
  structural rule
  zero (0)

morphine (street names)
  cotton brothers
  dope
  double yoke
  dreamer
  emsel
  first line
  God's drug
  hows
  M
  Miss Emma
  morpho
  mister blue
  morf
  M.S.
  New Jack Swing
  unkie
  white stuff
morphine-like action
morphinism
morphinomania
"morpho" (morphine)
"morpho moron" (hard drug user)
morphological rules
morphometric analysis
morphophonemic component
"mortal combat" (heroin)
mortality rate
Moses and monotheism
"mosquitos" (cocaine)
MOST (Modern Occupational Skills
  Test)
Mot (motility-related)
"mota/moto" (cannabis)
Mot-dysphagia patient
"moth-eaten" teeth
"mother" (cannabis)
Mother Card
mother-child bond
Mother-Child Relationship Evaluation,
  The (MCRE)
mother fixation

mother-infant attachment
Mother/Infant Communication Screen-
    ing (MICS)
mother instinct
"mother's little helper" (barbiturate)
Mother Superior complex
mother, surrogate
motility-related (Mot)
motion
    brownian
    involuntary
    simple harmonic (SHM)
    voluntary
motion perception
motion rate
motion studies
motivating operation
motivation
    decreased
    expressed
    external incentive
    personal
    psychological
    suicide
Motivational Patterns Inventory
Motivation Analysis Test (MAT)
motivation for cross-dressing
motivation for self-injury
motivator
motive (pl. motives)
    achievement
    conflicting
    mastery
motor
    fine
    gross
motor ability (pl. abilities)
    disturbance in
    perceptual
motor activity
motor agraphia
motor alexia

motor aphasia
    afferent (kinesthetic)
    efferent (kinetic)
    subcortical
    transcortical
motor apraxia
motor area
motor aura
motor behavior
    catatonic
    driven
    nonfunctional
    nonfunctional and repetitive
motor center
motor coordination
motor cortex
motor deficit
motor development
motor disinhibition
motor disorder
motor evoked potential (MEP)
Motor-Free Visual Perception Test
    (MVPT)
motor function
motor functioning
motoria
motorically
motoric immobility
motoric phenomenon
motor image
motor immobility
motor impairment
Motor Impersistence Test (MIT)
motor innervation
motor loss
motor movement
motor nerve
motor nerve conduction
motor neuron
motor paralysis
motor pathways disease
motor performance

motorphobia
motor planning
motor restlessness
motor skill disturbances
motor skills disorder
motor speed
Motor Steadiness Battery
motor symptoms
motor system
motor tic
    complex
    simple
motor tic disorder
motor type of symptom
motor-verbal tic disorder (Tourette)
motor vocalization
motor-vocal tic disorder
mourn
mourning
mouth breathing
mouthing movement
mouth, nothing by (NPO, n.p.o.)
"mouth worker" (re: drug user)
movement
    abnormal
    adventitious
    anomalous
    arcuate
    athetoid
    ballistic
    bodily
    brownian
    cardinal ocular
    choreiform
    clonic
    compensatory
    complex whole body
    coreoathetoid
    dyskinetic
    dyspractic
    dysrhythmic
    dystonic

movement *(cont.)*
    extraneous
    false perceptions of
    fetal
    flapping
    following
    free mandibular
    freezing of
    functional
    hemiballismic
    intentional stereotyped
    involuntary
    irregular
    jerking
    low-complexity
    mandibular
    medication-induced
    mouthing
    muscle
    myoclonic
    non-rapid eye (NREM)
    nonrhythmic stereotyped motor
    oscillatory
    paucity of
    perseverative
    poverty of
    purposeful
    purposeless
    purposive
    pursuit
    quasipurposive
    random
    rapid
    rapid-alternating (RAM)
    rapid eye (REM)
    rapid fine
    rapid repetitive
    reflex eye
    reflexive
    repetitive
    repetitive imitative
    rhythmic

movement *(cont.)*
   rhythmic slow eye
   roving eye
   roving ocular
   saccadic eye
   stereotyped
   stereotyped body
   stereotyped motor
   stereotypical
   synkinetic motor
   tonic-clonic
   tremulous
   vermicular
   vestibular
   visual pursuit
   volitional
   volitional oral
   voluntary
   voluntary muscle
   withdrawal
movement abnormality
movement disorder
   abnormal involuntary (AIMD)
   hysterical
   medication-induced
   neuroleptic-induced acute
   neuropsychiatric
   stereotypic
Movement Disorder Questionnaire
movement of tongue
movement peculiarities
movement scale
movement symptoms
movement toward the community
"movie star drug" (cocaine)
"mow the grass" (re: cannabis use)
Moynahan syndrome
MPCL (Mooney Problem Check List)
MPD (Measures of Psychosocial Development)
MPD (Minnesota Percepto-Diagnostic)
MPD (multiple personality disorder)

MPDT (Minnesota Percepto-Diagnostic Test)
MPI (Multiphasic or Multivariate Personality Inventory)
MPO (maximum power output)
MPPP (analog of meperidine)
MPS (Management Philosophies Scale)
MPTP (analog of meperidine)
MQ (memory quotient)
MRS (mania rating scale)
MRT (major role therapy)
MRT (Metropolitan Readiness Tests, Fifth Edition)
MRT Español
MRU (mean relational utterance)
"M.S." (morphine)
MSAS (Mandel Social Adjustment Scale)
MSAT (Minnesota Scholastic Aptitude Test)
MSCA (McCarthy Scales of Children's Abilities)
MSCS (Multidimensional Self Concept Scale)
MSDI (Martin S-D [suicide-depression] Inventory)
MSE (mental status examination)
MSER (Mental Status Examination Record)
MSL (mean sentence length)
MSLT (Multiple Sleep Latency Test)
MSN (Master of Science in Nursing)
MSQ (Managerial Style Questionnaire)
MSQ (Mental Status Questionnaire)
MSQ (Minnesota Satisfaction Questionnaire)
MSRPP (multidimensional scale for rating psychiatric patients)
MSRT (Minnesota Spatial Relations Test)
MSS (mental status schedule)
MSS (Minnesota Satisfaction Scales)

MSSST (Meeting Street School Screening Test)
MSW (Master of Social Work)
MT (music therapy)
MTAI (Minnesota Teacher Attitude Inventory)
MTP (Multidisciplinary Treatment Plan)
MTR (Music Therapist, Registered)
"M.U." (cannabis)
"mud" (heroin)
mucoid otitis media
mu opiate receptors
mu receptors
muffled voice
"muggie" (cannabis)
mugging
"mujer" (cocaine)
"mule" (re: drug dealing)
Mullen Scales of Early Learning
multiaxial evaluation
multiaxial system
MULTICROS (contralateral routing of signals)
multicultural environment
Multidimensional Aptitude Battery
Multidimensional Assessment of Gains in School (MAGS)
Multidimensional Assessment of Philosophy of Education (MAPE)
multidimensional scale for rating psychiatric patients (MSRPP)
Multidimensional Self Concept Scale (MSCS)
multidisciplinary group psychiatry
multidisciplinary management of aggressive behavior
multidisciplinary management of violence
Multidisciplinary Treatment Plan (MTP)
multidrug

Multifactor Leadership Questionnaire (MLQ)
multifocal leukoencephalopathy
multi-infarct dementia
multi-infarct psychosis
multi-item index
multi-item test
Multilevel Informal Language Inventory
Multilingual Aphasia Examination (MAE)
Multiphasic Environmental Assessment Procedure (MEAP)
Multiphasic Personality Inventory (MPI)
multiple analysis
multiple cognitive deficits
multiple distinct identities
multiple ego state
multiple focus
multiple life difficulties
multiple operations syndrome
multiple personality and gender
multiple personality crime
multiple personality disorder (MPD)
multiple psychotherapy
multiple regression technique
multiple sclerosis
multiple sclerosis-type organic psychosis
Multiple Sleep Latency Test (MSLT)
multiple therapy
multiplication table test
Multiscore Depression Inventory (MDI)
multisensory
multistep task
multisyllable word
Multivariate Personality Inventory (MPI)
multi-word phrase
mumbling automatism

Munchausen syndrome
Munchausen syndrome by proxy
"murder 8" (fentanyl)
"murder one" (heroin and cocaine)
murmuring, voice
Murphy-Meisgeier Type Indicator for
    Children (MMTIC)
Murray Valley viral encephalitis
muscarine cholinergic receptor for
    acetylcholine
muscarine receptors, blockade of
muscle (pl. muscles) of larynx, palate,
    pharynx, respiration, and tongue
    (see Appendix II)
muscle contraction headache
muscle disorder
muscle imbalance
muscle movement
muscle reflex
muscle relaxants
muscle rigidity
muscle strength
muscle tone
muscle twitch/twitching
muscular dystrophy
muscular relaxation
muscular rigidity
muscular tension
musculoskeletal disorder
"mushroom" (psilocin/psilocybin)
Music Achievement Tests 1, 2, 3,
    and 4 (MAT)
musical agraphia
musical alexia
Musical Aptitude Profile (MAP)
musical stimulus
musicogenic epilepsy
musicomania
musicophobia
musomania
musophobia
Music Therapist, Registered (MTR)

music therapy (MT)
"musk" (psilocybin/psilocin)
mussitans, delirium
mutation voice
mute, deaf
"mutha" (cannabis)
mutilate
mutilation, sadistic
mutism
    akinetic
    catatonic
    elected
    elective
    hysterical
    relative elective
    selective
    voluntary
mutism adjustment reaction, elective
muttering delirium
mutual affective responsiveness
mutualism
"muzzle" (heroin)
MVII (Minnesota Vocational Interest
    Inventory)
MVPT (Mertens Visual Perception
    Test)
MVPT (Motor-Free Visual Perception
    Test)
MWLT (Modified Word Learning
    Test)
MWMT (Monotic Word Memory
    Test)
myasthenia gravis
myasthenic facies
mydriasis
myelination
myelinization
myelin metabolism
Myers-Briggs psychological test
Myers-Briggs Type Indicator (MBTI)
Myerson reflex
mylohyoid muscle

myoclonic convulsion
myoclonic movements
myoclonic seizure
myoclonus, nocturnal
myoelastic-aerodynamic theory of
  phonation
myofunctional therapy
myopathic facies
myopathic paralysis
myopic insight
myotatic irritability
myotatic reflex
myotonic facies

myringitis
myringoplasty
myringotomy
myrinx
mysophilia
mysophobia
mysophobic
mystical experience
mythomania
mythophobia
myths, sexual (SM)
myxophobia

N, n

N (newton)
NA (Narcotics Anonymous)
N/A (not applicable)
NAA (N-acetyl-aspartate)
N-acetyl-aspartate (NAA)
n-Ach (achievement need)
NAD (no acute distress)
nadir
"nail" (cannabis cigarette)
nail-biting
"nailed" (arrested)
Nalline test
name, categorical
Names Learning Test (NLT)
name the date test
NAMI (National Alliance for the
    Mentally Ill)
naming common objects test
naming intact
naming test
N&V (nausea and vomiting)
"nanoo" (heroin)
napping phenomenon
Nar-Anon
narcissistic personality
narcissistic personality disorder
narcissistic rage

narcissistic tendencies
narcissistic vulnerability
narcoanalysis
narcohypnosis
narcolepsy
narcolepsy cataplexy syndrome
narcolepsy experience
narcoleptic
narcoma
narcomania
narcoplexy
narcose
narcosis
narcosomania
narcostimulant
narcosynthesis
narcotherapy
narcotic agonist drug
narcotic blockade
narcotic blocking drugs (narcotic
    antagonists)
narcotic chemical intoxication
narcotic drug dependence
narcotic hunger
Narcotics Anonymous (NA)
narcotics, toxic effects of
narcotic withdrawal

narcotism
narcotize
nares constriction
naris (pl. nares)
narrative speech
narrative therapy
narrow-band noise
narrow-based gait
narrow phonetic transcription
narrow-range audiometer
narrow-set eyes
narrow transcription
narrow vowel
NART (National Adult Reading Test), Second Edition)
nasal ala (pl. alae)
nasal bone
nasal cavity
  nasal bone
  inferior
  medial
  superior
  supreme
nasal concha (pl. nasal conchae)
  inferior
  medial
  superior
  supreme
nasal consonant
nasal consonant formation
nasal coupling
nasal emission
nasal escape
nasality
  assimilated
  excessive
  mixed
nasality voice disorder
nasalization of vowels
nasalized vowels
nasal lisp
nasal polyps

nasal port
nasal resonance
nasal respiration
nasal rustle
nasal septum
nasal skull bones
nasal snort
nasal sounds
nasal tract
nasal turbulence
nasal twang
nasal uncoupling
nasolabial folds
naso-ocular
naso-oral
nasopalatine
nasopharyngeal pathology
nasopharyngeus meatus
nasopharyngoscope
nasopharynx
NASW (National Association of Social Workers)
NAT (Non-Verbal Ability Tests)
NAT (Numerical Attention Test)
natal
NATB (Nonreading Aptitude Test Battery)
National Adult Reading Test, Second Edition (NART)
National Alliance for the Mentally Ill (NAMI)
National Association for Mental Health
National Association for the Deaf
National Association for the Visually Handicapped
National Association of Social Workers (NASW)
National Association of Veterans Affairs Chiefs of Psychiatry (NAVACP)
National Business Competency Tests

National Center for Health Statistics (NCHS)
National Council of Community Mental Health Centers (NCCMHC)
National Council of Stutterers (NCS)
National Depressive and Manic Depressive Association (NDMDA)
National Educational Development Tests
national epithets
National Institute on Aging (NIA)
National Institute on Alcohol Abuse and Alcoholism (NIAAA)
National Institute on Drug Abuse (NIDA)
National Institutes of Health (NIH)
National Institute of Mental Health (NIMH)
National Institute of Neurological and Communicative Disorders and Stroke (NINCDS)
National Medical Association (NMA)
National Mental Health Association (NMHA)
National Multiple Sclerosis Society (NMSS)
National Occupation Competency Testing (NOCTI)
National Police Officer Selection Test (POST)
National Stuttering Project (NSP)
National Training Laboratories
native language
nativist theory
natural class sounds
natural disasters as major childhood stressors
natural environment
natural environment type
natural frequency
natural group
natural phonological processes

natural pitch
Natural Process Analysis
nature versus nurture
nausea and vomiting (N&V)
nausea/vomiting
NAVACP (National Association of Veterans Affairs Chiefs of Psychiatry)
Naylor-Harwood Adult Intelligence Scale (NHAIS)
NBAS (Neonatal Behavioral Assessment Scale)
NBAS-K (Neonatal Behavioral Assessment Scale with Kansas Supplements)
NCCMHC (National Council of Community Mental Health Centers)
NCHS (National Center for Health Statistics)
NCS (National Council of Stutterers)
NDMDA (National Depressive and Manic Depressive Association)
NDT (noise detection threshold)
NEAT (Norris Educational Achievement Test)
neatly groomed
"nebbies" (pentobarbital)
necessary task
neck loop
neck pain, psychogenic
necromania
necromimesis
necrophilia
necrophilism
necrophilous
necrophily
necrophobia
necrosadism
necrosis negation
need (pl. needs)
    achievement (n-Ach)
    affective

need *(cont.)*
  emotional
  excessive
  inner
  instrumental
  psychological
  repressed (theory in stuttering)
  unmet
  unmet dependency
need a sentence test
need for admiration
need for approval
need for care, excessive
Need for Cognition Scale
need to control others
needless repetition
needle track
needs
nefazodone
neg (negative)
negation
  delusion of
  necrosis
negative (neg)
negative affect
negative behavior
negative body image
negative command
negative conditioning for sleep
negative correlation
negative effect of drug
negative emotion
negative emotionality
negative evaluation
negative factor
negative factor in schizophrenia
negative feedback
negative feelings
negative ion
negative judgments
negative life event
negative mood induction

negative mood state
negative practice
negative predictive power
negative qualities
negative reinforcement
negative reinforcer
negative relationship
negative response
negative scotoma
negative self-comparison
negative self-image
negative spike wave
negative symptoms of schizophrenia
negative transference
negative variation
negative voices
negativism
  catatonic
  command
  extreme
negativistic behavior
negativistic personality disorder
neglect
  auditory
  basic health
  child
  elder adult
  family
  household duties
  perceived
  pleasurable activities
  problems related to
  responsibilities
  school work
  spatial
  unilateral
  unilateral organic
  unilateral spatial
  unilateral visual
  victim of child
  visual
neglectful

neglect syndrome
negotiating goals skills
negotiating language
negotiating routines skills
negotiating rules skills
negotiation, problem-solving
Negrophobia
"nemmies" (barbiturate)
neocortex
NEO Five Factor Inventory
NEO Personality Inventory, Revised
  (NEO-PI-R)
neolalia
neolalism
neologism
neonatal auditory response cradle
neonatal auditory response cradle
  audiometry
Neonatal Behavioral Assessment Scale
  (NBAS)
Neonatal Behavioral Assessment Scale
  with Kansas Supplements (NBAS-K)
neonatal familial seizure
neonate
neophobia
neophrenia
NEO-PI-R (Revised NEO Personality
  Inventory)
nepenthic
nephophobia
nerve
  acoustic
  afferent
  alveolar
  cochlear
  cranial
  efferent
  facial
  glossopharyngeal
  hypoglossal
  motor
  olfactory

nerve *(cont.)*
  sensory
  vagus
  vestibulocochlear
nerve cell death
nerve cell destruction
nerve cell survival
nerve deafness
nerve fiber
nerve force
nerve growth factor (NGF)
nerve impulse
nerve loss
nerve tumor
nervosa
  anorexia
  bulimia
  dysphagia
nervous breakdown
nervous debility
nervous depression
nervous disease
nervous exhaustion
nervous fatigue
nervous gastritis
nervous giggling
nervousness
nervous stomach
nervous system
  autonomic (ANS)
  central (CNS)
  parasympathetic (PNS)
  peripheral (PNS)
  sympathetic (SNS)
  third
  visceral
nervous tension
nest
network (pl. networks)
  cortical
  delusional
  interpersonal

network therapy
neural deafness
neural deficit
neural efficiency
neuralgia, trigeminal
neuralgic pain
neurasthenia
neurasthenic neurosis
neurasthenic psychoneurosis
neurasthenic psychoneurotic reaction
neurasthenic reaction
neurinoma
neuroadaptation
neuroanatomy of aging
Neurobehavioral Cognitive Status
 Examination
Neurobehavioral Rating Scale
neurobehavioral syndrome
neurobiology
 behavioral
 molecular
neurobiology in aging
neurocirculatory asthenia
neurocirculatory disorder
neurocognitive disorder
neurodegenerative disease
neuroendocrine challenge
neuroendocrine function
neurofeedback training (NT)
neurofibrillary tangle
neurogenic claudication
neurogenic hyperventilation
neurogenic reaction
neurogenic shock
neurogenic shock syndrome
neurogenic stuttering
neuroimaging
neuroleptic (pl. neuroleptics)
 butyrophenone-based
 phenothiazine-based
neuroleptic agent (drug)

neuroleptic dose-dependent akathisia
neuroleptic-induced acute akathisia
neuroleptic-induced acute dystonia
neuroleptic-induced acute movement
 disorder
neuroleptic-induced akinesia
neuroleptic-induced parkinsonism
neuroleptic-induced parkinsonian
 tremor
neuroleptic-induced postural tremor
neuroleptic-induced tardive dyskinesia
neuroleptic malignant syndrome
 (NMS)
neuroleptic medication-induced
 postural tremor
neuroleptic-resistant schizophrenic
neuroleptic treatment
neurolinguistic programming
neurolinguistics
neurologic deficit
neurologic deterioration
neurologic disability
neurologic disturbance
neurologic signs
 focal
 focal nonextrapyramidal
neurological conditions
neurological control
neurological deficit
neurological dysfunction
Neurological Dysfunctions of Children
neurological evaluation
neurological examination
neurological functioning
neurological signs
neurological soft sign
neurology, behavioral
neuroma, acoustic
neurometric analysis
neurometrics
neuromotor

neuromuscular
neuron (pl. neurons)
  cholinergic
  locus ceruleus
  motor
  presynaptic
  serotonergic
neuronal circuit
neuronal degeneration
neuronal loss
neuronal metabolism
neuro-ophthalmologic history
neuro-otology
neuropathology of aging
neuropathy
  autonomic
  peripheral autonomic
neuropeptide
neurophonia
neurophysiological assessment
neurophysiological findings
neurophysiological heterogeneity
neurophysiological testing
neuropsychiatric disorder
neuropsychiatric movement disorder
neuropsychiatrist
neuropsychiatry, geriatric
neuropsychic
neuropsychological assessment
neuropsychological evaluation of
  dementia
neuropsychological findings
neuropsychological impairment
Neuropsychological Screening Exam
Neuropsychological Status Examination
neuropsychological test
neuropsychological testing
neuropsychologic battery of tests
neuropsychologic disorder
neuropsychologic evaluation
neuropsychologist

neuropsychology
neuropsychometric test
neuropsychopathy
neuropsychopharmacology
neuropsychosis
neurosis (pl. neuroses)
  accident
  actual
  anancastic
  anxiety
  association
  asthenic
  battle
  cardiac
  cardiovascular
  character
  climacteric
  combat
  compensation
  compulsive
  conversion
  craft
  depersonalization
  depressive
  environmental
  expectation
  experimental
  family
  fatigue
  fixation
  functional
  homosexual
  hypochondriacal
  hysterical
  impulsive
  military
  mixed
  neurasthenic
  obsessional
  obsessive-compulsive
  occupational
  oedipal

neurosis *(cont.)*
  pension
  phobic
  postconcussion
  posttraumatic
  professional
  psychasthenic
  railroad
  regression
  senile
  sexual
  situational
  transference
  traumatic
  vegetative
  war
neurosis tarda
neurosyphilis, dementia in
neurotherapy
neurotica
neurotic anxiety state
  atypical
  generalized
  panic attack
neurotic delinquency
  adolescent
  juvenile
neurotic depression
neurotic depressive reaction
neurotic depressive state
neurotic direction profile
neurotic disorder
  anxiety state
  compensation neurosis
  depersonalization
  depression
  dysthymic
  hypochondriasis
  hysteria
  neurasthenia
  obsessive-compulsive
  occupational

neurotic disorder *(cont.)*
  personality
  phobic
  sexual deviation
  somatization
neurotic features
neurotic hysteria disorder
  conversion type
  dissociative type
  factitious type
neuroticism
neurotic manifestation
neurotic mental disorder
neurotic personality disorder
  affective
  antisocial
  avoidant
  borderline
  compulsive
  dependent
  explosive
  histrionic
  narcissistic
  paranoid
  passive-aggressive
  schizoid
Neurotic Personality Factor Test
  (NPFT)
neurotic process
neurotic reaction
neurotic reaction brain syndrome
neurotic rumination
neurotic state with depersonalization
  episode
Neuroticism Scale Questionnaire
  (NSQ)
neurotization
neurotogenic
neurotransmission, serotonergic
neurotransmitter, catecholamine
  (norepinephrine)
neurotransmitter metabolics

neurotransmitter systems
neutralization rules
neutralization, vowel
neutralize an obsession
neutralized anxiety
neutralizing mechanism
neutral stimulus
neutral vowel
neutroclusion of teeth
nevoid amentia
"new acid" (phencyclidine)
"New Jack Swing" (heroin and morphine)
New Jersey Test of Reasoning Skills
"new magic" (phencyclidine)
new memory encoding
New Mexico Attitude Toward Work Test (NMATWT)
New Mexico Career Planning Testing (NMCPT)
New Mexico Job Application Procedures Test (NMJAPT)
New Mexico Knowledge of Occupations Test (NMKOT)
new-onset seizure
new responsibilities
news of death
New Sucher-Allred Reading Placement Inventory
newton (N)
new-work effort
New York University Parkinson's Disease Scale
NGF (nerve growth factor)
NHAIS (Naylor-Harwood Adult Intelligence Scale)
NIA (National Institute on Aging)
NIAAA (National Institute on Alcohol Abuse and Alcoholism)
niacin-deficiency
"nice and easy" (heroin)

"nickel bag" (heroin; $5 worth of drugs)
"nickel deck" (heroin)
"nickel note" (re: currency)
nicotine addiction
nicotine dependence
nicotine intoxication
nicotine-related disorder
nicotine use disorder
nicotine withdrawal
nicotinic cholinergic receptor for acetylcholine
nicotinic receptors, blockade of
NIDA (National Institute on Drug Abuse)
"niebla" (phencyclidine)
Niemann-Pick disease
night (noc), every (q.h.s.)
night hospital
nightmare disorder
nightmares (dream anxiety attacks), recurrent
night pain
night terrors (pavor nocturnus)
nighttime activity
nighttime agitation
nighttime sleep
    alcohol-induced
    fragmented
nigrostriatal tract
NIH (National Institutes of Health)
NIH Stroke Scale
nihilism, therapeutic
nihilistic delusion
NIL (noise interference level)
"nimbies" (barbiturate)
NIMH (National Institute of Mental Health)
NIMH data
NIMH-OC (National Institute of Mental Health Global Obsessive Compulsive Scale)

NINCDS (National Institute of Neurological and Communicative Disorders and Stroke)
nine-digit SDL task (SD9)
Ninjitsu
nitrate inhalant
  amyl
  butyl
  isobutyl
nitric oxide
nitrite headache
nitrous oxide (street names)
  buzz bomb
  laughing gas
  nitrous
  shoot the breeze
  whippets
"nix" (re: stranger in the group)
NL (normal libido)
NLC & C (normal libido, coitus, and
climax)
NLT (Names Learning Test)
NMA (National Medical Association)
NMATWT (New Mexico Attitude
Toward Work Test)
NMCPT (New Mexico Career
Planning Testing)
NMDA receptor alterations
NMHA (National Mental Health
Association)
NMI (no mental illness)
NMJAPT (New Mexico Job
Application Procedures Test)
NMKOT (New Mexico Knowledge of
Occupations Test)
NMS (neuroleptic malignant syndrome)
NMSS (National Multiple Sclerosis
Society)
no acute distress (NAD)
noc (night)

NOCTI (National Occupation Competency Testing) Teacher Occupational Competency Test:
Child Care and Guidance
Mechanical Technology
noctimania
noctiphobia
nocturnal confusion
nocturnal drinking syndrome
nocturnal eating syndrome
nocturnal emission
nocturnal enuresis
nocturnal epilepsy
nocturnal hallucination
nocturnal myoclonus
nocturnal panic attacks
nocturnal paroxysmal dystonia
nocturnal penile tumescence (NPT)
nocturnal polydipsia
nocturnal sleep
  insufficient
  undisturbed
nocturnal sleep duration
nocturnal sleep episodes
nocturnus, pavor (night terrors)
"nod" (re: heroin reaction)
nodding off
node (pl. nodes)
  Ranvier
  singer's
  speaker's
nodosa, chorditis
nodularity
nodule
  polyploid vocal
  sessile vocal
  vocal
no-echo chamber
noetic anxiety
"noise" (heroin)

noise
  acoustic
  ambient
  background
  complex
  extraneous
  feedback
  gaussian
  narrow-band
  pink
  random
  saw-tooth
  sixty-cycle hum
  speech
  speech discrimination in
  speech reception in
  startling
  thermal
  tone in (TIN)
  white
  wide-band
noise analyzer
noise detection threshold (NDT)
noise exposure meter
noise factor
noise figure
noise generator
noise hum
noise-induced deafness
noise-induced hearing loss
noise interference level (NIL)
noise level
noise limiter
noise pollution
noise proof
noise ratio
noise suppressor
nomatophobia
nomenclature, psychiatric
no mental illness (NMI)
nominal aphasia
nominal compound

nominalization
nominative case
nominative, predicate
nonability, cognitive
nonbarbiturate
nonbenzodiazepine
non-bizarre delusion
noncognitive subscale
noncoital stimulation
noncomplementary role
noncompliance with hospital regulations
noncompliance with treatment
noncompliant
nonconformity
nonconfrontive therapy
nonconsanguineous marriage
nonconsenting adult
nonconsenting partner
noncontrastive distribution
noncontributory
nonconvulsive status epilepticus
nondependent adult abuse
nondepressed mood
nondirectional microphone
nondirective approach
nondirective psychotherapy
nondirective therapy
nondistinctive features
nondominant hand
nonelaborative speech
nonexistence
nonextrapyramidal neurologic signs
nonfluency
nonfluent aphasia
nonfluent aphasic speech
nonfunctional and repetitive actions
  fiddling with fingers
  hand waving
  head banging
  hitting one's own body
  motor behavior

nonfunctional actions *(cont.)*
  picking at bodily orifices
  picking at skin
  playing with hands
  rocking
  self-biting
  twirling of objects
nonfunctional motor behavior
nongeneral phobic
nongenetic hearing loss
non grata, persona
noninvasive operation
nonjudgmental
Non-Language Learning Test
Non-Language Multi-Mental Test
nonlinear distortion
NONM (nonobstructive nonmotility-
  related)
NONM-dysphagia patient
non-narcotic analgesics
non-nasal sound
non-neuroleptic-induced tremor
nonnormative hair loss
nonobstructive nonmotility-related
  (NONM)
nonobtrusive text
nonoccluding earmold
nonorganic deafness
nonorganic origin
nonorganic psychosis
  acute paranoid reaction
  depressive type
  excitative type
  psychogenic paranoid
  reactive confusion
no-no tremor
nonparametric tests of significance
nonparaphilic behavior
nonparkinsonian tremor
nonpathological amnesia
nonpathological anxiety
nonpathological reaction to stress

nonpathological sexual fantasy
nonpathological substance use
nonperiodic wave
nonpharmacologically induced tremor
nonplussed
nonprescribed drugs
nonprescription drugs
nonproblematic drinking
nonproductive activity
nonpropositional speech
nonpsychotic anxiety
nonpsychotic brain syndrome
nonpsychotic severity psychoorganic
  syndrome
nonpsychotic symptoms
nonpulsating headache
nonpurging methods
non-rapid eye movement (NREM)
non-rapid-cycling pattern
Nonreading Aptitude Test Battery
  (NATB)
Non-Reading Intelligence Tests,
  Levels 1-3 (NRIT)
nonrecurrent
non-reduplicated babbling
non-REM (rapid eye movement)
    sleep stages
  deep sleep
  drowsiness
  light sleep
  very deep sleep
nonresponsive state
nonrestorative sleep
nonrestrictive modifier
nonrhythmic stereotyped motor movement
nonrhythmic stereotyped motor vocalization
nonsense syllable
nonsense syndrome
nonsense word
nonsensical speech

nonsensical statement
nonsensical words
non sequitur
nonsexual boundary violations
nonsmoker (NS)
nonspecific language
nonspecific syndrome
nonspeech sounds
nonstandard language
non-substance-induced mental disorder
non-substance-related episodes
nonsuffocation panicker
nonsuppression, dexamethasone
nonsuppurative otitis media
nonsyllabic speech sounds
nonsystematized delusion
"nontoucher" (re: affectionless crack
   user)
nontoxic lithium tremor
nontrivial value
nonturning against self (NTS)
non-24-hour sleep-wake pattern
non-24-hour sleep-wake syndrome
Non-Verbal Ability Tests (NAT)
nonverbal abstractive ability
nonverbal behavior
nonverbal communication
nonverbal information
nonverbal intellectual capacity
Non-Verbal Reasoning
nonverbal synthesizing ability
nonverbal tasks
nonvocal communication
noogenic neurosis
noothymopsychic ataxia
noradrenergic system
norepinephrine (catecholamine neurotransmitter)
norm (pl. norms)
   adaptive scale
   cultural
   deviation from physiological

norm (cont.)
   group
   physiological
   societal
   subculture
   violation of age-appropriate
      societal
normal activities of daily living
normal affect
normal development
normal distribution
normal fluency of speech
normal libido (NL)
normal libido, coitus, and climax
   (NLC & C, NL C/C1)
normal limits
normal mentation
normal muscle tone
normal neurological functioning
normal-pressure hydrocephalus (NPH)
normal probability curve
normal sleep duration
normal swallowing habit
normal transition
normal voluntary napping phenomenon
norm-assertive stance
Normative Adaptive Behavior
   Checklist
normative aging process
normative behavior
normative data
normative phonetics
norm-referenced tests
Norris Educational Achievement Test
   (NEAT)
North American Depression Inventories for Children and Adults
Northwestern Syntax Screening Test
   (NSST)
Northwestern University Children's
   Perception of Speech Test

Northwick Park Index of Independence in ADL
NOS (not otherwise specified)
"nose" (heroin)
"nose candy" (cocaine)
nose cleft
"nose drops" (liquified heroin)
"nose powder" (cocaine)
"nose stuff" (cocaine)
NOSIE (Nurses' Observation Scale for Inpatient Evaluation)
nosomania
nosophilia
nosophobia
nostalgia
nostomania
nostophobia
nostril
not applicable (N/A)
notched wave
nothing by mouth (n.p.o., NPO)
noticeable difference
noticeable hair loss
notoriety
notorious
not otherwise specified (NOS) disorder
not prisoner of war (NPOW)
Nottingham Extended ADL Index
Nottingham Health Profile
Nottingham Ten-Point ADL Scale
noun (parts of speech)
noun phrase
noun, predicate
novel setting
novel stimulus
novelty seeking
noxious responsibilities
noxious stimulus
NPFT (Neurotic Personality Factor Test)
NPH (normal pressure hydrocephalus)

n.p.o., NPO (nothing by mouth)
NPOW (not prisoner of war)
NPT (nocturnal penile tumescence)
NREM (nonrapid eye movement) sleep
NRIT (Non-Reading Intelligence Tests, Levels 1-3)
NS (nonsmoker)
NSP (National Stuttering Project)
NSQ (Neuroticism Scale Questionnaire)
NSST (Northwestern Syntax Screening Test)
NT (neurofeedback training)
NTS (nonturning against self)
NU Auditory Test Lists 4 and 6
nuance
"nubs" (mescaline)
nuchal rigidity
nuclear family
nucleus (pl. nuclei)
    dorsal cochlear
    ventral cochlear
nudomania
nudophobia
"nugget" (amphetamine)
"nuggets" (crack)
null hypothesis
"number" (cannabis cigarette)
number dysgnosia
"number 8" (heroin)
"number 4" (heroin)
"number 3" (cocaine, heroin)
number 3 traced on patient's palm test
numbers, series of
numb, feeling
numbing
    emotional
    psychic
    sense of
numbing sensation
numbness
    feeling of
    psychic

numerical aptitude (N)
Numerical Attention Test (NAT)
numerical cipher method
numerical reasoning skills
numerical symbols
nurse
   Licensed Vocational (LVN)
   psychiatric
   Registered (RN)
Nurse Aide Practice Test
nurse-patient relations
Nurses' Observation Scale for Inpatient
   Evaluation (NOSIE)
nursing
nurturance
   excessive need for
   lack of

nurture, nature versus
nurturer
nurturing environment
nutritional deficiency
nutritional insults
nyctophilia
nyctophobia
nympholepsy
nymphomania
nymphomaniac
nymphomaniacal
nystagmus
   horizontal
   toxic
   vertical

O, o

"O" (opium)
OA (object assembly) subtest
O-A (Objective-Analytic)
O/A (Overeaters Anonymous)
OADMT (Oliphant Auditory Discrimination Memory Test)
OAPs (Occupational Ability Patterns)
OARS Multidimensional Functional Assessment Questionnaire (OMFAQ)
OASIS-2 AS (Occupational Aptitude Survey and Interest Schedule, Second Edition, Aptitude Survey)
OASIS-2 IS (Occupational Aptitude Survey and Interest Schedule, Second Edition, Interest Survey)
OAST (Oliphant Auditory Synthesizing Test)
OAT (Optometry Admission Testing Program)
OBE (out-of-body experience)
obedient behavior
obfuscate
O'Brien Vocabulary Placement Test
object (pl. objects)
    analytic
    avoidance of an
    cued by an

object (cont.)
    direct
    exposure to an
    feared
    fetish
    good
    halo around
    indirect
    irrational fear of an
    love
    moving
    paraphiliac
    perception of
    sex
    substitute
    transitional
object agnosia
object assembly (OA) subtest
object attachment
object blindness
Object Classification Test (OCT)
object concept
object constancy
object "halos"
objective (pl. objectives)
    behavioral
    elements of performance

objective *(cont.)*
  instructional
  operational
  performance
  predicate
  principal
Objective-Analytic (O-A)
Objective-Analytic Batteries
objective case (parts of speech)
objective complement
objective quantity
objective psychology
objective symptoms of impairment
objective test (OT)
object libido
object of a delusion
object of sexual fantasy
object permanence
Object Relations Technique
object relations theory
object shadow
Object Sorting Scales (OSS)
object sorting test (OST)
objects test
  misplaced
  naming common
obligations, major role
obligatory occurrence
oblique arytenoid muscle
oblique muscle of abdomen
  external
  internal
oblongata, medulla
OBS (organic brain syndrome)
obscure vowel
observable disability
observation
  around-the-clock
  continuous
  direct
  longitudinal
  serial

observation audiometry
observer position
obsession (pl. obsessions)
  alien
  erotic
  guilt
  inappropriate quality of
  inhibitory
  intrusive quality of
  neutralize an
  revenge
  rotted
  trigger an
obsessional idea
obsessional impulse
obsessional mental image
obsessional neurosis
obsessional personality
obsessional phobia
obsessional psychoneurosis
obsessional rumination
obsessional state
obsessional syndrome
obsessional thoughts
obsession psychasthenia
obsession syndrome
obsessive behavior
obsessive-compulsive behavior
obsessive-compulsive disorder (OCD)
obsessive-compulsive features
obsessive-compulsive neurosis
obsessive-compulsive personality
obsessive-compulsive personality
  disorder
Obsessive-Compulsive Personality
  Disorder Subscale from Millon
  Clinical Multiaxial Inventory-II
obsessive-compulsive psychoneurosis
obsessive-compulsive reaction
Obsessive Compulsive Subscale of the
  Comprehensive Psychopathological
  Rating Scale

obsessive disorder
obsessive psychoneurotic reaction
obsessive reaction
Obst (obstruction)
Obst-dysphagia patient
obstreperous
obstructionism
obstruction (Obst), visual
obstructive apnea
obstructive hydrocephalus
obstructive sleep apnea
obstructive sleep apnea syndrome
obstruent consonant formation
obstruent omission
obstruent singleton omissions
obtrusive text
obtundation, mental
obtunded mentally
obturator
Occam's Razor
occasional (occ)
occipital bone
occipital lobe
occipital sulcus
occluded lisp
occlusion effect
occult cleft palate
occult head trauma
occulta, amentia
occupancy, receptor
Occupational Ability Patterns (OAPs)
occupational activity
Occupational Aptitude Survey and
    Interest Schedule, Second Edition—
    Aptitude Survey (OASIS-2 AS)
Occupational Aptitude Survey and
    Interest Schedule, Second Edition—
    Interest Survey (OASIS-2 IS)
Occupational Check List (OCL)
occupational deafness
occupational disorder

Occupational Environment Scales,
    Form E-2
occupational exposure
occupational function
occupational functioning
occupational history (OH)
occupational impairment
occupational interaction
Occupational Interests Explorer (OIE)
Occupational Interests Surveyor (OIS)
occupational neurosis
occupational psychoneurosis
occupational psychiatry
Occupational Roles Questionnaire
    (ORQ)
Occupational Safety and Health Act
    (OSHA)
occupational skill training
Occupational Stress Indicator (Research
    Version) (OSI)
Occupational Test Series—Basic Skills
    Tests
occupational therapist
Occupational Therapist, Registered
    (OTR)
occupational therapy (OT)
occupational tic
occurrence, obligatory
OCD (obsessive compulsive disorder)
ochlomania
ochlophobia
ochophobia
OCI (Organizational Culture Inventory)
OCL (Occupational Check List)
OCT (Object Classification Test)
"octane" (phencyclidine laced with
    gasoline)
octave-band analyzer
octave-band filter
octave filter
octave twist

ocular apraxia
ocular migraine headache
ocular movement
  cardinal
  roving
oculogyric crisis
oculomotor (cranial nerve III)
oculomotor apraxia
oculomotor disturbance
OD (overdose)
odd behavior
odd beliefs
odd-eccentric cluster
odd-even method reliability coefficient
oddity
oddly
odd speech
odd thinking
odontophobia
odor
  body
  distorted perception of
ODS (Operation Desert Storm)
odynophobia
oecophobia
oedipal behavior
oedipal conflict
oedipal neurosis
oedipal phase
oedipism
Oedipus complex
OEM (open-end marriage)
oenophobia
oestromania
off-balance
off effect
offender, sex (SO)
offending agent
Offer Self-Image Questionnaire
  (OSIQ)
Offer Parent-Adolescent Questionnaire

Offer Self-Image Questionnaire,
  Revised (OSIQ-R)
Offer Self-Image Questionnaire for
  Adolescents
off-glide
office seclusion
Office Skills Test
officer
  police
  probation (p.o.)
"ogoy" (heroin)
ogre
OH (occupational history)
Ohio Tests of Articulation and Per-
  ception of Sounds (OTAPS)
Ohio Vocational Interest Survey
  (OVIS), Second Edition
Ohio Work Values Inventory (OWVI)
ohm
Ohm's law
OHS (Overcontrolled Hostility Scale)
OI (Orientation Inventory)
OIE (The Occupational Interests
  Explorer)
oikomania
oikophobia
"oil" (heroin; phencyclidine)
oinophobia
OIS (The Occupational Interests
  Surveyor)
OISE Picture Reasoning Test (PRT)
"O.J." (cannabis)
old-age imbecility
old-age psychiatry
"Old Steve" (heroin)
olfactophobia
olfactory (cranial nerve I)
olfactory amnesia
olfactory area
olfactory aura
olfactory hallucination

olfactory psychomotor seizure
olfactory sensory modality
oligodontia
oligomania
oligophrenia
   moral
   phenylpyruvic
   polydystrophic
oligophrenic
oligopsychia
Oliphant Auditory Discrimination
   Memory Test (OADMT)
Oliphant Auditory Synthesizing Test
   (OAST)
olivopontocerebellar degeneration
OLMAT (Otis-Lennon Mental Ability
   Test)
OLSIDI (Oral Language Sentence
   Imitation Diagnostic Inventory)
OLSIST (Oral Language Sentence
   Imitation Screening Test)
ombrophobia
OMC (short orientation-memory-
   concentration test)
Omega sign (+ or − for suicide)
omen formation
OMFAQ (OARS Multidimensional
   Functional Assessment Questionnaire)
omission
   obstruent
   postvocalic obstruent singleton
omission articulation
ommatophobia; ommetaphobia
Omnibus Personality Inventory (OPI)
omnidirectional microphone
omnipotence
omnipotent
omnipresent
omniscience
omohyoid muscle
   anterior
   posterior

"on a mission" (re: crack acquisition)
onanism
"on a trip" (re: drug influence)
once a day (1/d; q.d.)
"one and one" (re: cocaine use)
"one box tissue" (one ounce of crack)
on edge, feeling
on effect
"one-fifty-one" (crack)
oneiric
oneirism
oneiroanalysis
oneirocritical
oneirodynia activa
oneirodynia gravis
oneirogenic
oneirogmus
oneiroid state
oneirology
oneiroanalysis
oneirophobia
oneirophrenia
oneiroscopy
one-on-one supervision
one's own control
one-to-one situation
"one way" (lysergic acid diethylamide)
on-glide
"on ice" (in jail)
ongoing treatment
oniomania
only child
on-off effect of L-dopa
on-off phenomenon
onomatomania
onomatophobia
onomatopoeia
onomatopoetic words
onomatopoiesis
onset
   abrupt
   adolescent

onset *(cont.)*
  age at
  insidious
  pattern of
onset during withdrawal
onset episode
onset of agitation
onset of dementia
onset of illness
onset of pain
onset of schizophrenia
  early
  late
  pathophysiological significance of
    age at
onset of sleep
onset of symptoms
onset time
on-task behavior
"on the bricks" (walking the streets)
"on the go"
"on the nod" (re: drug influence)
ontogenesis
ontogenic
ontogeny
"on top of the world"
onychotillomania
OOB (out of bed)
OOC (out of control)
OP or O/P (outpatient)
"O.P." (opium)
"ope" (opium)
open (parts of speech)
open-bite malposition of teeth
open-class word
open earmold
open-end marriage (OEM)
open-ended interview
open-ended session
open hospital
open juncture

openness, lack of
openness to experience
open place
open posture
open quotient
open seclusion restrictions
open syllable
open vowel
open-ward status
operant
  autoclitic
  echoic
  tact
  textual
  verbal
operant conditioning audiometry
operant learning
operant level
operant procedures
operant therapy
operation (pl. operations)
  effector
  formal
  logical
  invasive
  motivating
  noninvasive
  sensor
operational definition
operational objectives
operational signs
Operation Desert Storm (ODS)
operations period
  concrete
  formal
operators, modal
ophidiomania
ophidiophobia
ophiophobia
ophresiophobia
OPI (Omnibus Personality Inventory)

opiate receptors
  delta
  kappa
  mu
opinion, public
Opinions Toward Adolescents (OTA)
opioid (pl. opioids)
opioid abuse
opioid dependence
opioid intoxication
opioid intoxication delirium
opioid problem
opioid-related disorder
opioid-type drug dependence
opioid use disorder
opioid withdrawal
opiomania
opisthotonos
opium (O), descriptive terms
  Boston
  denarcotized
  deodorized
  granulated
  powdered
  pudding
opium (street names)
  ah-pen-yen
  big O
  black hash
  black pill
  Black Russian
  chandoo/chandu
  Chinese molasses
  Chinese tobacco
  chocolate
  dopium
  Dover's powder
  dream gum
  dreams
  dream stick
  easing powder
  fi-do-nie

opium *(cont.)*
  gee
  God's medicine
  goma
  gondola
  gong
  Goric
  great tobacco
  gum
  guma
  hocus
  hop/hops
  Indonesian bud
  joy plant
  licorice
  midnight oil
  mira
  O
  O.P.
  ope
  pen yan
  PG
  pin gon
  pin yen
  pox
  skee
  tar
  tout
  toxy
  when-shee
  Yen Shee Suey
  zero
opium addiction
opium dependence
"O.P.P." (phencyclidine)
Oppenheim reflex
opportunities for intervention
opportunity
  educational
  sexual
opposite affect state
opposite phase

opposite sex
opposites
    polar
    relational
oppositional attitude
oppositional-defiant disorder
oppositional disorder of adolescence
oppositional disorder of childhood
opposition breathing
opposition respiration
opsomania
OPT (outpatient)
optic (cranial nerve II)
optic agraphia
optical alexia
"optical illusions" (lysergic acid
    diethylamide)
optic aphasia
opticochiasmatic depression
optimal development
optimal method
optimal relational functioning
optimal therapeutic intervention
optimism
optimistic atmosphere
optimistically
oral apraxia
oral atresia
oral-aural method
oral cavity
oral character
oral dyskinesia
oral eroticism
oral form recognition
oral inaccuracy
oralism
orality
Oral Language Evaluation, Second
    Edition
Oral Language Sentence Imitation
    Diagnostic Inventory (OLSIDI)

Oral Language Sentence Imitation
    Screening Test (OLSIST)
oral manometer
Oral-Motor/Feeding Rating Scale
oral movement
oral-nasal acoustic ratio, the
    (TONAR)
oral peripheral examination
oral phase
oral respiration
oral sensory abilities
oral sensory discrimination
oral sounds
oral-stage psychosexual development
oral stereognosis
oral steroid
    anadrol
    anavar
    maxibolin
    methyltestosterone
    proviron
    winstrol
oral stimulation
Oral Verbal Intelligence Test (OVIT)
oral vowels
"orange barrels" (lysergic acid
    diethylamide)
"orange crystal" (phencyclidine)
"orange cubes" (lysergic acid diethyl-
    amide)
"orange haze" (lysergic acid diethyl-
    amide)
"orange micro" (lysergic acid diethyl-
    amide)
"oranges" (amphetamine)
"orange sunshine" (lysergic acid
    diethylamide)
"orange wedges" (lysergic acid
    diethylamide)
orbicularis, tic
orchidomania

order
  birth
  community treatment
  preoccupation with
  rank
ordering of sounds
Ordinal Scales of Psychological
  Development
ordinary demands of life
organic affective disorder
organic affective syndrome
organic amnesia
organic amnestic syndrome
organic anxiety syndrome
organic articulation disorder
organic brain dysfunction
organic brain syndrome (OBS)
organic brain syndrome with
  psychosis
organic deafness
organic delirium
organic delusional syndrome
organic disease
organic epilepsy
organic hallucinosis syndrome
organic impairment
Organic Integrity Test
organicity screening
organic mental disorder
organic mental syndrome
organic mood syndrome
organic neglect
organic personality syndrome, drug-
  induced
organic psychiatry
organic psychosis
  addiction
  alcoholism
  anergastic
  arteriosclerotic
  brain disease
  cerebrovascular disease

organic psychosis (cont.)
  childbirth
  dependence
  endocrine disease
  epilepsy
  Huntington chorea
  infection
  intoxication
  ischemia
  Jakob-Creutzfeldt disease
  liver disease
  metabolic disease
  mixed paranoid/affective
  multiple sclerosis
  physical condition
  posttraumatic
  senility
  status epilepticus
  transient
  trauma
organic psychosyndrome
  focal
  partial
organic psychotic state
  mixed paranoid/affective
  presenile
  senile
  transient
organic psychotic condition
organic reaction
  acute
  subacute
organization
  action
  care
  disrupt sleep
  preoccupation with
  psychic
  social welfare
  spatial
  temporal
Organizational Climate Index

Organizational Culture Inventory
(OCI)
organizational plan
organizational skills
organizational structure
Organizational Test for Professional
Accounting
Organizational Value Dimensions
Questionnaire (OVDQ)
Organization Health Survey
organized activity
organized-care psychiatry
organizing principle
organ language
organ of Corti
organophosphate insecticide
organ, vocal
orgasm
coital
inhibited female
inhibited male
sensation of
orgasmic capacity
orgasmic disorder
acquired-type female
acquired-type male
female
generalized-type female
generalized-type male
lifelong-type female
lifelong-type male
male
situational-type female
situational-type male
orgasmic disorder due to combined
factors
female
male
orgasmic disorder due to psychological factors
female
male

orgasmic dysfunction
orgasmic phase of sexual response
cycle
orgasmic problems
orgastic release
orientation
biological
bisexual
coronal
disturbed
ego-dystonic
heterosexual
homosexual
impaired
lack of goal
loss of
psychodynamic
reality (RO)
sagittal
same-sex
sexual
spatial
temporal
transverse
orientation reflex audiometry
oriented and alert times four (x 4)
(to person, place, time, and
future plans)
oriented and alert times three (x 3)
(to person, place, time)
oriented; awake, alert and (AAO)
oriented in all spheres
orienting reflex (OR)
orifices, body
origin
culture of
undetermined (UO)
original trauma
originaria, paranoia
Orleans-Hanna Algebra Prognosis
Test
ornery

ornithomania
ornithophobia
orobuccal dyskinesia
orofacial muscle imbalance
orolingual
oronasal
oro-ocular
oropharyngeal dystonia
oropharynx
ORQ (Occupational Roles Question-
    naire)
orthographic
orthography
orthomolecular psychiatry
orthomolecular therapy
orthomolecular treatment
orthophrenia
orthopsychiatry
orthostatic hypotension
OSBCL (Ottawa School Behavior
    Check List)
oscillating tremor
oscillation, laryngeal
oscillations of attachment
oscillator, bone-conduction
oscillatory movement
oscilloscope
OSHA (Occupational Safety and
    Health Act)
OSI (Occupational Stress Indicator),
    Research Version
OSIQ (Offer Self-Image Question-
    naire)
OSIQ-R (Offer Self-Image Question-
    naire, Revised)
osmophobia
osphresiophobia
osphresis
osphretic
OSS (Object Sorting Scales)
osseous labyrinth
ossicle

ossicular chain
OST (object sorting test)
osteoma (pl. osteomas, osteomata)
ostracism, peer
OT (objective test)
OT (occupational therapy)
OTA (Opinions Toward Adolescents)
OTAPS (Ohio Tests of Articulation
    and Perception of Sounds)
other-directed person
other people's boundaries
other position
other, significant
other substances
other type personality disorder
Otis-Lennon Mental Ability Test
    (OLMAT)
Otis-Lennon School Ability Test
Otis Quick Scoring Mental Abilities
    Tests
otitis media
    adhesive
    chronic suppurative
    mucoid
    nonsuppurative
    serous (SOM)
    suppurative
otitis media push-back
otological screening
otologist
otology
otorhinolaryngology
otosclerosis
otoscope
otoscopy
ototoxic
OTR (Occupational Therapist,
    Registered)
Ottawa School Behavior Check List
    (OSBCL)
ouranophobia

outburst
  aggressive
  angry
  temper
  violent
outburst of anger
outcast, social
outcome
  long-term
  well-formed
"outerlimits" (crack and lysergic acid
  diethylamide)
outflow tremor
outlandish
outlook, futural
out of bed (OOB)
out-of-body experience (OBE)
out-of-body sensation
out of character
out-of-control (OOC)
  feeling
  sense of being
out-of-control drinking behavior
out-of-control subjectivity
out-of-mind sensation
out of phase
out of the blue
outpatient (OP, O/P, OPT)
outpatient-based psychiatry
outpatient patient populations
outpatient physical therapy
outpatient setting
output
  articulatory
  HF average SSPL
  maximum acoustic
  maximum power (MPO)
  saturation
outrageous
outside control
outside force

outside stimulus
ovalis, fenestra
oval window
OVDQ (Organizational Value
  Dimensions Questionnaire)
overabstract speech
overall severity of illness
overall severity of psychiatric
  disturbance
overall sound level
overanxious disorder of adolescence
overanxious disorder of childhood
overanxious reaction
overbearance, phallic
overbite malposition of teeth
overbreathing, voluntary hysterical
Overcoming Depression software
overcompensation
overconcern with sleep
overconcrete speech
overconscientious personality disorder
Overcontrolled Hostility Scale (OHS)
overdependency
over-dependent attitude
overdetermination
overdose (OD), talk down from
Overeaters Anonymous (O/A)
overeating, marked
over-elaborate speech
overflow incontinence
overinclusiveness
overindependence
overinvolvement
overjut, horizontal
overjut of teeth
overlapping
overlay
  emotional
  psychogenic
  supratentorial
overlearning

overload
   fluid
   role
overprotectiveness
overreaction, emotional
overreact, tendency to
overresponse
oversleeping
overstatement (figure of speech)
overstimulation
overtalkative
overt behavior
overt compliance masking covert
   resistance
overt criticism
over-the-counter drug-related disorder
overt homosexuality
overt message
overt response
overtone, psychic
overuse of medication
overvaluation
overvalued idea

overwhelmed, sense of being
overwhelmed subjectivity
overwhelming depression
OVIS (Ohio Vocational Interest
   Survey)
OVIT (Oral Verbal Intelligence Test)
"Owsley" (lysergic acid diethylamide)
"Owsley's acid" (lysergic acid diethylamide)
OWVI (Ohio Work Values Inventory)
Oxford STA scale
oxidants
oxide
   nitric
   nitrous
oxycephalic idiocy
oxygen-carrying capacity
oxygen-deprived sexual arousal
oxygen-depriving activities
oxyhemoglobin saturation
"Oz" (inhalant)
"ozone" (phencyclidine)

P, p

P (form perception)
P (psychiatrist, psychiatry)
P (psychosis)
"P" (mescaline; phencyclidine)
PA (passive aggressive)
PA (picture arrangement) subtest
PA (Psychiatric Assistant)
PA (psychoanalysis, psychoanalyst)
PA (psychogenic aspermia)
PAAT (Parent as a Teacher Inventory)
PAB (Positive Attention Behavior)
PAC (parent-adult-child)
PAC (Progress Assessment Chart of Social and Personal Development)
PACE (Professional and Administrative Career Examination)
Paced Auditory Serial Addition Test (PASAT)
pace, future
pacemaker, endogenous circadian
PACG (Prevocational Assessment and Curriculum Guide)
PACG Inventory
pacing
  ceaseless
  restless
pacing behavior

"pack" (cannabis; heroin)
"pack of rocks" (cannabis cigarette)
packs per day (PPD, Ppd, p.p.d.)
PACL (Personality Adjective Check List)
P-ACT
PAD (Pain and Distress score)
PAD (primary affective disorder)
PAD (psychoaffective disorder)
paddling
paganism
PAI (Pair Attraction Inventory)
PAI (Personality Assessment Inventory)
pain (pl. pains)
  anatomical site of
  atypical
  atypical face
  burning
  causalgic
  dream
  mind
  neuralgic
  night
  phantom
  physical manifestation of
  posttraumatic

pain *(cont.)*
  psychogenic
  psychological
  psychosocial
  sexual
  unexplained
Pain and Distress score (PAD)
Pain Apperception Test (PAT)
pain avoidance
pain behavior
pain complaints
pain disorder
  psychogenic
  sexual
  somatoform
pain dysfunction syndrome (PDS)
painful affect
painful consequences
painful stimulus
painful symptom
painful thoughts
pain management
pain-pleasure principle
pain presentation
pain questionnaire (see *test*)
pain sensation, loss of
pain symptoms
pain syndromes
painter's encephalopathy
pain threshold
PAIR (Personal Assessment of
  Intimacy in Relationships)
Pair Attraction Inventory (PAI)
paired associate learning
paired syllables
PAIS (Psychosocial Adjustment to
  Illness Scale)
"Pakalolo" (cannabis)
"Pakistani black" (cannabis)
palatal area consonant placement
palatal fronting

palatal glide
palatal insufficiency
palatal lift
palatal paralysis
palatal sounds
palate
  bilateral cleft
  classifications of the cleft
  cleft
  complete cleft
  hard
  incomplete cleft
  occult cleft
  partial cleft
  primary
  secondary
  soft
  submucous cleft
  subtotal cleft
  total cleft
  unilateral cleft
palate cleft, soft
palate muscles
palatine bones
palatine raphe
palatine skull bones
palatine tonsil
palatoglossus muscle
palatogram
palatography
palatopharyngeal muscle
paleophrenia
paliacusis
palikinesia
palilalia
palingraphia
palinmnesis
palinopsia
palinphrasia palipraxia
PALST (Picture Articulation and
  Language Screening Test)

palsy
    ataxic cerebral
    Bell
    bilateral gaze
    cerebral
    cranial nerve
    dyskinetic cerebral
    Erb
    gaze
    ipsilateral
    lateral gaze
    progressive
    progressive supranuclear
    pseudobulbar
    shaking
    spastic cerebral
    supranuclear gaze
    vertical-gaze
    "Panama cut" (cannabis)
    "Panama gold" (cannabis)
    "Panama red" (cannabis)
    "panatella" (cannabis cigarette)
    "pancakes and syrup" (glutethimide
        and codeine cough syrup)
pandemic
pandysmaturation
P & N, P&N (psychiatry and neurol-
    ogy)
P & SH (personal and social history)
"pane" (lysergic acid diethylamide)
panencephalitis, subacute sclerosing
panendoscopy
"Pangonadalot" (heroin)
panic
    acute homosexual
    homosexual
"panic" (unavailability of drugs)
panic-agoraphobic syndrome
panic attack
    full
    nocturnal
    recurrent

panic attack *(cont.)*
    situationally bound (cued)
    situationally predisposed
    unexpected (uncued)
panic disorder
panic disordered patient
panicker
    nonsuffocation
    suffocation
panicky
panic state
panic-stricken
panic symptomatology
panic-type anxiety
panic-type anxiety neurosis
panophobia
panphobia
panphobic melancholia
PANSS (Positive and Negative
    Syndrome Scale)
pantomime
Pantomime Recognition Test (PRT)
pantophobia
pantophobic
PAP (passive-aggressive personality)
papaphobia
"paper acid" (lysergic acid diethyl-
    amide)
"paper bag" (re: drug container)
"paper blunts" (re: cannabis cigarettes)
"paper boy" (heroin dealer)
Papez circuit
papilla, acoustic
papilloma (pl. papillomas, papillomata)
papillomatosis, juvenile
PAQ (Personal Attributes Question-
    naire)
PAQ (Position Analysis Questionnaire)
PAR (Proficiency A ssessment Report)
PAR Admissions Testing program
parabolin (veterinary steroid)
paracentesis

paracentral scotoma
"parachute" (crack and phencyclidine
   smoked; heroin)
paracusis
   false
   localis
   Willis
paradigm
   transference
   word
paradigmatic response
paradigmatic shift
paradigmatic word
"paradise" (cocaine)
"paradise white" (cocaine)
paradoxical intervention
paradoxical sleep
paraesthetica, pseudomelia
parafunction
parafunctional
parageusia
parageusic
paragraphia
paragraph recall test
parahypnosis
paralalia
paralambdacism
paralanguage
paraldehyde
paralepsy
paralexia
paralexic errors
paralgesia
paralgesic
paralinguistics
paralipophobia
parallel distribution
parallel play
Parallel Spelling Tests
parallel talk
paralogia, thematic
paralogism

paralysis
   abductor
   adductor
   Bell
   bulbar
   conversion
   cricothyroid
   facial
   flaccid
   general
   labioglossolaryngeal
   labioglossopharyngeal
   laryngeal motor
   laryngeal sensory
   leaden
   lingual
   myopathic
   palatal
   postdormital sleep
   predormital sleep
   pseudobulbar
   pseudolaryngeal
   psychogenic
   sensory
   sleep
   spastic
   unilateral
   unilateral abductor
   unilateral adductor
   vocal cord
   vocal fold
paralysis agitans
paralytic dementia
   juvenilis
   syphilitic
   tabetic form
paralytic disorder
paralytic idiocy
paralytic ileus
paralyzed
paramania
parameter, chance-response

parametric study
parametric tests of significance
paramimia
paramnesia
paranoia
    alcoholic
    hallucinatory
    litigious
    querulous
    senile
paranoiac
paranoia originaria
paranoia querulans
paranoia scale
Paranoia "6" Scale
paranoica, aphonia
paranoic psychosis
paranoid/affective organic psychosis,
    mixed
paranoid behavior
paranoid belief system
paranoid delusion
paranoid disorder
    induced
    shared
paranoid fears
paranoid features
paranoid grandiose delusion
paranoid ideation
paranoid involutional reaction
paranoidism
paranoid personality disorder
paranoid psychosis
    alcoholic
    climacteric
    chronic
    involutional
    menopausal
    protracted reactive
    psychogenic
    schizophrenic
    senile

paranoid reaction
    acute
    chronic
    climacteric
    involutional
    menopausal
    senile
    simple
paranoid schizophrenia
Paranoid Sensitivity Profile
paranoid state
    alcohol-induced
    arteriosclerotic
    climacteric
    drug-induced
    involutional
    menopausal
    paranoia
    paranoia querulans
    paraphrenia
    senile
    sensitiver Beziehungswahn
    simple
paranoid tendencies
paranoid traits
paranoid trends
paranoid-type alcoholic psychosis
paranoid-type arteriosclerotic dementia
paranoid-type arteriosclerotic
    psychosis
paranoid-type presenile dementia
paranoid-type psycho-organic
    syndrome
paranoid-type senile dementia
paranoid-type senile psychosis
paranomia
paraphasia
    extended jargon
    literal
    phonemic
    thematic
    verbal

paraphasic speech
paraphasis
paraphemia
paraphernalia
  drug
  paraphiliac
  shared drug
paraphia
paraphilia
  exhibitionism
  fetishism
  frotteurism
  pedophilia
  transvestism
  troilism
  voyeurism
paraphiliac behavior
paraphiliac fantasy
paraphiliac focus
paraphiliac imagery
paraphiliac objects
paraphiliac paraphernalia
paraphiliac pornography
paraphiliac preferences
paraphiliac stimulus
paraphilic behavior
paraphobia
paraphora
paraphrases, lexical
paraphrasia
paraphrenia
  climacteric
  involutional
  late
  menopausal
paraphrenia confabulans
paraphrenia expansiva
paraphrenia phantastica
paraphrenia systematica
paraphrenic dementia
paraphrenic schizophrenia
paraplegic idiocy

parapraxia
parapraxis
parapsychology
parapsychosis
parasexuality
parasigmatism (lisp)
parasitophobia
parasomnia-type sleep disorder due to
  epilepsy
parasomnia-type sleep disorder due to
  general medical condition
parasomnia-type substance-induced
  sleep disorder
parasomniac conscious state
parasuicidal behavior
parasuicide
parasympathetic nervous system
  (PNS)
parataxic distortion
parathyroid disease
parent (pl. parents)
  biological
  ineffectual
  rejecting
  single
  surrogate
  ungiving
  weak
Parent-Adolescent Communication
  Scale
parent-adult-child (PAC)
Parental Acceptance-Rejection
  Questionnaire
parental control problem, leaving
parental loss
parental rejection
parental rights
Parent as a Teacher Inventory
  (PAAT)
Parent Attachment Structured
  Interview
Parent Attitude Scale (PAS)

Parent Awareness Skills Survey
(PASS)
parent-child conflict
parent-child conflict counseling
parent-child dyad
parent-child relational problem
Parent Effectiveness Training (PET)
parenthetical expression
parenthetical remarks
parentified role
parenting
    erratic
    positive
Parent Interview for Child Syndrome
(PICS)
Parenting Stress Index
parent language
parent-offspring bond
Parent Opinion Inventory
Parent Perception of Child Profile
(PPCP)
Parent Rating of Student Behavior
Parent-Teacher Questionnaire (PTQ)
paresis, general
paresthesia, laryngeal
paresthetic conversion reaction
paretic melancholia
parietal association area
parietal lobe dysfunction
parietal skull bones
parieto-occipital aphasia
parietotemporal area
Parkinson disease
    dementia due to
    primary
parkinsonian crisis
parkinsonian dysarthria
parkinsonian facies
parkinsonian gait
parkinsonian muscular rigidity
parkinsonian signs and symptoms
parkinsonian speech

parkinsonian tremor
parkinsonism
    drug-induced (pseudoparkinsonism)
    neuroleptic-induced
parkinsonism-dementia complex of
    Guam
parkinsonism-like effect
"parlay" (crack)
parousiamania
paroxysmal activity
paroxysmal convulsion
paroxysmal dystonia
paroxysmal migraine headache
paroxysmal phenomenon
paroxysmal psychosis
paroxysmal tachycardia, psychogenic
parrotlike speech pattern
parry
PARS (Personal and Role Skills)
"parsley" (cannabis, phencyclidine)
parthenophobia
partial agonist
partial amnesia
partial complex seizure
partial cross-dressing
partial disability
partial epilepsy
partial hospitalization
partial hospital patient populations
partial hospital setting
partial insanity
partial laryngectomy, anterior
partial nominal aphasia
partial permanent disability
partial recruitment
partial reinforcement
partial remission
    early
    sustained
partial seizure
    complex (CPS)
    repetitive

partial seizure *(cont.)*
  simple
  upper
partial sensory seizure
partial tone
partial tonic seizure
partial visual loss
participle (parts of speech)
particle velocity
particular grammar
particular identity
particular task
particulate
partner
  consenting
  nonconsenting
partner relational problem
Partner Relationship Inventory (PRI)
part-object manner
parts of speech
  accusative case
  adjective
  adverb
  conjoiner
  conjunction
  dative case
  factitive case
  genitive case
  gerund
  infinitive
  instrumental case
  interjection
  locative case
  nominative case
  noun
  objective case
  open
  participle
  pivot grammar
  possessive case
  preposition
  pronoun

parts of speech *(cont.)*
  subjective case
  verb
PAS (Parent Attitude Scale)
PAS (personality assessment system)
PAS (Prevocational Assessment
  Screen)
PASAT (Paced Auditory Serial
  Addition Test)
PASES (Performance Assessment of
  Syntax Elicited and Spontaneous)
PASS (Parent Awareness Skills
  Survey)
PASS (Perception of Ability Scale for
  Students)
passage comprehension
passages, memory pass-band filter
passionelle, psychose
passive accommodation
passive-aggressive (PA)
passive-aggressive acting out
passive-aggressive personality (PAP)
passive-aggressive personality disorder
passive-aggressive reaction
passive bilingualism
passive-dependent
passive-dependent personality (PDP)
passive-dependent reaction
passive influence
passive learning
passively
passive personality
passive reaction
passive sentence
passive therapist
passive therapy
passive voice
passivism
passivity
  active
  delusion of
passivity in anger expression

"paste" (crack)
past history (PH)
past-life hypnotic regression
pastoral care
pastoral counseling
pastoral counselor
past-oriented
past perfect progressive tense
past perfect tense
past progressive tense
past tense
past tics
"Pat" (cannabis)
PAT (Pain Apperception Test)
PAT (Photo Articulation Test)
PAT (Predictive Ability Test)
PAT (psychoacoustic testing)
patchy amnesia
patent medicines
paternal behavior
paternal deprivation
pathematic aphasia
pathogenic care
pathognomonic signs
pathognomonic symptoms of schizophrenia
pathological behavior
pathological care
pathological character formation
pathological communication
pathological drunkenness
pathological emotionality
pathological gambling
pathological intoxication
   alcohol
   drug
pathological liar
pathological lying
pathological personality
pathological preoccupation
pathological process

pathological sensitivity to perceived
   interpersonal rejection
pathological sexual fantasy
pathological sexuality
pathological substance use
pathologic condition
pathologic reflex
pathologist
   language
   speech
   voice
pathology
   aural
   Axis II
   brain
   central nervous system
   character
   cigarette-related
   language
   manifestations of
   nasopharyngeal
   pelvic
   psychosocial
   speech
   speech and language
   structural
pathology/audiology, speech (SPA)
pathomania
pathomimesis
pathomimia
pathomimicry
pathoneurosis
pathophobia
pathophysiological mechanism
   direct causative
   specific
pathophysiological process
pathophysiological significance of age
   at onset of schizophrenia
pathophysiology
pathopsychology

pathopsychosis
pathway
  auditory
  cerebellar
pathway stimulation
"patico" (crack)
patient
  abused
  agitated
  aphasic
  comatose
  combative
  disoriented
  hypnotic-dependent
  incoherent
  insomniac
  lethargic
  panic-disordered
  peregrinating
  posttraumatic
  self-destructive
  stuporous
  target
  unresponsive
patient acceptance of health care
Patient and Family Services (PFS)
patient compliance
patient encounter
patient populations
  clinic
  consultation/liaison
  inpatient
  outpatient
  partial hospital
  primary care
  private practice
Patient Rated Anxiety Scale (PRAS)
Patient Rated Disability Scale
Patient Rated Impairment Scale
Patient Rated Overall Life Impairment
patient resistance
"patient" role in factitious disorder

patient satisfaction
PATLC (Progressive Achievement Tests of Listening Comprehension)
PATM (Progressive Achievement Test of Mathematics), Revised
patriophobia
patronizing manner
pattern (pl. patterns)
  advanced sleep phase
  auditory
  autosomal dominant
  avoidance
  behavior
  binge eating
  changing sleep-wake
  characteristic
  chronically disabling
  communication
  continued drinking
  disturbed sleep
  enduring
  familial
  feminine speech
  habit
  inflexible
  irregular sleep
  irregular sleep-wake
  Kindling
  long-term
  maladaptive
  moderate drinking
  mood disorder with seasonal
  non-rapid-cycling
  non-24-hour sleep-wake
  parrotlike speech
  personality
  pervasive
  pressure
  prototypical course
  rapid-cycling
  reflex
  repetitive

pattern *(cont.)*
  role
  seasonal
  sleep
  speech time
  stable
  stable sleep-wake
  stress
  stuttering
  symptom
  symptom response
  syndromal
  syndrome
Patterned Elicitation Syntax Screening
  Test (PESST)
Patterned Elicitation Syntax Test
pattern-induced epilepsy
patterning of speech
pattern in speech
pattern of behavior
pattern of conduct
pattern of electroencephalogram (EEG)
pattern of language
pattern recognition
paucity of movement
paucity of speech content
paucity of verbalizations
pauses in speech
  filled
  involuntary
  unfilled
pauses, unfilled
Pavlov, Ivan Petrovich (1849-1936)
Pavlov method
pavor nocturnus (night terrors)
Paykel Life Events Scale
"paz" (phencyclidine)
P-BAP (Behavioral Assessment of Pain
  Questionnaire)
PB max score
PBQ (Preschool Behavior Questionnaire)

PB words (phonetically balanced
  words)
p.c. (after meals)
PC (Phrase Construction)
PC (picture completion) subtest
PCAS (Psychotherapy Competence
  Assessment Schedule)
PCE (analog of phencyclidine)
PCG (Planning Career Goals)
PCI (Premarital Communication
  Inventory)
PCL-R (Hare Psychopathy Checklist,
  Revised)
PCP, PCPA (phencyclidine) (see
  phencyclidine, street names)
PCP (Personal Communication Plan)
PCP (primary care physician)
PCPy (analog of phencyclidine)
PCS (Priority Counseling Survey)
pcs. (preconscious)
PCT (Physiognomic Cue Test)
PD (problem drinker)
PD (process diagnostic)
PD (psychopathic deviate)
PD (psychotic depression)
PDI Employment Inventory
"P-dope" (20-30% pure heroin)
PDP (passive-dependent personality)
PDR (*Physicians' Desk Reference*)
PDRT (Portland Digit Recognition
  Test)
PDS (pain dysfunction syndrome)
PDT (Phoneme Discrimination Test)
PE (pharyngoesophageal)
PE or P.E. (physical examination)
Peabody Developmental Motor Scales
  and Activity Cards
Peabody Individual Achievement Test
  (PIAT)
Peabody Mathematics Readiness Test
Peabody Picture Vocabulary Test
  (PPVT)

"peace" (lysergic acid diethylamide; phencyclidine)
peacemaker role
"peace pills" (phencyclidine)
"peace tablets" (lysergic acid diethylamide)
"peace weed" (phencyclidine)
"peaches" (amphetamine sulfate)
peak acoustic gain
peak amplitude
peak and trough levels
peak clipping
peak frequency
peak level of drug
peak-to-peak amplitude
"peanut butter" (phencyclidine mixed with peanut butter)
"peanuts" (barbiturate)
PEAQ (Personal Experience and Attitude Questionnaire)
"pearl" (cocaine)
"pearls" (amyl nitrite)
"pearly gates" (morning glory seeds; lysergic acid diethylamide)
"pears" (amyl nitrite)
"pebbles" (crack)
peccatiphobia
pecking order
pectoral muscle
   greater
   smaller
peculiar behavior
peculiar thoughts and language
peculiarities of language
pedagogical grammar
"peddlar" (drug supplier)
pederast
pederasty
pediatric audiology
Pediatric Early Elementary Examination

Pediatric Examination of Educational Readiness at Middle Childhood
Pediatric Extended Examination at Three (PEET)
pediatric growth chart
Pediatric Speech Intelligibility Test
pediculophobia
pediophobia
pedophile
pedophilia
   heterosexual
   homosexual
pedophilic behavior
pedophilic homosexuality
pedophilic stimuli
pedophobia
peduncular hallucinosis
"peep" (phencyclidine)
peeping tom
peer (pl. peers)
   age
   to emulate
peer group
peer interaction
peer interactional situation
peer likability
peer messages
Peer Nomination Inventory of Depression
peer ostracism
peer pressure
Peer Profile
peer relationships
peer review
PEET (Pediatric Extended Examination at Three)
"Pee Wee" ($5 worth of crack)
PEF (Psychiatric Evaluation Form)
"Peg" (heroin)
pejorative voices
Pelizaeus-Merzbacher disease

pellagra
pellagral
pellagraphobia
pellagrin
pellagroid
pellagrous
"pellets" (lysergic acid diethylamide)
pelvic pain, psychogenic
pelvic pathology
pelvic thrusting
pelvis, vasocongestion of
penalty, frustration, anxiety, guilt,
   hostility (PFAGH)
penectomy
peniaphobia
penile arousal
penile blood pressure
penile plethysmography
penile tumescence, nocturnal (NPT)
penis envy
penis pain, psychogenic
pense, tic de
pension, disability (DP)
pension neurosis
pentobarbital (street names)
   nebbies
   yellow bullets
   yellow dolls
"pen yan" (opium)
people
   aggression to
   "using"
peotillomania
PEP (Psychiatric Evaluation Profile)
PEP (Psycho-Epistemological Profile)
PEPAP (analog of meperidine)
"pep pill" (amphetamine)
PEP-R (Psychoeducational Profile
   Revised)
"Pepsi habit" (re: drug use)
peptic ulcer, psychogenic
per (according to)

per day (/d)
perceived attack on one's character
perceived emotional abandonment
perceived interpersonal rejection
perceived neglect
perceived noise level (PNdB)
perceived poor performance
percentile rank
perception
   auditory
   body-image
   central auditory
   color
   cross-modality
   depth
   distance
   distorted
   disturbance of
   disturbances in
   exaggerated
   extrasensory (ESP)
   family (DAF)
   figure-ground
   form
   gravity
   haptic
   inferential
   internal world of
   kinesthetic
   loudness
   LSD-type
   motion
   phonetic
   pitch
   proprioceptive
   sensory
   size
   social
   space
   speech
   stereognostic
   substance-induced

perception *(cont.)*
  tactile
  time
  touch
  true
  visual
  weight
perception deficit
perception disorder
Perception of Ability Scale for
  Students (PASS)
perception of being touched
Perception of Illness Scale
perception of objects
perception of odor
perception of physical sensations
Perception-of-Relationships-Test
  (PORT)
perception of self
perception of sound
perception of taste
perception of environment
perception of external world
perception of visual sensations
perceptions due to a psychotic
  disorder
perceptions due to drug effect
perceptions of external reality
perceptions of movement
perceptive deafness
perceptive epilepsy
perceptive hearing loss
perceptivity
perceptual abilities
perceptual analysis
perceptual closure
perceptual consistency
perceptual defense
perceptual disorder
perceptual distortion
perceptual disturbance
perceptual expansion

perceptual filter
perceptual immaturity
perceptually handicapped
perceptual masking
Perceptual Maze Test
perceptual-motor ability
Perceptual-Motor Assessment for
  Children & Emotional/Behavior
  Screening Program (P-MAC/ESP)
perceptual-motor impairment
perceptual-motor match
perceptual-motor skills
Perceptual Organization Deviation
  Quotient (PODQ)
perceptual psychology
perceptual retardation
perceptual set of disturbances
perceptual skills
perceptual symptoms, reexperiencing
peregrinating patient
"Perfect High" (heroin)
perfectionism, preoccupation with
perfectionist
perfectionistic
perfection, state of
perfect negative relationship
perfect performance
perfect positive relationship
perfect tense
performance
  academic
  impaired
  job
  linguistic
  motor
  perceived poor
  perfect
  poor work
  public
  psychomotor
  school
  sexual

performance *(cont.)*
  standards of
  task
performance abnormality
performance and analysis
performance anxiety
Performance Assessment of Syntax
  Elicited and Spontaneous (PASES)
performance characteristics
Performance Efficiency Test
performance fear
Performance Intelligence Quotient
  (PIQ)
performance-intensity function
Performance I.Q. Score
Performance Levels of a School
  Program Survey
performance objective
Performance Scale Scores
performance score
performance situation
performance task
performance test (see *test*)
"Perico" (cocaine)
perimeter earmold
perinatal development
perinatal hearing loss
period
  apneic
  apneustic
  childraising
  concrete operations
  decay
  depression
  developmental
  drinking
  endogenous circadian
  formal operations
  growth
  ictal
  illness
  interictal

period *(cont.)*
  learning
  non-REM
  preoperational thought
  prodromal
  refractory
  REM
  sadness
  sensorimotor intelligence
  sleep onset REM
periodical mania
periodic insanity
periodicity
periodic wave
period prevalence
perineometer
  electromyographic (EMG)
  rectal
perioral tremor
peripheral autonomic neuropathy
peripheral dysarthria
peripheral electromyographic activity
peripheral epilepsy
peripheral examination
peripheral field images
peripheral masking
peripheral nervous system
peripheral sensation
peripheral sensory loss
peripheral sympathomimetic effect
peripheral vascular disease
periphery
peritraumatic dissociation
periventricular white matter
Perley-Guze Hysteria Checklist
permanence, object
permanent disability, partial
permanent dominant idea
permanent epilation
permanently damaged
permanent residual impairment
permanent teeth

permanent threshold shift (PTS)
permutation
per os (p.o. or PO)
"perp" (re: fake crack)
perpetuating factors
perpetuator of abuse
perplexed-type manic-depressive
    psychosis
Perry sensor for vaginismus
persecution
    delusion of
    idea of
    social
persecution complex
persecutory delusional system
persecutory-type delusions
persecutory-type schizophrenia
perseverate
perseveration
    infantile
    verbal
perseverative movements
perseverative response
Persian Gulf War
persisting amnestic disorder
    alcohol-induced
    substance-induced
persisting dementia
    alcohol-induced
    substance-induced
persisting disorder
persisting perception disorder
person
    dominant
    inner-directed
    other-directed
    single
    time, place and (TP & P)
persona
Personal and Role Skills (PARS)
personal and social history (P & SH)
personal assault

Personal Assessment of Intimacy in
    Relationships (PAIR)
Personal Attributes Questionnaire
    (PAQ)
personal care
Personal Communication Plan (PCP)
personal construct theory
personal control
personal counselor
personal data inventory
Personal Experience and Attitude
    Questionnaire (PEAQ)
Personal Experience Screening
    Questionnaire (PESQ)
personal function
personal gain, desire for
personal growth laboratory
personal history (PH)
personal hygiene
    impaired
    minimal
personal identity
personal information
Personal Inventory of Needs
personality
    affective
    aggressive
    alexithymic
    allotropic
    alternating
    amoral
    anancastic
    antisocial (ASP)
    asocial
    asthenic
    authoritarian
    avoidant
    basic
    borderline
    coarctated
    compulsive
    cyclothymic

personality *(cont.)*
  cycloid
  dependent
  depressive
  disturbed
  double
  dual
  dyssocial
  eccentric
  epileptoid
  explosive
  fanatic
  histrionic
  hypomanic
  hysterical
  hysteroid
  immature
  inadequate
  introverted
  maladaptive
  masochistic
  multiple
  narcissistic
  obsessional
  obsessive-compulsive
  paranoid
  passive
  passive-aggressive (PAP)
  passive-dependent (PDP)
  pathological
  premorbid
  prepsychotic
  presenting
  psychoinfantile
  psychoneurotic
  psychopathic
  sadistic
  schizoid
  schizotypal
  seclusive
  self-defeating
  shut-in

personality *(cont.)*
  sociopathic
  split
  stable
  syntonic
  theory of
  type A
  type B
  unstable
  Personality Adjective Check List
    (PACL)
  personality and gender
  Personality Assessment Inventory
    (PAI)
  personality assessment system (PAS)
  personality change
  personality characteristics
  Personality Diagnostic Questionnaire-
    Revised (PDQ-R)
  personality disorder
    aggressive-type
    antisocial
    apathetic-type
    associated
    avoidant
    borderline
    cluster A
    cluster B
    cluster C
    combined-type
    dependent
    dependent-passive
    depressive
    disinhibited-type
    drug treatment for
    dyssocial
    emotional instability
    histrionic
    hyperthymic
    hypothymic
    labile
    moral deficiency

personality disorder *(cont.)*
  multiple (MPD)
  narcissistic
  negativistic
  obsessive-compulsive
  overconscientious
  paranoid
  passive-aggressive
  pseudosocial
  schizoid
  schizoid-schizotypal (SSPD)
  schizotypal
  seductive
  unspecified-type
personality disturbance
Personality Factor Questionnaire
  (PFQ)
personality features
personality formation
personality functioning
personality impoverishment
personality integration
personality inventory
Personality Inventory for Children
  (PIC), Revised
personality pattern
personality psychoneurosis
personality questionnaire (see *test*)
Personality Rating Scale (PRS)
personality reaction
Personality Research Form (PRF)
personality style
  extratensive
  introintensive
personality syndrome
  drug-induced organic
  organic
personality test (see *test*)
personality trait stability
personality traits
  cognitive
  interpersonal
  intrapsychic

personality type
personalized interpretation
Personal Locus of Control (PLC)
personal motivation
personal needs
Personal Orientation Inventory (POI)
Personal Preference Scale (PPS)
Personal Problems Checklist for
  Adolescents (PPC)
Personal Relationship Inventory (PRI)
Personal Resource Questionnaire
  (PRQ)
personal responsibility
personal satisfaction
Personal Skills Map
personal space
Personal Strain Questionnaire (PSQ)
Personal Style Inventory (PSI)
Personal Values Abstract (PVA)
personal values inventory (PVI)
persona non grata
person's culture
person deixis
personification (figure of speech)
Personnel Reaction Blank
Personnel Security Preview (PSP)
Personnel Selection Inventory
personnel, service
personnel test (see *test*)
Personnel Tests for Industry (PTI)
personologic psychotherapy
personology
person who stutters (PWS)
perspective, categorical
persuasive communication
"Peruvia" (cocaine)
"Peruvian" (cocaine)
"Peruvian flake" (cocaine)
"Peruvian lady" (cocaine)
persuasion
pervasive and persistent maladaptive
  personality traits
pervasive anxiety

pervasive developmental disorder
pervasive disinhibited type of developmental disorder
pervasive disorder
pervasive distrust
pervasive impairment of development
pervasive pattern
pervasive pessimism
pervasive proneness to guilt
pervasive self-criticism
pervasive unhappiness
perversion, polymorphic
perverted logic
perverted sexuality
pervert, sexual
pervigilium
PES (Psychiatric Emergency Service)
PESQ (Personal Experience Screening
  Questionnaire)
pessimism
  feelings of
  patterns of pervasive
pessimist
pessimistic
PESST (Patterned Elicitation Syntax
  Screening Test)
PET (Parent Effectiveness Training)
PET (positron emission tomography)
  scan for schizophrenia
PET (Professional Employment Test)
PET (Psychiatric Emergency Team)
"Peter Pan" (phencyclidine)
"peth" (barbiturate)
petit mal epilepsy
petit mal seizure
petit mal status
petit mal variant (Lennon-Gastaut)
  seizure
petulant
"peyote" (mescaline)
peyote dependence
PFAGH (penalty, frustration, anxiety,
  guilt, hostility)

PFAGH stuttering
PFQ (Personality Factor Questionnaire)
PFS (Patient and Family Services)
"P-funk" (crack; phencyclidine;
  heroin)
"PG" (tincture of opium)
PGR (psychogalvanic response)
PGSR (psychogalvanic skin resistance)
PGSR (psychogalvanic skin response)
PGSRA (psychogalvanic skin response
  audiometry)
PGT (play group therapy)
PH (past history)
PH (personal history)
phagomania
phagophobia
phallic overbearance
phallic phase
phallic stage psychosexual development
phalliform
phalloid
phallus
phaneromania
phantasia
phantasm
phantasmatomoria
phantasy
phantom limb
phantom pain
phantom sensation
phantom speech
pharmaceutical alternative
pharmaceutical equivalent
pharmacodynamic changes
pharmacodynamics
pharmacokinetic changes
pharmacokinetics
pharmacological aspects
pharmacological management

pharmacological provocation
pharmacological testing
pharmacological therapy
pharmacological treatment of dementia
pharmacology, serotonergic
pharmacomania
Pharmacopeia, United States (USP)
pharmacophilia
pharmacophobia
Pharmacopoeia, British (BP, B.Ph.)
pharmacopsychosis
pharmacotherapy
pharyngeal constrictor
  inferior
  middle
  superior
pharyngeal flap
pharyngeal motor activity
pharyngeal psychophysiologic reaction
pharyngeal raphe
pharyngeal reflex
pharyngeal speech
pharyngeal tonsil
pharynges
pharyngitis
pharyngoesophageal (PE) junction
pharyngoesophageal (PE) segment
pharyngopalatine arch
pharyngopalatine muscle
pharyngoplasty
pharynx (pl. pharynges)
pharynx muscles
phase
  anal
  delayed sleep
  dementia
  depressive
  developmental
  endogenous circadian rhythm
  excitement
  follicular
  genital

phase *(cont.)*
  group
  illness
  insomnia
  late luteal
  latency
  luteal
  manic
  oedipal
  opposite
  oral
  out of
  phallic
  pregenital
  pre-oedipal
  prodromal
  residual
  schizophrenia
  separation-individuation
  sleep
  stuttering
phase-advance sleep-wake hours
phase disparities
phase lag on EEG
phase of life problem
phase of schizophrenia
  active
  prodromal
  residual
phase of seizure
phase of sexual response cycle
  desire
  excitement
  orgasmic
  resolution
phase reversal on EEG
phase shift of sleep-wake cycle
phase spike on EEG
phasic REM activity
phasmophobia
Ph.D. (Doctor of Philosophy)

Phelps Kindergarten Readiness Scale
  (PKRS)
phencyclidine (street names)
  ace
  AD
  amoeba
  angel
  angel dust
  angel hair
  angel mist
  Angel Poke
  animal trank
  animal tranquilizer
  beam me up Scottie
  belladonna
  black whack
  blue madman
  boat
  bohd
  busy bee
  butt naked
  Columbo
  Cozmo's
  crazy coke
  Crazy Eddie
  crystal joint
  crystal T
  cycline
  cyclones
  D
  Detroit pink
  devil's dust
  dipper
  do it Jack
  DOA
  domes
  drink
  dummy dust
  dust
  dusted parsley
  dust joint
  dust of angels

phencyclidine *(cont.)*
  el diablito
  elephant
  elephant tranquilizer
  embalming fluid
  energizer
  erth
  fairy dust
  fake STP
  flakes
  fresh
  fuel
  good
  goon
  goon dust
  gorilla biscuits
  gorilla tab
  green
  green leaves
  green tea
  HCP
  heaven and hell
  herms
  Hinkley
  hog
  horse tracks
  horse tranquilizer
  ice
  jet fuel
  juice
  K
  kaps
  K-blast
  killer
  killer weed
  KJ
  koller joints
  kools
  krystal
  krystal joint
  KW
  LBJ

phencyclidine *(cont.)*
  leaky bolla
  leaky leak
  lemon 714
  lethal weapon
  little ones
  live ones
  log
  loveboat
  lovely
  mad dog
  madman
  magic
  magic dust
  mean green
  mint leaf
  mint weed
  missile basing
  mist
  monkey dust
  monkey tranquilizer
  more
  new acid
  new magic
  niebla
  O.P.P.
  octane
  oil
  orange crystal
  ozone
  P
  parachute
  parsley
  paz
  PCP
  PCPA
  peace
  peace pills
  peace weed
  peanut butter
  peep
  Peter Pan

phencyclidine *(cont.)*
  P-funk
  Pig Killer
  pit
  polvo
  polvo de angel
  polvo de estrellas
  puffy
  purple rain
  red devil
  rocket fuel
  scaffle
  scuffle
  sernyl
  sheets
  shermans
  sherms
  skuffle
  smoking
  snorts
  soma
  space base
  space cadet
  space dust
  spores
  stardust
  stick
  STP
  super
  Super Grass
  super joint
  super kools
  super weed
  surfer
  synthetic cocaine
  synthetic THT
  taking a cruise
  T-buzz
  tea
  tic
  tic tac
  tish

phencyclidine *(cont.)*
  titch
  tragic magic
  trank
  TT1
  TT2
  TT3
  wack
  water
  weed
  whack
  white horizon
  white powder
  wobble weed
  wolf
  worm
  yellow fever
  yerba mala
  zombie
  zombie dust
  zombie weed
  zoom
phencyclidine dose-related signs of
  withdrawal
phencyclidine intoxication delirium
phencyclidine-like substance
phencyclidine-related disorder
phengophobia
"phennies" (phenobarbital)
"pheno" (phenobarbital)
phenobarbital (street names)
  phennies
  pheno
  purple hearts
phenomenological features
phenomenological subgroups
phenomenology
phenomenon (pl. phenomena)
  Bell
  clasp-knife
  dissociative
  Doppler

phenomenon *(cont.)*
  freezing
  hesitation
  interactive
  motoric
  normal voluntary napping
  on-off
  paroxysmal
  psychic
  psychomotor
  Raynaud's
  split screen
  tip-of-the-tongue
  Wever-Bray
phenothiazine-based neuroleptics
phenothiazine-based tranquilizer
phenothiazine derivative
phenotype
phenylketonuria (PKU)
phenylpyruvic amentia
phenylpyruvic imbecility
phenylpyruvic oligophrenia
pheochromocytoma
pheromone
PHI (physiological hyaluronidase
  inhibitor)
Philadelphia Head Injury Questionnaire (PHIQ)
philander
philanderer
philandering
philopatridomania
philosophobia
philtrum (pl. philtra)
PHIQ (Philadelphia Head Injury
  Questionnaire)
phlegmatic
phobia (pl. phobias) (see also *fear of*)
  acarophobia (itching; mite or tick
    infestation)
  acerophobia (sour or sharp taste)
  achluophobia (darkness)

phobia *(cont.)*

acousticophobia (sounds; noise)
acrophobia (heights)
aelurophobia (cats)
aeroacrophobia (open high places)
aeronausiphobia (vomiting
 secondary to airsickness)
aerophobia (air; drafts; flying)
agliophobia (pain)
agoraphobia (open spaces)
agraphobia (sexual abuse)
agrizoophobia (wild animals)
agyiophobia (streets)
aichmophobia (pointed objects;
 knives)
ailurophobia (cats)
albuminurophobia (kidney disease)
alcoholophobia (alcoholism)
alektorophobia (chickens)
algophobia (pain)
alliumphobia (garlic)
allodoxaphobia (opinions)
altophobia (heights)
amathophobia (dust)
amaxophobia (vehicles)
ambulophobia (walking)
amnesiphobia (amnesia)
amychophobia (being scratched;
 scratches)
anablephobia (looking up)
androphobia (men, males)
anemophobia (wind; drafts)
anginophobia (angina pectoris
 attack)
Anglophobia (England/anything
 English)
angrophobia (becoming angry)
animal phobia
animal-type specific phobia
ankylophobia (joint immobility)
anthophobia (flowers)

phobia *(cont.)*

anthropophobia (human companionship; people)
antlophobia (flood)
apeirophobia (infinity)
aphephobia (touching; being
 touched)
apiphobia (bees)
apotemnophobia (persons with
 amputations)
aquaphobia (water)
arachibutyrophobia (peanut butter
 sticking to roof of mouth)
arachnephobia (spiders)
arachnophobia (spiders)
arithmophobia (numbers)
arrhenphobia (men)
asthenophobia (being weak; weakness)
astraphobia (thunder and lightning)
astrapophobia (thunder and lightning)
astrophobia (celestial space; stars)
ataxiophobia (disorder)
ataxophobia (disorder)
atelophobia (imperfection)
atephobia (personal ruin; reckless
 impulse)
atomosophobia (atomic explosions)
atychiophobia (failure)
aulophobia (flutes)
aurophobia (gold)
auroraphobia (dawn; northern
 lights)
automysophobia (uncleanliness;
 being dirty; personal body odor)
autophobia (self; solitude; being
 alone)
aviatophobia (flying)
aviophobia (flying)
bacillophobia (bacilli; germs)

phobia *(cont.)*
  bacteriophobia (bacteria; germs)
  ballistophobia (missiles)
  bathmophobia (walking)
  bathophobia (deep spaces)
  barophobia (gravity)
  batonophobia (plants)
  batophobia (being on tall buildings;
    high objects)
  batrachophobia (frogs and toads)
  belonephobia (sharp objects; pins
    and needles)
  bibliophobia (books)
  blennophobia (slime)
  bogyphobia (demons and goblins)
  bromidrosiphobia (body odors;
    sweat)
  brontophobia (thunder; thunder-
    storms)
  bufonophobia (toads)
  cacophobia (ugliness)
  cainophobia (novelty)
  cainotophobia (novelty)
  caligynephobia (beautiful women)
  cancerophobia (cancer; malig-
    nancy)
  carcinophobia (cancer; malignancy)
  cardiophobia (heart disease)
  carnophobia (flesh; meat)
  catapedaphobia (jumping from high
    or low places)
  categelophobia (ridicule)
  cathisophobia (sitting down)
  catoptrophobia (mirrors)
  Celtophobia (Celts; anything Celtic)
  cenophobia (open spaces; barren-
    ness; emptiness)
  ceraunophobia (thunder and light-
    ning)
  chaetophobia (hair)
  cheimaphobia (cold)
  chemophobia (chemicals)

phobia *(cont.)*
  cherophobia (gaiety)
  chionophobia (snow)
  chiroptophobia (being touched)
  cholerophobia (cholera)
  chorophobia (dancing)
  chrematophobia (wealth)
  chromatophobia (colors)
  chromophobia (colors)
  chronometrophobia (clocks)
  chronophobia (time)
  cibophobia (food)
  claustrophobia (confinement;
    enclosed space; being locked in)
  cleisiophobia (being locked in an
    enclosed place)
  cleithrophobia (being locked in an
    enclosed place)
  cleptophobia (loss through thievery)
  climacophobia (climbing; stairs)
  clinophobia (going to bed)
  clithrophobia (being locked in)
  cnidophobia (insect stings)
  coimetrophobia (cemeteries)
  coitophobia (sexual intercourse)
  cometophobia (comets)
  coprophobia (excrement; feces;
    rectal excreta)
  coprostasophobia (constipation)
  coulrophobia (clowns)
  counterphobia (confronting one's
    phobias)
  cremnophobia (precipices)
  cryophobia (ice; frost)
  crystallophobia (glass)
  cyberphobia (computers)
  cyclophobia (bicycles)
  cymophobia (waves; wavelike
    motion)
  cynophobia (dogs; pseudorabies)
  cypridophobia (sexual intercourse;
    venereal disease)

phobia *(cont.)*

cypriphobia (venereal disease)
decidophobia (making decisions)
defecalgesiophobia (painful bowel movements)
deipnophobia (dining; dinner conversations)
dementophobia (insanity)
demonophobia (demons and devils; spirits)
demophobia (people; crowds)
dendrophobia (trees)
dentophobia (dentists)
dermatophobia (skin disease)
dermatopathophobia (skin disease)
dermatosiophobia (skin disease)
dextrophobia (objects on the right side of the body)
diabetophobia (diabetes)
didaskaleinophobia (going to school)
dikephobia (justice)
dinophobia (whirlpools)
diplopiaphobia (double vision)
dipsophobia (drinking)
domatophobia (home)
doraphobia (animals skins; fur; skins of animals)
dromophobia (crossing streets)
dysmorphophobia (deformity; becoming deformed)
dystychiphobia (accidents)
ecclesiophobia (churches)
ecophobia (home environment and surroundings; home life)
eicophobia (home)
eisoptrophobia (mirrors)
electrophobia (electricity)
eleutheraphobia
elurophobia (cats)
emetophobia (vomiting)
enetophobia (pins)

phobia *(cont.)*

enochlophobia (crowds)
enosiophobia (unpardonable sin)
entomophobia (insects)
eosophobia (dawn)
epistaxiophobia (nosebleeds)
epistemophobia (knowledge)
equinophobia (horses)
eremiophobia (or eremophobia) (deserted places; solitude; being alone; aloneness)
ereuthrophobia (blushing; color red)
ergasiophobia (working; functioning)
ergophobia (work)
erotophobia (physical love; sexual feelings)
erythrophobia (blushing; color red)
euphobia (good news)
eurotophobia (female genitalia)
examination
febriphobia (fever)
felinophobia (cats)
fibriphobia (fibers)
Francophobia (France/anything French)
frigophobia (cold)
galeophobia (cats)
Gallophobia (France/anything French)
gamophobia (marriage)
gatophobia (cats)
geliophobia (laughter)
geniophobia (chins)
genophobia (sexual intercourse)
genuphobia (knees)
gephyrophobia (crossing a bridge)
gerascophobia (growing old)
Germanophobia (Germany/ anything German)
gerontophobia (the elderly; old people)
geumophobia (taste; flavors)

phobia *(cont.)*
  glossophobia (speaking; talking)
  gnosiophobia (knowledge)
  graphophobia (writing)
  gringophobia (white strangers in
    Latin America)
  gymnophobia (nakedness)
  gynephobia (women)
  gynophobia (women)
  hadephobia (the underworld;
    the dead; hell)
  hagiophobia (sacred objects; saints)
  hamartophobia (sin; error)
  hamaxophobia (vehicles)
  haphephobia (being touched;
    touching)
  haphophobia (being touched;
    touching)
  haptophobia (being touched;
    touching)
  harpaxophobia (robbers)
  hedonophobia (pleasure)
  heliophobia (sun's rays; sunlight)
  hellenologophobia (Greek terms;
    complex scientific terms)
  helminthophobia (worms)
  hematophobia (blood; bleeding)
  hemophobia (blood; bleeding)
  hereiophobia (challenges to official
    doctrine; radical deviation)
  heresyphobia (challenges to official
    doctrine; radical deviation)
  herpetophobia (reptiles; amphib-
    ians)
  heterophobia (opposite sex)
  hierophobia (religious objects;
    sacred objects)
  hippophobia (horses)
  hodophobia (traveling)
  homichlophobia (fog)
  homilophobia (sermons)
  hominophobia (men)

phobia *(cont.)*
  homophobia (homosexuality)
  hoplophobia (firearms)
  hormephobia (rapid motion; shock)
  hyalophobia (glass)
  hydrargyophobia (mercurial medi-
    cines)
  hydrophobia (choking/gagging on
    liquids; water)
  hydrophobophobia (fear of rabies)
  hygrophobia (dampness; moisture;
    liquids esp. wine, water)
  hylephobia (forests; wood)
  hypegiaphobia (responsibility)
  hypengyophobia (responsibility)
  hypnophobia (sleep)
  hypsiphobia (heights)
  hypsophobia (heights)
  iatrophobia (going to the doctor)
  ichthyophobia (fish)
  ideophobia (ideas)
  illyngophobia (vertigo; dizziness
    when looking down)
  insectophobia (insects)
  iophobia (being poisoned; rusty
    objects)
  isolophobia (solitude; being alone)
  isopterophobia (termites)
  ithyphallophobia (an erect penis)
  Japanophobia (Japan/everything
    Japanese)
  Judaeophobia (Jews, Jewish culture)
  Judophobia (Jews, Jewish culture)
  kainophobia (newness; change;
    novelty)
  kakorrhaphiophobia (failure; defeat)
  katagelophobia (ridicule)
  kathisophobia (sitting down)
  kenophobia (emptiness; open spaces;
    barrenness; voids)
  keraunophobia (thunder and light-
    ning)

phobia *(cont.)*

kinesophobia (movements; motions)
kleptophobia (loss through thievery)
koinoniphobia (rooms)
kolphophobia (genitalia, particularly female)
koniophobia (dust)
kopophobia (fatigue)
kosmikophobia (cosmic phenomena)
kymophobia (waves)
kynophobia (pseudorabies)
kyphophobia (stooping)
lachanophobia (vegetables)
laliophobia (speaking; talking)
lalophobia (speaking; talking)
leprophobia (leprosy)
leukophobia (the color white)
levophobia (objects on the left side of the body)
ligyrophobia (loud noises)
lilapsophobia (tornadoes; hurricanes)
limnophobia (lakes)
linonophobia (string)
logophobia (words)
luiphobia (lues; syphilis)
lygophobia (darkness)
lyssophobia (rabies; insanity)
mageirocophobia (cooking)
maieusiophobia (pregnancy)
malaxophobia (love play)
maniaphobia (insanity)
marked and excessive specific
marked and persistent specific
marked and unreasonable specific
mastigophobia (whipping)
mechanophobia (machinery)
medomalacuphobia (losing an erection)
medorthophobia (an erect penis)
megalophobia (large objects)
melissophobia (bees)

phobia *(cont.)*

melophobia (music)
meningitophobia (meningitis; brain disease)
menophobia (menstruation)
merinthophobia (being bound)
metallophobia (metal objects)
metathesiophobia (change)
meteorophobia (weather; climate; meteors)
methyphobia (alcohol)
metrophobia (poetry)
microbiophobia (microbes; microorganisms; germs)
microphobia (small objects)
misophobia (contamination by dirt)
mnemophobia (memories)
molysmophobia (infection; contamination)
monopathophobia (a specific diseased body part)
monophobia (solitude; being alone; aloneness)
motorphobia (motor vehicles)
mottephobia (moths)
musicophobia (music)
musophobia (mice)
myctophobia (darkness)
myrmecophobia (ants)
mysophobia (dirt; infection; contamination; filth)
mythophobia (myths; stating an untruth; stories)
myxophobia (slime)
nebulaphobia (fog)
necrophobia (corpses; death)
negrophobia (black people)
nelophobia (glass)
neopharmaphobia (new drugs)
neophobia (novelty; newness; innovation)
nephophobia (clouds)

phobia *(cont.)*
  noctiphobia (night; darkness)
  nomatophobia (names)
  nosocomephobia (hospitals)
  nosophobia (illness; disease)
  nostophobia (returning to home)
  nucleomituphobia (nuclear
     weapons)
  nudophobia (nudity; being unclothed)
  numerophobia (numbers)
  nyctophobia (darkness; night)
  obesophobia (gaining weight)
  obsessional
  ochlophobia (crowds)
  ochophobia (vehicles)
  octophobia (the figure 8)
  odontophobia (teeth)
  odynophobia (pain)
  oenophobia (wine)
  oikophobia (home; family)
  oinophobia (wine)
  olfactophobia (odors; smells)
  ombrophobia (rain; rainstorms)
  ommatophobia (eyes)
  ommetaphobia (eyes)
  oneirophobia (dreams)
  onomatophobia (names; certain
     words)
  ophidiophobia (snakes; reptiles)
  ophiophobia (snake venom)
  ophthalmophobia (being stared at)
  optophobia (opening one's eyes)
  ornithophobia (birds)
  orthophobia (property)
  osmophobia (odors; smells)
  osphresiophobia (body odors)
  ostraconophobia (shellfish)
  ouranophobia (heaven)
  pagophobia (ice; frost)
  panophobia (general anxiety;
     nonspecific fear)

phobia *(cont.)*
  panphobia (general anxiety;
     nonspecific fear)
  panthophobia (suffering; disease)
  pantophobia (general anxiety;
     nonspecific fear; everything)
  papaphobia (the Pope)
  papyraphobia (paper)
  paralipophobia (omission of duty;
     neglect of duty)
  paraphobia (sexual perversion)
  parasitophobia (parasites)
  parthenophobia (young girls)
  pathophobia (disease)
  patriophobia (hereditary disease)
  peccatiphobia (sinning)
  pediculophobia (lice)
  pediophobia (children; dolls)
  pedophobia (children; dolls)
  peladophobia (bald people)
  pellagraphobia (rough skin)
  peniaphobia (poverty)
  phagophobia (eating; swallowing)
  phalacrophobia (becoming bald)
  phallophobia (an erect penis)
  pharmacophobia (drugs; medicines)
  phasmophobia (ghosts)
  phengophobia (daylight)
  philemaphobia (kissing)
  philemataphobia (kissing)
  philophobia (falling/being in love)
  philosophobia (philosophers)
  phobanthropy (human companion-
     ship)
  phobophobia (phobias; being afraid;
     fearing)
  phonophobia (voices; sounds;
     noise; one's own voice)
  photalgiophobia (fear of photalgia)
  photaugiaphobia (glare of light)
  photophobia (light)

phobia *(cont.)*

phronemophobia (mind; thoughts; thinking)
phthiriophobia (lice)
phthisiophobia (tuberculosis)
placophobia (tombstones)
plutophobia (wealth)
pluviophobia (rain; being rained on)
pneumatiphobia (spirits)
pneumatophobia (air; breathing)
pnigerophobia (choking; smothering)
pnigophobia (choking; smothering)
pocrescophobia (gaining weight)
pogonophobia (beards)
poinephobia (punishment)
politicophobia (politicians)
polyphobia (many things)
ponophobia (fatigue; overwork)
potamophobia (rivers)
potophobia (drinking)
proctophobia (rectal disease; the rectum)
prosophobia (progress)
psychoneurosis
psychophobia (mind)
psychrophobia (cold temperatures)
pteromerhanophobia (flying)
pteronophobia (feathers)
pyrexiophobia (fever)
pyrophobia (fire)
radiophobia (radiation; x-rays)
ranidophobia (frogs)
rectophobia (rectal disease; rectum)
rhabdophobia (being beaten; punishment by rod)
rhypophobia (filth; dirt; defecation; feces)
rhytiphobia (becoming wrinkled)
rupophobia (filth; dirt)
Russophobia (Russia/anything Russian)
sarmassophobia (love play)

phobia *(cont.)*

Satanophobia (Satan; things satanic)
scabiophobia (scabies)
scatophobia (excrement; using obscene language)
scelerophobia
sciophobia (shadows)
scoleciphobia (worms)
scolionophobia (school)
scopophobia (being stared at)
scotomaphobia (visual-field blindness)
scotophobia (darkness)
scriptophobia (writing in public)
selaphobia (flash of light)
selenophobia (the moon)
seplophobia (decaying matter)
sesquipedalophobia (long words)
sexophobia (opposite sex)
siderodromophobia (railway; trains)
siderophobia (iron; stars)
simple
sinistrophobia (things to the left, left-handed)
Sinophobia (China; anything Chinese)
sitiophobia (eating; food)
sitophobia (eating; food)
snakephobia (snakes)
social
social phobia (being viewed negatively in social situations)
sociophobia (society; people)
somniphobia (sleep)
sophophobia (learning)
soteriophobia (depending on others)
spacephobia (outer space)
spectrophobia (seeing one's image in a mirror; phantoms)
spermatophobia (loss of semen)

phobia *(cont.)*
  spermophobia (germs)
  sphecidophobia (wasps)
  spheksophobia (wasps)
  stasibasiphobia (attempting to stand and/or walk)
  stasiphobia (standing still)
  staurophobia (a cross or crucifix)
  stenophobia (narrow things; narrow places)
  stygiophobia (hell)
  suriphobia (mice)
  symbolophobia (perceptions; symbolism)
  symmetrophobia (symmetry)
  syphilophobia (being infected with syphilis)
  tabophobia (wasting sickness)
  tachophobia (speed)
  taeniophobia (tapeworms)
  taphephobia (being buried alive; graves)
  taphophobia (being buried alive; graves)
  tapinophobia (small things)
  taurophobia (bulls)
  technophobia (technology)
  telephonophobia (telephone)
  teleophobia (teleology)
  teratophobia (bearing a deformed child)
  testophobia (taking tests)
  tetanophobia (lockjaw; tetanus)
  Teutonophobia (Germany, things German)
  Teutophobia (Germany, things German)
  textophobia (certain fabrics)
  thaasophobia (sitting)
  thalassophobia (the sea)
  thanatophobia (death)
  theatrophobia (theaters)

phobia *(cont.)*
  theologicophobia (theology)
  theophobia (God; religion)
  thermophobia (heat)
  thixophobia (shaking)
  tocophobia (childbirth)
  tomophobia (surgery)
  tonitrophobia (thunder)
  topophobia (places)
  toxicophobia (poison)
  toxiphobia (poison)
  toxophobia (poison)
  traumatophobia (trauma; wounds; injury)
  tremophobia (trembling)
  trichinophobia (trichinosis)
  trichopathophobia (hair abnormalities and disease)
  trichophobia (loose hair on clothing, etc.)
  tridecaphobia (the number 13)
  triskaidekaphobia (the number thirteen)
  tropophobia (moving; making changes)
  trypanophobia (injections)
  tuberculophobia (tuberculosis)
  tyrannophobia (morbid cruelty; tyrants)
  uranophobia
  urophobia (passing urine)
  vaccinophobia (vaccination)
  venereophobia (venereal disease)
  venustraphobia (beautiful women)
  verbophobia (words)
  vermiphobia (worms)
  verminophobia (germs)
  wicaphobia (witches; witchcraft)
  xenophobia (strangers; foreigners)
  xerophobia (dry places; deserts)
  xylophobia (wooden objects; forests)

phobia *(cont.)*
  zelophobia (jealousy)
  zoophobia (animals)
phobic
  generalized
  nongeneral
  social
phobic avoidance of situations
phobic disorder
phobic neurosis
phobic obsessional neurosis
phobic psychoneurotic reaction
phobic reaction
phobic situation
phobic state
phobic stimulus
phobic trends
phobophobia
phonasthenia
phonation
  maximum duration of
  myoelastic-aerodynamic theory of
  reverse
  ventricular
  voice disorders of
phonation break
phonatory disorder
phonatory seizure
phoneme
  back
  compact
  diffuse
  front
  grave
  lax
  lenis
  segmental
  suprasegmental
  tense
Phoneme Discrimination Test (PDT)
phoneme/grapheme association
phonemic analysis

phonemic articulation error
phonemic awareness
phonemic paraphasia
phonemic regression
phonemic representation
phonemic synthesis
phonemic transcription
phonemics
Phonetically Balanced Kindergarten
  Word Lists
phonetically balanced words (PB
  words)
phonetic alphabet
phonetic-analysis skills
phonetic articulation error
phonetic context
phonetic features
phonetician
phoneticization
phonetic perception
phonetic placement
phonetic power
phonetic representation
phonetics
  acoustic
  articulatory
  auditory
  impressionistic
  linguistic
  normative
  physiologic
phonetic skills
phonetic sound segments
phonetic symbols
phonetic transcription
  close
  narrow
phonetic variations
phoniatrician
phoniatrics
phoniatrist
phonics, vocal

phonogram
phonological agraphia
phonological analysis
phonological conditioning
phonological disorder
phonological impairment
Phonological Process Analysis (PPA)
phonological processes
    developmental
    natural
phonological rules
phonology
phonomania
phonophobia
phonosurgery
phonotactics
phosphatidylinositol (PI)
phosphene
phosphodiesterase inhibitors
phosphoinositide cascade
photalgiophobia
photaugiaphobia
photic epilepsy
Photo Articulation Test (PAT)
photogenic seizure
photomania
photon-counting hypothesis of seasonal
    affective disorders
photophobia
photosensitive epilepsy
phrasal category
phrase (pl. phrases)
    absolute construction of
    carrier
    endocentric construction of
    exocentric construction of
    incomplete
    multi-word
    noun
    prepositional
    verb
phrase construction (PC)

phrase level
phrase repetition
phrase stress
phrase structure grammar
phrenetic
phrenic
phrenocardia
phrenology
phrenotropic
phronemomania
phronemophobia
PHSQ (Psychosocial History Screening
    Questionnaire)
phthiriomania
phthiriophobia
phyloanalysis
phylogenesis
phylogenetic
phylogeny
physical abuse
physical activity
physical aggression
physical agitation
Physical and Architectural Features
    Checklist
physical appearance
physical attack
physical bondage (restraint)
physical change
physical concomitant of anxiety
physical condition
physical defect
physical disorder
physical environment
physical examination (P.E. or PE)
physical experience
physical fights
physical harm
physical health
physical independence
physically endangered
physical manifestation of pain

physical problem
physical sensations
physical signs and symptoms
physical strain
physical support
physical symptoms
  adjustment reaction
  psychogenic
physical tension
physical therapy
Physical Tolerance Profile (PTP)
physical trauma
physician
  family
  primary care (PCP)
physician-patient relations
Physicians' Desk Reference (PDR)
physician's role
physiogenic
Physiognomic Cue Test (PCT)
physiological basis
physiological dependence
  substance dependence with
  substance dependence without
physiological effect
physiological factor
physiological functional variation
physiological hyaluronidase inhibitor
  (PHI)
physiological intoxication
physiological manifestations
physiological measurements
physiological norm
physiological process
physiological psychologist
physiological psychology
physiological reactivity
physiological response
physiological signs of withdrawal
physiological sleepiness
physiological tremor
physiologic mechanism

physiologic phonetics
physiologic psychology
physiologic tremor
physiology
  auditory
  vestibular
physiology of successful aging
physiopsychic
PI (phosphatidylinositol)
PI (present illness)
PI (proactive inhibition)
Piaget cognitive development stages
Piaget, Jean (1896-1980)
"pianoing" (re: crack acquisition)
PIAPACS (psychological information,
  acquisition, processing and control
  system)
PIAT (Peabody Individual Achieve-
  ment Test)
piblokto (culture-specific syndrome)
PIC (Personality Inventory for
  Children)
pica
PICA (Porch Index of Communicative
  Ability)
PICAC (Porch Index of Communica-
  tive Ability in Children)
Picha-Seron Career Analysis (PSCA;
  PSCA-CP; PSCA-OP; PSCA-PP)
Pick disease, dementia in
Pickford Projectives Pictures (PPP)
picking at bodily orifices
picking at skin
PICS (Parent Interview for Child
  Syndrome)
PICSI (Picture Identification for
  Children-Standardized Index)
PICSYMS (picture symbols)
pictographs
pictorial aphasia
Pictorial Test of Intelligence (PTI)
picture arrangement (PA) subtest

Picture Articulation and Language
    Screening Test (PALST)
picture assembly
picture, clinical
picture completion (PC) subtest
Picture Identification for Children-
    Standardized Index (PICSI)
Picture Identification Test (PIT)
Picture Interest Exploration Survey
    (PIES)
Picture Sound Discrimination Test
Picture Speech Discrimination Test
Picture Spondee Threshold Test
Picture Story Language Test (PSLT)
picture test
picture with perceptual disturbances
PICU (Psychiatric Intensive Care
    Unit)
pidgin sign English (PSE)
"piece" (1 ounce)
"piedras" (crack)
Pierre Robin syndrome
Piers-Harris Children's Self-Concept
    Scale
PIES (Picture Interest Exploration
    Survey)
PIF (premorbid inferiority feeling)
"Pig Killer" (phencyclidine)
Pike dementia
PIL (Purpose in Life) test
"piles" (crack)
pill-rolling tremor
piloerection
"pimp" (cocaine)
"pimp your pipe" (re: crack equip-
    ment)
Pimsleur Language Aptitude Battery
"pin" (cannabis)
pine
Pinel, Phillipe (1746-1826)
"ping-in-wing" (re: drug injection)
"pin gon" (opium)

pining
"pink blotters" (lysergic acid diethyl-
    amide)
"pink hearts" (amphetamine)
"pink lady" (secobarbital)
"Pink Panther" (lysergic acid diethyl-
    amide)
"pink robots" (lysergic acid diethyl-
    amide)
"pinks" (secobarbital)
"pink wedges" (lysergic acid diethyl-
    amide)
"pink witches" (lysergic acid diethyl-
    amide)
pinna (pl. pinnae) of ear
pinning and piercing (infibulation)
pinpoint pupils
pins-and-needles sensation
pins-sticking sensation
Pin Test
"pin yen" (opium)
PIP (Psychotic Inpatient Profile)
"pipe" (re: cannabis equipment; crack
    equipment; drug injection; mixed
    drugs)
piperidine derivative
"pipero" (re: crack user)
pipe smoking, straight
PIQ (Performance Intelligence
    Quotient)
PIT (Picture Identification Test)
"pit" (phencyclidine)
pitch
    basal
    downdrift
    habitual
    natural
pitch brake
    descending
    ascending
pitch discrimination
pitch perception

pitch range
pitch shift
pithecoid idiot
pivot grammar (parts of speech)
pivot word
"pixies" (amphetamine)
PK (psychokinesis)
PK (psychokinetic)
PKRS (Phelps Kindergarten Readiness
   Scale)
PKSAP (Psychiatric Knowledge and
   Skills Self-Assessment Program)
PKU (phenylketonuria)
PL (psychosocial-labile)
place
   articulation
   closed
   crowded
   open
   oriented as to
   unfamiliar
placebo
placebo effect
placebo medication trial
place deixis
place hearing theory
place identity
placement
   alveolar consonant
   bilabial area consonant
   glottal area consonant
   labiodental area consonant
   lingua-alveolar area consonant
   linguadental area consonant
   palatal area consonant
   phonetic
   sense of
   velar area consonant
place theory
placid disposition
plagiocephalic idiocy

plan
   action
   formulate a
   homicidal
   management
   meticulously detailed
   organizational
   realistic
   suicidal
   suicide
   treatment (TrPl)
plane
   axial
   coronal
   frontal
   horizontal
   median sagittal
   sagittal
planigraphy
planned pregnancy
Planning Career Goals (PCG)
planning, motor
"plant" (re: drug concealment)
plantar response
plaque, senile
plasma cortisol
plasma homovanillic acid (HVA)
plasma HVA levels in schizophrenia
plasma protein metabolism
plateau in improvement
plateau masking technique
plateau method
platonic friendship
platonic relationship
plausible
play
   expression of traumatic themes
      through repetitive
   fantasy
   group
   imaginative

play *(cont.)*
   make-believe
   parallel
   rough-and-tumble
   symbolic
   verbal
play audiometry
play group therapy (PGT)
play hunches
playing, role
playing with hands
playmate, imaginary
play therapy
play vocal range
PLC (Personal Locus of Control)
plea for help
pleasure in everyday activities
pleasure in few activities
pleasure-pain principle
pleasure principle
pleasure-seeking
pleasure, sexual
pleasuring
pleonexia
plethysmography, penile
plosive consonant formation
plosive-injection method
PLS (Preschool Language Scale)
pluralism
plus juncture
plutomania
PM, P.M., p.m. (afternoon)
PMA (analog of amphetamine/
   methamphetamine)
P-MAC/ESP (Perceptual-Motor
   Assessment for Children and
   Emotional/Behavior Screening
   Program)
PMPQ (Professional and Managerial
   Position Questionnaire)
PMS (premenstrual syndrome)
PMT (Porteus Maze Test)

PN (Psychiatry-Neurology)
PN (psychoneurologist)
PN (psychoneurology)
PN (psychoneurotic)
PNAvQ (positive-negative ambivalent
   quotient)
PNdB (perceived noise level)
pneumatic artificial larynx
pneumatophobia
pneumogram
pneumograph
pneumotachogram
pneumotachograph
PNI (psychoneuroimmunology)
pnigerophobia
pnigophobia
PNP (psychogenic nocturnal polydipsia)
PNS (parasympathetic nervous
   system)
PNS (peripheral nervous system)
p.o. (per os)
p.o. (probation officer)
POBE (Profile of Out-of-Body
   Experiences)
"pocket rocket" (cannabis)
"pod" (cannabis)
PODQ (Perceptual Organization
   Deviation Quotient)
pogonophobia
POI (Personal Orientation Inventory)
poinephobia
point
   activity
   articulation
point of subjective equality (PSE)
point prevalence
poise, tough
"poison" (fentanyl; heroin)
poisoning
   acute alcohol
   lead

"poke" (cannabis)
pokeweed mitogen
polar opposites
polarities, sorting
polarity response
police power
Policy and Program Information Form
political values
politicomania
politicophobia
Politte Sentence Completion Test
Pollack-Branden Inventory:
    For Identification of Learning
    Disabilities, Dyslexia and Class-
    room Dysfunction
Pollyanna-like view
"polvo" (heroin; phencyclidine)
"polvo blanco" (cocaine)
"polvo de angel" (phencyclidine)
"polvo de estrellas" (phencyclidine)
polyarteritis nodosa
polydipsia
polydrug abuse
polydystrophic oligophrenia
Polyfactorial Study of Personality
polygenic inheritance
polyglot
polygraph
polymorphemic utterances
polymorphic perversion
polyneuritic psychosis
polyneuropathy
polyphagia
polyphasic potential
polyphasic wave
polyphobia
polyphyria
polyp, nasal
polypoid degeneration of the true
    folds
polypoid vocal nodules
polysemous

polysemy
polysomnographic abnormalities
polysomnographic study
polysomnography
polysubstance-related disorder
polysurgical addiction
polysyllabic word
polytomography
POMS (Profile of Mood States)
ponophobia
PONS (Profile of Nonverbal Sensi-
    tivity)
"pony" (crack)
"poor man's pot" (inhalant)
"pop" (re: cocaine use)
"poppers" (amyl nitrite)
"poppy" (heroin)
population setting
populations, community
POR (problem oriented record)
Porch Index of Communicative
    Ability (PICA)
Porch Index of Communicative
    Ability in Children (PICAC)
poriomania
pornographomania
pornography dependence
porphyria
porphyrin metabolism
port
    nasal
    velopharyngeal
PORT (Perception-of-Relationships
    Test)
Portable Mental Status Questionnaire,
    Short (SPMSQ)
Porteus Maze Test (PMT)
Portland Digit Recognition Test
    (PDRT)
Portland Problem Behavior Checklist,
    Revised
portmanteau word

Portuguese Speaking Test (PST)
pos (positive)
position
  body
  cortical thumb
  final consonant
  first
  initial consonant
  intervocalic consonant
  medial consonant
  medically related
  observer
  other
  postvocalic consonant
  prevocalic consonant
  seated
  second
  sustained
  third
positional tremor
Position Analysis Questionnaire
  (PAQ)
positioning of distal limbs
position of responsibility
positive (pos)
positive ability
Positive and Negative Syndrome Scale
  (PANSS)
Positive Attention Behavior (PAB)
positive communication skills
positive comparison
positive correlation
positive emotion
positive emotionality
positive events
positive feeling
positive frontal release signs
positive incentive
positive ion
positive-negative ambivalent quotient
  (PNAvQ)
positive parenting

positive predictive power
positive reinforcement
positive reinforcer
positive relationship
positive response
positive schizophrenic symptoms
  disorganization dimension of
  psychotic dimension of
positive speech content
positive spike-waves
positive symptoms of schizophrenia
positive transference
positivity
positron-emission tomography (PET)
  scan
possessing agent
possession, drug
possession trance state
possession trance symptom
possessive case
possessor-possession
possible effect
POST (National Police Officer
  Selection Test)
postanalytic supervision
postanoxic encephalopathy
postanoxic epilepsy
postcentral gyrus
postcentral sulcus
postconcussion disorder
postconcussion headache
postconcussion neurosis
postconcussion syndrome
postconcussive amnesia
postconsonantal vowel
postcontusion brain syndrome
postdormital sleep paralysis
postencephalitic syndrome
posterior alexia
posterior cricoarytenoid muscle
posterior digastric muscle
posterior vertical canal

posthypnotic amnesia
posthypnotic psychosis
posthysterectomy depression
postictal confusion
postictal depression phase of seizure
postictal state
post-incident care for the assaulted
staff
postinfectious psychosis
postleukotomy syndrome
postlingual deafness
postlobotomy syndrome
postmortem studies of suicide victims
postoperative confusion
postoperative confusional state
postoperative psychosis
postoperative status
postpartum depression
postpartum major depression
postpartum psychosis
postpsychotic depression
postponements
postprandial (P.P.)
postpsychotic depressive disorder of
schizophrenia
postpubertal
postpuberty
postpubescence
postpubescent
poststroke depression
postsynaptic receptor
posttermination, boundaries
posttraumatic amnesia (PTA)
posttraumatic amnestic syndrome
posttraumatic brain syndrome
nonpsychotic
psychotic
posttraumatic cerebral syndrome
posttraumatic chronic disability
posttraumatic cortical dysfunction
posttraumatic delirium
posttraumatic dementia

posttraumatic encephalopathy
posttraumatic epilepsy
posttraumatic headache
posttraumatic neurosis
acute
chronic
situational
posttraumatic organic psychosis
acute
subacute
posttraumatic pain
posttraumatic psychopathic constitution
posttraumatic seizure
posttraumatic stress disorder (PTSD)
acute
brief
chronic
delayed
prolonged
posttraumatic stress disorder by proxy
Posttraumatic Stress Disorder Scale
posttraumatic stress syndrome
postulates, conversational
postural awareness
postural seizure
postural tremor
caffeine-induced
fine
medication-induced
neuroleptic-induced
stimulant-induced
posture
bent
bizarre
body
fetal position
inappropriate
rigid
sagging
unusual sleep
posturing, catatonic
Post-Viet Nam Psychiatric Syndrome
(PVNPS)

postvocalic consonant position
postvocalic obstruent singleton omissions
"pot" (cannabis)
potamophobia
"potato" (lysergic acid diethylamide)
"potato chips" (crack cut with benzocaine)
potency
potential
   acoustic evoked
   acting out
   action
   auditory event-related
   auditory evoked (AEP)
   biphasic
   brain stem auditory evoked
     (BAEP)
   brain stem evoked
   cerebral
   cortical evoked
   early latency
   EEG
   electrical
   estimated-learning (ELP)
   event-related
   evoked
   glossokinetic
   high-tolerance
   leadership
   low-tolerance
   motor-evoked (MEP)
   polyphasic
   resting
   sensory-evoked (SEP)
   suicidal
   visual-evoked (VEP)
potential adverse effects
potential energy
potential evaluation by others
potential external awards
potential external rewards

Potential for Addiction Index
potential for injury
potential for painful consequences
potential impact
potential impairment of immune functioning
potential intellectual capacity
potential positive events
potential problems
potential risks for malnutrition
potential secondary gain
potential targets
potentiometer
potomania
potophobia
"potten bush" (cannabis)
pounding pain
poverty, delusion of
poverty of content
poverty of ideas
poverty of movement
poverty of speech
poverty of speech content
poverty of thought
POW (prisoner of war)
Powassan viral encephalitis
"powder" (amphetamine; heroin)
"powder diamonds" (cocaine)
powdered opium
power (pl. powers)
   distribution of
   inflated
   instantaneous
   manipulative behavior to attain
   mind
   negative predictive
   phonetic
   police
   positive predictive
power CROS (contralateral routing of
   signals)
power density, sound

powerful emotion
powerless
powerlessness
power output
"power puller" (re: crack equipment)
power struggle (leadership pattern)
power test
"pox" (opium)
P.P. (postprandial)
PPA (Phonological Process Analysis)
PPC (Personal Problems Checklist for
    Adolescents)
PPCP (Parent Perception of Child
    Profile)
PPD, Ppd, p.p.d. (packs per day)
PPMS (Purdue Perceptual-Motor
    Survey)
PPP (Pickford Projectives Pictures)
PPS (Personal Preference Scale)
PPSRT (Printing Performance School
    Readiness Test)
PPVT (Peabody Picture Vocabulary
    Test)
PR (psychotherapy responder)
"P.R." (Panama Red)
practical aspects of assaultive client
    care
Practical Math Assessments
practical reasoning
practical social judgment score
practice
    family
    negative
    psychology
practice effects
praecox, dementia
pragmatic aphasia
Pragmatics Profile of Early Commu-
    nication Skills
Pragmatics Screening Test
pragmatic structures
pragmatic text

PRAS (Patient Rated Anxiety Scale)
pre-article
PREB (Pupil Record of Education
    Behavior)
precautions, suicide
precentral gyrus
precentral seizure
precentral sulcus
precipitant exposure, common
precipitate
precipitating crisis
precipitating event
precipitating factor
precipitating stress
precipitating tremor
precipitation of epilepsy
precipitation of seizure
precipitous mood shifts
precision therapy
precocious
precocity
precognition
preconscious (pcs.)
preconsciousness
preconsonantal vowel
precordial pain, psychogenic
predators, sexual
predicate
    complete
    simple
predicate adjective
predicate nominative
predicate noun
predicate objective
predicate truncation
prediction from the acoustic reflex
prediction of consequence variables
prediction of dangerousness
Predictive Ability Test (PAT)
Predictive Screening Test of Articula-
    tion
predictive validity

predictor, psychometric
predictor variable
predispose
predisposed, situationally
predisposed panic attacks
predisposing factor
predisposition, biological
predominant affect
predominant current defense level
predominant defense level
predominantly hyperactive-impulsive attention-deficit/hyperactivity disorder
predominantly inattentive-type attention-deficit/hyperactivity disorder
predominantly predormital sleep paralysis
predominant mood disturbance
predominant symptom presentation
predominate
preepisode status
preexisting cognitive variables
preexisting condition
preexisting dementia
preexisting illness
preexisting mental disorder
preexisting tremor
preexisting underlying emotional issues
preference (pl. preferences)
    conditioned place (CPP)
    consonant-vowel
    paraphiliac
    risk
preferred method
preferred representational system
prefix
prefixation
prefrontal lobotomy
pregenital phase
pregnancy
    accidental
    hysterical

pregnancy *(cont.)*
    planned
    psychosis in
    unplanned
    unwanted
prejudice
Preliminary Diagnostic Questionnaire
prelingual deafness
prelogical thinking
Premarital Communication Inventory (PCI)
premature death
premature ejaculation
premaxilla
premeditation
premenstrual dysphoric disorder
premenstrual syndrome (PMS)
premolar teeth
premonition of seizure
premonitory sign
premorbid ability
premorbid adjustment
premorbid asociality
premorbid functioning
premorbid history
premorbid inferiority feeling (PIF)
premorbid intellectual function
premorbid level of functioning
premorbid personality
premorbid state
premotor area
preoccupation
    control
    death
    defect
    details
    homicidal
    lists
    orderliness
    organization
    perfectionism
    pathological
    rules

preoccupation *(cont.)*
  schedules
  suicidal
  unshakable
preoccupied
pre-oedipal phase
preoperational thought period
prepalatal
preparatory set
preposition (parts of speech)
prepositional phrase
Pre-Professional Skills Test
prepsychotic personality
prepsychotic psychosis
prepsychotic schizophrenia
prepubertal borderline psychosis
prepubertal child
prepubertal psychopathology
prepuberty
prepubescence, prepubescent
preputial sensation
Pre-Reading Expectancy Screening
  Scales (PRESS)
presbyacusis
presbyophrenia
presbyophrenic psychosis
Preschool and Kindergarten Interest
  Descriptor
Preschool Behavior Questionnaire
  (PBQ)
preschool child
Preschool Development Inventory
Preschool Language Assessment
  Instrument (PLAI)
Preschool Language Scale (PLS)
Preschool Language Screening Test
Preschool Screening Test
Preschool Speech and Language
  Screening Test
prescience
prescribed treatment
prescription (Rx)

"prescription" (cannabis cigarette)
prescription drug-related disorder
prescriptive grammar
Prescriptive Reading Inventory (PRI)
presenile dementia
  confusional-state
  delirium in
  delusional-type
  depressed-type
  paranoid-type
  simple-type
  uncomplicated
presenile mental disorder
presenile psychosis
presenilis
  anxietas
  dementia
presenility
presentation
  atypical
  catatonic
  clinical
  equivalent symptomatic
  historical
  mixed
  pain
  predominant symptom
  psychotic
  substance-induced
  subthreshold
  symptom
present illness (PI)
presenting personality
presenting problem
presenting psychopathology
presenting symptom
present-oriented
present perfect progressive tense
present perfect tense
present progressive tense
Present State Examination (PSE)
present tense

presidents test
pre-speech tension
press
  glossopharyngeal
  tongue
"press" (crack; cocaine)
PRESS (PreReading Expectancy
  Screening Scales)
pressing thoughts
press limits
pressure
  environmental
  group
  intraoral
  intrapleural
  intrapulmonic
  intrathoracic
  minimum audible (MAP)
  peer
  pulmonary
  systolic
  time
pressured behavior
pressured speech
pressure level
  saturation sound (SSPL)
  sound (SPL)
pressure level range
pressure of speech
pressure pattern
pressure wave
presumed causality
presupposition
presynaptic neuron
"pretendica" (cannabis)
"pretendo" (cannabis)
pretentious
prevalence
  period
  point
prevalence of insomnia
prevalence of schizophrenia

prevalent
prevention
  anxiety
  exposure and response
  primary
  relapse (RP)
  response
  secondary
  stress
  tertiary
prevention of disclosure
prevention of extrapyramidal symptoms
prevention of physical harm
prevention of weight gain
prevention of withdrawal
preventive intervention
preventive psychiatry
previous history
previously stabilizing social situations
prevocalic consonant position
prevocalic singleton
prevocalic voicing of consonants
Prevocational Assessment and
  Curriculum Guide (PACG)
Prevocational Assessment Screen
  (PAS)
prevocational deafness
PRF (Personality Research Form)
PRI (Partner Relationship Inventory)
PRI (Personal Relationship Inventory)
PRI (Prescriptive Reading Inventory)
priapism
pride, excessive
pride of place
primal father
primal scene
primal therapy
primary affective disorder (PAD)
primary anxiety disorder
primary auditory cortex
primary autism

primary caregiver
primary care patient populations
primary care physician (PCP)
primary care setting
primary case
primary complaint
primary degenerative dementia
primary dementia
  acute
  degenerative
primary drive
primary function
primary gain
primary hypersomnia
primary identity
primary insomnia
Primary Language Screen, The (TPLS)
Primary Measures of Music Audiation
primary mental disorder
primary mood disorder with psychotic features
primary narcissism
primary oppositional attitude
primary palate
primary Parkinson disease
primary prevention
primary process
primary process thinking
primary psychotic disorder
primary reinforcement
primary reinforcer
primary responsibility
primary schizophrenia
primary seizure
Primary Self-Concept Inventory (PSCI)
primary sex characteristics
primary sexual deviation
primary sleep disorder
primary stress
primary support group

Primary Test of Cognitive Skills (PTCS)
primary tic
Primary Visual Motor Test (PVMT)
primes
primitive auditory segregation
"primo" (cannabis and crack)
primobolan (injectable and oral steroid)
"primos" (cigarettes laced with cocaine and heroin)
Prince, Morton (1854-1929)
principal clause
principal diagnosis
principal focus
principal investigation
principal objective
principle
  authority
  binary
  organizing
  pain-pleasure
  pleasure
  pleasure-pain
  psychophysiologic
  rebus
  reality
  talion (or talion law)
Printing Performance School Readiness Test (PPSRT)
prints, voice
prion diseases
prior history
prioritize
Priority Counseling Survey (PCS)
prior to admission (PTA)
prisoner of war (POW)
prison psychosis
private material
private practice patient populations
private psychiatric hospital
privilege

privileged communication
privileges, bathroom (BRP)
p.r.n., PRN (as necessary)
proactive inhibition (PI)
probability curve
probability learning
probability of success
proband, autistic
probation officer (p.o.)
probe microphone measurements
probe tube microphone
problem (pl. problems)
  academic
  acculturation
  adolescent identity
  age-related cognitive decline
  alcohol
  behavior
  career change
  cocaine
  concurrent psychiatric
  developmental learning (DLP)
  disturbing
  divorce
  drug
  economic
  educational
  emotional
  environmental
  erectile
  expressive language
  faith conversion
  gait
  gender identity
  health
  housing
  identity
  immediate gratification
  impulse-control
  individuation
  leaving parental control
  leaving school

problem (cont.)
  life circumstance
  loss of faith
  marriage
  memory
  new career
  occupational
  opioid
  orgasmic
  parent-child relational
  partner relational
  phase of life
  physical
  potential
  presenting
  psychological
  psychosocial
  questioning faith
  real-life
  receptive language
  relational
  religious
  retirement
  school change
  school discipline
  school drop-out
  school entering
  separation
  sexual arousal
  sexual desire
  sibling relational
  sleep
  spiritual
  stress-related psychophysiological
  substance-related
  word-finding
  work-related
problem-based learning
problem categories
problem drinker (PD)
Problem Experiences Checklist
problem-oriented record (POR)

problem solving
  difficulties with
  interpersonal cognitive (ICPS)
  visuo-spatial
problem-solving communication
Problem Solving Inventory
problem-solving negotiation
problem-solving skills
problem-solving strategies
problem-solving style
procedure (pl. procedures) (see *test*)
Procedures for the Phonological
  Analysis of Children's Language
proceedings, care and protection
process (pl. processes)
  automatic psychological
  biological
  bizarre thought
  central auditory
  clinical evaluation
  closure
  comprehensive identification
  computational
  concrete thought
  decision-making
  dementia
  dementing
  developmental phonological
  disease
  egocentric thought
  empirical
  escalative
  evidence-based
  explicit
  fantasy
  feature contrasts
  free access to
  goal-oriented
  harmony
  idiosyncratic
  imaginal
  mastoid

process *(cont.)*
  maxilla
  mental
  monosyllabic
  natural phonological
  neurotic
  normative aging
  pathological
  pathophysiological
  phonological
  physiological
  primary
  psychosocial
  psychotic
  revision
  schizophrenic
  secondary
  systematic
  therapeutic
  thought
  transition
Process Diagnostic (PD)
Process for the Assessment of
  Effective Student Functioning
processing
  auditory
  higher integrative language
  language
  speech
  temporal auditory
  visuo-spatial
processing disorder, central auditory
processing of affective experience
processing of dissociative states and
  disorders
processing of language, auditory
processing of traumatic experience
Processing Word Classes
process issues
Process Skills Rating Scales (PSRS)
process thinking
process words

procrastination
proctophobia
procursiva, aura
procursive epilepsy
prodromal period
prodromal phase
prodromal phase of schizophrenia
prodromal schizophrenia
prodromal symptoms
prodrome of schizophrenia
prodrome, visual
production
  constricted vocal
  divergent
  language
  speech sound
  stressful word
production of symptoms
productivity of speech
productivity of thought
product moment
Professional and Administrative Career
  Examination (PACE)
Professional and Managerial Position
  Questionnaire (PMPQ)
professional burnout
professional counselor
professional distance
Professional Employment Test (PET)
professional exploiters
professional-family relations
professional gambler
professional neurosis
professional-patient relations
Professional Sexual Role Inventory
  (PSRI)
Professional Standards Review
  Organization (PSRO)
profile
  adaptability
  anxiety
  clinical

profile *(cont.)*
  criminal
  employment
  left-out sibling
  mood
  neurotic direction
  psychotic direction
  risk
  spiked
Profile of Adaptation to Life
Profile of Mood States (POMS)
Profile of Nonverbal Sensitivity
  (PONS)
Profile of Out-of-Body Experiences
  (POBE)
profound amnesia
profound hearing impairment
profound hearing loss
profound idiocy/idiot
profoundly retarded
profound mental retardation
  I.Q. under 20
  idiocy
profound mental subnormality
prognathic
prognosis (Px, px), long-term
Prognostic Value of Imitative and
  Auditory Discrimination Tests
program (pl. programs) (see *test*)
  behavior modification
  therapeutic
  treatment
  twelve-step (12-step)
  weight-control
Program for Assessing Youth Employment Skills
programmable hearing aid
programmed therapy
programming
  articulation
  neuro-linguistic

Progress Assessment Chart of Social
and Personal Development (PAC)
Progressive Achievement Tests of
Listening Comprehension
(PATLC)
Progressive Achievement Test of
Mathematics [Revised] (PATM)
Progressive Achievement Tests of
Reading [Revised]
progressive assimilation
progressive disease
progressive disability
progressive muscular relaxation
progressive relaxation
progressive tense
  future perfect
  past perfect
project (pl. projects)
projection, delusional
Projective Assessment of Aging
Method
projective identification
projective technique
projective test
prolabium
prolongation
  sound
  syllable
prolonged depressive reaction
prolonged episode
prolonged grief reaction
prolonged nocturnal sleep episodes
prolonged posttraumatic stress
disorder
prolonged prodrome of schizophrenia
prolonged sleep episodes
prolonged sleep latency
prolonged sleep treatment
prolonged speech elements
prominence, laryngeal
prominent anxiety
prominent deterioration

prominent grimacing
prominent hallucination
prominent irritable mood
prominent mood symptoms
prominent negative symptoms of
schizophrenia
promiscuity, protracted
promiscuous sexual behavior
prompting
prone, accident
proneness to addiction
pronoun (parts of speech)
  anaphoric
  bound
  exophoric
  reflexive
  unbound
pronunciation
proof, incontrovertible
propaganda
property, semantic
prophylactic treatment
proportions, delusional
proposed treatment
propositional speech
proprioception
proprioceptive feedback
proprioceptive perception
prosodic feature
prosodic phonology
prosody of speech
Prosody-Voice Screening Profile
(PVSP)
prosopagnosia
prospective (experimental study
designs)
prosthesis (pl. prostheses), indwelling
low pressure voice
prosthetic management of cleft palate
prosthodontist
prostitution
prostrate

prostration
protection device
  canal caps hearing
  circumaural hearing
  earmuffs hearing
  earplugs hearing
  hearing (HPD)
  insert hearing
  semiaural hearing
protection proceedings
protective survival strategy
"protector" identity
protector role
protein
  beta-amyloid
  Crk
  heterotrimeric G
proteinphobia
protest
prothrombin time (pro-time or PT)
pro time (prothrombin time)
protocol, test
protolanguage
prototaxic
prototypical case
prototypical course patterns
protoword
protracted difficulties
protracted promiscuity
protracted reactive paranoid psychosis
protrusion lisp
protrusion, tongue
proverb interpretation test
proverbs test
provider, day-care
proviron (oral steroid)
provocation
  aggression without
  pharmacological
provocative behavior
provoke
provoked anxiety

provoking stimulus
prowess, sexual
proxemia
proxemic
proxy
  factitious disorder by
  Munchausen disease by
PRP (Psychotic Reaction Profile)
PRQ (Personal Resource Questionnaire)
PRS (Personality Rating Scale)
PRS (Pupil Rating Scale: Screening
  for Learning Disabilities)
PRT (Picture Reasoning Test), OISE
PRT (Pantomime Recognition Test)
prude
prudish
pruritic disorder
PS (psychiatric)
PSAn, PsAn (psychoanalysis)
PSAn, PsAn (psychoanalyst)
PSCA (Picha-Seron Career Analysis)
PSCI (Primary Self-Concept Inventory)
PSE (pidgin sign English)
PSE (point of subjective equality)
PSE (Present State Examination)
psellism
pseudoaggression
pseudoagraphia
pseudoauthenticity
pseudobulbar palsy
pseudobulbar paralysis
"pseudocaine" (re: adulterated crack)
pseudocollusion
pseudocombat fatigue
pseudocyesis
pseudodelirium
pseudodementia
pseudodepression
pseudogeusia
pseudographia

pseudohallucination
  ego-dystonic
  manipulative
pseudohermaphrodite
pseudohermaphroditism
pseudoinsomnia
pseudolaryngeal paralysis
pseudologia
pseudomania
pseudomasturbation
pseudomelia paraesthetica
pseudomemory
pseudonarcotic
pseudonarcotism
pseudoneurological symptoms
pseudoneurotic schizophrenia
pseudoparaplegia
pseudoplegia
pseudopsia
pseudopsychopathic schizophrenia
pseudopsychosis
pseudoseizure
pseudosmia
pseudosocial personality disorder
pseudostuttering
pseudotumor cerebri
PSI (Personal Style Inventory)
PSI (Psychological Screening Inventory)
PSI Basic Skills Test for Business, Industry, and Government
PSI (psychosomatic inventory)
psilocybin/psilocin (street names)
  boomers
  business man's acid
  caps
  God's flesh
  hombrecitos
  las mujercitas
  little smoke
  magic
  magic mushroom

psilocybin/psilocin *(cont.)*
  Mexican mushroom
  mushroom
  musk
  sacre mushroom
  shrooms
  Silly Putty
  Simple Simon
PSLT (Picture Story Language Test)
PSMed (Psychosomatic Medicine)
PSP (Personnel Security Preview)
PSQ (Personal Strain Questionnaire)
PSRI (Professional Sexual Role Inventory)
PSRO (Professional Standards Review Organization)
PSRS (Process Skills Rating Scales)
PSS (Psychiatric Services Section)
PSS (Psychiatric Status Schedule)
PST (Portuguese Speaking Test)
PSTO (Purdue Student-Teacher Opinionaire)
PSV (psychological, social, and vocational)
Psy, psy (psychiatry, psychology)
psych or PSYCH (psychiatric, psychiatry)
psychagogy
psychalgia
psychalgic
psychalia
psychanalysis
psychanopsia
psychasthenia
  compulsive
  mixed compulsive states
  obsession
psychasthenia scale
Psychasthenia "7" Scale
psychasthenic-type neurosis
psychataxia
psyche

psycheclampsia
psychedelic agent dependence
psychedelic therapy
psychentonia
psychiat. (psychiatric, psychiatry)
psychiatric (PS, psych)
psychiatrically disabled
Psychiatric Assistant (PA)
psychiatric brain disorders
psychiatric case history
psychiatric chemistry
psychiatric comorbidity
psychiatric consequences of stroke
psychiatric deviance
psychiatric diagnosis and assessment
Psychiatric Diagnostic Interview
psychiatric disability
psychiatric disease
psychiatric disorder
psychiatric disturbance
psychiatric drug
psychiatric education
Psychiatric Emergency Service (PES)
Psychiatric Evaluation Form (PEF)
Psychiatric Evaluation Profile (PEP)
psychiatric examination
psychiatric factors affecting medical
   conditions
psychiatric genetics
psychiatric ghetto
psychiatric history
psychiatric hospital
psychiatric illness
psychiatric illness during pregnancy
psychiatric inpatient
Psychiatric Intensive Care Unit
   (PICU)
psychiatric interview
Psychiatric Knowledge and Skills
   Self-Assessment Program (PKSAP)
psychiatric manifestations
psychiatric nomenclature

psychiatric nurse
psychiatric nursing
psychiatric problems, concurrent
psychiatric rating scale
psychiatric reacting scale
Psychiatric Services Section (PSS)
psychiatric setting
psychiatric social work
psychiatric social worker
psychiatric somatic therapies
Psychiatric Status Rating Scale
Psychiatric Status Schedule (PSS)
psychiatric syndrome
   anger and violence
   anxiety-related
   apathy and failure to rehabilitate
   dementia-related
   depression-related
   disinhibition
   gender difference
   pain, touch, and stroke
   paranoia and delusions
   sex and stroke
   speaking and understanding
psychiatric system interface disorder
psychiatric treatment
psychiatric unit
psychiatric ward
psychiatrist (P)
   board-certified
   board-eligible
   child
   forensic
   public
   social
psychiatry (P, psy, PSYCH, psych,
   psychiat.)
   academic
   addiction
   administrative
   adolescent
   adulthood

psychiatry *(cont.)*
  analytic
  biologic
  child (CHP, CP)
  Clunis inquiry forensic
  community
  consultation liaison
  contractual
  cross-cultural
  descriptive
  dynamic
  existential
  forensic
  geriatric
  hospital and community
  hospital-based
  industrial
  legal
  military
  multidisciplinary group
  occupational
  old age
  organic
  organized-care
  orthomolecular
  outpatient-based
  preventive
  prison
  psychoanalytic
  psychopharmacologic
  public
  rehabilitation
  rural
  schools of
  small-city
  social
  speech and language disorders in
  staff HMO-based
  transcultural
  urban
psychiatry and neurology (P & N,
  P&N)

Psychiatry Emergency Team (PET)
Psychiatry-Neurology (PN)
psychiatry of stroke
psychic censor
psychic determinism
psychic disorder
psychic disturbance
psychic epilepsy
psychic equivalent
psychic experience
psychic factor
psychic numbing
psychic numbness
psychic organization
psychic overtone
psychic phenomena
psychic seizure
psychinosis
psychism
psychoacoustic testing (PAT)
psychoactive disorder
psychoactive drugs
psychoactive effects
psychoactive medication
psychoactive substance abuse
psychoactive substance-induced
  organic mental disorder
psychoaffective disorder (PAD)
psychoallergy
psychoanaleptic
psychoanalysis (PA, PSAn, PsAn)
  active
  adlerian
  boundaries in
  boundary violations in
  freudian
  jungian
psychoanalysis and character disorder
psychoanalysis and depression
psychoanalysis and neuroses
psychoanalysis and object relations
psychoanalysis and paranoid states

psychoanalysis and pathological
   character formation
psychoanalysis and psychopathology
psychoanalysis and psychosomatics
psychoanalysis and schizophrenia
psychoanalysis and self-psychology
psychoanalysis and sexual disorders
psychoanalysis and symptom formation
psychoanalyst (PA, PSAn, PsAn)
psychoanalytic group psychotherapy
psychoanalytic interpretation
psychoanalytic psychiatry
psychoanalytic psychotherapies
psychoanalytic technique
psychoanalytic theorists
   Abraham
   Adler
   Fenichel
   Freud
   Hartmann
   Horney
   Jung
   Klein
   Reich
psychoanalytic therapy
psychoasthenics
psychoauditory
psychobiological process
psychobiology, clinical
psychocatharsis
psychocentric
psychochemistry
psychochrome
psychochromesthesia
psychocortical
psychocutaneous
psychodiagnosis
psychodiagnostics
psychodometer
psychodometry
psychodrama

psychodynamic approach
psychodynamic concepts
psychodynamic conflicts
psychodynamic formulations
psychodynamic interpretation and
   treatment
psychodynamic orientation
psychodynamic research orientation
psychodynamic treatments
psychodysleptic
Psycho-Educational Evaluation
Psychoeducational Profile, Revised
   (PEP-R)
psychoendocrinology
psychoepileptic episode
Psycho-Epistemological Profile (PEP)
psychoexploration
psychogalvanic response (PGR)
psychogalvanic skin resistance
   (PGSR)
psychogalvanic skin response (PGSR)
psychogalvanic skin response audiometry (PGSRA)
psychogalvanometer
psychogender
psychogenesis
psychogenetic
psychogenic air hunger
psychogenic alopecia
psychogenic amnesia
psychogenic aphagia
psychogenic aspermia (PA)
psychogenic asthenia
psychogenic ataxia
psychogenic backache
psychogenic cardiospasm
psychogenic confusion
psychogenic constipation
psychogenic cough
psychogenic deafness
psychogenic depression
psychogenic dermatitis

psychogenic diarrhea
psychogenic disorder
  allergic
  anxiety
  appetite
  blood
  cardiovascular
  compulsive
  cutaneous
  digestive
  dyspneic
  endocrine
  esophagus
  eye
  feeding
  functional
  gastric
  gastrointestinal functional
  genitourinary
  heart
  hemic
  hypochondriacal
  hysterical
  intestinal
  joint
  learning
  limb
  low back
  lymphatic
  menstrual
  micturition
  monoplegic
  motor
  muscle
  musculoskeletal
  neurocirculatory
  obsessive
  occupational
  phobic
  physical
  rectal
  respiratory

psychogenic disorder *(cont.)*
  rheumatic
  sexual
  skin
  sleep
  stomach
psychogenic dysmenorrhea
psychogenic dyspareunia
psychogenic dyspepsia
psychogenic dysuria
psychogenic eczema
psychogenic effort syndrome
psychogenic enuresis
psychogenic excitation
psychogenic fatigue
psychogenic fugue
psychogenic headache
psychogenic hearing loss
psychogenic hiccough
psychogenic hyperventilation
psychogenic nocturnal polydipsia
  (PNP)
psychogenic oculogyric crisis
psychogenic origin
psychogenic overlay
psychogenic pain
psychogenic pain disorder
psychogenic painful coitus
psychogenic painful erection
psychogenic painful menstruation
psychogenic paralysis
psychogenic paranoid psychosis
psychogenic paroxysmal tachycardia
psychogenic physiological manifestations
psychogenic psychosis
psychogenic reaction
psychogenic retention
psychogenic rumination
psychogenic seizure
psychogenic stupor
psychogenic stuttering

psychogenic tic
psychogenic torticollis
psychogenic twilight state
psychogenic ulcer
psychogenic urticaria
psychogenic vomiting
psychogenic yawning
psychogeny
psychogeriatrics
psychogeusic
psychognosis
psychognostic
psychogogic
psychogram
psychograph
psychographic disturbance
Psycho-Graphic Z software
psychography
psychohistory
psychoimmunology
psychoinfantile personality
psychokinesia
psychokinesis (PK)
psychokinetic (PK)
psychokym
psycholagny
psycholepsy
Psycholinguistic Rating Scale
psycholinguistic theories
psychological abuse
psychological adjustment
psychological basis
psychological changes
psychological defense system
psychological disorder affecting GMC
psychological distress
Psychological Distress Inventory
psychological dysfunction
    manifestation of
    symptoms of
psychological evaluation
psychological examination

psychological factors, unspecified
psychological interventions
psychological interview
psychological loner
psychologically meaningful
psychologically mediated response
psychological management of
    dementia
psychological mindedness
psychological models
psychological motivation
psychological needs
psychological pain
psychological problems
psychological procedure
psychological process
psychological reaction
psychological refractory period
psychological related symptoms
psychological response
Psychological Screening Inventory
    (PSI)
psychological signs and symptoms
psychological, social, and vocational
    (PSV)
psychological strain
psychological stress
psychological symptoms
psychological syndrome
psychological techniques
psychological tests
psychological theory
psychological therapy
psychological trauma depressive
    psychosis
psychological warfare (PW)
psychologic desensitization
psychologic tests
psychologist
    clinical
    licensed
    motor learning

psychology (psy, psych)
  abnormal
  adlerian
  adolescent
  analytic
  analytical (Anal. Psychol.)
  animal
  applied
  atomistic
  behavioristic
  child (CP)
  clinical
  cognitive
  community
  comparative
  constitutional
  counseling
  criminal
  depth
  developmental
  dynamic
  educational
  environmental
  existential
  experimental
  forensic
  genetic
  gestalt
  holistic
  humanistic
  individual
  industrial
  medical
  military
  objective
  perceptual
  physiologic
  physiological
  schizophrenic
  social
  subjective
psychology of deceit

psychology practice
psychometer
psychometric evaluation
psychometrician
psychometric performance characteristics
psychometric predictor
psychometric skew
psychometric test (testing)
psychometry
psychomotor activity
psychomotor agitation
psychomotor attacks
psychomotor behavior
psychomotor changes
psychomotor convulsion
psychomotor development
psychomotor disorder
psychomotor disturbance stress
  reaction
psychomotor epilepsy
psychomotor excitement
psychomotor fit
psychomotor intelligence
psychomotor measurement
psychomotor performance
psychomotor phenomenon
psychomotor restlessness
psychomotor retardation
psychomotor seizure
psychomotor slowing
psychomotor stimulant
psychomotor symptom
psychoneural
psychoneuroimmunology (PNI)
psychoneurologist (PN)
psychoneurology (PN)
psychoneurosis
  anxiety
  climacteric
  compensation
  compulsion

psychoneurosis *(cont.)*
  conversion
  depersonalization
  depressive-type
  dissociative
  hypochondriacal
  hysteria
  mixed
  neurasthenic
  obsessional
  obsessive-compulsive
  occupational
  personality
  phobia
  senile
psychoneurotic (PN)
psychoneurotic depressive reaction
psychoneurotic disorder
  mental
  mixed
psychoneurotic personality
psychoneurotic reaction
  anxiety
  compulsive
  conversion
  depersonalization
  depressive
  dissociative
  hypochondriacal
  hysterical
  neurasthenic
  obsessive
  phobic
  tension state
psychonomics
psychonomy
psychonosis
psychonosology
psychonoxious
psycho-optical reflex controls

psycho-organic syndrome
  acute
  brain
  depressive type
  hallucinatory type
  nonpsychotic severity
  paranoid type
  subacute
psychopath, criminal sexual (CSP)
psychopathia martialis
psychopathia sexualis
psychopathic constitution, posttraumatic
Psychopathic Deviance "4" Scale
psychopathic deviate (PD)
psychopathic inferiority
psychopathic personality
  amoral trends
  antisocial trends
  asocial trends
  mixed types
psychopathic state
psychopathist
psychopathologist
psychopathology
  impulsive/compulsive
  levels of
  prepubertal
  presenting
  psychoanalysis and
  related
psychopathology and non-mendelian
  inheritance
psychopathology of gender
psychopathy
psychopharmaceutical intervention
psychopharmacological therapy
psychopharmacological treatment
psychopharmacologic psychiatry

psychopharmacology
  clinical
  gender-sensitive
psychopharmacology in child
  psychiatry
psychophobia
psychophonasthenia
psychophysical
psychophysiological change
psychophysiological disorder
psychophysiological insomnia
psychophysiological problem
psychophysiological test
psychophysiologic correlates
psychophysiologic disorder
psychophysiologic manifestation
psychophysiologic principle
psychophysiologic reaction
  laryngeal
  pharyngeal
psychophysiology
psychoplegia
psychoplegic
psychopneumatology
psychoprophylaxic
psychoprophylaxis
psychoreaction
psychorelaxation
psychorhythmia
psychormic
psychorrhea
psychorrhexis
psychosedation
psychosedative
psychosensorial
psychosensory aphasia
psychosensory epilepsy
psychosensory stimulus/stimuli
psychosensory symptom
psychose passionelle
psychosexual development
  anal stage
  gender identity

psychosexual development *(cont.)*
  latency period
  oral stage
  phallic stage
psychosexual disorder
psychosexual dysfunction
  functional dyspareunia
  functional vaginismus
  inhibited female orgasm
  inhibited male orgasm
  inhibited sexual desire
  premature ejaculation
psychosexual gender identity disorder
psychosexual history
psychosexual identity disorder
  adult-life
  childhood
psychosexual sphere
psychosexual symptoms
psychosis (pl. psychoses)
  acute
  acute delusional
  affective
  alcoholic
  alternating
  amnestic
  amphetamine
  anergastic
  arteriosclerotic
  atypical
  bipolar
  borderline
  brief reactive
  Cheyne-Stokes
  child
  childhood
  chronic
  circular
  climacteric
  confusional
  depressive
  disintegrative
  drug

psychosis *(cont.)*
  dysmnesic
  epileptic
  excitative
  exhaustion
  exogenous
  febrile
  functional
  gestational
  hypomanic
  hysterical
  idiophrenic
  incipient
  induced
  infantile
  infective
  infection-exhaustion
  interactional
  involutional
  Korsakoff
  manic
  manic-depressive
  menopausal
  mixed schizophrenic/affective
  multi-infarct
  organic
  organic brain syndrome with
  paranoic
  paranoid
  paroxysmal
  polyneuritic
  posthypnotic
  postinfectious
  postoperative
  postpartum
  prepsychotic
  presbyophrenic
  presenile
  prison
  psychogenic
  puerperal
  reactive

psychosis *(cont.)*
  scale of (SP)
  schizoaffective
  schizophrenia
  schizophrenic
  schizophreniform
  senile
  situational
  stigmata
  subacute
  symbiotic infantile
  toxic
  transient
  traumatic
  unipolar
  windigo
  zoophil
psychosis due to physical condition
psychosis in childbirth
psychosis in pregnancy
psychosis in puerperium
psychosis of childhood
Psychosocial Adjustment to Illness
  Scale (PAIS)
psychosocial and environmental
  problem
psychosocial aspects of schizophrenia
psychosocial complications
psychosocial deprivation
psychosocial development
psychosocial dwarfism
psychosocial event
psychosocial factors
psychosocial functioning
Psychosocial History Screening
  Questionnaire (PHSQ)
psychosocial-labile (PL)
psychosocial pathology
psychosocial problem
psychosocial process
psychosocial setting
psychosocial stigma

psychosocial stress
psychosocial stressor
psychosocial treatments
psychosomatic disorder
  paralytic
  pruritic
psychosomatic illness
psychosomatic inventory (PSI)
Psychosomatic Medicine (PSMed)
psychosomatic reaction
psychosomatics
psychosomatic symptom
psychostimulant dependence
psychosuggestive
psychosuggestivity
psychosurgeon
psychosurgery
psychosyndrome
psychosynthesis
psychotechnics
psychotherapeutic measures
psychotherapeutic treatments
psychotherapy
  activity-interview group (A-IGP)
  adlerian
  anaclitic
  analytic
  autonomous
  behavioral
  brief
  client-centered
  cognitive
  contractual
  crisis-intervention group
  directive
  dyadic
  dynamic
  existential
  family and systemic
  freudian
  gestalt
  group
  group analytic

psychotherapy *(cont.)*
  heteronomous
  hypnotic
  individual
  insight-oriented
  intensive
  interpersonal (IPT)
  marathon group
  multiple
  nondirective
  personologic
  psychoanalytic group
  rational
  rational-emotive
  reconstructive
  regressive-inspirational group
  structured interactional group
  suggestive
  supportive
  transactional
Psychotherapy Competence Assessment
  Schedule (PCAS)
psychotherapy responder (PR)
Psychotherapy Supervisory Inventory
psychothymia
psychothymic
psychotic attack
psychotic brain syndrome
psychotic denial
psychotic depression (PD)
  reactive
  recurrent episode
  single episode
psychotic dimension of positive schizophrenic symptoms
psychotic dimension of schizophrenia
psychotic disease
psychotic disorder
  brief
  primary
  shared
  substance-induced

psychotic disorder with delusions
   alcohol-induced
   amphetamine-induced
   cannabis-induced
   cocaine-induced
psychotic disorder with hallucinations
   alcohol-induced
   amphetamine-induced
   cannabis-induced
   cocaine-induced
psychotic disorganization
psychotic distortion
psychotic disturbance
psychotic drug
psychotic exacerbation
psychotic features
   mood-congruent
   mood-incongruent
psychotic illness
Psychotic Inpatient Profile (PIP)
psychoticism
psychotic manifestation
psychotic mental disorder, senile
psychotic presenile mental disorder
psychotic presentation
psychotic process
psychotic reaction
   brief
   confusional
   depressive
   excitation
   involutional
   recurrent episode
   single episode
Psychotic Reaction Profile (PRP)
psychotic speech
psychotic state
psychotic symptom
   active
   residual
psychotic symptomatology
psychotic symptoms

psychotic trigger reaction (PTR)
psychotogenic
psychotomimetic agent dependence
psychotropic drug (PTD)
psychotropic effects of thyroid axis
   manipulation
psychovisual therapy
pt (patient)
PTA (posttraumatic amnesia)
PTA (prior to admission)
PTCS (Primary Test of Cognitive
   Skills)
PTD (psychotropic drug)
pteronophobia
PTI (Personnel Tests for Industry)
PTI (Pictorial Test of Intelligence)
PTO (Purdue Teacher Opinionaire)
PTP (Physical Tolerance Profile)
PTQ (Parent-Teacher Questionnaire)
PTR (psychotic trigger reaction)
PTS (permanent threshold shift)
PTSD (posttraumatic stress disorder)
   aging and
   complex
   early-age trauma and
   elder maltreatment and
   late-age trauma and
pubertal
puberty
puberty melancholia
pubescence
pubescent
public display of affection
public display of emotion
public health
public opinion
public performance
public psychiatrist
public psychiatry
public urination
pudding opium
puerile

puerperal convulsion
puerperal delirium
puerperal mania
puerperal melancholia
puerperal psychosis
puerperium
"puff the dragon" (re: cannabis use)
"puffer" (re: crack user)
"puffy" (phencyclidine)
"pulborn" (heroin)
"pullers" (re: crack user)
pull out
pulsated voice
pulsating headache
pulsating pain
pulsation
pulse
   alternating
   chest
   glottal
pulse waveform
"pumping" (re: crack dealing)
punch-drunk encephalopathy
punctuation
puncture
   lumbar (LP)
   tracheoesophageal
punishment, deserved
Pupil Rating Scale: Screening for
   Learning Disabilities (PRS)
Pupil Record of Education Behavior
   (PREB)
pupillary reaction
pupils
   constricted
   dilated
   nonreactive
   pinpoint
   reactive
   unreactive
Purdue Pegboard Dexterity Test

Purdue Perceptual-Motor Survey
   (PPMS)
Purdue Student-Teacher Opinionaire
   (PSTO)
Purdue Teacher Opinionaire (PTO)
"pure" (heroin)
pure agraphia
pure alexia
pure aphasia
pure aphemia
pure chance
"pure love" (lysergic acid diethylamide)
pure tone
pure-tone air conduction
pure-tone air-conduction threshold
pure-tone audiometer
pure-tone audiometry (AC; BC)
pure-tone average
pure-tone bone conduction
pure-tone bone-conduction threshold
pure vowel
pure wave
pure word deafness
purgation
purge, bulimic
purging methods
purine metabolism
purists, language
"purple" (ketamine)
"purple barrels" (lysergic acid
   diethylamide)
"purple flats" (lysergic acid diethylamide)
"purple haze" (lysergic acid diethylamide)
"purple hearts" (amphetamine; barbiturate; lysergic acid diethylamide;
   phenobarbital)
"purple microdot" (lysergic acid
   diethylamide)

"purple ozoline" (lysergic acid
   diethylamide)
"purple rain" (phencyclidine)
purposeful behavior
Purpose in Life Test (PIL)
purposeless agitation
purposeless motor activity
purposeless movement
purposes, educational
purposive movement
pursuits, family
purulent otitis media
"push" (re: drug dealing)
"pusher" (drug dealer)
"push shorts" (re: drug dealing)
PVA (Personal Values Abstract)
PVI (personal values inventory)
PVMT (Primary Visual Motor Test)
PVNPS (Post-Viet Nam Psychiatric
   Syndrome)
PVS (Beery Picture Vocabulary
   Screening Series)

PVS (persistent vegetative state)
PVSP (Prosody-Voice Screening
   Profile)
PVT (Beery Picture Vocabulary Test)
PW (psychological warfare)
PWS (person who stutters)
Px, px (prognosis)
pyloric stenosis, congenital hypertrophic
pyramidal cerebral palsy (CP)
pyramidal system
pyramidal tract
Pyramid Scales
pyrexiophobia
pyrimidine metabolism
pyrolagnia
pyromania
pyromaniac
pyrophobia

Q, q

"Q" (barbiturate)
Q (clerical perception)
Q (clerical response)
Q (coulomb)
q (every)
QA (Quality Assurance)
q.d. (every day)
q.h.s. (every night)
q.i.d. (four times a day)
QLQ (Quality of Life Questionnaire)
q.n.s. (quantity not sufficient)
q.o.d. (every other day)
QPS (Quick Phonics Survey)
QPVT (Quick Picture Vocabulary Test)
q.s. (sufficient quantity)
q-sort
QSP (Quick Screen of Phonology)
qt (quiet)
QT (Quick Test)
q.2h. (every 2 hours)
"quad" (barbiturate)
quadrangular therapy
quadrilateral, vowel
quadriplegia
qualifier
qualitative difference
qualitative impairment in communication

quality
 poor form
 sound
 subjective
quality of caring
Quality of Life Questionnaire (QLQ)
quality of life rehabilitation assessment
quality of obsessions
 inappropriate
 intrusive
quality of performance
quality of sexual functioning
quality of sleep
Quality of Well-Being Scale
quality speech
quality time
quantified cognitive assessment
quantifier, universal
quantitative electroencephalography
quantitative variable
quantity
 absolute
 objective
 relative
 subjective
 sufficient (q.s.)

451

quantity not sufficient (q.n.s.)
quarrelsomeness
"quarter" (1/4 ounce or $25 worth of
   drugs)
"quarter bag" (re: cocaine; $25 worth
   of drugs)
"quarter moon" (hashish)
"quarter piece" (1/4 ounce)
quartile
"quartz" (smokable speed)
"quas" (barbiturate)
quasi contract
quasipurposive movement
"Queen Anne's lace" (cannabis)
querulous paranoia
questioning faith problem
questioning, socratic
questionnaire (see *test*)
Questionnaire of Basic Personality
   Supports
Questionnaire on Resources and Stress
   for Families with Chronically
   Ill or Handicapped Members
Quick Neurological Screening Test
Quick Phonics Survey (QPS)
Quick Picture Vocabulary Test
   (QPVT)
Quick-Score Achievement Test
Quickscreen
Quick Screening of Mental Develop-
   ment

Quick Screen of Phonology (QSP)
"quicksilver" (isobutyl nitrite)
Quick Test (QT)
Quick Word Test
quiescent
quiet (qt), wakefulness
quiet sleep
"quill" (cocaine; heroin; methamphetamine)
quinolone (injectable steroid)
quotient
   achievement (AQ)
   adolescent language
   custody
   educational (EQ)
   expressive language
   grammar language
   intelligence (I.Q.)
   listening language
   memory (MQ)
   open
   positive-negative ambivalent
   reading language
   receptive language-processing
   social (SQ)
   speed
   spoken language
   verbal language
   vocabulary language
   written language

R, r

R or r (roentgen)
"racehorse charlie" (cocaine; heroin)
racial epithets
racing thoughts
radiation
   acoustic
   visual
radiation-induced mental deterioration
radical mastoidectomy
radicals, free
radioimmunoassay
radioligand
radiophobia
RADS (Reynolds Adolescent Depression
   Scale)
rageful feelings
rage, road
"ragweed" (cannabis; heroin)
"railroad weed" (cannabis)
"rainy day woman" (cannabis)
rambling flow of thought
rambling speech
"Rambo" (heroin)
Ramsay Hunt syndrome
Rand Functional Limitations Battery
random activity
random movement

random noise
RAND Patient Satisfaction Questionnaire
Rand Physical Capacities Battery
"rane" (cocaine; heroin)
range
   age
   audible
   central speech
   dynamic
   emotional
   frequency
   maximum frequency
   most comfortable loudness (MCLR)
   pitch
   tolerance
   T-score
range of affect
range of emotional expression
range of emotions
range of feelings
"Rangood" (wild cannabis)
rankian theory
rankian therapy
rank order
rank, percentile

"rap" (criminal charge; to talk with
  someone)
rape, sadistic act of
raphe
  lingual
  median longitudinal
  palatine
  pharyngeal
rapid alternating movements (RAM)
rapid change in activity
rapid cycling
rapid-cycling course
rapid-cycling pattern
rapid eye movement (REM)
rapid eye movement latency
rapid eye therapy
rapid fine movements
rapidity of analyzing information
rapidity of assimilating information
rapidity of reinforcement
Rapidly Alternating Speech Perception
  Test (RASP)
rapidly shifting emotion
rapid movement
rapid repetitive movements
rapid shifting of emotions
rapid speech
rapid tremor
rapist
rapport, poor interpersonal
raptus of attention
rare clefts
rarefaction
rash
  glue sniffer's
  breast
RASP (Rapidly Alternating Speech
  Perception Test)
"raspberry" (re: crack prostitute)
"rasta weed" (cannabis)

rate
  alterating the speech
  alternate motion (AMR)
  alternation in speech
  death
  decay
  fluency
  language development
  maturation
  mentation
  metabolic
  response
rate control
Rathus Assertiveness Scale
Rating Inventory for Screening
  Kindergartners (RISK)
rating scale (see test)
Rating Scale of Communication in
  Cognitive Decline (RSCCD)
rating, subjective unit of distress
  (SUDS)
ratio
  characteristic sex
  equal sex
  high affectivity
  the oral-nasal acoustic (TONAR)
  signal to noise (S/N)
rational/cognitive coping
rational-emotive psychotherapy
rational filter
rational psychotherapy
rational suicide
ratio reinforcement schedule
  fixed
  variable
"rave" (re: hallucinogenic drug use)
"raw" (crack)
raw score
Raynaud phenomenon
"razed" (re: drug influence)
RBH Test of Learning Ability (TLA)

RBMT (Rivermead Behavioral
Memory Test)
RCDS (Revised Children's Depression Scale)
RCDS (Reynolds Child Depression
Scale)
RCS (Reality Check Survey)
RDI (Retirement Descriptive Index)
reaction
angry
anniversary
arrest
catastrophic
dangerous behavior
doll's eye
emotional
escape
idiosyncratic
justifiable
manic
nonpathological
pain
psychological
pupillary
stress
toxic
reaction time
reaction to death
reaction to minor stimuli
reactive attachment disorder
disinhibited type
inhibited type
reactive inhibition
reactive psychosis
reactive response
reactive, symptomatically
reactivity
affective
physiological
reactivity to environment

readiness
academic
developmental
reading
school
readiness inventory (see *test*)
readiness scale (see *test*)
Readiness Scale—Self Rating and
Manager Rating Forms
readiness test
reading
choral
mind
reading achievement
reading aphasia, speech
Reading Comprehension Battery for
Aphasia
reading comprehension impairment
Reading Comprehension Inventory
reading disorder
reading epilepsy
Reading/Everyday Activities in Life
reading inventory (see *test*)
reading readiness
reading test (see *test*)
"ready rock" (cocaine; crack; heroin)
real abandonment
real-life circumstances
real-life problems
realistic plan
reality
abnormal perceptions of external
external
external world of
inconsistent contact with
map of
reality ability testing
Reality Check Survey (RCS)
reality testing
diminished
gross impairment in

reality testing ability (Rorschach)
reanalysis, data
reanalysis strategy
reanalyzed data
reasonable fear
reasoning
    disturbance in
    formal
    nonverbal
    practical
    verbal
Reasons for Living Inventory (RLI)
reassignment
    hormonal sexual
    surgical sexual
reassurance
    excessive need for
    need for
re-attribute
rebound, REM sleep
rebus principle
recalcitrant pain
recall
    auditory
    body image
    dream
    inconsistent
    memory
recalled information
recall 5 items after 5 minutes test
recall of information test
    forward digital span
    paragraph
    reverse digit span
receiver
    air-conduction
    bone-conduction
reception audiometry
reception in noise
reception, speech (SR)
reception threshold (SRT)
receptive development

Receptive-Expressive Emergent
    Language Test, Second Edition
    (REEL-2)
receptive-expressive language
    disorder
Receptive-Expressive Observation
    Scale (REO)
receptive language development
receptive language disorder
receptive language problem
Receptive One Word Picture
    Vocabulary Test (ROWPVT)
receptor
    delta
    delta opiate
    kappa
    kappa opiate
    mu
    mu opiate
    opiate
    sensory
receptor alterations
receptor functioning
reciprocal assimilation
reciprocal communication
reciprocal social interaction
reciprocity, emotional
reckless behavior
reckless driving habits
recklessness, tendency toward
recognition
    facial
    speech
    visual pattern
recognition memory
Recognition Memory Test
recognition vs. recall
recollection of trauma
recompensated
"recompress" (re: cocaine processing)
reconstitute

record
  candidate profile
  functional performance
  manager profile
  supervisory profile
recovery
  full interepisode
  spontaneous
recreation
recreational use of cannabis
recruitment
  complete
  incomplete
  partial
rectal bleeding, self-inflicted
rectal fissure
rectal pain
rectal perineometer
rectovaginal fistula
recurrence of a memory
recurrent brief depressive disorder
recurrent respiratory papillomatosis
recursion
recursive autoassociative memory
"recycle" (lysergic acid diethylamide)
"red" (re: drug influence)
"red and blue" (barbiturate)
"red bullets" (barbiturate)
"red caps" (crack)
"red chicken" (heroin)
"red cross" (cannabis)
"red devil" (barbiturate, phencyclidine)
"red dirt" (cannabis)
"red eagle" (heroin)
"red phosphorus" (smokable amphetamine)
reduction
  anxiety
  cluster
  syllable
  trial of dosage

reduction of Adam's apple
redundancy rules
reduplicated babbling
reed artificial larynx
Reed report forensic psychiatry
REEL-2 (Receptive-Expressive Emergent Language Test, Second
  Edition)
reenactment, trauma-specific
reexacerbation
reexperienced traumatic event
reexperiencing perceptual symptoms
reexperiencing the trauma
reference
  standard
  transient ideas of
reference group
  cultural
  ethnic
  social
reference zero level
referential delusions
referential function
referential index
  shift
  switch
referential semantics
referred pain
reflected wave
reflex (pl. reflexes)
  absent
  acousticopalpebral
  auditory
  auditory-oculogyric
  auropalpebral (APR)
  Babinski
  brain stem
  brisk
  cochlear
  cochleo-orbicular
  cochleopalpebral (CPR)
  deep tendon

reflex *(cont.)*
  delayed
  depressed
  diminished
  doll's eye
  facial
  flexion
  gag
  intact
  intra-aural
  jaw-closing muscle
  laryngeal
  middle ear muscle
  Moro
  Myerson
  myotatic
  orienting (OR)
  pathological
  pharyngeal
  psycho-optical
  sensitivity prediction from the
    acoustic (SPAR)
  stapedial acoustic
  stapedius
  startle
  stretch
  swallow
reflex amplitude
reflex arc
reflex asymmetries
reflex audiometry
reflex changes
reflex controls
reflex convulsion
reflex decay
reflex eye movement
reflexive pronoun
reflex latency
reflex pattern
reflex seizure
reflex threshold
reflex time

re-focus
reform, thought
reformulation
refracted wave
refractory period
reframing
  context
  meaning
  six-step
refreshing sleep attacks
refusal to treat
regard
regional dialect
regions, brain
register
  loft
  vocal
  voice
register tones
regression
  hierarchial
  past-life hypnotic
  phonemic
regressive assimilation
regressive behavior
regressive speech
regular determiner
"regular P" (crack)
regulation
  impulse
  lack of impulse
rehabilitation
  bimodal aural
  combined aural
  lipreading aural
  simultaneous aural
  speech
  speechreading aural
  swallowing
  vocal
  vocational

rehabilitation assessment
rehabilitation behavior
rehabilitation counselor
rehabilitation evaluation
Rehabilitation Indicators (RIs)
rehabilitation psychiatry
rehabilitation treatment
rehabilitative audiology
Reid Report
"reindeer dust" (heroin)
reinforcement
   continuous
   differential
   frequency of
   partial
   primary
   rapidity of
   secondary
   social
   verbal
reinforcement schedule
reinforcer
   negative
   positive
   primary
   secondary
Reissner's membrane
Reitan Evaluation of Hemispheric
   Abilities and Brain Improvement
   Training
Reitan-Indiana Neuropsychological
   Test Battery for Adults
Reitan-Indiana Neuropsychological
   Test Battery for Children
rejecting parent
rejection
   fear of
   increased sensitivity to
   pathological sensitivity to perceived
      interpersonal
   perceived interpersonal
rejection sensitivity

re-label
relapse-prevention (RP) technique
related, transformational
related by marriage
relatedness
   developmentally inappropriate
     social
   disturbance in social
   disturbed social
   markedly disturbed social
   social
related position
related psychopathology
related sleep disorder
related symptoms
related to abuse
related to interaction with the legal
   system
related to neglect
related to the social environment
relation addiction
relational functioning
   competent
   disrupted
   dysfunctional
   optimal
relational opposites
relational problem
   parent-child
   partner
   sibling
relational unit
relational utterance
relational words
relations
   community-institutional
   extramarital
   family
   hospital-patient
   hospital-physician
   interdepartmental
   intergenerational

relations *(cont.)*
  interinstitutional
  interpersonal
  interprofessional
  nurse-patient
  physician-patient
  professional-family
  professional-patient
  semantic
  sibling
relationship (pl. relationships)
  addiction
  age
  apparent
  appropriate
  causal
  chronological
  clearly demarcated
  close
  doctor-patient
  dysfunctional
  early
  effect of trauma on
  etiological
  good
  incestual
  intense
  interpsychic
  intrafamilial
  lack of meaningful
  last
  long-term
  meaningful
  monogamous
  pattern of discomfort in close
  perfect negative
  perfect positive
  poor peer
  replacement
  sexual
  social
  special

relationship *(cont.)*
  stability in
  stress-strain
  temporal
  transference
  unstable
  working
relationship inventory (see *test*)
relationship therapy
relationship to a deity or famous
  person
relative elective mutism
relative lack of self-destructiveness
relative quantity
relatives, biological
relative scotoma
relative slow-wave sleep stability
relative stability of self-image
relativity, linguistic
relaxants, depolarizing muscle
relaxation
  differential
  progressive
  sense of muscular
relaxation technique training
release of sexual tension
release of tension
release sign
  frontal
  positive frontal
releasing consonant
relevant diagnostic criteria
reliability coefficient
  alternate forms
  comparable forms
  odd-even method
  split half
  test-retest
reliance, hemispheric
relief of tension
relief, sense of
religious activity

religious ecstasy
religious institution
religious problem
religious values
reliving an event
REM (rapid eye movements)
  REM activity
  REM-onset sleep
  REM period
  REM sleep behavior disorder
  REM sleep rebound
  REM stage of sleep
remarks, parenthetical
remedial intervention
remedial teaching
remission
  early full
  early partial
  long-term
  sustained full
  sustained partial
remitting dementia
remorse, lack of
remote memory test
removed affect
remuneration
  benefit
  financial
repeated heavy drinker
repeated painful experience
repeated substance self-administration
Repeated Test of Sustained Wakefulness (RTSW)
repeat tendency
repetition
  monosyllabic whole word
  phrase
  senseless imitative word
  sound and syllable
  word
repetition compulsion

repetition of sounds
repetition test
repetitious activity
repetitious speech elements
repetitive behavior
repetitive checking behavior
repetitive convulsion
repetitive imitative movement
repetitive impulse disorder
repetitive lying
repetitive motor behavior
repetitive movements
repetitive partial seizure
repetitive pattern of behavior
repetitive play
repetitive restricted behavior
repetitive speech
repetitive task
replacement relationship
report
  performance
  proficiency
representational system
representative sample
repressed feelings
repressed need (theory in stuttering)
repression, emotional
repression-sensitization scales
repressive behavior
reproductive function
reproductive hormonal measurement
reptilian stare
required task
research, comparative
research orientation
  behavioral
  biological
  cognitive
  family/system
  interpersonal
  psychodynamic

reserve air
reserve volume
   expiratory (ERV)
   inspiratory (IRV)
Resident and Staff Information Form
residential treatment
residual air
residual capacity
residual impairment
residual pain
residual period of illness
residual phase of schizophrenia
residual psychotic symptom
residual schizophrenia
residual schizophrenic
residual symptoms of schizophrenia
residual volume (RV)
resistance
   galvanic skin
   overt compliance masking covert
   patient
   therapist
resistant depression
resolution phase of sexual response
   cycle
resolving conflict skills
resonance
   facilitation of
   nasal
   vocal
   voice disorders or
resonance disorders
resonance spectroscopy in psychiatric
   brain disorders
resonance-volley theory
resonant frequency
resonator
   subglottic
   supraglottic
resource, health
resource state
respect

respiration
   abdominal-diaphragmatic
   bronchial
   Cheyne-Stokes
   clavicular
   cortical
   diaphragmatic-abdominal
   laryngeal
   nasal
   opposition
   oral
   thoracic
respiratory capacity
respiratory disorder
respiratory frequency
respiratory infection
respiratory system
respiratory tract
respiratory volume
respirometer
response (pl. responses)
   adaptive
   anxiety
   auditory brainstem (ABR)
   brain stem auditory evoked
     (BAER)
   catastrophic
   chaining
   clasp-knife
   clerical (Q)
   color
   conditioned
   covert
   culturally sanctioned
   culturally unsanctioned
   delayed
   differential
   disorders of sexual
   dyspnea
   emotional
   evoked (ER)
   evoked somatosensory

response *(cont.)*
    exaggerated startle
    expectable
    extensor plantar
    fabulized
    false-negative
    false-positive
    fight or flight
    frequency
    generalization
    hedonic
    hostile
    human movement
    latent
    long latency
    maladaptive
    mean length of (MLR)
    middle latency
    morbid
    negative
    overt
    paradigmatic
    pattern of
    perseverative
    polarity
    positive
    psychogalvanic skin
    psychological
    psychologically mediated
    reactive
    satiety
    sexual
    small detail
    space
    startle
    state
    stress
    stress-related physiological
    syntagmatic
    target
    texture
    treatment

response *(cont.)*
    unconditioned
    unexpected
    vibrotactile
    vista
    visual evoked (VER)
response audiometry
    auditory brain stem (ABR)
    average evoked (AERA)
    brain stem evoked (BSER)
    cardiac response (CERA)
    electric (ERA)
    electrodermal
    evoked (ERA)
    galvanic skin (GSRA)
    psychogalvanic skin
response cradle
response cradle audiometry
response curve
response cycle
response hierarchy
response magnitude
response pattern, symptom
response prevention
response rate
response set
response strength
response system
response test
response time
response to pain
response to speech dysfluencies
responsibility (pl. responsibilities)
    assigned
    avoidance of
    diminished
    generational
    greater
    homemaking
    household
    important
    increased

responsibility *(cont.)*
  individual
  interpersonal
  job
  lack of
  legal
  neglect of
  new
  noxious
  personal
  poor sense of
  position of
  primary
  sense of
  social
  serotonergic
Responsibility and Independence Scale
  for Adolescents (RISA)
responsiveness
  abnormal
  diminished
  emotional
  facial
  general
  mutual affective
  reduced
resting energy expenditure
resting potential
resting tremor
resting, wakefulness
restless behavior
restlessness
  feelings of
  motor
restraint (physical bondage)
restraints
  chemical
  four-point
  leather
  Posey
  soft
restricted affect

restricted behavior
  repetitive
  stereotyped
restricted diet
restricted range of affect
restricted range of emotional expression
restriction (pl. restrictions)
  activity
  building
  close watch
  gown
  mandibular
  open seclusion
  shoe
  unit (UR)
restrictive behavior
restrictive modifier
restructuring, cognitive
rest tremor
results
  field-trial
  inconsistent laboratory test
  knowledge of
  "resuscitative" snores
resynthesis, binaural
retardation
  idiopathic language
  perceptual
retarded
  educable
  educationally mentally (EMR)
  mentally
  moderately
  severely
retention
  fluid
  linguistic
  memory
  urinary
reticular formation
retino-neuropathy, toxic

Retirement Descriptive Index (RDI)
retirement problem
retribution, fear of
retrieval, method of
retrieval problem
retrieval task
retroauricular
retrocochlear deafness
retrocollis
retroflex consonant formation
retroflex vowel
retrognathic
retrograde amnesia
retrograde loss of memory
retropulsion of gait
retrospective gaps in memory
Rett syndrome
return of sensation
reuptake, dopamine
reuptake inhibitor
re-value
revenge, desire for
revenge obsession
reverberation room
reverberation time
reversal learning
reversal, letter
reversal test
   digit
   left-right
reverse digit span recall test
reverse phonation
reverse swallowing
reversible affective disorder syndrome
   (SADS)
reversible amnesia
reversible memory impairment
re-victimization
review
   comprehensive
   empirical
   systematic

review method
review of symptoms
Review of Test Results
Revised Behavior Problem Checklist
Revised Children's Depression Scale
   (RCDS)
Revised Denver Prescreening Devel-
   opment Questionnaire (R-PDQ)
Revised Diagnostic Interview for
   Borderlines
Revised Edinburgh Functional Com-
   munication Profile (EFCP)
Revised Evaluating Acquired Skills in
   Communication (EASIC)
Revised NEO Personality Inventory
   (NEO-PI-R)
Revised Token Test
Revised Ways of Coping Checklist
revision process
revivication
revulsion, sexual stimuli
reward
   potential external
   token economy
reward dependence
Reynell-Zinkin Scales: Developmental
   Scales for Young Handicapped
   Children, Part 1 Mental Develop-
   ment)
Reynolds Adolescent Depression Scale
   (RADS), Revised
Reynolds Child Depression Scale
   (RCDS)
Rey-Ostereith Complex Figure Test
rheobase
rheumatic pulmonary valve disease
"Rhine" (heroin)
rhinitis
rhinolalia aperta voice disorder
rhinolalia clausa voice disorder
rhinophonia
rhinoplasty

rhotacism
"rhythm" (amphetamine)
rhythm (pl. rhythms)
  alpha
  biologic
  circadian
  delta
  erratic speech
  speech
  stuttered
  theta
  ultradian
rhythmical twitch/twitching
rhythmic contraction
rhythmicity of tremor
rhythmic movement
rhythmic slow eye movement
rhythmic tremor
rhythm of speech
rhythm on EEG
rhythm phase
RI (retroactive inhibition)
RIAST (Reitan-Indiana Aphasia
  Screening Test)
RIBLS (Riley Inventory of Basic
  Learning Skills)
ribonucleic acid (RNA)
ridge
  alveolar
  bony tooth
  rugal
"riding the wave" (re: drug influence)
"rig" (re: drug injection)
right (rt) (pl. rights)
  parental
  visitation
"righteous bush" (cannabis)
"righteous weed" (cannabis)
right hemisphere cognitive skills
right hemisphere dominance
right-left confusion
Right-Left Orientation Test (RLO)

rights of others
right to refuse treatment
right to treatment
rigid attitude
rigid cerebral palsy (CP)
rigidity
  catatonic
  cogwheel
  "lead-pipe"
  muscle
  nuchal
  parkinsonian muscular
  ratchet
rigid posture
Riley Articulation and Language Test
  (RALT)
Riley Inventory of Basic Learning
  Skills (RIBLS)
Riley Motor Problems Inventory
Riley Preschool Developmental
  Screening Inventory (RPDSI)
Ring and Peg Tests of Behavior
  Development
"ringer" (re: crack use)
Rinne Hearing Conduction Test
RIPIS (Rhode Island Pupil Identification Scale)
"rippers" (amphetamine)
RIs (Rehabilitation Indicators)
RISA (Responsibility and Independence Scale for Adolescents)
RISB (Rotter Incomplete Sentences
  Blank), Second Edition
rising curve audiogram configurations
risk
  accidents
  attributable
  depression
  determining
  elevated
  health
  relative

risk *(cont.)*
  schizophrenia
  significant
  specific
  suicide
  violence
RISK (Rating Inventory for Screening Kindergartners)
risk activities
risk behavior
risk factors for mental disorders
risk for malnutrition
risk indicators
risk of suicide attempts
risk preference
risk reduction
risk rescue rating (RRR)
risk-taking
  sex-related
  sexual
risk-taking behavior
risus sardonicus
ritual
  degrading
  handwashing
  masochistic
ritual abuse
ritual behavior
ritualistic behavior
ritualistic thinking
ritualized makeup application
ritualizer
rituals, healing
rivalry, sibling
Rivermead ADL Test
Rivermead Behavioral Memory Test (RBMT)
Rivermead Mobility Index
Rivermead Motor Assessment
Rivermead Perceptual Assessment Battery
RLE (Recent Life Events)

RLO (Right-Left Orientation Test)
RMI (Reading Miscue Inventory)
RN (Registered Nurse)
RNA (ribonucleic acid)
RO (reality orientation)
R/O (rule out)
"roach" (butt of cannabis cigarette)
"roach clip" (re: cannabis equipment)
"road dope" (amphetamine)
road rage
robbery
Robbins Speech Sound Discrimination and Verbal Imagery Type Tests
"Robby" (cough preparations with codeine)
Robert's Apperception Test for Children (RATC): Supplementary Test Pictures for Black Children
"roca" (crack)
"roche" (Rophynol)
Rochester method
"rock" (crack/cocaine)
"rock attack" (crack)
"rocket" (cannabis cigarette)
"rocket caps" (re: crack containers)
"rocket fuel" (phencyclidine; re: drug injection)
"Rockette" (re: female crack user)
"rock house" (crackhouse)
rocking, nonfunctional and repetitive
"rocks of hell" (crack)
"rock star" (re: crack prostitute)
"Rocky III" (crack)
Roeder Manipulative Aptitude Test
roentgen (R, r)
roentgenogram
roentgenography
rogerian therapy
Rogers Criminal Responsibility Scale
Rogers Personal Adjustment Inventory–UK Revision
"roid range" (re: steroid use)

Rokeach Value Survey (RVS)
rolandic epilepsy
Rolando, fissure of
role (pl. roles)
    adultomorphic behavior
    alternating
    attacker
    caretaking
    complementary
    contributing
    cross-sex
    cultural
    follower
    gender
    helper
    important
    intangible benefits of the "sick"
    interpersonal
    interpreter
    leader
    leadership
    minimal
    interpreter
    leader
    leadership
    physician's
    protector
    sick
    significant
    social
    social stereotypical gender
    thematic
    therapeutic
    victim
role ambiguity
role boundary
role conflict
role deviance
role disorder, false
role function
role insufficiency
role obligations

role of giving
role overload
role pattern
role-play activity
role pattern
role therapy
"roller" (re: drug injection)
roller-coaster emotions
"rollers" (police)
"rolling" (methylenedioxymetham-
    phetamine)
romantic fantasy
Romberg Test
"roofies" (Rophynol)
room
    dead (no-echo chamber)
    reverberation
"rooster" (crack)
"root" (cannabis)
rooted obsession
root of the tongue
roots
    addiction
    cultural
    developmental
root signs
root word
"rope" (cannabis)
Rophynol (street names)
    roche
    roofies
    roples
    ruffles
"roples" (Rophynol)
Ror (Rorschach)
Rorschach cards
Rorschach Content Test (RCT)
Rorschach Inkblot Test
Rorschach Projective Technique
Rorschach test (Exner Scoring
    System)
ROS (Review of Systems)

"Rosa" (amphetamine)
"Rose Marie" (cannabis)
Rosenberg Self-esteem Scale (RSES)
Rosenzweig Picture-Frustration Study
(RPFS)
"roses" (amphetamine)
Ross Information Processing Assessment
Ross Test of Higher Cognitive
Processes
Roswell-Chall Auditory Blending Test
Roswell-Chall Diagnostic Reading
Test of Word Analysis Skills:
Revised and Extended
rotation test
rote learning
rote memory
Rothwell-Miller Interest Blank
Rotter Incomplete Sentences Blank,
Second Edition (RISB)
Rotter Sentence Completion Test
(RSCT)
rotunda, fenestra
rough-and-tumble play
rough hoarseness
round window
rounded vowel
rounding, lip
routine (pl., routines)
hospital
family
routine skills
routing of signals
bilateral contralateral (BICROS)
contralateral (CROS)
focal contralateral (FOCALCROS)
front (FROS)
hearing aid contralateral (CROS)
ipsilateral (IROS)
ipsilateral frontal (IFROS)
roving eye movement
roving ocular movement

ROWPVT (Receptive One Word
Picture Vocabulary Test)
"rox" (crack)
"Roxanne" (cocaine; crack)
"royal blues" (lysergic acid diethyl-
amide)
"Roz" (crack)
RP (relapse therapy)
R-PDQ (Revised Denver Prescreening
Development Questionnaire)
RPDSI (Riley Preschool Develop-
mental Screening Inventory)
RPFS (Rosenzweig Picture-Frustration
Study)
RPI (Racial Perceptions Inventory)
RRR (risk rescue rating)
RRT (Registered Recreation Thera-
pist)
RSCCD (Rating Scale of Communi-
cation in Cognitive Decline)
RSCT (Rotter Sentence Completion
Test)
RSES (Rosenberg Self-esteem Scale)
RSPM (Raven Standard Progressive
Matrices)
rt (right)
RT (rational therapy)
RTAVI (Risk-Taking, Attitude,
Values Inventory)
RTSW (Repeated Test of Sustained
Wakefulness)
rubral tremor
Rucker-Gable Educational Program-
ming Scale (RGEPS)
"ruderalis" (cannabis)
"ruffles" (Rophynol)
ruga (pl. rugae)
rule (pl. rules)
as a general
assimilation
base
disregard for

rule *(cont.)*
  dissimilation
  Durham
  ground
  group
  M'Naghten
  morphological
  neutralization
  phonological
  preoccupation with
  redundancy
  semantic
  sequencing
  serious violation of
  syntactic
  Tarasoff
  transformational
rule bending
Rule Eleven Psych Evaluation
rule in a diagnosis
rule of thumb
rule out (R/O)
rule out a diagnosis
rules of syntax
rules skills
ruminate
rumination
  homicidal
  morbid
  neurotic
  obsessional
  psychogenic
  suicidal

rumination disorder
ruminative, introspective and
runaway from home
runaway reaction
  socialized
  undersocialized
run, cocaine
"runners" (re: drug dealers)
"running" (methylenedioxymetham-
    phetamine)
running commentary
running speech
runs in family
rupophobia
ruptures, gastric
rural psychiatry
"rush" (butyl nitrite)
rush (noun)
Rush, Benjamin (1745-1813)
"rush snappers" (isobutyl nitrite)
Russell Version Wechsler Memory
    Scale
"Russian sickles" (lysergic acid
    diethylamide)
Russomania
Russophobia
Rust Inventory of Schizotypal Cogni-
    tions
rustle, nasal
Rutler-Graham Psychiatric Interview
Rutter-B questionnaire
RVS (Rokeach Value Survey)
Rx (prescription; therapy; treatment)

S, s

S (schizophrenia)
S (spatial aptitude)
S (systems)
SA (self-analysis)
SA (sensory awareness)
SA (social acquiescence)
SA (social age)
SA (suicide attempt)
sabotage
saboteur
saccadic eye movements
sac, alveolar
saccule
"sack" (heroin)
SACL (Sales Attitude Check List)
SACQ (Student Adaptation to College Questionnaire)
"sacrament" (lysergic acid diethylamide)
"sacre mushroom" (psilocybin)
SAD (seasonal affective disorder)
SAD (Self-Assessment Depression) scale
SAD (separation anxiety disorder)
SAD (social avoidance and distress)
SADD (Standardized Assessment of Depressive Disorders)
SADL (simulated activities of daily living)

sadism and masochism (S&M)
sadism, sexual
sadist
sadistic act of rape
sadistic behavior
sadistic mutilation
sadistic personality
sadomasochism (SM, S/M)
sadomasochistic relationship
SADQ (Self-Administered Dependency Questionnaire)
SADS (seasonal affective disorder syndrome)
SADS (Shipman Anxiety Depression Scale)
SADS (Schedule for Affective Disorders and Schizophrenia, Third Edition)
SADS-C (Schedule for Affective Disorders and Schizophrenia–Change)
SADS-L (Schedule for Affective Disorders and Schizophrenia–Lifetime, Third Edition)
SAE (Standard American English)
"safe" situation

Safran Student's Interest Inventory
(SCII), Third Edition
SAGES-P (Screening Assessment for
Gifted Elementary Students,
Primary)
sagging posture
sagittal orientation
sagittal plane
SAI (Social Adequacy Index)
SAI (Student Adjustment Inventory)
salaam convulsion
salad, word
Salamon-Conte Life Satisfaction in the
Elderly Scale (LSES)
Sales Attitude Check List (SACL)
Sales Personality Questionnaire (SPQ)
Sales Style Diagnostic Test
salience
Salience Inventory (Research Edition)
(SI)
saliva smearing
"Salmon River Quiver" (cannabis)
salpingopharyngeal muscle
"salt" (heroin)
"salt and pepper" (cannabis)
SAL (sensorineural acuity level) test
SALT-P (Slosson Articulation Language Test with Phonology)
"Sam" (federal narcotics agent)
SAM (sex arousal mechanism)
same-sex marriage
same-sex orientation
sample
language
random
SAMS (Study Attitudes and Methods
Survey)
sanatorium
"sancocho" (to steal)
sanctioned behavior, culturally
sanctioned response, culturally

sanctions
imposition of legal
imposition of social
Sander disease
S&H (speech and hearing)
S&M (sadism and masochism)
"sandos" (lysergic acid diethylamide)
S&R (seclusion and restraint)
"sandwich" (re: layers of cocaine and
heroin)
SANS (Scale for the Assessment of
Negative Symptoms)
"Santa Marta" (cannabis)
SAPD (self-administration of psycho-
active drugs)
sapphism
SAPS (Scale for the Assessment of
Positive Symptoms)
SAQ (School Atmosphere Question-
naire)
SAQ (Substance Abuse Questionnaire)
SAQ-Adult Probation
SAR (sexual attitude reassessment)
SAR (sexual attitude restructuring)
sarcasm
sarcastic
sardonic
sardonicus, risus
SAS (School Assessment Survey)
SAS (School Attitude Survey)
SAS (self-rating anxiety scale)
SAS (Social Adaptation Status)
"sasfras" (cannabis)
SAS-RS (Social Adjustment Self-
Report Scale)
SASSI (Substance Abuse Subtle
Screening Inventory)
SAT (Scholastic Aptitude Test)
SAT (School Ability Test)
SAT (School Attitude Test)
SAT (Senior Apperception Technique)
SAT (Shapes Analysis Test)

SAT (speech awareness threshold)
SAT (Stanford Achievement Test)
SAT (systematized assertive therapy)
SAT (systemic assertive therapy)
SATA (Scholastic Abilities Test for Adults)
satanic worship
Satanophobia
"satan's secret" (inhalant)
SATB (Special Aptitude Test Battery)
"satch" (re: drug smuggling)
"satch cotton" (re: drug injection)
satiation
satiety response
satisfaction
    job
    patient
    personal
satisfaction with life
"sativa" (cannabis)
saturation output
saturation, oxyhemoglobin
satyriasis
satyromania
savant, linguistic
saw-tooth noise
SB, S-B (Stanford-Binet [intelligence test])
SBAI (Social Behavior Assessment Inventory)
S bar
SBD (Supervisory Behavior Description)
SBIS (Stanford-Binet Intelligence Scale)
SBQ (Smoking Behavior Questionnaire)
SBS (social-breakdown syndrome)
scabiophobia
"scaffle" (phencyclidine)
scaffolded language-learning environment

"scag" (heroin)
SCAL (Self-Concept as a Learner)
scale
scala (pl. scalae)
scala media
scala tympani
scala vestibuli
scale (pl. scales) (see also test)
    ADLs (activities of daily living)
    anxiety
    behavior rating
    coma
    communication
    content
    depression
    developmental
    disability status (DSS)
    ego development
    experiences
    family evaluation
    intelligence
    internal versus external (I-E Scale)
    language
    mania rating (MRS)
    masculinity-femininity
    memory
    psychasthenia
    rating
    reading
    repression-sensitization
    school readiness
    self-esteem
    self-rating anxiety (SAS)
    sensory
    sexual differentiation (SDS)
    TMJ (temporomandibular joint)
    verbal (VS)
    vocabulary
SCALE (Scaled Curriculum Achievement Levels Test)
SCALE (Scales of Creativity and Learning Environment)

Scaled Curriculum Achievement Levels
Test (SCALE)
Scale for Assessment of Negative
Symptoms (SANS)
Scale for Assessment of Positive
Symptoms (SAPS)
Scale for Early Communication Skills
(SECS) for Hearing-Impaired
Children
Scale for Emotional Blunting (SEB)
scale for rating psychiatric patients
scalene muscle
    anterior
    middle
    posterior
scale norms
Scale of Independent Behavior
scale of psychosis (SP)
Scale of Social Development
scale questionnaire (see *test)*
scale score (see *test)*
SCAMIN (Self-Concept and Motivation
Inventory)
scan
    computerized axial tomography
        (CAT)
    computerized tomography (CT)
    positron emission tomography
        (PET)
    single photon emission computed
        tomography (SPECT)
SCAN (suspected child abuse/neglect)
scanning communication board
scanning, eye
scanning quality speech
scanning speech
scanning-type speech
scanning visage
SCAN-TRON Reading Test
S-CAPE (Spanish Computerized
    Adaptive Placement Exam)
scapegoated subsystem

scapegoating (communication pattern)
scaphocephalic idiocy
Scarlett O'Hara "V"
"scat" or "scate"(heroin)
SCAT (School and College Ability Test)
scatophobia
scatter, intratest
scelerophobia
scenario
scene, primal
Schaie-Thurstone Adult Mental Abilities
    Test
schedule (see also *test)*
    abnormal sleep-wake
    continuous reinforcement
    extinction reinforcement
    fixed interval reinforcement
    fixed ratio reinforcement
    intermittent reinforcement
    mental status (MSS)
    preoccupation with
    reinforcement
    shifting sleep-work
    variable interval reinforcement
    variable ratio reinforcement
    vocational interest (VIS)
Schedule for Affective Disorders and
    Schizophrenia–Change (SADS-C)
Schedule for Affective Disorders and
    Schizophrenia for School Age
    Children (K-SADS-P)
Schedule for Affective Disorders and
    Schizophrenia, Third Edition (SADS)
Schedule for Affective Disorders and
    Schizophrenia–Lifetime, Third Edition
    (SADS-L)
Schedule of Growing Skills
Schedule of Recent Experience
Scheibe deafness
schema (pl. schemata)
Schilder, Paul (1886-1940)
schiz. (schizophrenia)

schizoaffective disorder
schizoaffective episode
schizoaffective psychosis
schizoaffective schizophrenia
  depressed
  excited
schizocaria
schizoid features
schizoid personality
  introverted
  schizotypal
schizoid personality disorder
schizophasia, glossomanic (subtype)
schizophrenia (S, schiz., SZ)
  abnormal frontotemporal interactions
    in
  ambulatory
  atypical
  borderline (BS)
  burned-out anergic
  catalepsy
  catatonic-type
  cenesthopathic
  childhood-type
  chronic
  coenesthesiopathic
  cyclic
  disorganized-type
  dissolution of cerebral cortical
    mechanisms in
  erotomanic-type
  flexibilitas cerea
  grandiose-type
  hebephrenic-type
  incipient
  insights from neuroimaging into
  jealous-type
  latent
  mixed-type
  nuclear
  paranoid-type
  paraphrenic

schizophrenia (cont.)
  persecutory-type
  prepsychotic
  primary
  process
  prodromal
  pseudoneurotic
  pseudopsychopathic
  reactive
  residual-type
  restzustand
  schizoaffective-type
  schizophreniform-type
  simple-type
  somatic-type
  subchronic
  undifferential-type
Schizophrenia "8" Scale
schizophrenia index
schizophrenia psychosis
schizophrenia simplex
schizophrenia spectrum (SS)
schizophrenia with premorbid asociality
  (SPA)
schizophrenic affect
schizophrenic/affective psychosis
schizophrenic attack
schizophrenic catalepsy
schizophrenic catatonia
schizophrenic disorder
schizophrenic disturbance of speech
  and language
schizophrenic episode
schizophrenic process
schizophrenic psychology
schizophrenic psychosis
  incipient
  paranoid
schizophrenic reaction (SR, S/R)
  acute paranoid (SR/AP)
  acute undifferentiated (SR/AU)
  chronic paranoid (SR/CP)

schizophrenic reaction *(cont.)*
   chronic undifferentiated (SR/CU)
   latent
schizophrenic, residual
schizophrenic residual state (SRS)
schizophrenic speech and language
   disorder
schizophrenic symptoms
   disorganization dimension of
      positive
   psychotic dimension of positive
schizophrenic syndrome of childhood
schizophrenic thought disorder
   Descartes' "cogito" as
   linguistic analysis of
schizophreniform attack
schizophreniform disorder
schizophreniform psychosis
   affective
   confusional
schizophreniform-type schizophrenia
schizophrenoides, delirium
schizothemia
schizothymia
   introverted
   schizotypal
schizotypal personality
schizotypal personality disorder
schizotypal schizoid personality
"schmeck" (cocaine)
Schmidt syndrome
Schneider list of first-rank symptoms
Scholastic Abilities Test for Adults
   (SATA)
Scholastic Aptitude Test (SAT)
school achievement
school adjustment
School Administrator Assessment
   Survey
school-age children
School and College Ability Tests
   (SCAT) II and III

School Apperception Method
School Assessment Survey (SAS)
School Atmosphere Questionnaire
   (SAQ)
School Attitude Survey (SAS)
School Attitude Test (SAT)
school aversion
"schoolboy" (cocaine; cough preparations with codeine)
School Climate Inventory
"schoolcraft" (crack)
school discipline problem
school drop-out
school dysfunction
school entering problems
school environment, inadequate
School Environment Preference Survey
school functioning impairment
School Handicap Condition Scale
   (SEH)
School Interest Inventory
school language
School Library/Media Skills Test
School Motivation Analysis Test
   (SMAT)
school of psychiatry
school performance
school phobia
School Problem Screening Inventory
   (SPSI)
School Readiness Screening Test
School Readiness Survey
School Situation Survey (SSS)
School Social Skills Rating Scale (S3
   Rating Scale)
school truancy
school/work activities
"schoolcraft" (crack)
Schreber case
Schubert General Ability Battery
Schutz Measures
schwa

Schwabach Test
schwannoma
SCID (Structured Clinical Interview
   for DSM-IV)
SCID-CV (Structured Clinical Interview for DSM-IV Axis I Disorders: Clinician Version)
SCID-D (Structured Clinical Interview
   for DSM-IV Dissociative Disorders, Revised)
SCID-PD (Structured Clinical Interview for DSM-IV: Psychotic
   Disorders)
SCID-II (Structured Clinical Interview
   for DSM-IV Axis II Personality
   Disorders)
science (pl. sciences)
   behavioral
   cognitive
   communication
   hearing
   speech
   speech and hearing
science of aging
Science Research Associates (SRA)
   Mechanical Aptitudes
scientific grammar
SCII (Strong-Campbell Interest Inventory)
scintillating scotoma
sciophobia
"scissors" (cannabis)
SCL-90-R (Symptom Checklist-90-
   Revised)
sclerosing panencephalitis, subacute
sclerosis
   amyotrophic lateral (ALS;
      Lou Gehrig's disease)
   multiple (MS)
   tuberous
sclerotic area
sclerotome area

scoleciphobia
scopophobia
"score" (purchase drugs)
score (pl. scores) (see also *test*)
   APGAR
   coma
   clinical performance (CPS)
   elevated
   finger-tapping
   intelligence
   high
   K-corrected raw
   practical social judgment
   raw
   standard
   subtest scale
   test
score discrimination
"scorpion" (cocaine)
scotoma (pl. scotomata)
   absolute
   bilateral
   cecocentral
   central
   dense
   fortification
   homogenous scintillating
   mental
   negative
   paracentral
   relative
   scintillating
scotophobia
"Scott" (heroin)
"Scottie" or "Scotty" (cocaine)
Scott Mental Alertness Test
"scramble" (crack)
"scratch" (currency)
screen; screening (see also *test*)
   blank
   blood drug
   drug

screen *(cont.)*
 heavy metal
 organicity
 otological
 THC elevation
 urine drug
SCREEN (Screening Children for Related Early Educational Needs)
screen memory
screen out irrelevant stimuli
screener (see *test*)
screening articulation test
Screening Assessment for Gifted Elementary Students–Primary (SAGES-P)
screening audiometry
Screening Children for Related Early Educational Needs (SCREEN)
Screening Deep Test of Articulation
screening examination (see *test*)
Screening Instrument for Targeting Educational Risk (SIFTER)
screening inventory (see *test*)
Screening Kit of Language Development (SKOLD)
Screening Procedure for Emotional Disturbance (Draw A Person) (DAP:SPED)
Screening Speech Articulation Test
screening test (see *test*)
Screening Test for Assignment of Remedial Treatments (START)
Screening Test for Auditory Comprehension of Language (STACL)
Screening Test for Auditory Perception
Screening Test for Auditory Processing Disorders
Screening Test for Developmental Apraxia of Speech
Screening Test for Educational Prerequisite Skills (STEPS)

Screening Test for Identifying Central Auditory Disorders (SCAN)
Screening Test for Young Children and Retardates (STYCAR)
Screening Test of Academic Readiness
Screening Test of Adolescent Language
scribblemania
scribomania
"scrubwoman's kick" (naphtha)
scrutinize
scrutiny
"scruples" (crack)
scrupulous
scrutiny, fear of
SCS (Social Climate Scales)
SCT (Sentence Completion Test)
SCT (Sexual Compatibility Test)
SCT-B (Short Category Test, Booklet Format)
"scuffle" (phencyclidine)
scurrile
SD (speech discrimination)
SD (standard deviation)
SD, Sd (stimulus drive)
SD (suicide-depression)
S-D (suicide-depression)
S-D Proneness Checklist
SDAT (senile dementia, Alzheimer-type)
SDD (specific developmental disorder)
SDL (Serial Digit Learning Test)
SDL task, nine-digit (SD9)
SDMT (Symbol Digit Modalities Test)
SDPC (Suicide-Depression Proneness Checklist)
SDQII (Self-Description Questionnaire II)
SDS (Self-Directed Search)
SDS (Self-Rating Depression Scale)
SDS (sensory deprivation syndrome)
SDS (sexual differentiation scale)

SDS (speech discrimination score)
SDS (Student Disability Survey)
SDT (speech detection threshold)
SEA (Survey of Employee Access)
search
    self-directed
    transderivational
    word
SEARCH: A Scanning Instrument for
    the Identification of Potential
    Learning Disability
searing pain
Seashore Rhythm Test
seasonal affective disorder (SAD)
seasonal affective disorder syndrome
    (SADS)
seasonal headache
seasonal migraine headache
seasonal mood disorder
seasonal pattern
Seasonal Pattern Assessment Ques-
    tionnaire (SPAQ)
seasonal-related psychosocial stressors
seated position
SEB (Scale for Emotional Blunting)
secandi, mania
"seccy" (secobarbital)
seclusion
    locked
    office
seclusion and restraint (S&R)
seclusive personality
secobarbital (street names)
    Christmas trees
    double trouble
    pink lady
    pinks
    rainbows
    red devils
    reds
    seccy
    tooies

secondary articulation
secondary drive
secondary gain
secondary palate
secondary prevention
secondary process
secondary reinforcement
secondary sex characteristics
secondary verb
secretary, unit (US)
secretion, cortisol
secretive manner
SECS (Scales for Early Communica-
    tion Skills for Hearing-Impaired
    Children)
Section, Psychiatric Services (PSS)
secure environment
security unit, maximum
sedation, daytime
sedative drug dependence
sedative effect
sedative-hypnotic agent (drug)
sedative-hypnotic use
sedative-hypnotic withdrawal symptom
sedative-induced anxiety
sedative intoxication delirium
sedative-related disorder
sedative-type withdrawal
sedative use disorder
sedative withdrawal delirium
sedentary lifestyle
seduce
seducer
seductive behavior
seductive personality disorder
seductive tendency
seductiveness
seductress
SEE (Seeing Essential English)
SEE (Signing Exact English)
SEED Developmental Profiles
"seeds" (cannabis)

seekers, care
seeking, novelty
Seeking of Noetic Goals Test
"seggy" (barbiturate)
segmental analysis
segmental phoneme
segment, pharyngoesophageal (PE)
SEH (severe emotional handicap)
SEI (Self-Esteem Index)
SEI (Self-Esteem Inventory)
seizure (pl. seizures) (also *convulsion*)
  absence
  acute
  akinetic
  alcoholic
  alcohol-related
  alcohol withdrawal
  aphasic
  apneic
  apoplectiform
  asteric
  asymptomatic
  atonic absence
  atypical absence
  audiogenic
  auditory
  benign neonatal familial
  bilateral myoclonic
  brain
  cardiovascular
  central
  centrencephalic
  cephalic
  cerebellar fits
  cerebral
  cerebrospinal
  clonic
  clonic-tonic-clonic
  complex partial (CPS)
  continuing petit mal
  conversion
  convulsive

seizure *(cont.)*
  coordinate
  cryptogenic
  diencephalic
  drug-induced
  drug-withdrawal
  eclamptic
  epilepsia partialis continua
  epileptic
  epileptiform
  essential
  febrile
  generalized
  generalized tonic-clonic convulsion
    (GTC)
  grand mal (tonic-clonic)
  hysterical
  iatrogenic
  ictal confusional
  infantile
  jacksonian
  Lennon-Gastaut
  local
  major motor
  maximal electroshock (MES)
  mimetic
  mimic
  myoclonic
  new-onset
  olfactory psychomotor
  paroxysmal
  partial complex
  partial sensory
  partial tonic
  petit mal (typical absence)
  petit mal variant
  phonatory
  photogenic
  post-traumatic
  postural
  precentral
  primary

seizure *(cont.)*
  psychic
  psychogenic
  psychomotor
  puerperal
  recurrent
  reflex
  repetitive
  repetitive partial
  salaam
  sensory-evoked
  simple partial
  situation-related
  sleep-related
  somatosensory
  spasmodic
  spontaneous
  subclinical
  symptomatic
  tetanic
  tonic
  tonic-clonic (grand mal)
  traumatic
  typical
  typical absence (petit mal)
  uncinate
  unilateral
  uremic
  vertiginous
  visual
  withdrawal
seizure epilepsy
seizure frequency (SF)
seizure resistant (SR)
seizure seconds
seizure sensitive (SS)
seizure-type of symptom
selaphobia
selection
  hearing aid
  treatment
selection bias

selection communication board, direct
selection of sounds
selective amnesia
selective attachments
selective auditory agnosia
selective focusing on environmental
  stimuli
selective inattention
selective listening
selective memory
selective mutism
Selective Reminding Test
self
  aniled sense of
  disturbed sense of
  effect of trauma on
  experience of the
  perception of
  sense of
  turning against (TAS)
self-absorbed tendencies
self-absorption
Self-Administered Dependency Questionnaire (SADQ)
self-administered penectomy
self-administration of drugs
self-administration of psychoactive
  drugs (SAPD)
self-aggrandizing
self-analysis (SA)
self-assertion
Self-Assessment Depression (scale)
  (SAD)
Self-Assessment in Writing Skills
self-assurance
self-assured
self-awareness
self-biting
  nonfunctional and repetitive
  severe
self-care activity
self-care dysfunction

self-care skills
self-castration
self-centered attitude
self-centeredness
Self-Concept and Motivation
    Inventory (SCAMIN)
Self-Concept as a Learner (scale)
    (SCAL)
Self-Concept Scale
self-condemning
self-confidence, low
self-conflict, undisciplined
Self-Consciousness Scale
Self-Control Inventory
self-criticism, patterns of pervasive
self-damaging behavior
self-damaging impulsivity
self-defeating personality
self-deprecating thoughts
self-deprecation
self-deprivation
self-derogatory concepts
self-derogatory content
self-derogatory themes
Self-Description Questionnaire II
    (SDQII)
self-destructive behavior
    direct (DSDB)
    indirect (ISDB)
self-destructive hallucination
self-destructiveness
Self-Directed Search (SDS)
self-discipline
self-disclosure
self-discovery
self-disgust
self-dramatization
self-dramatizing behavior
self-esteem
    denigrated
    lack of
    low
    negative

Self-Esteem Index (SEI)
Self-Esteem Questionnaire
self-evaluation
self-evident
self-harm(ing)
self-hate
self-help group
self-help skills
self-hypnosis training
self-identity
self-image
    relative stability of
    splitting of
    unstable
self-importance, sense of
self-imposed high standards of perfor-
    mance
self-individuation
self-induced alopecia
self-induced hair loss
self-induced injury
self-induced vomiting
self-inflicted (SI)
self-inflicted bodily injury
self-inflicted gunshot wound
self-inflicted rectal bleeding
self-inflicted wound (SIW)
self-initiated activity
self-injurious behavior (SIB)
self-injury
self-interest
selfishness
self-limited
self-loathing
self-love
self-management
self-medication
self-mutilating behavior
self-mutilation (SM)
self-observation
Self-Perception Inventory (SPI)
Self-Perception Profile for Children
self-pity

self-portrait
self-position/index
self-preservation
self-pressuring
self-propagation
self-psychology, psychoanalysis and
self-punish
self-punishing behavior
self-rating anxiety scale (SAS)
self-rating test
self-realization
self-regard
self-regulatory capacity
self-reliance
self-report measure of social adjustment measure
self-report personalities inventories
self-reproach
self-responsibility, lack of
self-righteous
self-role concept
self-sacrifice
self-seeking
self-starvation
self-stimulation behavior
self-stimulatory behaviors in sensory
   deficit individuals
self-stimulatory behaviors in the young
self-sufficiency
self-sufficient
self-support
self-supportive
self-treatment
self-understanding
self-worth
Selz and Reitan rules to assess learning
   disorders
semantic aphasia
semantic argument (communication
   pattern)
semantic constraints
semantic dementia

semantic differential
semantic feature
semantic implication
semantic interference
semantic memory
semantic pragmatic disorder
semantic relationships
semantic rule
semantics
   behavioral
   extension
   generative
   intention
   referential
semantics of autism
semantic substitution
semen loss
semiaural hearing protection device
semiautomatic action
semi-autonomous systems concept of
   brain function
semicircular canal
semiology
semipurposeful behavior
semistarvation
semi-vowel consonant formation
Semon law
Semon-Rosenbach law
"sen" (cannabis)
senescence
Senf Comrey Ratings of Extra
   Educational Needs
"seni" (mescaline)
senile affective psychosis
senile brain syndrome
senile chorea
senile delirium
senile dementia
   acute confusional state
   Alzheimer-like (ALSD)
   Alzheimer-type (SDAT)
   delusional-type

senile dementia *(cont.)*
  depressed-type
  exhaustion
  paranoid-type
  simple-type
  uncomplicated
senile depression
senile epilepsy
senile imbecility
senile insanity
senile mania
senile melancholia
senile memory
senile neurosis
senile osteoporosis
senile paranoia
senile paranoid reaction
senile paranoid state
senile paroxysmal psychosis
senile plaque
senile psychoneurosis
senile psychosis
  delusional-type
  depressed-type
  paranoid
  simple deterioration
senile psychotic mental disorder
senile tremor
senile-type organic psychosis
Senior Apperception Technique
Senior Apperception Test (SAT)
sensation (pl. sensations)
  altered
  buzzing
  creeping-crawling
  decreased peripheral
  deep
  diminished
  dysesthesic
  ejaculatory inevitability
  electric shock
  facial

sensation *(cont.)*
  fetal movement
  fine tactile
  floating
  flying
  foreskin
  hearing
  impaired
  insect infestation
  lack of control
  light touch
  loss of
  numbing
  orgasm
  out-of-body
  out-of-mind
  pain
  phantom
  physical
  pins-and-needles
  pins sticking
  reduced preputial
  scalp
  slowed time
  smell
  superficial
  tactile
  taste
  temperature
  tingling
  touch
  vibration/vibratory
  visual
  wakefulness
  well-being
sensation level (SL)
Sensation-Seeking Scale (SSS)
sensation unit (SU)
sense
  aniled
  apprehension
  arousal

sense *(cont.)*
 common
 detachment
 foreshortened future
 kinesthetic
 time
senseless imitative word repetition
sense of:
 being out of control
 being overwhelmed
 difficulty concentrating, subjective
 emptiness
 entitlement
 frustration
 identity
 impending doom
 muscular relaxation
 numbing
 other people's boundaries
 personal identity
 placement
 reality
 relief
 reliving an event
 responsibility
 self-importance
 sexual pleasure
 tension
 time
 well-being (Wb)
Sense of Coherence Questionnaire
sensibility
sensitive Beziehungswahn
sensitive, seizure (SS)
sensitivity
 contrast
 rejection
sensitivity group
sensitivity prediction from the acoustic
 reflex (SPAR)
sensitivity reaction of adolescence
sensitivity reaction of childhood

sensitivity to perceived interpersonal
 rejection
sensitivity to rejection
sensitivity-training group (T-group)
sensitization, covert
sensor operation
sensorial epilepsy
sensorial idiocy
sensorimotor act
sensorimotor arc
sensorimotor intelligence period
sensorimotor system
sensorineural acuity level masking
 technique
sensorineural deafness
sensorineural hearing loss
sensorium
 clear
 cloudy
sensory acuity
sensory alexia
sensory anesthesia
sensory aphasia, transcortical
sensory apraxia
sensory ataxia
sensory aura
sensory awareness (SA)
sensory-based
sensory bondage (blindfolding)
sensory charge
sensory cortex
sensory deficit
sensory deprivation syndrome (SDS)
sensory difficulties
sensory discrimination
sensory dissociation
sensory disturbance
sensory environment
sensory epilepsy
sensory evoked potential (SEP)
sensory-evoked seizure
sensory extinction

sensory function
sensory impairment
sensory-induced epilepsy
Sensory Integration and Praxis Tests
   (SIPT)
sensory level
sensory loss
   central
   cortical
   dense
   dissociated
   level of
   peripheral
   stocking-glove
sensory modality (pl. modalities)
   auditory
   gustatory
   olfactory
   tactile
   visual
sensory/motor behavior
sensory nerve
sensory paralysis
sensory pathway stimulation
sensory perception
sensory receptor
sensory scale
sensory seizure
sensory shock
sensory stimulation
sensory stimulus
sensory symptoms
sensory testing
sensory threshold
sensual dysarthria
sentence (pl. sentences)
   brief
   complex
   compound
   compound-complex
   constituent
   declarative

sentence (cont.)
   derivation of a
   derived
   embedded
   exclamatory
   imperative
   interrogative
   kernel
   matrix
   performative
   shortened
   simple
sentence classification
sentence closure task
Sentence Closure Test
sentence completion test (see test)
sentence constituents
sentence copying errors
sentence derivation
sentence length
sentence repetition (SR)
Sentence Repetition Test
sentence test (see test)
sentence types
sentimental value
SEP (somatosensory evoked potential)
   brain test
separation
   binaural
   family
   fear of
   marital
   traumatic
separation agreement
separation anxiety disorder (SAD)
separation anxiety of infancy and
   childhood
separation-individuation phase
separation of ideas from feelings
separation problem
separator state
septal area

septum
   alveolar
   deviated
   nasal
sequence
   syllable
   ungrammatical
   word
Sequenced Inventory of Language
   Development (SILD)
sequence memory
sequence of sounds and memory
sequencing, auditory
sequencing rules of syntax
Sequential Assessment of Mathematics
   Inventories: Standardized Inventory
sequential multiple analysis (SMA)
Sequential Tests of Educational
   Progress, Series III (STEP-III)
SER (somatosensory evoked response)
   brain test
serial content speech
Serial Digit Learning Test (SDL)
serial epilepsy
serial killers
serial learning
serial list learning
serial observation
serial sevens (7's) test
serial sexual killers
serial threes (3's) test
seriatim speech
seriation skills
series (see *test*)
series of numbers
serious assaultive acts
serious traumatic stress
serious violation of rules
"sernyl" (phencyclidine)
serotonergic anxiolytic
serotonergic neuron
serotonergic neurotransmission

serotonergic pharmacology
serotonin reuptake inhibitor
serotonin-specific reuptake inhibitor
   antidepressant medications
serous otitis media (SOM)
"Serpico 21" (cocaine)
serratus anterior muscle
serratus posterior-inferior muscle
serratus posterior-superior muscle
serum calcium level
serum levels
"server" (crack dealer)
service (pl. services)
   ACT Evaluation/Survey(ESS)
   armed
   community mental health
   Consultation-Liaison (CLS)
   Crisis Evaluation Referral (CERS)
   disability determination (DDS)
   Educational Testing (ETS)
   general hospital consultation/liaison
   health care
   hospital consultation/liaison
   medical
   Memphis Educational Model
      Providing Handicapped Infant
      (MEMPHIS)
   Patient and Family (PFS)
   Psychiatric Emergency (PES)
   Social and Rehabilitation (SRS)
   System to Plan Early Childhood
      (SPECS)
   U.S. Department of Health and
      Human (DHHS)
   U.S. Employment (USES)
   U.S. Public Health (USPHS)
   Vocational Rehabilitation (VRS)
service agency, social
service personnel
services of prostitutes
servomechanism
"sess" (cannabis)

sessile vocal nodules
session
  dyadic
  fixed-ended
  group
  open-ended
set (pl. sets)
  criteria
  data
  preparatory
  response
  single criteria
  word
"set" (drug-buying place)
SET (support, empathy, truth) therapy
setback
set of disturbances
  affective
  attentional
  behavioral
  cognitive
  linguistic
  perceptual
set of procedures
set system, symbol
setter, fire (FS)
setting
  clinical
  community
  cultural
  educational
  fire
  general population
  group
  home
  inpatient psychiatric
  institutional
  novel
  outpatient
  partial-hospital
  psychosocial
  residential
  social

"Seven-up" (cocaine; crack)
"sewer" (re: drug injection)
sex
  anal
  assigned
  biological
  forced
  indeterminate
  opposite
  promiscuous
  trading
  unprotected
  "wrong"
sex acts, criminal
sex addiction
sex arousal mechanism (SAM)
sex characteristics
  primary
  secondary
sex chromosomes
sex clinic
sex counseling
sex for drugs
sex headache
Sex Knowledge and Attitude Test
  (SKAT)
sex object
sex offender (SO)
sexology
sexopathy
sex ratio
  characteristic
  equal
sex-reassignment, hormonal
sex-reassignment surgery
sex-related risk-taking
sex-role behavior
sex therapy
sexual abstinence
sexual abuse
  adult
  childhood
  problems related to

sexual abuse as major childhood
    stressor
sexual acting out
sexual activity
sexual and gender identity disorder
sexual anesthesia
sexual arousal
    oxygen-deprived
    problems with
sexual arousal disorder
    acquired-type female
    female
    generalized-type female
    lifelong-type female
    situational-type female
sexual arousal problems
sexual assault
sexual attitude reassessment (SAR)
sexual attitude restructuring (SAR)
sexual aversion disorder
    acquired-type
    generalized-type
    lifelong-type
    situational-type
sexual behavior
    cultural-related standards of
    inappropriate
    intense
    masochistic
    promiscuous
    unusual
    voyeuristic
sexual boundary violations
sexual climax
sexual coercion
Sexual Compatibility Test (SCT)
sexual contact
sexual, contrary
sexual desire
    absent
    deficient
    hyperactive

sexual desire (cont.)
    hypoactive
    inhibited
    loss of
    low
sexual desire disorder
    acquired-type hypoactive
    generalized-type hypoactive
    hypoactive
    lifelong-type hypoactive
    situational-type hypoactive
sexual development
sexual deviance
sexual deviance disorder
sexual deviant
sexual deviation
sexual differentiation scale (SDS)
sexual disorder
sexual drive
sexual dysfunction
    acquired
    alcohol-induced
    amphetamine-induced
    cocaine-induced
    generalized
    life-long
    situational
    substance-induced
sexual dysfunction due to general
    medical condition
sexual encounters
    frequency of
    indiscriminate
    types of
sexual erethism
sexual escapade
sexual excitement
    adequate
    inhibited
sexual experience
sexual expression

sexual fantasy
  female object of
  intense
  masochistic
  nonpathological
  pathological
sexual favors
sexual fears
sexual frigidity
sexual function
sexual functioning
Sexual Functioning Index (SFI)
sexual gratification
sexual harassment (SH)
sexual history
sexual identity
sexual identity disorder
sexual impotence
sexual inappropriateness
sexual indifference
sexual indiscretion
sexual instinct
sexual interaction
sexual intercourse
sexual interest
  diminished
  low
sexuality
  infantile
  pathological
  perverted
  psychopathic
Sexuality Preference Profile (SPP)
sexual life
sexually addictive behavior
sexually arousing behavior
sexually arousing fantasies
sexually seductive behavior
sexually transmitted disease (STD)
sexual maladjustment
sexual masochism
sexual maturity

sexual maturity rating, Tanner
sexual melancholia
sexual misconduct in the helping
  professions
sexual mores
sexual myths (SM)
sexual neurosis
sexual opportunity
sexual orientation
sexual pain
sexual pain disorder
sexual performance
sexual physiology
sexual pleasure
sexual promiscuity
sexual prowess
sexual psychopath
sexual reassignment
  hormonal
  surgical
sexual relationships
sexual response
sexual response cycle
  desire phase of
  excitement phase of
  orgasmic phase of
  resolution phase of
sexual responsibility
sexual risk-taking
sexual sadism
sexual stimulation
sexual stimuli
sexual stimuli revulsion
sexual symptoms
sexual tension
sexual urges
  intense
  masochistic
  voyeuristic
sexual values
"sezz" (cannabis)
SF (seizure frequency)

SFA (Stuttering Foundation of America)
SFI (Sexual Functioning Index)
SFI (Social Function Index)
SFLE (Stress from Life Experience)
SFS (stutter-free speech)
SFT (stutter fluently therapy)
SH (sexual harassment)
SH, S.H. (social history)
"shabu" (methamphetamine hydrochloride)
shading, emotional
shadow curve
shadow effect
shadowing masking technique
shadowing method
shadow, object
"shake" (cannabis)
"shaker/baker/water" (re: cocaine use; shaker bottle, baking soda, water)
shaking palsy
shaking tremor
shaking voice
shaky voice
shallow affect
shallow expression of emotion
shaman
shamanism
shamed, fear of being
shame, feelings of
shameful
shape
   body
   syllable
Shapes Analysis Test (SAT)
shared delusional belief (folie a deux)
shared mechanism
shared paranoid disorder
shared phenomenological features
shared psychotic disorder
shared understanding

sharing drug paraphernalia
sharing of values
sharp, intellectually
"sharps" (needles; razor blades)
"she" (cocaine)
"sheet rocking" (crack and lysergic acid diethylamide)
"sheets" (phencyclidine)
sheet sign
shell earmold
shell shock
Sheltered Care Environment Scale
sheltered home
sheltered life
sheltered workshop
"shermans" (phencyclidine)
"sherms" (crack; phencyclidine)
shield, ideational
shift
   Doppler
   gradual topic
   method threshold
   paradigmatic
   permanent threshold (PTS)
   pitch
   precipitous mood
   temporary threshold (TTS)
   voice
shift ability
shifting of emotions
shifting sleep-work schedule
shift in mood
shift masking technique
shift of sleep-wake cycle
shift referential index
shift work-type dyssomnia
shimmer, amplitude
Shipley Institute of Living Scale (SILS)
Shipley Personal Inventory (SPI)
Shipman Anxiety Depression Scale (SADS)

SHM (simple harmonic motion)
"shmeck/schmeek" (heroin)
shock
  auditory
  culture
  electrical
  neurogenic
  psychic
  sensory
  spinal
shock syndrome
  psychic
  neurogenic
shock therapy (ST)
shock treatment
shock exhibitionism
shock treatment, Metrazol
shoe restrictions
"shooting gallery" (drug-using place)
shooting pain
"shoot/shoot up" (re: drug injection)
"shoot the breeze" (nitrous oxide)
"shopaholic" (oniomaniac)
shoplift
shoplifting
shopping spree
short cycle
Short Employment Tests
Shortened Edinburgh Reading Tests
Short Imaginal Processes Inventory
  (SIPI)
Short Increment Sensitivity Index
  (SISI)
short-lived schizophrenic affect
Short Michigan Alcoholism Screening
  Test (SMAST)
short orientation-memory-concentration test (OMC)
Short Portable Mental Status Questionnaire (SPMSQ)
short REM latency
short sleep duration

short sleep latency
short sleeper
Short Term Auditory Retrieval and
  Storage (STARS) test
short-term goals (STG)
short-term memory (STM)
Short Test for Use with Cerebral Palsy
  Children
"shot" (re: drug injection)
"shot down" (re: drug influence)
shoulders, stooped
shower collar, laryngectomee
shrinking retrograde amnesia
shrinking retrograde amnesic
"shrooms" (psilocybin/psilocin)
SHSS (Stanford Hypnotic Susceptibility
  Scale)
SHT (STYCAR Hearing Tests)
shuffling gait
shuffling steps
shunting
shut-in personality
shy behavior
  culturally appropriate
  developmentally appropriate
shyness disorder of childhood
SI (Salience Inventory, Research
  Edition)
SI (self-inflicted)
SI (social introversion)
SI (structure of intellect)
SIB (self-injurious behavior)
sibilant consonant formation
sibling jealousy
sibling lifestyle
sibling profile
sibling relational problem
sibling relations
sibling rivalry
sibship
Sickness Impact Profile (SIP) test
sickness, sleeping

"sick" role
"Siddi" (cannabis)
side effect
    anticholinergic
    autonomic
    extrapyramidal
    medication
side effects of treatment
siderodromomania
siderodromophobia
siderophobia
SIFTER (Screening Instrument for
    Targeting Educational Risk)
"sightball" (crack)
sign
    arithmetic
    autonomic
    autonomic hyperactivity
    Babinski
    brain stem
    cerebellar
    cerebral
    Claude hyperkinesis
    focal neurologic
    focal nonextrapyramidal neurologic
    frontal release
    increased autonomic
    neurological soft
    Omega (+ or – for suicide)
    operational
    pathognomonic
    positive frontal release
    premonitory
    psychological
    root
    sheet
    soft neurological
    withdrawal
    vital (VS)
signal
    acoustic
    speech

signal anxiety
signal detection
signal speech
signal, therapeutic error (TES)
signal-to-noise ratio (S/N)
sign depression
signed English
signed out against medical advice
    (SOAMA)
significance
    nonparametric tests of
    parametric tests of
    statistical
significance level
significance of age at onset of schizo-
    phrenia
significant differences
significant loss
significant other
Signing Exact English (SEE)
Sign Language
    American (ASL) (Ameslan)
    American Indian (Amerind)
sign linguistics
sign marker
sign systems
signs of withdrawal
    anchor
    phencyclidine dose-related
    physiological
sign word
sign writing
SIL (speech interference level)
SILD (Sequenced Inventory of Lan-
    guage Development)
silence (communication pattern)
silence, tyranny of
silent blocking in speech
silent speech blocking
silent speech elements
silliness, childlike
silly affect

"Silly Putty" (psilocybin/psilocin)
SILS (Shipley Institute of Living
    Scale)
similarities mental status test
similarities subtest
similarities test
similarity disorders of aphasia
similar shared features
simile (figure of speech)
Similes Test
simple alcoholic drunkenness
simple aphasia
simple deterioration senile psychosis
simple deteriorative disorder
simple drunkenness
simple figures
simple future progressive tense
simple future tense
simple hallucination
simple harmonic motion (SHM)
simple motor tics
simple paranoid reaction
simple paranoid state
simple partial seizure
simple past progressive tense
simple past tense
simple phobia
simple predicate
simple present progressive tense
simple present tense
simple schizophrenia
simple sentence
"Simple Simon" (psilocybin/psilocin)
simple sound source
simple subject
simple syllabic vowel
simple task
simple tense
simple tone
simple-type arteriosclerotic psychosis
simple-type presenile dementia
simple-type schizophrenia

simple vocal tics
simple wave
simple word
simplex, melancholia
simulated activities of daily living
    (SADL)
simultanagnosia
simultaneous auditory feedback
simultaneous aural rehabilitation
simultaneous insanity
simultaneous method sine wave
simultaneous nerve impulse
sine wave
sine wave ECT (electroconvulsive
    therapy)
sine wave unilateral ECT (electrocon-
    vulsive therapy)
singer's formant frequency
Singer-Loomis Inventory of Personality
    (SLIP)
singer's nodes
Single and Double Simultaneous
    Stimulation Test
single criteria set
single person
singleton omissions
singleton, prevocalic
singsong fashion
sinistral
sinistrality
Sinophobia
"sinse" (cannabis)
"sinsemilla" (cannabis)
sinsemillan marijuana
sinusoidal wave
SIP (Sickness Impact Profile)
SIPI (Short Imaginal Processes
    Inventory)
SIPT (Sensory Integration and Praxis
    Tests)
SIRS (Structured Interview of Reported
    Symptoms)

SIs (Status Indicators)
SIS (Stress Impact Scale)
SISI (Short Increment Sensitivity
    Index)
sissyish behavior
SIT (Slosson Intelligence Test)
sitiophobia (also sitophobia)
sitomania
sitophobia (also sitiophobia)
SIT-R (Slosson Intelligence Test
    [1991 Edition])
sitting balance
situational depression
    acute
    brief
    prolonged
situational disturbance, acute
situational insomnia
situationally appropriate atmosphere
situationally bound (cued) panic attack
situationally optimistic atmosphere
situationally predisposed panic attack
situational neurosis
situational posttraumatic neurosis
situational psychosis
situational reaction
    acute maladjustment
    acute stress
    adjustment
    depressive
situational sexual dysfunction
situational stressor
situational-type dyspareunia
situational-type female orgasmic
    disorder
situational-type female sexual arousal
    disorder
situational-type hypoactive sexual
    desire disorder
situational-type male erectile disorder
situational-type male orgasmic
    disorder

situational-type sexual aversion
    disorder
situational-type vaginismus
situation anxiety
situation-related epilepsy
situation-related seizure
SIV (Survey of Interpersonal Values)
SIW (self-inflicted wound)
Sixteen Personality Factor Question-
    naire (16PF), Fifth Edition
sixth sense
"sixty-two" (re: drug injection)
size
    body
    chunk
size perception
"skag" (heroin)
SKAT (Sex Knowledge and Attitude
    Test)
"skee" (opium)
"skeeger/skeezer" (re: crack user)
skeleton earmold
skeptic
skepticism
"sketching" (re: drug withdrawal)
"skid" (heroin)
skid row bum
skid row derelict
"skied" (re: drug influence)
skill (pl. skills)
    activities of daily living (ADLS)
    age-appropriate self-help
    assertiveness
    assessment of
    attentional
    auditory
    basic
    calculation
    communication
    comprehension
    conceptual
    cross-dressing

skill *(cont.)*
  decision-making
  decoding
  ego-coping
  encoding
  individual
  intellectual
  interpersonal
  leisure
  linguistic
  mathematical
  memory
  minimum acceptable
  negotiating goals
  negotiating routines
  negotiating rules
  numerical reasoning
  organizational
  perceptual
  perceptual-motor
  phonetic
  phonetic-analysis
  problem-solving
  resolving conflict
  self-care
  seriation
  social
  socialization
  stress adaptability
  verbally mediated
  visual-perceptual
  word-attack
  wordfinding
skill domains, adaptive
Skill Indicators (SKIs)
Skill Scan for Management Development
SKILLSCOPE for Managers
skill training
  occupational
  social
"skin popping" (re: cocaine; drug injection)

skin resistance
  galvanic
  psychogalvanic (PGSR)
skin response audiometry
  galvanic (GSRA)
  psychogalvanic
skin response, galvanic (GSR)
skipping
SKIs (Skill Indicators)
Sklar Aphasia Scale: Revised
"skuffle" (phencyclidine)
skull asymmetry
"skunk" (cannabis)
"Skunk Number 1" (cannabis)
SL (sensation level)
SL (sublingual)
"slab" (crack)
"slam" (re: drug injection)
"slanging" (re: drug dealing)
SLC (Sociopolitical Locus of Control)
sleazy
sleep
  active
  alcohol-induced nighttime
  circadian phase of
  confusional arousals from
  consolidated
  daytime
  decreased
  deep
  depth of
  difficulty maintaining
  disorder of initiating and maintaining (DIMS)
  disordered
  disrupted
  disturbed
  dreamless
  environmental disturbances of
  fitful
  forced
  fragmented nighttime

sleep *(cont.)*
  increased
  increased arousal from
  indeterminate
  lack of excessive
  negative conditioning for
  non-REM
  nonrestorative
  NREM (nonrapid eye movement)
  paradoxical
  quiet
  REM (rapid eye movement)
    REM onset
    REM stage of
  slow-wave (SWS)
  stage 1-4 NREM
  stage of REM
  stage W (wakefulness)
  timing of
  transitional
  undisturbed nocturnal
  unintended
  unrefreshing
  very deep
  very light
sleep abnormalities
sleep and wakefulness
  identifiable pattern of
  pattern of
sleep apnea syndrome
  adult obstructive
  central
  mixed
  obstructive
sleep architecture
sleep arousal
sleep attacks
  refreshing
  sudden
  uncontrollable
sleep behavior disorder
sleep complaint

sleep continuity
  better
  specific
  worse
sleep continuity disturbance(s)
sleep cycle
sleep deprivation
sleep difficulty
sleep disorder
  alcohol-induced
  amphetamine-induced
  breathing-related
  caffeine-induced
  circadian rhythm
  cocaine-induced
  gender differences in
  insomnia-type caffeine-induced
  insomnia-type substance-induced
  medical/psychiatric
  parasomnia-type substance-induced
  primary
  psychogenic
  related
  substance-induced
sleep disorder insomnia
sleep disruption, increased
sleep disturbance
  breathing-related
  chronic
"sleep drunkenness"
sleep duration
  nocturnal
  normal
  reduced
  short
sleep efficiency
sleep epilepsy
sleep episodes
  daytime
  prolonged
  prolonged nocturnal
  unintentional daytime

"sleeper" (barbiturate; heroin)
sleeper
   long
   short
"sleepers" (sleeping pills)
sleep hygiene
sleepiness
   daytime
   excessive
   index of physiological
   physiological
sleeping, difficulty
sleeping erection
"sleeping pill" (barbiturate or nonbarbiturate)
sleeping sickness
sleep latency
   mean
   prolonged
   short
sleepless
sleeplessness
sleep loss
sleep-onset episode
sleep-onset insomnia
sleep onset REM period (SOREMP)
sleep organization
sleep paralysis
   postdormital
   predormital
sleep pattern
   disturbed
   irregular
sleep phase dyssomnia
sleep phase pattern
sleep phase syndrome
   advanced
   delayed
sleep postures
sleep problems
sleep rebound, REM
sleep-related epilepsy

sleep-related hallucination
sleep-related seizures
sleep spindles (on EEG)
sleep stability
sleep stage
sleep state misperception
sleeptalking
sleep tendency
sleep terror disorder
sleep terror episodes
sleep-terror event
sleep therapy
sleep treatment
sleep-wake abnormality
sleep-wake cycle
sleep-wakefulness cycle
sleep-wake hours
sleep-wake pattern
   changing
   irregular
   non-24-hour
   stable
sleep-wake schedule
sleep-wake syndrome
sleep-wake system
sleep-wake timing mechanisms
sleep-wake transition
sleepwalking disorder
sleepwalking behavior
"sleet" (crack)
SLES (Speech and Language
   Evaluation Scale)
SLI (speech and language impaired)
"slick superspeed" (methcathinone)
"slime" (heroin)
Slingerland College-Level Screening
   for the Identification of Language
   Learning Strengths and Weaknesses
Slingerland Screening Tests (SST) for
   Identifying Children with Specific
   Language Disability

SLIP (Singer-Loomis Inventory of Personality)
"slip off the track"
slip, freudian
slip of the tongue
slit fricative consonant formation
sloppy appearance
Slosson Articulation Language Test with Phonology (SALT-P)
Slosson Children's Version Family Environment Scale
Slosson Drawing Coordination Test
Slosson Intelligence Test for Children and Adults
Slosson Intelligence Test–Revised (SIT-R)
Slosson Oral Reading Test–Revised (SORT-R)
Slosson Test of Reading Readiness (STRR)
slow-acting viral encephalitis
slowed reaction time
slowed time, sensation of
slow eye movement
slow-frequency (delta) EEG activity
slowing activity
slowing, psychomotor
slowness, articulatory
slow rate of language development
slow release drug (SR)
slow speech
slow-wave activity
slow-wave sleep (SWS)
slow-wave sleep stability
SLP (speech-language pathologist)
SLSQ (Speech and Language Screening Questionnaire)
SLT (STYCAR Language Test)
slurred speech
slurring
SM, S/M (sadomasochism)
SM (self-mutilation)

SM (sexual myths)
SMA (sequential multiple analysis)
"smack" (heroin)
smacking, lip
small-amplitude rapid tremor
small-city psychiatry
small detail responses
small shuffling steps
SMAST (Short Michigan Alcoholism Screening Test)
SMAT (School Motivation Analysis Test)
smearing, saliva
"smears" (lysergic acid diethylamide)
smell sensation
SMH (state mental hospital)
SMI (severely mentally impaired)
SMI (Style of Mind Inventory)
smile, social
Smith-Johnson Nonverbal Performance Scale
"smoke" (cannabis; crack; heroin and crack)
"smoke Canada" (cannabis)
"smoke-out" (re: drug influence)
smoker's syndrome
"smoking" (phencyclidine)
smoking
   marijuana
   straight pipe
Smoking Behavior Questionnaire (SBQ)
smoking cessation
"smoking gun" (heroin and cocaine)
S/N (signal to noise) ratio
"snap" (amphetamine)
"snappers" (amyl nitrite)
"sniff" (inhalant; methcathinone; re: cocaine use)
sniffing death
sniff method of esophageal speech
"snop" (cannabis)

snores, "resuscitative"
"snort" (re: cocaine use; inhalant use)
snorting
snort, nasal
"snorts" (phencyclidine)
"snot" (re: amphetamine use)
"snot balls" (burned rubber cement)
snout reflex
"snow" (amphetamine; cocaine;
    heroin)
"snowball" (cocaine and heroin)
"snowbirds" (cocaine)
"snowcones" (cocaine)
"snow pallets" (amphetamine)
"snow seals" (cocaine and ampheta-
    mine)
"snow soke" (crack)
"Snow White" (cocaine)
SNS (sympathetic nervous system)
SO (sex offender)
SOAMA (signed out against medical
    advice)
sober
sobriety
    long-term
    "white knuckling"
    Youth Enjoying (YES)
SOC (state of consciousness)
sociability
social acquiescence (SA)
social activities
social adaptation
Social Adaptation Status (SAS)
Social Adequacy Index (SAI)
social adjustment measures
Social Adjustment Scale II
Social Adjustment Self-Report Scale
    (SAS-RS)
social age (SA)
social alienation
Social and Occupational Functioning
    Assessment Scale (SOFAS)

Social and Prevocational Information
    Battery (SPIB)
Social and Rehabilitation Service (SRS)
social anxiety disorder
social apprehensiveness
social attachment
social avoidance and distress (SAD)
social awkwardness
social babbling
Social Behavior Assessment Inventory
    (SBAI)
Social Behavior Assessment Schedule
social breakdown syndrome (SBS)
social class
Social Climate Scales (SCS)
social competence
social conformity
social control
social cripple
social deprivation
social desirability
social detachment
social deviance
social dialect
social disability
social distance
social dominance
social drinking
social dysfunction
Social-Emotional Dimension Scale
social-emotional functioning
social facilitation
Social Function Index (SFI)
social functioning
    anxiety-induced impaired
    frustration-induced impaired
    impairment in
    level of
    marked distress in
social gambling
social gesture speech
social hierarchy

social history (SH, S.H.)
social identification
social immaturity
social inappropriateness
social ineptness
social inhibition
social insecurity
social instinct
social integration
Social Intelligence Test
social interaction
  impaired
  impairment in reciprocal
Social Interaction Scale
social introversion (SI)
Social Introversion Scale
social isolate (noun)
social isolation
socialite
socialization
socialization skills
socialized childhood truancy
socialized conduct disorder
socialized disturbance
socialized runaway reaction
social judgment score
social learning theory
socially acceptable (or unacceptable)
  behavior
socially disruptive environment
social network therapy
social outcast
social persecution
social perception
social phobia experience
social phobic-like behavior
social psychiatrist
social psychiatry
social psychology
social quotient (SQ)
Social Readjustment Rating Scale
  (SRRS)

social reference group
social reinforcement
social relatedness
  developmentally inappropriate
  disturbance in
  disturbed
social relationship
social relations test (SRT)
social responsibility
Social Reticence Scale
social role
social sanctions, imposition of
Social Security (Soc Sec, SS)
Social Security Administration (SSA)
Social Security Disability (SSD)
social service agency
social service consultation
social services (SS)
social setting
social situations
Social Skills Rating System (SSRS)
social skill training
social smile
social standards
social status
social stereotypical behavior
social stereotypical gender roles
social stimulation
social strata
social stress and functionability
  inventory (SSFI)
social support
social tension
social therapy
social values
social welfare organization
social withdrawal of childhood
Social Work
  Bachelor of (BSW)
  Master of (MSW)
  psychiatric

social worker
  certified (CSW)
  psychiatric
societal bias
societal norms, age-appropriate
societal structure
society (see list under *association*)
  majority
  marginal member of
  traditional
"society high" (cocaine)
Society of Teachers of Family Medicine (STFM)
sociobiology
sociocentric
sociocentrism
sociocosm
sociocultural
sociocultural background
sociodemographic features
socioeconomic group
socioeconomic life change
socioenvironmental status
socioenvironmental therapy
sociogram
sociolinguistics
sociologic
sociology, medical
sociometric distance
sociometrist
sociometry
sociopath
sociopathic disturbance
sociopathic personality
sociopathy
Sociopolitical Locus of Control (SLC)
sociotherapy
sociotropy scale
socratic questioning
"soda" (injectable cocaine)
sodium amytal
sodium excretion feedback

sodium lactate avoidance in posttraumatic stress disorder
sodomize
sodomy
SOFAS (Social and Occupational
  Functioning Assessment Scale)
SOFT (Sorting of Figures Test)
"softballs" (barbiturate)
soft neurological signs
soft palate
soft palate cleft
soft sign, neurological
soft speech
software
  Overcoming Depression
  Psycho-Graphic
soft whisper
SOI (Student Opinion Inventory)
SOI-Learning Abilities Test:
  Screening Form for Gifted
solemn affect
SOLER (squarely [face person], open
  [posture], lean [toward person],
  eye [contact], relaxed)
"soles" (hashish)
solitariness
solitary activities
solitary aggressive-type conduct
  disorder
solitary stealing
SOLST (Stephens Oral Language
  Screening Test)
solution analysis
solvent (inhalation) dependence
SOM (serous otitis media)
"soma" (phencyclidine)
somatic complaint
somatic delusion
somatic focus
somatic hallucination
Somatic Inkblot Series
somatic symptoms

somatic therapy
Somatic "3" Scale
somatic treatment for depression
somatic-type delusions
somatic-type schizophrenia
somatization disorder
somatization gastrointestinal symptom
somatization pain symptoms
somatization pseudoneurological
   symptoms
somatization reaction
somatization sexual symptoms
somatization, tendency toward
somatizing clinical depression
somatoform disorder, atypical
somatoform interface disorder
somatoform pain disorder
somatomotor epilepsy
somatosensory epilepsy
somatosensory response
somatosensory seizure
somatron table
somesthetic area
somesthetic dysarthria
somnambulism
somnolence, daytime
somnolent
SOMPA (System of Multicultural
   Pluralistic Assessment)
SOMT (Spatial Orientation Memory
   Test)
sonant consonant formation
sone unit of loudness
sonogram
sonorants
sonority
"sopers" (barbiturate)
sophomania
soporific drug dependence
"sopors" (methaqualone)
SOQ (Suicide Opinion Questionnaire)
SOREMP (sleep onset REM period)

sorter, Keirsey Temperament
Sorting of Figures Test (SOFT)
sorting polarities
SORT-R (Slosson Oral Reading Test),
   Revised
SOS (Student Orientations Survey)
SOT (stream of thought)
"soul loss"
sound (pl. sounds)
   affricative
   air-blade
   aspirated
   attention to
   consonantal
   coronal
   developmentally expected speech
   discrimination of
   distorted perception of
   embedded
   errors of ordering of
   errors of selection of
   fricative
   gross
   liquid
   nasal
   natural class
   non-nasal
   nonspeech
   nonsyllabic speech
   palatal
   prolongation of
   repetition of
   speech
   syllabic speech
   unaspirated
sound analysis
sound and syllable repetition
sound blending
sound changes, conditioned
sound development, speech
sound discrimination, speech
sound field

sound flow, speech
sound intensity
sound, interdental
sound level
sound localization
sound power density
sound pressure level (SPL)
sound pressure level range
sound pressure wave
sound-produced sensation of color
sound production, speech
sound prolongation
sound quality
sound quantity
sounds and memory, sequence of
sounds and symbols, association of
sound segments, phonetic
sound source
sound spectrogram
sound spectrograph
sound spectrum
sound-symbol association
sound symbolism
sound tolerance
sound wave
sound writing
source language
source of information
sources, collateral
Southern California Motor Accuracy
    Test, Revised
Southern California Postrotary
    Nystagmus Test
Southern California Sensory Integra-
    tion Tests
SP (scale of psychosis)
S/P (status post)
SP (systolic pressure)
SPA (ACT Study Power Assessment
    and Inventory)
SPA (schizophrenia with premorbid
    asociality)

SPA (speech pathology/audiology)
"space base" (cigar laced with phen-
    cyclidine and crack; crack dipped
    in phencyclidine)
"space cadet" (crack dipped in phen-
    cyclidine)
"space dust" (crack dipped in phency-
    clidine)
space perception
space, personal
space responses
"space ship" (re: crack equipment)
spacing, interpersonal (communication
    pattern)
Spadafore Diagnostic Reading Test
span
    attention
    auditory memory
    comprehension
    digit (DS)
    life
    memory
    visual memory (VMS)
Spanish Computerized Adaptive
    Placement Exam (S-CAPE)
span recall test
SPAR (sensitivity prediction from the
    acoustic reflex)
SPAR Spelling and Reading Tests,
    Second Edition
"spark it up" (re: cannabis use)
"sparkle plenty" (amphetamine)
"sparklers" (amphetamine)
sparsity of verbalizations
spasm
    habit
    hemifacial
    laryngeal-pharyngeal
spasmodic convulsion
spasmodic laryngitis
spasmodic syndrome, winking
spasms and tics, compulsive

spasm tic
   chronic
   transient disorder of childhood
spasmus nutans
spastic amaurotic axonal idiocy
spastic cerebral palsy (CP)
spastic dysarthria
spastic dysphonia
spastic paralysis
spastic speech
spastic state
spasticity
SPAT-D (Structured Photographic
   Articulation Test Featuring Dudsberry)
spatial ability
spatial agraphia
spatial aptitude (S)
spatial balance
spatial behavior
spatial disorganization
spatial disorientation
spatial distortion
spatial neglect
spatial organization
Spatial Orientation Memory Test
   (SOMT)
speaker's nodes
speaking avoidance
speaking capacity
speaking, choral
Special Aptitude Test Battery (SATB)
special caution
"special "K"" (ketamine)
"special la coke" (ketamine)
specialized language assessment
specific age features
Specific Aptitude Test Battery
specific culture features
specific developmental disorder
   (SDD)
specific diagnosis (provisional)

specific gender features
specificity
specific phobia
   animal-type
   marked and excessive
   marked and persistent
   marked and unreasonable
specific risk
specific situational stressor
specific sleep continuity
specific treatment
SPECS (System to Plan Early
   Childhood Services)
spectin, brain
spectrogram (or spectrograph), sound
spectrophobia
spectrum (pl. spectra or spectrums)
   acoustic
   band
   schizophrenia (SS)
   sound
   tonal
SPECTRUM–I: A Test of Adult
   Work Motivation
SPECT scan
speech
   accelerated
   agrammatic
   alaryngeal
   aphasic
   articulate
   ataxic
   atoxic
   audible blocking in
   automatic
   Bell's Visible
   blocked
   breathing method of esophageal
   buccal
   cerebellar scanning quality
   cerebellar scanning-type
   circumlocution of

speech *(cont.)*
  circumstantial
  clipped
  cold-running
  compressed
  confabulation of
  confused
  connected
  conversational
  cued
  dactyl
  deaf
  delayed
  deviant
  digressive
  disconnected
  disfluent
  disorganized
  displaced
  disturbance in normal fluency of
  disturbance in time patterning of
  droning
  dysarthric
  dysrhythmic
  echo
  egocentric
  emotive
  erratic rhythm of
  esophageal
  excessive
  excessively impressionistic
  executive
  explosive
  fast
  festinant quality in parkinsonian
  filled pauses in
  filtered
  flaccid
  fluent
  fluent aphasic
  fluent paraphasic
  halting

speech *(cont.)*
  helium
  high-stimulus
  hyperkinetic
  hypokinetic
  impaired
  impoverished
  impressionistic
  incessant
  incoherent
  incomprehensible
  indistinct
  infantile
  inner
  internal
  involuntary pauses in
  irrelevant
  labored
  limited
  loud
  manic
  metaphorical
  mimetic
  mimic
  minimal prosody of
  mirror
  monosyllabic
  monotone
  narrative
  nonelaborative
  nonfluent aphasic
  nonpropositional
  nonsensical
  odd
  over-abstract
  over-concrete
  over-elaborate
  paraphasic
  phantom
  pharyngeal
  poverty of
  pressured

speech *(cont.)*
  productivity of
  propositional
  psychotic
  rambling
  rapid
  rate of
  regressive
  repetitive
  rhythm of
  running
  scanning
  serial content
  seriatim
  silent blocking in
  slow
  slurred
  social gesture
  soft
  spastic
  spontaneous
  staccato
  stereotyped
  subvocal
  tangential
  telegraphic
  thickened
  tolerance threshold for
  tracheoesophageal
  tremulous
  underproductive
  unfilled pauses in
  unintelligible
  unvoiced
  vague
  visible
  well-articulated
speech acts
speech analysis, aerodynamic
speech and hearing (S&H)
speech and hearing science
speech and language behavior

speech and language characteristics of
  cleft palate
speech and language clinician
speech and language disorder
speech and language disorders in
  psychiatry
Speech and Language Evaluation
  Scale (SLES)
speech and language impaired (SLI)
Speech and Language Screening
  Questionnaire (SLSQ)
speech apraxia
speech articulation
speech aspects
speech assessment
speech audiometry
speech awareness threshold (SAT)
speech behavior
speech blocking
  audible
  silent
speech breakdown
speech breathing
speech center
speech community
speech conservation
speech content
  paucity of
  positive
  poverty of
speech correction
speech defect
speech derailment
speech detection threshold (SDT)
speech developmental disorder
speech difficulty
speech disability
speech discrimination (SD)
speech discrimination audiometry
Speech Discrimination in Noise
speech disfluency
speech disintegration

speech disorder
speech disruption
speech distortion
speech disturbance
speech dysfluencies
  avoidance of
  emotional response to
speech education
speech elements
  audible
  involuntary
  prolonged
  repetitious
  silent
speech frequency (ies)
speech impairment
Speech Improvement Cards
speech inflection
speech innateness theory
speech in schizophrenia
speech intelligibility
speech interference level (SIL)
speech interruption
speech/language behavior
speech-language pathologist (SLP
Speech-Language Pathology
  Evaluation Assessment
speech mannerism
speech mechanism
speech-motor deficit
speech-motor function
speech noise
speech pathology/audiology (SPA)
speech pattern
  feminine
  parrotlike
speech perception deficit
speech processing
speech production
Speech Questionnaire
speech range
speech reaction time

speech-reading aphasia
speech-reading aural rehabilitation
speech reception (SR)
speech reception audiometry
speech reception threshold (SRT)
speech recognition
speech rehabilitation
speech-related struggle
speech rhythm
speech science
speech signal
speech sound (pl. sounds)
  developmentally expected
  nonsyllabic
  standard
  syllabic
speech sound development
speech sound discrimination
speech sound flow
Speech Sound Memory Test
speech sound production
Speech-Sounds Perception Test
speech synthesis
speech test (see *test*)
speech therapist
speech therapy
speech time patterns
speech training units
speech understanding
speech visualization
Speech with Alternating Masking
  Index (SWAMI)
speed
  information processing
  motor
  Verbal Perceptual
  Visual Perceptual
  word identification
"speed" (amphetamine; methamphetamine hydrochloride)
"speedball" (amphetamine; heroin and
  cocaine)

"speed boat" (cannabis, phencyclidine, and crack)
"speed for lovers" (methylenedioxymethamphetamine)
"speed freak" (re: methamphetamine user)
speed of information processing
speed of thought
speed quotient
"speed runs"
spell-a-word-backwards test
spell backwards test
spelling dyspraxia
Spelling Grade Equivalent
Spelling Grade Rating
Spelling Scale (British Ability Scales)
SPELT-P (Structured Photographic Expressive Language Test-II)
spermatophobia
spermophobia
sphecidophobia
sphenoid bone
sphenoidal nasal concha
sphenoidal turbinated bone
sphere, psychosexual
spheres, oriented in all
SPI (ACT Study Power Assessment and Inventory)
SPI (Self-Perception Inventory)
SPI (Shipley Personal Inventory)
SPIB (Social and Prevocational Information Battery)
"spider blue" (heroin)
Spielberger Anxiety Inventory
Spielberger State–Trait Anger Expression Inventory
"spike" (needle; re: drug injection)
spike and wave complex
spike, diphasic
spiked profile
spike-like waves
spike on EEG

spike waves
  negative
  six hertz positive
spina bifida
spinal accessory nerve (cranial nerve XI)
spinal shock
spindle on EEG, sleep
spinocerebellar degeneration
spiral effect of stuttering
spirant consonant formation
spirits, controlling external
spiritual aspects of the body
spiritual counselor
spiritual function
spiritual possession
spiritual problem
Spiritual Well-Being Scale (SWBS)
spirometer
spite reaction
SPL (sound pressure level)
"splash" (amphetamine)
"spliff" (cannabis cigarette)
"splim" (cannabis)
"split" (half and half; to leave)
split half reliability coefficient
split personality
splitting behavior
splitting of self-image
split word
"splivins" (amphetamine)
SPMSQ (Short Portable Mental Status Questionnaire)
spoken language quotient
spondee word
spontaneity
  lack of
  loss of
spontaneous convulsion
spontaneous imitation
spontaneous recovery
spontaneous speech

"spoon" (1/16 ounce of heroin)
"spores" (phencyclidine)
"sporting" (re: cocaine use)
spot
   blind
   figurative blind (scotoma)
spousal abuse
spouse abuse
SPP (Sexuality Preference Profile)
SPQ (Sales Personality Questionnaire)
SPR (Society for Psychotherapy Research)
"spray" (inhalant)
spring-summer viral encephalitis, Russian
"sprung" (re: drug user)
SPSI (School Problem Screening Inventory)
SPT (Supervisory Practices Test)
SPT (Symbolic Play Test)
SQ (social quotient)
sq, subcu, or subq (subcutaneous)
SQ3R (survey, question, read, review, recite)
squandermania
squarely (face person), open (posture), lean (toward person), eye (contact), relaxed (SOLER)
"square mackerel" (cannabis)
"square time Bob" (crack)
squatting
squeeze technique (of penis)
"squirrel" (re: cocaine, cannabis and PCP use)
SR, S/R (schizophrenic reaction)
SR (seizure resistant)
SR (sentence repetition)
SR (slow release)
SR (speech reception)
SRA (Science Research Associates)
SRA Achievement Series: Forms 1-2
SRA Arithmetic Test
SRA Nonverbal Form
SRA Pictorial Reasoning Test
SRA Reading Test
SRA Verbal Form
SR/AP (schizophrenic reaction, acute, paranoid)
SR/AU (schizophrenic reaction, acute, undifferentiated)
SRC (Student Reactions to College)
SR/CP (schizophrenic reaction, chronic, paranoid)
SR/CU (schizophrenic reaction, chronic, undifferentiated)
SRF (Stuttering Resource Foundation)
SRRS (Social Readjustment Rating Scale)
SRS (schizophrenic residual state)
SRS (Social and Rehabilitation Service)
SRS (Symptom Rating Scale)
SRT (social relations test)
SRT (speech reception threshold)
SS (schizophrenia spectrum)
SS (seizure sensitive)
SS (Social Security)
SS (social services)
SSA (ACT Study Skills Assessment and Inventory)
SSA (Social Security Administration)
SSC (Stein Sentence Completion) test
SSD (Social Security Disability)
SSFI (social stress and functionability inventory)
SSHA (Survey of Study Habits and Attitudes)
SSI (ACT Study Skills Assessment and Inventory)
SSI (Supplemental Security Income)
SSIAM (Structured and Scaled Interview to Assess Maladjustment)
SSII (Safran Student's Interest Inventory)

SSOP (Standard System of Psychiatry)
SSPD (schizoid-schizotypal personality disorder
SSPL (saturation sound pressure level)
SSPL output HF average
SSRI (selective serotonin reuptake inhibitor)
SSRS (Social Skills Rating System)
SSS (School Situation Survey)
SSS (Sensation-Seeking Scale)
SST (Slingerland Screening Tests)
SST for Identifying Children with Specific Language Disability
ST (shock therapy)
ST (standardized test)
stabbing pain
stability
  emotional
  family
  marital
  personality trait
  relative slow-wave sleep
stability in relationships
stability of self-image
stability of vocational functioning
stabilization
stabilizing social situations
stable ego structure
stable, emotionally
stable personality
stable pattern
stable sleep difficulty
stable sleep-wake pattern
STABS (Suinn Test Anxiety Behavior Scale)
staccato speech
"stack" (cannabis)
"stacking" (taking prescription steroids)
stacking anchors
STACL (Screening Test for Auditory Comprehension of Language)

Staff Burnout Scale for Health Professionals
staff HMO-based psychiatry
stage (pl. stages)
  anal
  anesthesia
  cognitive development
  dementia
  developmental
  group
  oral
  phallic
  Piaget cognitive development
  REM sleep
  sleep
  stuttering
  two-word
stage I of non-REM (drowsiness)
stage II of non-REM (light sleep)
stage III of non-REM (deep sleep)
stage IV of non-REM (very deep sleep)
stage fright
stage W (wakefulness) sleep
stage whisper
staggering gait
STAI (State-Trait Anxiety Inventory)
STAIC (State-Trait Anxiety Inventory for Children)
stalker
stalking behavior
stammering
stamp, digit
stance
  approach-avoidance
  defensive adultomorphic
  norm-assertive
standard (pl. standards)
  foreign
  performance
  sexual behavior
  sexual performance
  social

Standard American English (SAE)
standard community psychotherapy
(SCP)
standard deviation (SD)
standard earmold
standard error
Standardized Assessment of Depressive Disorders (SADD)
standardized cognitive assessment
techniques
standardized test (ST)
Standardized Test of Computer
Literacy (STCL)
standard language
standard of living
standard of performance
self-imposed high
strict
Standard Progressive Matrices
standard reference
standard score
standard speech sound
Standard System of Psychiatry (SSOP)
standard word
standing balance
standing trial
standing wave
Stanford Achievement Test (SAT)
Stanford Achievement Test (SAT),
Abbreviated Version, 8th Edition
Stanford-Binet Intelligence Scale
(SBIS): Form L-M
Stanford Diagnostic Mathematics Test
Stanford Early School Achievement
Test, Second Edition
Stanford Hypnotic Clinical Scale for
Children
Stanford Hypnotic Susceptibility Scale
(SHSS)
Stanford Profile Scales of Hypnotic
Susceptibility, Revised
Stanton Survey

stapedectomy
stapedial acoustic reflex
stapes (pl. stapes) mobilization
"star" (methcathinone)
starch-eating
"stardust" (cocaine, phencyclidine)
stare
    blank
    empty
    reptilian
staring eyes
staring face
staring facial expression
STAR Profile (Student Talent and
    Risk Profile)
STARS (Short Term Auditory
    Retrieval and Storage)
"star-spangled powder" (cocaine)
START (Screening Test for the
    Assignment of Remedial Treat-
    ments)
startle reaction
startle reflex
startle response
startling noise
startling stimulus
starvation fasting
STAS (State-Trait Anger Scale)
"stash" (re: drug storage)
"stash areas" (re: drug storage)
stasibasiphobia
stasiphobia
"stat" (methcathinone)
stat or STAT (immediately)
STAT (Suprathreshold Adaptation
    Test)
state
    acute confusional (ACS)
    affective and paranoid
    agitated
    alert-awake
    alertness

state *(cont.)*
    alpha
    altered
    amnesic
    amnestic
    anxiety (AS)
    anxiety-tension (ATS)
    apprehension
    borderline
    break
    catatonic
    central excitatory
    clouded
    confusional
    consciousness
    constitutional psychopathic (CPS)
    convulsive
    crepuscular
    current
    delirium-like
    depressive
    disequilibrium
    dissociative
    dream
    dreamy
    ego
    emotional
    epileptic confusional (ECS)
    epileptic fugue
    euthymic
    feeling
    fugue
    full wakefulness
    hallucinatory
    heightened attention
    heightened awareness
    hyperdopaminergic
    hypnagogic
    hypnoid
    hypnopompic
    hypnotic
    hysterical

state *(cont.)*
    hysteric coma-like
    hysterical fugue
    identity
    lacunar
    locked in
    mental
    mind
    mixed-mood
    moribund
    multiple ego
    negative mood
    neurotic
    nonresponsive
    obsessional
    oneiroid
    organic psychotic
    panic
    paranoid
    parasomniac conscious
    perfection
    persistent vegetative (PVS)
    phobic
    possession trance
    postictal
    premorbid
    psychotic
    rapid eye movement
    resource
    schizophrenic residual (SRS)
    separator
    sleep
    spastic
    subacute confusional (SCS)
    subjectively experienced feeling
    substance-induced
    tension
    toxic-confusional
    trance
    transient mental
    twilight
    unresponsive

state *(cont.)*
  vegetative
  vulnerability to life's stressors
  wakeful
  withdrawal
state dependent memory
state licensing board
state markers of heavy drinking (GGT)
state mental hospital (SMH)
state response
State-Trait Anger Expression Inventory (STAXI)
State-Trait Anger Scale (STAS)
State-Trait Anxiety Index
State-Trait Anxiety Inventory (STAI)
State-Trait Anxiety Inventory for Children (STAIC)
State-Trait Personality Inventory (STPI)
stated desire
statements, "I"
static acoustic impedance
static dementia
static encephalopathy
static tremor
stationary focus
statistical deviation
statistical inference
statistical information
statistical significance
statistics, psychiatric
status
  absence
  altered mental
  ambulatory
  clinical
  confident
  current cognitive
  disordered mental
  elopement (ES)
  grand mal

status *(cont.)*
  hostage
  immigrant
  marital
  mental
  open-ward
  petit mal
  postoperative
  preepisode
  social
  Social Adaptation (SAS)
  socioenvironmental
  symptomatic
  temporal lobe
status aura
status dysgraphicus
status epilepsy
status epilepticus
  convulsive
  nonconvulsive
status epilepticus organic psychosis
status examination
status index (see *test*)
Status Indicators (SIs)
status inventory (see *test*)
status post (S/P)
status questionnaire (see *test*)
status scale
status schedule
status value
STAXI (State-Trait Anger Expression Inventory)
stay on task
STCL (Standardized Test of Computer Literacy)
STD (sexually transmitted disease)
steady rhythmicity of tremor
stealing an anchor
stealing, solitary
"steerer" (re: drug dealing)
Stegreiftheater (Theater of Spontaneity)

Stein Sentence Completion (SSC) test
Stekel, Wilhelm (1868-1940)
"stem" (re: crack equipment)
"stems" (cannabis)
Stenger Test
Stenographic Skill-Dictation Test
stenosis (pl. stenoses)
  carotid artery
  congenital hypertrophic pyloric
  urethral
"step on" (dilute drugs)
Step Fa (stepfather)
stepfather (Step Fa)
Stephens Oral Language Screening
  Test (SOLST)
Step Mo (stepmother)
stepmother (Step Mo)
STEPS (Screening Test for Educational Prerequisite Skills)
steps in therapy
Steps Up Developmental Screening
  Program
STEP-III (Sequential Tests of Educational Progress, Series III)
stepwise deterioration
stereognosis, oral
stereognostic perception
stereotyped repetition
stereotyped activity
stereotyped behavior
stereotyped body movements
stereotyped interests
stereotyped motor movement
stereotyped motor vocalization
stereotyped movements
stereotyped restricted behavior
stereotyped speech
stereotyped stress
stereotypical gender roles
stereotypical movements
stereotypical social behavior
stereotypic behavior

stereotypic motor movement
stereotypic movement disorder
stereotypic sex-role behavior
stereotypy/habit disorder
Stern alcoholic amentia
sternoclavicular muscle
sternocleidomastoid muscle
sternohyoid muscle
sternothyroid muscle
steroid, anabolic
STFM (Society of Teachers of Family
  Medicine)
STG (short-term goals)
S3 Rating Scale (School Social Skills
  Rating Scale)
"stick" (cannabis, phencyclidine)
sticking sensation
stigma, psychosocial
stigmata of psychosis
stimulant
  CNS (central nervous system)
  psychomotor
stimulant challenge test
stimulant effect
stimulant-induced postural tremor
stimulating environment
stimulating experience
stimulation
  auditory
  environmental
  epileptogenic
  external
  genital
  insufficient
  lack of
  linguistic
  manual
  noncoital
  oral
  sensory
  sensory pathway
  sexual

stimulation *(cont.)*
  social
  subliminal
  synesthetic
  tactile
  tactile genital
  visual
stimulation fatigue
stimuli revulsion, sexual
stimulus (pl. stimuli)
  alerting
  appropriate
  auditory
  aversive
  conditioned
  emotional
  emotionally provoking
  emotion-related feedback
  environmental
  epileptogenic
  erotic
  external
  fatness
  frightening
  internal
  minor
  musical
  neutral
  novel
  noxious
  outside
  painful
  paraphiliac
  pedophilic
  phobic
  psychosensory
  screen out irrelevant
  sensory
  sexual
  startling
  tactile
  terrifying

stimulus *(cont.)*
  thermal
  threshold of
  triggering
  unconditioned
  visual
  visuo-spatial
stimulus control
stimulus drive (SD, Sd)
stimulus generalization
Stimulus Recognition Test
stimulus-response
stimulus substitution
stimulus therapy
stinging pain
"stink weed" (cannabis)
stirrup
STM (short-term memory)
stocking-glove anesthesia
stocking-glove distribution
stocking-glove sensory loss
stoma (pl. stomas or stomata)
stoma blast
stoma button
stomach disorder, psychogenic
Stone and Neale Daily Coping Assessment
  ment
"stoned" (re: drug influence)
"stoner" (drug user)
"stones" (crack)
stooped shoulders
stop-and-think technique
stop consonant formation
stop, glottal
"stoppers" (barbiturate)
stopping of fricatives
"stop, look, and listen" intervention
storage, auditory
stormed defense
Story Articulation Test
storylike dream sequence

STP (analog of amphetamine/metham-
  phetamine)
"STP" (phencyclidine)
STPI (State-Trait Personality Inventory)
straight pipe smoking
strain (pl. strains)
  alpha-wave
  interpersonal
  physical
  psychological
  vocational
straitjacket
stranger anxiety
strata, social
strategies
  bibliotherapeutic
  conflict-resolution
  coping
  problem-solving
strategy
  data reanalysis
  gambling
  protective survival
Strauss syndrome
"straw" (cannabis cigarette)
"strawberries" (barbiturate)
"strawberry" (re: crack prostitute)
"strawberry hill" (lysergic acid
  diethylamide)
stream
  breath
  misdirected urinary
stream of consciousness
stream of mental activity
stream of thought (SOT)
street-drug culture
street drugs (see *drugs, street*)
street person
Street Survival Skills Questionnaire
strength
  antagonistic muscle
  ego

strength *(cont.)*
  fatigue
  response
Strength of Grip Test
strephosymbolia
stress
  biology of
  breakdown under
  catastrophic
  causative
  chronic
  combat
  contrastive
  coping with
  disabling
  emotional
  excessive
  family
  fatigue
  iambic
  identifiable
  Level of Psychosocial (Axis IV)
  life
  medical
  phrase
  precipitating
  primary
  psychological
  psychosocial
  secondary
  serious traumatic
  severe life
  social
  stereotyped
  temporary
  tertiary
  trochaic
  war-related
  wax-weak
  weak
stress adaptability skills
stress and functionability inventory
Stress Audit

stress disorder, posttraumatic (PTSD)
stressed syllable
stressed vowel
Stress Evaluation Inventory
stress exposure
Stress from Life Experience (SFLE)
stressful life experiences
stressful word production
stress immunity
Stress Impact Scale (SIS)
stress-induced reactive bowel
stress management
stressor (pl. stressors)
  childhood
  external
  extreme
  identifiable
  internal
  major
  psychosocial
  seasonal-related psychosocial
  specific situational
  state of vulnerability to life's
  traumatic
stress patterns
stress precipitating tremor
stress prevention
stress reaction
  acute
  chronic
  consciousness
  emotions
  gross
  group
  mixed
  psychomotor
stress reduction
stress-related disturbance
stress-related paranoid ideation
stress-related physiological responses
stress-related psychophysiological
  problem

Stress Response Scale
stress situational reaction
stress-strain relationship
stress syndrome
stretch reflex
stria, acoustic
striatal dopaminergic system
striatal hypometabolism
striatocerebral tremor
strict standards of performance
stricture, vaginal
stridency deletion
strident lisp
stridor
stridulous laryngitis
string
  initial
  intermediate
  terminal
stroboscope
stroke (CVA)
  brain stem
  glottal
  lacunar
Strong-Campbell Interest Inventory
  (SCII)
strong emotion
Strong Interest Inventory [Fourth
  Edition] (SVIB-SCII)
strongly held idea
Stroop Color and Word Test
STRR (Slosson Test of Reading
  Readiness)
structural abnormality
structural ambiguity
Structural Analysis of Social Behavior
structural atrophy
structural brain abnormalities
structural brain imaging
structural linguistics
structural pathology
structural rule morpheme

structure
  abnormal brain
  base
  external
  functional superego
  grammatical
  group
  hierarchial
  intermediate
  lack of
  language
  organizational
  performative pragmatic
  pragmatic
  stable ego
  substituted-phenylethylamine
  surface
  syllable
  underlying
  word
Structured and Scaled Interview to
  Assess Maladjustment (SSIAM)
Structured Clinical Interview for DSM-
  IV Axis I Disorders: Clinician
  Version (SCID-CV)
Structured Clinical Interview for DSM-
  IV Axis II Personality Disorders
  (SCID-II)
Structured Clinical Interview for
  DSM-IV Dissociative Disorders
  (SCID-D), Revised
structured hallucination
structured interactional group psycho-
  therapy
Structured Interview of Reported
  Symptoms (SIRS)
structured milieu
Structured Photographic Articulation
  Test Featuring Dudsberry (SPAT-D)
Structured Photographic Expressive
  Language Test-II (SPELT-P)

structured task
structure grammar
structure of intellect (SI)
Structure of Intellect Learning Abilities
  Test, Form P (Primary)
structure word
struggle, speech-related
"strung out" (re: drug addiction)
strychnine
student (pl. students)
  above-average
  average
  below-average
student dropouts
Student Opinion Inventory (SOI)
Student Orientations Survey (SOS)
Student Talent and Risk Profile (STAR
  Profile)
study (pl. studies)
  community
  double-blind
  electrodiagnostic
  epidemiological
  genetic linkage
  hospital-based
  hysteria
  nerve conduction
  nocturnal penile tumescence
  parametric
  polysomnographic
  systematic
  time and motion
Study Attitudes and Methods Survey
  (SAMS)
study case
study design
Study of Values (SV)
"stuff" (heroin)
"stumbler" (barbiturate)
stump hallucination

stupor
  catatonic
  psychogenic
stupor mania
stuporous melancholia
stuporous patient
stuporous-type manic-depressive
  psychosis
stuttered rhythm
stutter
stutterer
stutter fluently therapy (SFT)
stutter free speech (SFS)
stuttering (see also *stuttering, theory in*)
  developmental
  exteriorized
  fixation in
  hysterical
  implicit
  incipient
  interiorized
  internal
  jaw dysfunction
  laryngeal
  lip dysfunction
  neurogenic
  PFAGH
  phases of
  primary
  psychogenic
  secondary
  spiral effect
  stages of
  tongue dysfunction
  transitional
Stuttering Foundation of America
  (SFA)
stuttering gait
stuttering modification therapy
stuttering pattern
Stuttering Resource Foundation (SRF)

stuttering, theory in
  anticipatory-struggle
  breakdown under stress
  cybernetic
  laterality
  learning
  neurotic
  repressed need
STYCAR (Screening Tests for Young
  Children and Retardates)
STYCAR Hearing Test (SHT)
STYCAR Language Test (SLT)
STYCAR Vision Tests (SVT)
stygiophobia
style (pl. styles)
  cognitive
  coping
  deception
  extratensive coping
  extratensive personality
  introtensive
  introtensive personality
  introversive problem-solving
Style of Leadership and Management
Style of Leadership Survey
Style of Management Inventory
Style of Mind Inventory (SMI)
styloglossus muscle
stylohyoid muscle
stylopharyngeal muscle
SU (sensation unit)
subacute confusional state (SCS)
subacute psychosis
subacute sclerosing panencephalitis
subarachnoid hemorrhage
subaverage academic functioning
subaverage intellectual functioning
subaverage motor coordination
subchronic schizophrenia
subclassification
subclavian muscle

subclinical score
subclinical seizure
subcoma insulin treatment
subconscious memory
subcortical alexia
subcortical aphasia
subcortical brain involvement
subcortical dementia
subcortical encephalopathy
subcortical motor aphasia
subcortical white matter
subcu (subcutaneous)
subcultural language
subculture norms
subcutaneous (subcu, sq)
subdural hemorrhage
subglottic laryngitis
subglottic resonator
subgroup
   cultural
   phenomenological
subject
   complete
   simple
subjective case
subjective drive
subjective equality
subjective insomnia complaint
subjective psychology
subjective experience
subjective fear
subjective feelings
subjectively experienced feeling state
subjective sensation
subjective symptoms
Subjective Treatment Emergent Side
   Effects Scale
subjective unit of distress rating (SUDS)
subjectivity
   out of control
   overwhelmed

subjects as their own control (experimental study designs)
subject-verb agreement
subjunctive mood
sublimation
subliminal behavior
subliminal stimulation
sublingual drug (SL)
submania
submissive behavior
submissiveness
submodalities, critical
submucous cleft palate
subnormality
   mental
   mild mental
   moderate mental
   profound mental
   severe mental
suboccipital headache
subordinate clause
subsequent amnesia
subsequent development
subsonic
substance (pl. substances)
   anxiolytic
   behavior-altering
   character of a
   high-dose use of
   illicit psychoactive
   mood-altering
   phencyclidine-like
   psychoactive
   sexual dysfunction due to a
substance abuse counselor
substance abuse disorder
Substance Abuse Problem Checklist
Substance Abuse Questionnaire (SAQ)
Substance Abuse Subtle Screening
   Inventory (SASSI)
substance abuser

substance dependence with physiological dependence
substance dependence without physiological dependence
substance group
substance-induced organic mental disorder
substance-induced state
substance intoxication delirium
substance-related causes
substance-related disorder
substance-related problems
substance-seeking behavior
substance self-administration
substance use
  compulsive
  escalating pattern of
  maladaptive pattern of
  pathological
  pattern of compulsive
  signs of compulsive
substance use disorder
substance-using friends
substance withdrawal
substance-withdrawal delirium
substance-withdrawal tremor
substandard language
substantive universals
substituted benzamide
substitution disorder
substitution, symptom
substituted-phenylethylamine structure
substituting behavior
substitute object
substitution
  semantic
  stimulus
  word
substitution analysis
substitution articulation
substitutional lisp
subsyndromal depressive symptoms

subsystem
  depreciated
  individuals
  parents
  scapegoated
  siblings
  spouses
subsystem boundaries
subtest (on WAIS-R)
  arithmetic
  block design
  comprehension
  digit span
  information
  object assembly (OA)
  picture arrangement (PA)
  picture completion (PC)
  similarities
subtest scale scores
subthreshold presentations
subtotal cleft palate
subtotal laryngectomy
subtype
  diagnostic
  disorganized
subvocal speech
success, cumulative probability of (CPS)
success experience
successful suicide
successive approximation
succinimides
succinylcholine
sucking behavior
sucking technique
suck reflex
suction method of esophageal speech
sudden fear
sudden loss of vision
sudden-onset headache
sudden sleep "attack"
sudden sniffing death
SUDS (subjective unit of distress) rating

suffering death
sufficient quantity (q.s.)
suffix
suffixation
suffocating attachment
suffocation panicker
"sugar" (cocaine; heroin; lysergic
   acid diethylamide)
"sugar block" (crack)
"sugar cubes" (lysergic acid diethylamide)
"sugar daddys" (amphetamine)
"sugar lumps" (lysergic acid diethylamide)
"sugar weed" (cannabis)
suggestibility effect
suggestion hypnosis
suggestion therapy
suggestion under hypnosis, direct
   (DSUH)
suggestive psychotherapy
suicidal behavior
suicidal gestures
suicidal ideation
suicidal intent
suicidality, repetitious
suicidal melancholia
suicidal plan
suicidal potential
suicidal preoccupation
suicidal rumination
suicidal thoughts
suicidal thinking
suicide
   accidental
   adolescent
   altruistic
   assisted
   cluster
   completed
   half-hearted attempt at
   high risk for

suicide *(cont.)*
   rational
   risk factors for
   successful
   teenage
suicide act
suicide attempt (SA)
suicide-depression (SD)
Suicide-Depression Proneness Checklist (SDPC)
suicide gesture
Suicide Intervention Response Inventory
suicide motivation
Suicide Opinion Questionnaire (SOQ)
suicide plan
suicide precautions
Suicide Probability Scale
suicide risk
suicide-risk factor
suicide talk
suicide threat
suicide victims
Suinn Test Anxiety Behavior Scale
   (STABS)
sulcus (pl. sulci)
   callosal
   central
   frontal
   inferior frontal
   inferior temporal
   lateral
   lateral occipital
   median lingual
   middle frontal
   postcentral
   precentral
   superior frontal
   superior temporal
   terminal
   temporal
sulfate, morphine (MS)

Sullivan, Harry Stack (1892-1949)
summation, binaural
"sunshine" (lysergic acid diethylamide)
"super" (phencyclidine)
"super acid" (ketamine)
"super C" (ketamine)
superego control
superego structure
superficial affect
superficial charm
superficial idiot
superficial pain
superficial sensation
superficiality
"super grass" (cannabis; phencyclidine)
"super ice" (smokable methamphetamine)
superimposed delirium
superior constrictor muscle of pharynx
superior frontal sulcus
superior intelligence
superiority complex
superior laryngotomy
superior longitudinal muscle of tongue
superior manner
superior maxillary bone
superior nasal concha
superior nasal meatus
superior pharyngeal constrictor
superior temporal sulcus
superior to others
superior turbinate bone
"super joint" (phencyclidine)
"super kools" (phencyclidine)
superlative comparative
supernormal score
supernumerary teeth
superoxides
superstition
superstitious behavior

superstitiousness
Supervisory Behavior Description
(SBD)
Supervisory Practices Inventory
Supervisory Practices Test (SPT)
Supervisory Profile Record
"super weed" (phencyclidine)
supplemental air
Supplemental Security Income (SSI)
suppletion
support
child
community
emotional
empirical
environmental
informational
instrumental
limited
physical
social
support for assaulted staff
support group
supporting persons, significant
supportive psychotherapy
suppression, bone marrow
suppression test, dexamethasone
(DST)
suppressor, noise
suppurative otitis media
supraglottic resonator
suprahyoid extrinsic muscles
supramarginal gyrus
supranuclear gaze palsy
suprasegmental analysis
suprasegmental phoneme
supratentorial overlay
Suprathreshold Adaptation Test
(STAT)
suprathreshold ECT
supraversion of teeth
surd

surface structure
"surfer" (phencyclidine)
surgical reduction of Adam's apple
surgical sex-reassignment
surgical sexual reassignment
surliness
surly
surrogate father
surrogate mother
surrogate parent
surroundings
    familiar
    indifferent to
survey (see *test*)
survey data
Survey of Employee Access (SEA)
Survey of Interpersonal Values (SIV)
Survey of Organizations
Survey of Personal Values
Survey of School Attitudes
Survey of Study Habits and Attitudes
    (SSHA)
Survey of Work Values, Revised,
    Form U
survey, question, read, review, recite
    (SQ3R)
survival, nerve cell
survival strategy
survivor of child abuse
survivor of neglect
survivors of death
suspected disease
suspected child abuse/neglect (SCAN)
suspension laryngoscopy
suspicion of others' motives
suspicious ideation
suspiciousness
sustained belief
sustained blowing
sustained fatigue
sustained full remission

sustained manner
sustained partial remission
sustained position
sustention/intention tremor
SV (Study of Values)
SVT (STYCAR Vision Tests)
swallow method of esophageal speech
swallowing
    deviant
    difficulty
    infantile
    reverse
    visceral
swallowing automatism
swallowing dysfunction
swallowing habit
SWAMI (Speech with Alternating
    Masking Index)
swaying, body
swaying gait
SWBS (Spiritual Well-Being Scale)
swearing, compulsive
sweat gland activity
sweep-check test
"Sweet Jesus" (heroin)
"Sweet Lucy" (cannabis)
"sweets" (amphetamine)
"sweet stuff" (cocaine; heroin)
swelling of external genitalia
"swell up" (crack)
Swinging Story Test
swing phase control
swings, mood
swish
switching
switch referential index
SWS (slow-wave sleep)
Sx (symptoms)
sycophant
Sydenham chorea
syllabary

syllabic (pl. syllabics)
  complex
  simple
syllabic aphonia
syllabication
syllabic consonant
syllabic speech sound
syllabic vowel
syllabic writing
syllable (pl. syllables)
  closed
  consonant-vowel
  consonant-vowel-consonant
  nonsense
  open
  paired
  stressed
  vowel-consonant
syllable deletion
  unstressed
  weak
syllable duplication
syllable duration
syllable prolongations
syllable reduction
syllable repetition, sound and
syllable sequence
syllable shape
syllables, paired
syllable structure
Sylvius, fissure of
symbiosis
symbiotic attachment
symbiotic infantile psychosis
symbiotic psychosis
symbiotic psychosis of childhood
symbol (pl. symbols)
  association of sounds and
  digit (DS)
  letter
  mathematical
  numerical

symbol *(cont.)*
  phonetic
  Wing
Symbol Digit Modalities Test (SDMT)
symbolic elaboration
symbolic meaning
Symbolic Play Test (SPT), Second
  Edition
symbolic thinking
symbolic value
symbolism
  dream
  sound
symbolophobia
symbol set system
symmetromania
symmetrophobia
sympathetic dysfunction
sympathetic nervous system (SNS)
sympathetic vibration
sympathic mimetic addiction
sympathomimetic abuse
sympathomimetic addiction
sympathomimetic drug
sympathomimetic effect
symptom (pl. symptoms) (Sx);
  also, symptom of
  active psychotic
  active-phase
  anchor
  anxiety
  attention-deficit
  auditory
  avoidance
  baseline
  behavioral dysfunction
  biological dysfunction
  bodily signs and
  brain stem
  catatonic
  conversion
  deficit

symptom *(cont.)*
delusion
depression
dissociative
emotional
equivalent
extrapyramidal
fatigue
feigned
first rank (schneiderian) (FRS)
gastrointestinal
hypochondriacal
impairment
insomnia
intentionally produced
manic
minimal residual
mood
motor
movement
pain
painful
preexisting mental disorder
presenting
prodromal
prominent mood
pseudoneurologic
psychogenic physical
psychological dysfunction
psychomotor
psychosensory
psychosexual
psychosomatic
psychotic
reexperiencing perceptual
residual psychotic
schizophrenia
sensory
sexual
somatic
somatization
subsyndromal depressive
trance

symptom *(cont.)*
unintentionally produced
vegetative
visual
withdrawal
symptomatically reactive
symptomatic epilepsy
symptomatic presentation
symptomatic seizure
symptomatic status
symptomatic therapy
symptomatic treatment
symptomatology
depressive
mood
panic
psychotic
Symptom Checklist-90-Revised
(SCL-90-R)
symptom criteria
symptom diary
symptom formation
symptom free
symptom pattern
symptom presentation
symptom ratings
Symptom Rating Scale (SRS)
symptom relief through hypnosis
symptom response pattern
symptom substitution
synapse (pl. synapses)
synaptic cleft
synaptic plasticity
synchronic linguistics
syncopal
syncope
syncretic thoughts
syncretism
syndromal depression
syndromal pattern
syndrome
absence
acute brain

syndrome *(cont.)*
 acute organic brain
 adult obstructive sleep apnea
 advanced sleep phase
 alcohol abstinence
 alcohol amnestic
 alcohol dependence
 alcohol withdrawal
 Alice in Wonderland
 Alzheimer
 amnesic
 amnestic
 amnestic-confabulatory
 amotivational
 androgen insensitivity
 anxiety
 "approximate answers"
 Asperger
 asphyctic
 avoidance
 Avellis
 Bardet-Biedl
 battered child
 Beckwith-Weideman
 behavioral
 black-patch
 bradykinetic
 brain death
 brain stem
 Briquet
 Brissaud
 Brissaud-Marie
 Bristowe
 callosal disconnection
 Capgras
 cat cry (cri du chat)
 central alveolar hypoventilation
 central sleep apnea
 cerebellar
 characteristic
 characteristic withdrawal
 child abuse

syndrome *(cont.)*
 chromosome 21-trisomy
 chronic
 chronic alcoholic brain (CABS)
 chronic brain (CBS)
 chronic fatigue
 Claude
 Clerambault
 clumsiness
 Collet-Sicard
 concentration camp
 concussion
 confused language (CLS)
 contralateral neglect
 Cornelia de Lange
 Costen
 Cotard
 Creutzfeldt-Jakob
 cri-du-chat
 culturally bound
 culture-bound (CBS)
 culture-specific
 Cushing
 DaCosta
 Dejerine
 de Lange
 delayed sleep phase
 delusional
 dementia-aphonia
 denial visual hallucination
 Dennie-Marfan
 depersonalization
 depressive
 De Sanctis-Cacchione
 Ditthomska
 Down
 drug abstinence
 drug withdrawal
 dysmnesic
 dyspraxia
 effort
 empty nest

syndrome *(cont.)*
  epileptic
  evolution of the
  exhaustion
  extrapyramidal (EPS)
  fatigue
  fetal alcohol
  fragile X
  Franceschetti
  frontal lobe
  Ganser
  general adaptational (GAS)
  Gerstmann
  Gilles de la Tourette
  gray-out
  headache
  Heller
  hepatorenal
  hospital addiction
  Hunt
  Hurler
  hyperactive child
  hyperkinetic
  hyperventilation (HVS)
  intoxication
  irritable
  isolation
  Jackson
  jet lag
  Kallmann
  Kanner
  Kleine-Levin
  Klinefelter
  Klüver-Bucy
  Korsakoff
  lacunar
  Landau-Kleffner
  Lesch-Nyhan
  lobotomy
  Magenblase
  manic-depressive
  Marfan

syndrome *(cont.)*
  Menkes
  migrainous
  Mobius
  Moynahan
  multiple-operations
  Munchausen
  narcolepsy-cataplexy
  neglect
  neurobehavioral
  neuroleptic malignant (NMS)
  nocturnal drinking
  nocturnal eating
  nonsense
  nonspecific
  non-24-hour sleep-wake
  obsession
  obstructive sleep apnea
  organic affective
  organic aggressive
  organic amnestic
  organic anxiety
  organic brain (OBS)
  organic delusional
  organic hallucinatory and
    delusional
  organic hallucinosis
  organic mental
  organic mood
  organic personality
  pain
  pain dysfunction (PDS)
  panic-agoraphobic
  Pierre Robin
  postconcussion
  postcontusion
  postencephalitic
  postleucotomy
  postlobotomy
  posttraumatic
  posttraumatic brain
  posttraumatic cerebral

syndrome *(cont.)*
  posttraumatic stress
  Post-Viet-Nam Psychiatric
    (PVNPS)
  Prader-Willi
  premenstrual (PMS)
  psychological
  psycho-organic
  Ramsay Hunt
  rapid-time-zone change
  rapture-of-the-deep
  restless legs
  Rett
  Rubinstein-Taybi
  schizophrenic
  Schmidt
  reversible affective disorder
  seasonal affective disorder (SADS)
  Seckel
  sensory deprivation (SDS)
  sensory dissociation
  shock
  Sjögren-Larssen
  Smith-Lemli-Opitz
  smoker's
  social breakdown (SBS)
  Sotos
  spasmodic
  Strauss
  sudden unexplained nocturnal death
  Tabagism
  Tapia
  tardive Tourette
  temporomandibular joint
  time zone change
  Tourette (Gilles de la)
  Turner
  Usher
  velocardiofacial
  Vernet
  Wernicke-Korsakoff
  wet brain

syndrome *(cont.)*
  white-out
  Williams
  withdrawal
  wounded-victim
syndrome aphasia
syndrome pattern
synecdoche (figure of speech)
synesthesia
synesthetic stimulation
synkinesis
synkinetic motor movement
synonym
syntactical aphasia
syntonic personality
syntactic aphasia
syntactic categories
syntactic rule
syntagmatic response
syntagmatic word
syntax, rules of
syntaxic language
syntaxic thought
synthesis (pl. syntheses)
  auditory
  distributive analysis and
  phonemic
  speech
synthesizing ability
synthetic drug dependence
synthetic heroin (analog of fentanyl/
  meperidine) dependence
synthetic method
Synthetic Sentence Identification Test
"synthetic THT" (phencyclidine)
syntropy
syphilis
  CNS (central nervous system)
  tertiary
syphilitic meningitis
syphilitic paralytic dementia
syphilitic progressive dementia

syphilophobia
system (pl. systems) (S)
  aculturated into a
  auditory
  autonomic nervous
  categorical
  circadian
  classification
  coding
  delusional
  extrapyramidal (EPS)
  endocrine
  family support
  five-axis
  fixed delusional
  focus of delusional
  genitourinary
  haptic
  hearing aid
  integumentary
  lead
  legal
  limbic
  man-machine
  motor
  multiaxial
  nervous
  neuroendocrine
  neurotransmitter
  nigrostriatal
  peripheral nervous (PNS)
  peripheral vascular
  persecutory delusional
  personality assessment (PAS)
  preferred representational
  psychological defense

system (cont.)
  pyramidal
  representational
  respiratory
  response
  second-messenger
  sensorimotor
  sign
  sleep-wake
  striatal dopaminergic
  symbol set
  sympathetic nervous
  visceral nervous
  well-systematized delusional
System for Testing and Evaluation of
  Potential
System of Multicultural Pluralistic
  Assessment (SOMPA)
System to Plan Early Childhood
  Services (SPECS)
systematic desensitization
systematic method
systematic process
systematic review
systematic study
systematized amnesia
systematized assertive therapy (SAT)
systematized delusion
systemic assertive therapy (SAT)
systemic desensitization
systems agency, health (HSA)
systems interface disorders, psychiatric
systolic pressure (SP)
SZ (schizophrenia)
Szondi Test

T, t

"T" (cannabis; cocaine)
T (transformation)
TA (Transactional Analysis)
Tabagism syndrome
tabetic-form paralytic dementia
table, somatron
taboo
tabophobia
"tabs" (lysergic acid diethylamide)
tabular index
tabulation, allophone
tachistoscope
tachistoscopy viewing
tachophobia
tachycardia
tachylalia
tachylogia
tachyphemia
tachypnea
tachypneic
TACL (Test for Auditory Comprehension of Language)
TACL-R (Tests for Auditory Comprehension of Language–R)
tact
tactful
tactfully

tact operant
tactile agnosia
tactile alexia
tactile amnesia
tactile anomia
tactile aphasia
tactile feedback
Tactile Finger Recognition Test (TFRT)
Tactile Form Recognition Test (TFRT)
tactile genital stimulation
tactile hallucination
tactile illusion
tactile image
tactile information with motor activity
tactile kinesthetic perception
tactile perception
tactile sensation
tactile sensory difficulties
tactile sensory modality
tactile stimulation
tactile stimulus
tactless
Tactual Performance Test (TPT)
taeniophobia
taftian theory
taftian therapy

tag question
TAI (Teacher Attitude Inventory)
TAI (Test Anxiety Inventory)
"tail lights" (lysergic acid diethylamide)
tail, velar
"taima" (cannabis)
take pleasure in few activities
"taking a cruise" (phencyclidine)
taking control
"Takkouri" (cannabis)
talion law or principle
talk
  baby
  parallel
  suicide
talkative
talkativeness
talk-down from overdose
talk therapy
TALPS (Transactional Analysis Life Position Survey)
tangential associations
tangentiality
tangential speech
tangential thinking
tangible reinforcement operant conditioning audiometry (TROCA)
tangles
  Alzheimer
  neurofibrillary
"Tango & Cash" (fentanyl)
Tanner sexual maturity rating
tantrums, temper
TAP (Trainer's Assessment of Proficiency)
TAP-D (Test of Articulation Performance-Diagnostic)
tape-editing
taphophobia
Tapia syndrome
tapinophobia

tap reflex, glabella
TAP-S (Test of Articulation Performance, Screen)
"tar" (heroin; opium)
Tarasoff Decision
Tarasoff Rule
TARC Assessment System
tarda, neurosis
tardive dyskinesia
tardive dystonia
tardive oral dyskinesia
tardive orobuccal dyskinesia
tardive tic
tardive Tourette syndrome
"tardust" (cocaine)
tardy epilepsy
target language
target patient
target response
targets, potential
TAS (Test of Attitude Toward School)
TAS (turning against self)
task
  added purpose
  attend to
  complex
  complex multistep
  continuous performance (CPT)
  dichotic listening
  incomplete sentences
  instrumental
  manipulatory
  necessary
  nine-digit
  nonverbal
  particular
  repetitive
  required
  sentence-closure
  simple
  stay on

task *(cont.)*
  structured
  three-step
  visual memory span
  visual-motor
  word retrieval
task analysis
Task Assessment Scales
task completion
Tasks of Emotional Development
  (TED)
Task-Oriented Assessment
task-oriented group
task performance and analysis
"taste" (heroin; re: drugs dealing)
taste sensation
taste threshold
TAT (Thematic Apperception Test)
TAT (Thematic Aptitude Test)
taurophobia
tautologous
TAWF (Test of Adolescent/Adult
  Word Finding)
"taxing" (crackhouse entrance fee;
  re: drug dealing)
Taylor-Johnson Temperament
  Analysis
Taylor Manifest Anxiety Scale
  (TMAS)
Tay-Sachs disease
TBI (traumatic brain injury)
TBRS (Timed Behavioral Rating
  Sheet)
TBS (Transition Behavior Scale)
"T-buzz" (phencyclidine)
TCA (tricyclic antidepressant)
TCA (tricyclic antipsychotic)
TCMP (Thematic Content Modifica-
  tion Program)
TCP (analog of phencyclidine)
TCP (teacher-child-parent)
TCP (Test of Creative Potential)

TCSM (Test of Cognitive Style in
  Mathematics)
TCSW (Thinking Creatively with
  Sounds and Words)
TCU (Test of Concept Utilization)
TD (threshold of discomfort)
TDD (telephone device for the deaf)
TDE (thiamine deficiency encepha-
  lopathy)
TDF (Thinking Disturbance Factor)
"tea" (cannabis; phencyclidine)
Teacher Attitude Inventory (TAI)
teacher-child-parent (TCP)
Teacher Evaluation Scale (TES)
Teacher Feedback Questionnaire
Teacher Occupational Competency
  Test: Child Care and Guidance,
  NOCTI
Teacher Occupational Competency
  Test: Mechanical Technology,
  NOCTI
Teacher Opinion Inventory
Teacher School Readiness Inventory
  (TSRI)
Teacher Stress Inventory
teaching
  diagnostic
  remedial
teaching alphabet
teaching grammar
teaching hospital
Teaching Style Inventory
team
  interdisciplinary (IDT)
  psychiatry emergency (PET)
  two-person interview
Team Effectiveness Survey (TES)
team leader (TL)
team member (TM)
"tea party" (re: cannabis use)
"teardrops" (re: crack containers)
tearful

tearfulness, breakthrough
tears, esophageal
"tecate" (heroin)
"tecatos" (Hispanic heroin addicts)
technique
  ascending
  bounce (stuttering)
  cognitive-behavioral
  communicative
  compensatory
  corrective
  descending
  head-turn
  high-amplitude sucking (HAS)
  Hood
  Hood masking
  kinesthetic
  multiple regression
  object relations
  plateau-masking
  projective
  psychoanalytic
  psychological
  relapse-prevention
  relaxation
  Rorschach projective
  senior apperception
  sensorineural acuity level masking
  shadowing masking
  short-term psychotherapy
  squeeze (of penis)
  standardized cognitive assessment
  startle
  stop-and-think
  threshold shift-masking
  verbal
technique audiometry
  ascending
  descending
technological detection of deceit
TED (Tasks of Emotional Development)

TEEM (Test for Examining Expressive Morphology)
"teenage" (1/16 gram of methamphetamine)
teenage suicide
teenaged
teenager
"teeth" (cocaine; crack)
teeth
  auditory
  axioversion of
  bicuspid
  buccoversion of
  buck
  canine
  central incisor
  closed-bite malposition of
  cross-bite malposition of
  cuspid
  deciduous
  distoclusion of
  eye
  facioversion of
  first deciduous molar
  first premolar
  Hutchinson
  incisor
  infraversion of
  jumbling of
  labioversion of
  lateral incisor
  linguoversion of
  mesioclusion of
  mesioversion of
  molar
  neutroclusion of
  overbite malposition of
  overjet of
  permanent
  premolar
  second deciduous molar
  second premolar

teeth *(cont.)*
  supernumerary
  supraversion of
  torsiversion of
  transversion of
  underbite malposition of
  wisdom
teeth grinding
teeth malocclusion
teeth malpositions
TEL (Test of Economic Literacy,
  Second Edition)
TELD (Test of Early Language
  Development)
TELD-2 (Test of Early Language
  Development, Second Edition)
teleceptor
telegraphic speech
telegraphic utterance
teleophobia
telepathy, belief in
telephone device for the deaf (TDD)
telephone hearing theory
telephone sex
telephonophobia
telescoped words
television-induced epilepsy
Tell-Me-A-Story (TEMAS)
TEMAS (Tell-Me-A-Story)
Temperament and Values Inventory
Temperament Assessment Battery for
  Children
temperament trait
temperature
  body
  core body
temperature biofeedback
temperature measurement
temperature sensation
temper dyscontrol
temper outburst

temper tantrums
tempestuous
templates
Temple University Short Syntax
  Inventory [Revised] (TUSSI)
temporal association
temporal auditory processing
temporal bones
temporal characteristics of pain
temporal gyri
temporal headache
temporal lobe epilepsy
temporal lobe status
temporal organization
temporal orientation
temporal relationship
temporal skull bones
temporal sulcus (pl. sulci)
  inferior
  superior
temporarily disabled
temporary disability
temporary epilation
temporary habit
temporary stress
temporary threshold shift (TTS)
temporomandibular joint (TMJ)
temporoparietal aphasia
tenacity
tendency (pl. tendencies)
  acting-out
  antisocial
  central
  dependence
  destructive
  excitement-seeking
  familial
  hypomanic
  impulsive
  insightless
  introversive

tendency *(cont.)*
  paranoid
  repeat
  seductive
  self-absorbed
  sleep
  somatization
  tough-minded
tender-minded
Tennessee Self-Concept Scale (TSCS)
tense
  feeling
  future perfect
  future perfect progressive
  past perfect
  past perfect progressive
  perfect
  present perfect
  present perfect progressive
  progressive
  simple
  simple future
  simple future progressive
  simple past
  simple past progressive
  simple present
  simple present progressive
tense gaze
tenseness
tense phoneme
tense vowel
"tension" (crack)
tension
  combat
  inner
  laryngeal
  marked
  muscular
  nervous
  physical
  pre-speech

tension *(cont.)*
  sexual
  social
tension headache
tension migraine headache
tension state psychoneurotic reaction
tension-type headache
tension-vascular headache
tensor muscle of soft palate
TENVAD (Test of Nonverbal Auditory
  Discrimination)
TERA-D/HH (Test of Early Reading
  Ability—Deaf or Hard of Hearing)
teratophobia
terminal
  axon
  clause
terminal achievement behavior
terminal behavior
terminal dementia
terminal insomnia
terminal juncture
terminal lag
terminal string
terminal sulcus
terminal tremor
termination time, voice (VTT)
terms
  abstract
  generic
terrifying stimulus
territoriality
terrorism behavior
terrors
  day (pavor diurnus)
  night (pavor nocturnus)
tertiary prevention
tertiary stress
tertiary syphilis
TES (Teacher Evaluation Scale)
TES (Team Effectiveness Survey)
TES (Therapeutic error signal)

test, diagnostic—a quick-reference list,
including *analysis, appraisal,
assessment, battery, checklist,
evaluation, examination, index,
indicator, interview, inventory,
measurement, profile, question-
naire, scale, score, screen,
survey*
Abbreviated Conners Rating Scale
Abbreviated Conners Teacher
Questionnaire
ABC Inventory–Extended
ability test
Ability-to-Benefit Admissions Test
abnormal involuntary movement
scale (AIMS)
Academic Alertness (AA) test
Academic Aptitude Test (AAT)
Academic Instruction Measurement
System
Acceptance of Disability Scale
(AD Scale)
Access Management Survey
(AMS)
Accounting Program Admission
Test (APAT)
ACER Advanced Test B90, New
Zealand Edition
ACER Applied Reading Test
ACER Tests of Basic Skills–Blue
Series
ACER Tests of Basic Skills–Green
Series
ACER Test of Reasoning Ability
Ackerman-Schoendorf Scales for
Parent Evaluation of Custody
(ASPECT)
ACO: Improving Writing, Think-
ing, and Reading Skills
acoustic immittance measurement
ACT Evaluation/Survey Service
(ESS)

test *(cont.)*
ACT Study Power Assessment and
Inventory (SPA; SPI)
ACT Study Skills Assessment and
Inventory (SSA; SSI)
Activity Losses Assessment (ALA)
Activity Pattern Indicators (APIs)
Actualizing Assessment Battery I:
The Interpersonal Inventories
Actualizing Assessment Battery II:
The Interpersonal Inventories
Acute Panic Inventory
Adaptability Test
Adapted Sequenced Inventory of
Communication Development
(A-SICD)
Adaptive Behavior Evaluation
Scale (ABES)
Adaptive Behavior Inventory for
Children (ABIC)
Adaptive Behavior Scale (ABS)
ADAS noncognitive subscale
ADC Scale
ADD-H: Comprehensive Teacher's
Rating Scale, Second Edition,
(ACTeRS)
Addiction Severity Index (ASI)
Adjective Check List (ACL)
ADL (activities of daily living)
Adolescent Alienation Index
Adolescent-Coping Orientation for
Problem Experiences
Adolescent Diagnostic Interview
(ADI)
Adolescent Drinking Index (ADI)
Adolescent-Family Inventory of
Life Events and Changes
Adolescent Language Screening
Test
Adolescent Life Change Event
Questionnaire (ALCEQ)

test *(cont.)*

Adolescent Multiphasic Personality Inventory

Adolescent Separation Anxiety Test

Adult Basic Learning Examination (ABLE)

Adult Career Concerns Inventory (ACCI)

Adult Neuropsychological Questionnaire (ANQ)

Adult Performance Level Survey (APLS)

Adult Personal Adjustment and Role Skills

adult personal data inventory (APDI)

Adult Personality Inventory (API)

Adult Suicidal Ideation Questionnaire (ASIQ)

Advanced Measures of Music Audiation

Advanced Progressive Matrices

Affects Balance Scale

Age Projection Test (APT)

AGS Early Screening Profiles

AH4 Group Intelligence Test

AH5 Group Test of High Grade Intelligence

AH6 Group Test of High Level Intelligence

AICPA Orientation Test for Professional Accounting

Ainsworth Strange Situation

Alcadd Test

Alcohol Assessment and Treatment Profile

Alcohol Use Inventory (AUI)

Allied Health Professions Admission Test (AHPAT)

Alternate Binaural Loudness Balance (ABLB)

Alternate Lifestyle Checklist (ALC)

test *(cont.)*

Alternate Monaural Loudness Balance (AMLB)

Alzheimer Disease Assessment Scale (ADAS)

American Association of Teachers of Spanish and Portuguese National Spanish Examinations

American Drug and Alcohol Survey

American Law Institute (ALI) Formulation

American Law Institute (ALI) Test

American Occupational Therapy Association, Inc., Fieldwork Evaluation for the Occupational Therapist

amphetamine challenge test

Amytal interview

Analysis of Coping Style

analysis of homonymy

analysis of information

Analysis of Readiness Skills

analysis of transference

analysis of variance (ANOV, ANOVA)

Analytical Reading Inventory

Analytic Learning Disability Assessment

Andresen Six-Basic-Factors-Model (A-SBFM) Questionnaire

Animal and Opposite Drawing Technique (AODT)

Ann Arbor Learning Inventory and Remediation Program

Annett hand preference scale

Anomalous Sentences Repetition Test (ASRT)

Anorexic Behavior Scale

ANSER System

Anton Brenner Developmental Gestalt Test of School Readiness

Anxiety Scales for Children and Adults (ASCA)

test *(cont.)*

Anxiety Scale Questionnaire (ASQ)
Anxiety Disorders Interview
Schedule
anxiety status inventory (ASI)
APGAR Score (adaptability, part-
nership, growth, affection, and
resolve) in families
Aphasia Clinical Battery
Aphasia Language Performance
Scales (ALPS)
aphasia screening test
Appraisal of Language Distur-
bances (ALD)
apprehension test
Apraxia Battery for Adults (ABA)
Aptitude-Intelligence Test Series,
I.P.I.
Aptitude Interest Measurement
Aptitude Survey and Interest
Schedule, Second Edition,
Interest Survey (OASIS-2 IS)
Aptitude Tests for School Begin-
ners (ASB)
Arithmetic Grade Equivalent
Arithmetic Grade Rating
arithmetic subtest
Arizona Articulation Proficiency
Scale (AAPS), Revised
Arizona Battery for Communica-
tion Disorders of Dementia
(ABCD)
Arlin Test of Formal Reasoning
Armed Services Vocational Apti-
tude Battery
articulation index
A Sales Potential Inventory for
Real Estate (ASPIRE)
Assessing Specific Competencies
Assessing Specific Employment
Skill Competencies

test *(cont.)*

Assessment Link Between
Phonology and Articulation
Assessment in Mathematics
assessment of affect
Assessment of Basic Competencies
Assessment of Career Development
(ACT)
Assessment of Career Decision
Making (ACDM)
Assessment of Chemical Health
Inventory
Assessment of Children's Language
Comprehension (ACLC)
Assessment of Conceptual Organi-
zation (ACO)
Assessment of Core Goals (ACG)
Assessment of Intelligibility of
Dysarthric Speech
Assessment of Phonological
Processes, Revised (APP-R)
assessment of recurrent suicidal
behavior
Assessment of Suicide Potential
Assessment Program of Early
Learning Levels (APELL)
Association Adjustment Inventory
Athletic Motivation Inventory
(AMI)
Attention Deficit Disorder Behavior
Rating Scales (ADDBRS)
Attention Deficit Disorders Evalua-
tion Scale (ADDES)
Attitude Survey Program for
Business and Industry
Attitude to School Questionnaire
(ASQ)
Attitudes Toward Disabled Persons
(ATDP)
Attitudes Toward Mainstreaming
Scale (ATMS)

test *(cont.)*
- Attributional Style Questionnaire
- audiometric test
- Auditory Analysis Test
- Auditory Discrimination and Attention Test
- Auditory Pointing Test
- auditory screening test
- Auditory Test W-1/W-2; W-22
- Austin Spanish Articulation Test
- Autism Screening Instrument for Educational Planning
- Autistic Behavior Composite Checklist and Profile
- Automated Child/Adolescent Social History
- autonomy scale
- Balthazar Scales for Adaptive Behavior I: Scales of Functional Independence
- Balthazar Scales for Adaptive Behavior II: Scales of Social Adaptation
- Bankson-Bernthal Test of Phonology (BBTOP)
- Bankson Language Screening Test (BLST)
- Bankson Language Test-2 (BLT-2)
- Barber Scales of Self-Regard for Preschool Children
- Barclay Classroom Climate Inventory (BCCI)
- Barclay Learning Needs Assessment Inventory (BLNAI)
- Barranquilla Rapid Survey Intelligence Test (BARSIT)
- Barron-Welsh Art Scale (BWAS)
- Barry Five Slate System
- Barthel ADL Index
- Basic Achievement Skills Individual Screener
- Basic Concept Inventory

test *(cont.)*
- Basic Educational Skills Test
- Basic Inventory of Natural Language
- Basic Language Concepts Test
- Basic Occupational Literacy Test
- Basic Personality Inventory (BPI)
- Basic Reading Inventory, Fifth Edition (BRI)
- Basic School Skills Inventory (BSSI)—Diagnostic
- Basic School Skills Inventory—Screen
- Basic Screening and Referral Form for Children With Suspected Learning and Behavioral Disabilities
- Basic Skills Assessment Program
- Batelle Developmental Inventory
- Bay Area Functional Performance Evaluation, Second Edition (BaFPE; SIS; TOA)
- Bayley Scales of Infant Development
- Beck Depression Inventory (BDI)
- Beck Hopelessness Scale (BHS)
- Beck Questionnaire
- Bedside Evaluation and Screening Test of Aphasia
- Beery-Buktinica Developmental Test of Visual Motor Integration
- Beery Picture Vocabulary Test and Beery Picture Vocabulary Screening Series (PVS; PVT)
- Behavior Activity Profile (BAP)
- Behavioral Academic Self-Esteem
- Behavioral Assessment of Pain Questionnaire (BAP; P-BAP)
- behavioral avoidance tests (BATs) for OCD
- Behavioral Checklist
- Behavioral Deviancy Profile
- behavioral hearing test
- Behavioral Inattention Test (BIT)

test *(cont.)*

behavioral observation audiometry
(BOA)
Behavioral Observation Scale for
Autism
Behavior Assessment Battery, 2nd
Edition
Behavior Disorders Identification
Scale (BDIS)
Behavior Evaluation Scale–2
(BES-2)
Behavior Problem Checklist (BPC),
Revised
Behavior Rating Instrument for
Autistic and Other Atypical
Children
Behavior Rating Profile, Second
Edition (BRP-2)
Bellevue Index of Depression
Bell Object Relations-Reality
Testing Inventory
Bem Sex-Role Inventory
benchmarks
Bender Gestalt (BG)
Bender-Gestalt Visual Motor Test
Bender Visual Gestalt drawings
Bender Visual-Motor Gestalt Test
(BVMGT)
Bender Visual Retention Test
Bennett Mechanical Comprehension
Test
Benson-Geschwind classification of
aphasia
Benton Revised Visual Retention
Test
Benton Visual Retention Test
(BVRT)
Bexley-Maudsley Automated
Psychological Screening
Big Five Questionnaire (BFQ)
Bilingual Syntax Measure (BSM) II
Test

test *(cont.)*

Bingham Button Test (BBT)
Biographical Inventory Form U
Bipolar Psychological Inventory
Birth to Three Assessment and
Intervention System
Birth to Three Developmental
Scale
Blacky Pictures, The
Blessed Behavior Scale
Blessed Dementia Rating Scale
(BDRS)
Blessed Information-Memory-
Concentration Test
Blind Learning Aptitude Test
Block Survey and S.L.I.D.E.
blood level of illicit drugs test
blood screen for drugs
Bloom Analogies Test
Boder Test of Reading—Spelling
Patterns
Body Image and Eating Question-
naire
body mass index (BMI)
Boehm Test of Basic Concepts,
Revised
Boston Assessment of Severe
Aphasia (BASA)
Boston Classification System
Boston Diagnostic Aphasia
Examination (BDAE)
Boston Naming Test
Boston University Speech Sound
Discrimination Test
Botel Reading Inventory
Bracken Basic Concept Scale
brain electrical activity map (or
mapping) (BEAM)
brain stem auditory evoked poten-
tial (BAEP)
brain stem auditory evoked
response (BAER)

test *(cont.)*

brain stem evoked response audiometry (BSER)

Brief Aphasia Screening Examination (BASE)

Brief Cognitive Rating Scale (BCRS)

Brief Drinker Profile

Brief Life History Inventory (BLHI)

Brief Neuropsychological Mental Status Examination (BNMSE)

brief psychiatric rating scale (BPRS)

brief psychiatric reacting scale (BPRS)

Brief Symptom Inventory

Bristol Language Development Scales (BLADES)

Bristol Social Adjustment Guides

British Ability Scales: Spelling Scale (BAS)

Brook Reaction Test (BRT)

Bruininks-Oseretsky Standardized Test

Bruininks-Oseretsky Test of Motor Proficiency

Bryant-Schwan Design Test (BSDT)

Burks Behavior Rating Scale

Burns/Roe Informal Reading Inventory: Preprimer to Twelfth Grade, Third Edition (IRI)

Buschke Short-Term Recall

Buss-Durkee Hostility Inventory

Bzoch-League Receptive-Expressive Emergent Language Scale

CAGE alcohol use questionnaire (CAGE, an acronym for *cutting* down on drinking, *annoyance* at others' concern about drinking, feeling *guilty* about drinking,

test *(cont.)*

CAGE *(cont.)*

using drinking as an *eye-opener* in the morning)

Cain-Levine Social Competency Scale

calculation test

California Achievement Tests, Fifth Edition (CAT/5)

California Child Q-Set

California Consonant Test

California Critical Thinking Dispositions Inventory (CCTDI)

California Critical Thinking Skills Test (CCTST)

California Life Goals Evaluation Schedules

California Marriage Readiness Evaluation (CMRE)

California Motor Accuracy Test, Southern (Revised)

California Occupational Preference Survey (or System) (COPS)

California Personality Inventory (CPI)

California Phonics Survey

California Preschool Social Competency Scale (CPSCS)

California Psychological Inventory Test (CPIT)

California Q-Sort

California Relative Value Studies (CRVS)

California Short-Form Test of Mental Maturity (CTMM-SF)

California Test of Personality (CTP)

California Verbal Learning Test

Callier-Azusa Scale: G Edition

caloric stimulation test for vestibular function

Camelot Behavioral Checklist (CBC)

Campbell Leadership Index (CLI)

test *(cont.)*

Campbell Organizational Survey (COS)

Canadian Cognitive Abilities Test, Form 7 (CCAT)

Canadian Neurological Scale

Canadian Tests of Basic Skills (CTBS)

Canfield Instructional Styles Inventory

Canter Background Interference Procedure (BIP) for the Bender Gestalt Test

CAP Assessment of Writing

Career Assessment Inventory, Enhanced Version

Career Assessment Inventories: For the Learning Disabled

Career Beliefs Inventory (CBI)

Career Decision-Making (CDM)

Career Decision Scale

Career Development Inventory

Career Maturity Inventory (CMI)

Career Planning Program (CPP)

Career Problem Check List

Caregiver School Readiness Inventory (CSRI)

Caregiver Strain Index

Caring Relationship Inventory (CRI)

Carlson Psychological Survey

Carrell Discrimination Test

Carrow Auditory-Visual Abilities Test

Carrow Elicited Language Inventory (CELI)

Cattell Infant Intelligence Scale

Cattell Personality Factor Questionnaire

Cattell Scales

Center for Epidemiologic Studies Depression Scale (CES-D Scale)

test *(cont.)*

Central Institute for the Deaf Preschool Performance Scale

CERAD Assessment Battery

CFQ-for-others assessment

Change Agent Questionnaire (CAQ)

Charteris Reading Test

Child Abuse Potential Inventory

Child and Adolescent Adjustment Profile

Child Anxiety Scale

Child Assessment Schedule

Child "At Risk" for Drug Abuse Rating Scale (DARS)

Child Autism Rating Scale

Child Behavior Checklist

Child Care and Guidance (NOCTI Teacher Occupational Competency Test)

Child Care Inventory

Child Depression Inventory

Childhood Autism Rating Scale (CARS)

Child Neuropsychological Questionnaire (CNQ)

Child Personality Scale (CPS)

Children of Alcoholism Screening Test (CAST)

Children's Academic Intrinsic Motivation Inventory

Children's Adaptive Behavior Scale, Revised

Children's Affective Rating Scale (CARS)

Children's Apperception Test (CAT)

Children's Apperception Test—Human (CAT-H)

Children's Apperceptive Story-Telling Test (CAST)

Children's Articulation Test (CAT)

test *(cont.)*

Children's Attention and Adjustment Survey (CAAS)
Children's Auditory Verbal Learning Test-2 (CAVLT-2)
Children's Coma Score
Children's Depression Inventory
Children's Depression Rating Scale, Revised (CDRS-R)
Children's Depression Scale, Revised (RCDS)
Children's Depression Scale (CDS), Second Research Edition
Children's Diagnostic Inventory (CDI)
Children's Embedded Figures Test (CDFT)
Children's Hypnotic Susceptibility Scale
Children's Inventory of Self-Esteem (CISE)
Children's Language Battery
Children's Language Processes
Children's Manifest Anxiety Scale, Revised (RCMAS)
Children's Perception of Support Inventory (CPSI)
Children's Personality Questionnaire (CPQ)
Children's Psychiatric Rating Scale (CPRS)
Children's Self-Concept Scale (CSCS)
Children's Version/Family Environmental Scale
Chronic Family Invalid-Depressed (MMPI)
Chronicle Career Quest (R) (CCQ)
Chronological Drinking Record (CDR)
CID Preschool Performance Scale
city and state test

test *(cont.)*

Clarke Reading Self-Assessment Survey
Clark-Madison Test of Oral Language
Clark Picture Phonetic Inventory
Classroom Atmosphere Questionnaire (CAQ)
Classroom Environmental Scale (CES)
Classroom Environment Index
Claybury Selection Battery
Clifton Assessment Procedure for the Elderly
Clinical Analysis Questionnaire (CAQ)
Clinical Appraisal of Psychological Problems (CAPP)
Clinical Dementia Rating Scale (CDR)
Clinical Evaluation of Language Functions, Revised (CELF–R)
Clinical Global Impression of Change (CGIC)
Clinical Global Improvement Scale
Clinical Institute Withdrawal Assessment of Alcohol
clinical performance score (CPS)
Clinical Probes of Articulation Consistency (C-PAC)
Clinical Rating Scale (CRS)
Clinical Scales (MMPI)
Clinical Support System Battery
Clinician Global Rating Scale (CGRS)
Clinician Rated Anxiety Scale (CRAS)
Clinician Rated Overall Life Impairment
Clunis inquiry forensic psychiatry
Clyde Mood Scale (CMS)
Clymer-Barrett Readiness Test

test *(cont.)*

Coarticulation Assessment in Meaningful Language (CAML)
Cognitive Abilities Test (CAT)
Cognitive Behavior Rating Scales
Cognitive Control Battery
Cognitive Diagnostic Battery
Cognitive Observation Guide (COG)
Cognitive Skills Assessment (CSA) Battery
Cold-Running Speech Test
Collaborative Study Psychotherapy Rating Scale
College and University Environment Scales (CUES)
College Basic Academic Subjects Examination
College-Level Examination Program General Examination (CLEP)
College Major Interest Inventory (CMII)
College Student Questionnaires (CSQ)
College Student Satisfaction Questionnaire (CSSQ)
Collis-Romberg Mathematical Problem Solving Profiles
Colorado Educational Interest Inventory
combining power test (CPT)
complex thematic pictures test
Composite Psycholinguistic Age
Composite Risk Index (CRI)
Comprehending Oral Paragraphs
Comprehensive Ability Battery (CAB)
Comprehensive Assessment of Symptoms and History (CASH)
Comprehensive Assessment Program: Achievement Series

test *(cont.)*

Comprehensive Career Assessment Scale (CCAS)
Comprehensive Developmental Evaluation Chart
Comprehensive Drinker Profile
Comprehensive Identification Process (CIP)
Comprehensive Level of Consciousness Scale (CLCS)
Comprehensive Psychiatric Rating Scale (CPRS)
Comprehensive Psychopathological Rating Scale
Comprehensive Test of Adaptive Behavior
Comprehensive Test of Basic Skills, Forms U and V
Comprehensive Test of Visual Functioning (CTVF)
Compton Speech and Language Screening Evaluation
Computer Anxiety Index (Version AZ) (CAIN)
Computer Operator Aptitude Battery (COAB)
Computer Programmer Aptitude Battery (CPAB)
Comrey Personality Scales
concentration performance test
Concept Mastery Test (CMT)
Concept-Specific Anxiety Scale (CAS)
Conceptual Systems Test (CST)
Conditioned Place Preference (CPP)
Conflict in Marriage Scale (CIMS)
Conflict Management Appraisal (CMA)
Conflict Management Survey (CMS)
Conflicts Tactics Scale

test *(cont.)*

confrontation naming test
Conners Hyperkinesis Index–
   Parent Form
Conners Hyperkinesis Index–
   Teacher Form
Conners Parent Questionnaire
   (CPQ)
Conners Parent Rating Scale
   (CPRS-48, CPRS-93)
Conners Teacher Questionnaire
   (CTQ)
Conners Teacher Rating Scale
   (CTRS-28, CTRS-39)
Content Mastery Examinations for
   Educators (CMEE)
Content Scales (MMPI)
continuous performance task or test
   (CPT)
Continuous Performance tetanic
   facilitation test
Continuous Visual Memory Test
   (CVMT)
Conversion V (MMPI)
Cooperation Preschool Inventory,
   Revised
Cooperative Primary Tests (CPT)
Cooper-Farran Behavioral Rating
   Scales (CFBRS)
Cooper-MacGuire Diagnostic Word
   Analysis Test
Coping Operations Preference
   Enquiry (COPE)
Coping Resources Inventory (CRI)
Coping with Stress
Coping with Tests
COPSystem Interest Inventory
copy geometric designs test
copy intersecting pentagons test
Cornell Critical Thinking Tests—
   Level X and Level Z

test *(cont.)*

Cornell Learning and Study Skills
   Inventory (CLASSI)
Cornell Medical Index
Cornell Word Form (CWF)
Correctional Institutions Environ-
   ment Scale
Correctional Officers' Interest Blank
cortical testing
count backwards from 100 test
Couple's Pre-Counseling Inventory
Creativity Assessment Packet
Creativity Attitude Survey (CAS)
Creativity Checklist
Creativity Tests for Children (CTC)
criterion-referenced test
Criterion Test of Basic Skills
Critical Reasoning Tests (CRT)
Crowley Occupational Interests
   Blank (COIB)
Cultural Attitude Inventories (CAI)
Cultural Attitude Scales (CAS)
Cultural Literacy Test
Culture Fair Intelligence Test
   (CFIT)
Culture-Free Self-Esteem Inven-
   tories, Second Edition (CFSEI-2)
Culture-Free Self-Esteem Inventories
   for Children and Adults
Culture Shock Inventory
Current and Past Psychopathology
   Scales (CAPPS)
Curtis Completion Form
Curtis Interest Scale
Custody Quotient, The
Daberon Screening for School
   Readiness
DART Phonics Testing Program
   (Diagnostic and Achievement
   Reading Tests)
day of month test

test *(cont.)*

Death Anxiety Scale (DAS)
Death Personification Exercise
(DPE)
Decision Making Inventory
Decision-Making Organizer
Decoding Skills Test
deep articulation test
Defense Functioning Scale (DFS)
Defense Mechanism Inventory
(DMI)
Defensive Functioning Scale (DFS)
Degrees of Reading Power (DRP)
Del Rio Language Screening Test
(DRLST)
Del Rio Language Screening Test,
English/Spanish
Dementia Behavior Disturbance
Scale (DBD)
Dementia Mood Assessment Scale
(DMAS)
Dennis Test of Child Development
(DCD)
Denver Articulation Screening
Examination (DASE, D.A.S.E.)
Denver Developmental Screening
Test (DDST)
Denver Prescreening Development
Questionnaire, Revised (R-PDQ)
Denver II test
Depression Adjective Check List
(DACL)
Depression Rating
Depression "2" Scale
Depressive Experiences Question-
naire (DEQ)
Description of Body Scale
Determining Needs in Your Youth
Ministry
Detroit Test of Learning Aptitude–
Adult (DTLA-A)

test *(cont.)*

Detroit Test of Learning Aptitude–
Third Edition (DTLA-3)
Detroit Test of Learning Aptitude–
Primary, Second Edition (DTLA-
P:2)
Detroit Tests of Learning Aptitude
(DTLA)
Developing Skills Checklist (DSC)
Developmental Activities Screening
Inventory (DASI)
Developmental Articulation Test
(DAT)
Developmental Assessment of Life
Experiences (D.A.L.E. System)
Developmental Indicators for As-
sessment of Learning–Revised/
AGS Edition (DIAL-R)
Developmental Sentence Scoring
(DOS)
Developmental Test of Visual-Motor
Integration (VMI), Third Edition
Developmental Test of Visual Per-
ception (DTVP)
Devereux Adolescent Behavior
Rating Scale
Devereux Child Behavior Rating
Scale
Devereux Elementary School
Behavior Rating Scale II
(DESBRS-II)
dexamethasone suppression test
Diabetes Opinion Survey and Parent
Diabetes Opinion Survey
Diagnostic Achievement Battery,
Second Edition (DAB-2)
Diagnostic Achievement Test for
Adolescents
Diagnostic Analysis of Reading
Errors
Diagnostic and Therapeutic Tech-
nology Assessment (DATTA)

test *(cont.)*

diagnostic articulation test
Diagnostic Assessments of Reading (DAR)
Diagnostic Checklist for Behavior-Disturbed Children Form E-2
Diagnostic Employability Profile
Diagnostic Interview for Borderlines, Revised
Diagnostic Interview Schedule (DIS)
Diagnostic Mathematics Inventory (DMI)
Diagnostic Mathematics Profiles
Diagnostic Reading Scales: Revised
Diagnostic Skills Battery
Diagnostic Tests and Self-Helps in Arithmetic
Dichotic Consonant-Vowel Test
Dichotic Digits Test
Differential Ability Scales
Differential Aptitude Tests (DAT), Fifth Edition
Differential Aptitude Tests for Personnel and Career Assessment (DAT for PCA)
Differential Test of Conduct and Emotional Problems (DT/CEP)
Digital Finger Tapping Test (DFTT)
digit repetition test
digit reversal test
digit span (DS) subtest
digit symbol
diminished reality testing
disability status scale (DSS)
Dissociate Disorders Interview Schedule
Dissociative Experiences Scale (DES)
Diversity Awareness Profile (DAP)

test *(cont.)*

DMI Mathematics Systems Instructional Objectives Inventory
Dodd Test of Time Estimation
Dole Vocational Sentence Completion Blank
Doren Diagnostic Reading Test of Word Recognition Skills
Dos Amigos Verbal Language Scales
draw a clock face test
Draw-A-Family test
draw a house test
Draw A Person: Screening Procedure for Emotional Disturbance (DAP:SPED)
draw a picture from memory test
drawing test
Driver Risk Inventory (DRI)
drug screening test
Durrell Analysis of Reading Difficulty: Third Edition
Dyadic Parent-Child Interaction Coding System
Dynamic Personality Inventory (DPI)
Dyslexia Determination Test
Dyslexia Screening Survey, The
Early Child Development Inventory
Early Coping Inventory
Early Development Scale for Preschool Children
Early Language Milestone Scale
Early School Assessment (ESA)
Early School Personality Questionnaire (ESPQ)
Early Screening Inventory
Early Social Communication Scale (ESCS)
Early Speech Perception Test (ESP)
Early Years Easy Screen (EYES)

test *(cont.)*

Eating Disorder Inventory-2
(EDI-2)

Eating Disorder Inventory for
Children

Eating Inventory

Eby Elementary Identification
Instrument

Edinburgh Articulation Test (EAT)

Edinburgh Functional Communication Profile, Revised (EFCP)

Edinburgh Handedness Inventory

Edinburgh Picture Test

Edinburgh Reading Tests

Edinburgh Rehabilitation Status
Scale

Edinburgh-2 Coma Scale

Educational Development Series

Education Apperception Test (EAT)

Edwards Personal Preference
Schedule (EPPS)

Effective School Battery, The (ESB)

Effective Reading Tests

Egocentricity Index

Ego Development Scale (EDS)

Ego Function Assessment

Ego-Ideal and Conscience
Development Test (EICDT)

Ego State Inventory (ESI)

Eidetic Parents Test (EPT)

Eight State Questionnaire

Elicited Articulatory System Evaluation

Elihorn Maze Test

Elizur Test of Psycho-Organicity:
Children & Adults

Embedded Figures Test (EFT)

Emotional and Behavior Problem
Scale (EBPS)

Emotions Profile Index

Employability Inventory

Employee Aptitude Survey Tests

test *(cont.)*

Employee Attitude Inventory

Employee Effectiveness Profile

Employee Reliability Inventory
(ERI)

Endler Multidimensional Anxiety
Scales (EMAS; EMAS-P;
EMAS-S; EMAS-T)

English Language Institute Listening Comprehension Test

English/Spanish Del Rio Language
Screening Test

Enhanced ACT Assessment

Environmental Language Inventory
(ELI)

Environmental Pre-Language
Battery

Environmental Response Inventory
(ERI)

Erhardt Developmental Prehension
Assessment (EDPA)

Erhardt Developmental Vision
Assessment (EDVA)

Escala de Inteligencia Wechsler
para Adultos (EIWA)

Evaluating Acquired Skills in
Communication (EASIC),
Revised

Evaluating Communicative Competence: A Functional Pragmatic Procedure

Evaluating Educational Programs
for Intellectually Gifted Students

Evaluating Movement and Posture
Disorganization in Dyspraxic
Children

Evaluating the Participant's Employability Skills

Evaluation Disposition (Toward
the) Environment (EDEN)

Examining for Aphasia Test

Executive Profile Survey

test *(cont.)*

    Exner Scoring System (Rorschach test)

    Experiential World Inventory (EWI)

    Expressive One-Word Picture Vocabulary Test–Revised (EOWPVT-R)

    Expressive One-Word Picture Vocabulary Test–Upper Extension

    Extended Merrill-Palmer Scale

    Extended Personal Attributes Questionnaire (EPAQ)

    Eysenck Personality Inventory (EPI)

    Eysenck Personality Questionnaire (EPQ)

    Eysenck's Psychoticism Scale

    Facial Action Coding System (FACS)

    Family Adaptability and Cohesion Evaluation Scales III (FACES III)

    Family Apperception Test (FAT)

    Family Aptitudes Questionnaire (FAQ)

    Family Attitudes Test (FAT)

    Family Drawing Depression Scale (FDDS)

    Family Environment Scale, Second Edition (FES)

    Family Inventory of Life Events and Changes (FILE)

    Family Relationship Inventory

    Family Relations Test (FRT): Children's Version

    Family Satisfaction Scale

    Famous Sayings Test

    FAS Word Fluency Test

    Fear Survey Schedule (FSS) for Children–Revised

test *(cont.)*

    15-Item Memorization Test

    Figurative Language Interpretation Test (FLIT)

    Finger Localization Test (FLT)

    Finger Oscillation Test

    Fingertip Number Writing Perception

    Fisher-Logemann Test of Articulation Competence (FLTAC)

    Five P's: Parent Professional Preschool Performance Profile

    Flanagan Aptitude Classification Test (FACT)

    Flanagan Industrial Tests (FIT)

    Fleishman Job Analysis Survey (F-JAS)

    Flint Infant Security Scale (FISS)

    Florida International Diagnostic–Prescriptive Vocational Competency Profile

    Florida Kindergarten Screening Battery

    Flowers Auditory Screening Test (FAST)

    Flowers Auditory Test of Selective Attention (FATSA)

    Flowers-Costello Tests of Central Auditory Abilities

    Follow-up Drinker Profile

    Folstein Mini-Mental Status Examination

    Forer Structured Sentence Completion Test

    48-Item Counseling Evaluation Test (ICET)

    forward digital span recall test

    Foster Mazes

    Fourier analysis

    Four Picture Test

    Franck Drawing Completion Test (FDCT)

test *(cont.)*

Freedom from Distractibility Deviation Quotient (FDDQ)
Freeman Anxiety Neurosis and Psychosomatic Test (FANPT)
Freiburger Personality Inventory (FPI)
Frenchay Activities Index
Frenchay Aphasia Screening Test (FAST)
Frenchay Dysarthria Assessment
Frostig Developmental Test of Visual Perception (FDTVP)
Frostig Movement Skills Test Battery (FMSTB)
Frost Self-Description Questionnaire (FSDQ)
Fuld Object-Memory Evaluation
Fullerton Language Test for Adolescents
Full-Range Picture Vocabulary Test
Full Scale Broad Cognitive Ability
Full-Scale Intelligence Quotient (FSIQ)
Full-Scale Score Total (FSST)
Functional Assessment Inventory
Functional Independence Measure (FIM)
Functional Limitation Profile
Functional Needs Assessment (FNA)
Functional Performance Record (FPR)
Functional Pragmatic Procedure (Evaluating Communicative Competence)
Functional Status Questionnaire (FSQ)
Functional Time Estimation Questionnaire (FTEQ)

test *(cont.)*

Fundamental Interpersonal Relations Orientation–Behavior (FIRO-B)
Fundamental Interpersonal Relations Orientation–Feelings (FIRO-F)
fund of information test
GAF scale score
Galveston Orientation and Awareness Test (GOAT)
Gardner Analysis of Personality Survey (GAP)
Gates-MacGinitie Reading Test, Third Edition
Gates-McKillop-Horowitz Reading Diagnostic Tests
General Aptitude Test Battery (GATB)
General Clerical Test (GCT)
General Cognitive Index (GCI)
General Health Questionnaire (GHQ)
Geriatric Depression Scale
Gerontological Apperception Test (GAT)
Gesell Child Development Age Scale (GCDAS)
Gesell Developmental Schedules
Gesell Preschool Test
Gesell School Readiness Test
Gifted and Talented Screening Form
Gifted Evaluation Scale (GES)
Gifted Program Evaluation Survey
Gillingham-Childs Phonics Proficiency Scales: Series I and II
Gilmore Oral Reading Test
Glasgow Assessment Schedule
Glasgow Coma Scale (GCS)
Glasgow Outcome Scale

test *(cont.)*

Global Assessment of Functioning (GAF) Scale (Axis V)
Global Assessment of Relational Functioning (GARF) Scale
Global Assessment Scale (GAS)
Global Sexual Satisfaction Index (GSSI)
Goldberg Index
Goldman-Fristoe Test of Articulation
Goldman-Fristoe-Woodcock Auditory Skills Test Battery
Goldman-Fristoe-Woodcock Test of Auditory Discrimination
Goldstein-Scheerer Tests of Abstract and Concrete Thinking
Golombok Rust Inventory of Marital State (GRIMS)
Goodenough "Draw-A-Man"
Goodenough-Harris Drawings Test
Gordon Personal Inventory (GPI)
Gordon Personal Profile Inventory
Graded Naming Test
Graded Word Spelling Test
Graduate and Managerial Assessment
Graduate Records Examination (GRE)
Graduate Records Examination Aptitude Test (GREAT)
Grammatical Analysis of Elicited Language (GAEL)
Grassi Basic Cognitive Evaluation (GBCE)
Grassi Block Substitution Test
Gray Oral Reading Tests, Third Edition (GORT-3)
Gregorc Style Delineator
Grid Test of Schizophrenic Thought Disorder (GTSTD)
Grief Experience Inventory (GEI)

test *(cont.)*

Grip-Strength Test
Grooved Pegboard Test
Group Achievement Identification Measure
Group Embedded Figures Test (GEFT)
Group Environment Scale (GES)
Group Encounter Scale (GES)
Group Inventory for Finding Creative Talent
Group Reading Test, Third Edition (GRT)
Group Styles Inventory (GSI)
Group Tests of Musical Abilities
Guilford-Zimmerman Aptitude Survey (GZAS)
Guilford-Zimmerman Interest Inventory (GZII)
Guilford-Zimmerman (GZ) Personality Test
Guilford-Zimmerman Temperament Survey (GZTS)
Hahnemann Elementary School Behavior Rating Scale
Hahnemann High School Behavior Rating Scale
Hall Occupational Orientation Inventory (HOOI)
Halstead and Reitan Batteries
Halstead Aphasia Test (HAT)
Halstead Category Test
Halstead-Reitan Battery
Halstead-Reitan Neurological Battery and Allied Procedures
Halstead-Reitan Neuropsychologic Test Battery (HRNTB)
Halstead-Reitan Neuropsychological Test Battery for Adults
Halstead-Russell Neuropsychological Evaluation System (HRNES)

test *(cont.)*

Halstead-Wepman Aphasia Screening Test

Hamburg-Wechsler Intelligence Test for Children (HAWIC)

Hamilton Anxiety (scale) (HAMA)

Hamilton Anxiety Rating Scale (HARS)

Hamilton Depression (scale) (HAMD)

Hamilton Depression Rating Scale (HDRS)

Hamilton Rating Scale for Depression

Hand Test (HT)

Haptic Intelligence Scale (HIS)

Harding W87 Test

Hare Psychopathy Checklist–Revised (PCL-R)

Harrington-O'Shea Career Decision-Making System, Revised (CDM-R)

Harris-Lingoes Subscales–MMPI

Harvard Group Scale of Hypnotic Susceptibility (HGSHS)

Hawaii Early Learning Profile (HELP)

Haws Screening Test for Functional Articulation Disorders

Health Assessment Questionnaire (HAQ)

Health Care Questionnaire

Henderson-Moriarty ESL/Literacy Placement Test

Hendler Test for Chronic Pain (HTCP)

Henmon-Nelson Ability Test, Canadian Edition

Henmon-Nelson Tests of Mental Ability

Hereford Parental Attitude [survey] (HPA)

test *(cont.)*

Hess School Readiness Scale (HSRS)

Heston Personality Index (HPI)

Heterosexual Attitudes Toward Homosexuality [scale] (HATH)

High School Career-Course Planner (HSCCP)

High School Personality Questionnaire (HSPQ)

Hill Interaction Matrix (HIM)

Hilson Adolescent Profile

Hilson Personnel Profile/Success Quotient (HPP/SQ)

Hiskey-Nebraska Test of Learning Aptitude (HNTLA)

Hodkinson Mental Test (HMT)

Hogan Personality Inventory and Hogan Personnel Selection Series

Holtzman Inkblot Technique (HIT)

Home Environment Questionnaire

Home Observation for Measurement of the Environment

Home Screening Questionnaire

Hooper Visual Organization Test (VOT)

Hopkins Symptom Checklist-90 Total Score (HSCL-90 T)

Hospital Anxiety and Depression Scale

Hostility and Direction of Hostility Questionnaire (HDHQ)

house-tree-person test (HTP, H-T-P)

house-tree test (HT, H-T)

Houston Test for Language Development

Howell Prekindergarten Screening Test

How-I-See-Myself Scale (HISMS)

test *(cont.)*

Human Information Processing
Survey
Hundred Pictures Naming Test
(HPNT)
Hutchins Behavior Inventory (HBI)
Hymovich Chronicity Impact and
Coping Instrument (CICI)
Hypnotic Induction Profile (HIP)
IDEA Oral Language Proficiency
Test
IDEA Oral Language Proficiency
Test–II
IDEA System
I-E Scale (internal versus external
scale)
Illinois Children's Language As-
sessment Test
Illinois Test of Psycholinguistic
Abilities (ITPA)
Illness Behavior Questionnaire
immediate memory test
immittance testing
Impact Message Inventory, Re-
search Edition (IMI)
Impact of Event Scale
Improving Writing, Thinking, and
Reading Skills (ACO)
Impulsive Nonconformity Scale
Incomplete Sentences Survey
Incomplete Sentences Task
Independent Living Behavior
Checklist
Index of Well-Being (IWB)
Individual Career Exploration
(ICE)
Individualized Criterion Referenced
Testing (ICRT)
Individualized Criterion Referenced
Testing Reading (ICRTR)
Individualized Criterion Referenced
Testing Mathematics (ICRTM)

test *(cont.)*

Individual Phonics Criterion Test
Infant Reading Tests
Infant/Toddler Environment Rating
Scale (ITERS)
inferential behavioral monitoring
Inferred Self-Concept Scale
Informal Reading Comprehension
Placement Test
inkblot test (IBT)
Inpatient Multidimensional
Psychiatric Scale (IMPS)
Input Receptive Language
Processing
Inquiry Mode Questionnaire: A
Measure of How You Think
and Make Decisions (INQ)
Institute of Educational Research
(intelligence) Test (IER Test)
Institutional Functioning Inventory
(IFI)
Institutional Goals Inventory (IGI)
Instructional Environment Scale,
The (TIES)
Instructional Leadership Inventory
instrumental ADL measurement
Instrument Timbre Preference Test
Integrated Assessment System
(IAS)
intelligence test
Interest Check List
Intermediate Booklet Category Test
Intermediate Personality Question-
naire (IPQ)
internal versus external scale (I-E
Scale)
International Primary Factors (test
battery) (IPF)
International Test for Aphasia
International Version of the Mental
Status Questionnaire

test *(cont.)*

Interpersonal Cognitive Problem-Solving (ICPS)

Interpersonal Language Skills and Assessment (ILSA)

Interpersonal Language Skills Assessment: Final Edition

Interpersonal Perception Scale (IPS)

Interpersonal Reaction Test (IPRT)

Interpersonal Style Inventory

Inter-Person Perception Test (IPPT)

interpretation test

Intimacy Potential Quotient (IPQ)

Intra- and Interpersonal [Relations Scale] (IIP)

intracorporeal pharmacological testing

Intrex Questionnaires

Introvertive Anhedonia Scale

Inventory for Client and Agency Planning

Inventory for Counseling and Development

Inventory of Individually Perceived Group Cohesiveness

Inventory of Language Abilities and Inventory of Language Abilities II (ILA, ILA-II)

Inventory of Peer Influence on Eating Concerns

Inventory of Perceptual Skills (IPS)

Inventory of Psychosocial Development (IPD)

Inwald Personality Inventory (IPI), Revised

Iowa Algebra Aptitude Test, Fourth Edition (IAAT)

Iowa Conners Rating Scale

test *(cont.)*

Iowa Pressure Articulation Test (IPAT)

Iowa Severity Rating Scales for Speech and Language Impairments

Iowa Tests of Basic Skills, Forms G and H

Iowa Tests of Educational Development, Forms X-8 and Y-8

IPAT Anxiety Scale

IPAT Depression Scale

Irish Study of High-Density Schizophrenia Families

irresistible impulse test

Is This Autism? A Checklist of Behaviors and Skills for Children Showing Autistic Features

It Scale for Children (ITSC)

Jackson Evaluation System

Jackson Personality Inventory (JPI)

Jackson Vocational Interest Survey (JVIS)

James Language Dominance Test

Jansky Screening Index (JSI)

Jenkins Activity Survey (JAS)

Jenkins Non-Verbal Test

Jesness Behavior Checklist (JBC)

Jesness Inventory (JI)

Jette Functional Status Index

Jevs Work Sample Battery

Job Attitude Scale (JAS)

Job Descriptive Index (JDI)

Job Seeking Skills Assessment

Johnson-Kenney Screening Test (JKST)

Johnston Informal Reading Inventory (JIRI)

Jordan Left-Right Reversal Test

Joseph Pre-School and Primary Self-Concept Screening Test

test *(cont.)*

Judgment of Line Orientation
(JLO)

Judgment of Occupational
Behavior-Orientation

Junior Eysenck Personality Inventory (JEPI)

K-corrected raw score

Kahn Intelligence Tests (KIT)

Kahn Test of Symbol Arrangement
(KTSA)

Kasanin-Hanfmann Concept Formation Test

Katz Adjustment Scales (KAS)

Katz ADL Index

Kaufman Adolescent and Adult
Intelligence Test (KAIT)

Kaufman Assessment Battery for
Children (KABC)

Kaufman Brief Intelligence Test
(K-BIT)

Kaufman Development Scale

Kaufman Infant and Preschool
Scale

Kaufman Survey of Early Academic and Language Skills
(K-SEALS)

Kaufman Test of Education
Achievement

Keegan Type Indicator

Keirsey Temperament Sorter

Kendrick Cognitive Tests for the
Elderly

Kenny ADL Index

Kenny Self-Care Evaluation

Kenny Self-Care Questionnaire

Kent Infant Development Scale

Kerby Learning Modality Test,
Revised

KeyMath Revised: A Diagnostic
Inventory of Essential Mathematics

test *(cont.)*

Kindergarten Auditory Screening
Test (KAST)

Kindergarten Language Screening
Test (KLST)

Kindergarten Readiness Test
(KRT)

Kinetic Family Drawings (KFD)

Knowledge of Occupations Test
(KOT)

Knox's Cube Test

Kolbe Conative Index (KCI)

Koppitz Scoring System for
Organicity

Kuder General Interest Survey,
Form E

Kuder Occupational Interest
Survey (KOIS)

Kuder Preference Record-Vocational (KPR-V)

Lambeth Disability Screening
Questionnaire

Language Modalities Test for
Aphasia

Language Processing Test

Language Sampling, Analysis, and
Training

Language-Structured Auditory
Retention Span (LARS)

language test

Laterality Preference Schedule

Leader Behavior Analysis II
(LBAII)

Leader Behavior Description
Questionnaire (LBDQ)

Leadership Ability Evaluation

Leadership Evaluation and Development Scale (LEADS)

Leadership Opinion Questionnaire
(LOQ)

Leadership Practices Inventory
(LPI)

test *(cont.)*

Leadership Skills Inventory
Learning and Study Strategies Inventory (LASSI)
Learning Disability Evaluation Scale (LDES)
Learning Disability Rating Procedure
Learning Efficiency Test-II (LET-II)
Learning Inventory of Kindergarten Experiences (LIKE)
Learning Styles Inventory
Learning Style Profile (LSP)
Least Preferred Coworker Score
Leatherman Leadership Questionnaire (LLQ)
Leeds Scales for the Self-Assessment of Anxiety and Depression
Leisure Activities Blank (LAB)
Leisure Diagnostic Battery
Leiter Adult Intelligence Scale
Leiter International Performance Scale
Leiter Recidivism Scale
"Let's Talk" Inventory for Adolescents
letter cancellation test
level of demarcation in sensory testing
Levine-Pilowsky Depression Questionnaire
Leyton Obsessive Inventory (LOI)
Life Event Scale Adolescents
Life Event Scale Children
Life Experiences Checklist (LEC)
Life Satisfaction Index (LSI)
Life Skills, Forms 1 & 2
Life Styles Inventory (LSI)
Limon Self-Image Assessment

test *(cont.)*

Lincoln-Oseretsky Motor Development Scale
Lincoln-Oseretsky Motor Performance Test (LOMPT)
Lindamood Auditory Conceptualization Test (LACT)
Linguistic Analysis of Speech Samples (LASS)
Linguistic Awareness in Reading Readiness
Lista de Destrezas en Desarrollo (La Lista)
Listening Comprehension Test (LCT)
Loevinger's Washington University Sentence Completion Test
logical memory test
LOI (Leyton Obsessive Inventory)
Lollipop Test: A Diagnostic Screening Test of School Readiness
Lombard Test
London Psychogeriatric Scale (LPS)
Longitudinal Interval Follow-Up Evaluation
Look and Say Articulation Test
Lorge-Thorndike Intelligence Test/ Cognitive Abilities Test
LOTE Reading and Listening Tests
Louisville Behavior Checklist
Luria-Nebraska Neuropsychological Battery
Luria's Neuropsychological Investigation
Luria test
MacAndrew Addiction Scale (MAS)
Machover Draw-A-Person (MDAP) test

test *(cont.)*

Macmillan Graded Word Reading Test

Maferr Inventory of Masculine Values (MIMV)

Make-A-Picture-Story (MAPS)

making change (money) test

Male Impotence Test (MIT)

Management Appraisal Survey (MAS)

Management Development Profile

Management Inventory on Leadership, Motivation and Decision-Making (MILMD)

Management Philosophies Scale (MPS)

Management Position Analysis Test

Management Readiness Profile

Management Styles Inventory

Managerial Style Questionnaire (MSQ)

Manager Style Appraisal

Mandel Social Adjustment Scale (MSAS)

Mania "9" Scale

mania rating scale (MRS)

Marital Attitudes Evaluation (MATE)

Marital Communication Scale

Marital Satisfaction Inventory

Marlow-Crowne (Social Desirability) Scale (MCS)

Marriage Adjustment Inventory (MAI)

Marriage and Family Attitude Survey

Martin S-D (suicide-depression) Inventory (MSDI)

Martinez Assessment of the Basic Skills

Maryland Parent Attitude Survey

Masculinity-femininity "5" Scale

test *(cont.)*

Maslach Burnout Inventory (MBI), Second Edition

Matching Familiar Figures Test (MFFT)

Maternal Attitude Scale (MAS)

Math Achievement

Mathematics Anxiety Rating Scale (MARS)

Mathematics Anxiety Rating Scale Adolescents (MARS-A)

Matrix Analogies Test

Maudsley Obsessional Compulsive Inventory (MOCI)

Maudsley Personality Inventory

Maxfield-Buchholz Social Maturity Scale for Blind Preschool Children

McCarthy Scales of Children's Abilities (MSCA)

McCarthy Screening Test

McGill Pain Questionnaire

McMaster Health Index Questionnaire

Measurement of Language Development

Measures of Musical Abilities

Measures of Psychosocial Development (MPD)

Mechanical Technology (NOCTI Teacher Occupational Competency Test)

Meeting Street School Screening Test (MSSST)

Mega Test

Memory Assessment Scales (MAS)

Memory-for-Designs test (MFD)

memory for digits test

Menstrual Distress Questionnaire (MDQ)

Mental Deterioration Battery (MBD)

test *(cont.)*

mental status examination (MSE)
Mental Status Examination Record
(MSER)
mental status schedule (MSS)
mental status test
Mertens Visual Perception Test
(MVPT)
methylphenidate challenge
Metropolitan Achievement Tests,
Seventh Edition (MAT7)
Metropolitan Language Instruc-
tional Test
Metropolitan Readiness Tests,
Fifth Edition (MRT)
Meyer-Kendall Assessment Survey
(MKAS)
Michigan Alcoholism Screening
Test (MAST)
Michigan English Language
Assessment Battery
Michigan Picture Stories
Michigan Picture Test, Revised
Michigan Screening Profile of
Parenting
Miles ABC Test of Ocular
Dominance
Military Environment Inventory
Miller Analogies Test (MAT)
Miller Assessment for Preschoolers
Miller-Yoder Language Compre-
hension Test (Clinical Edition)
Mill Hill Vocabulary Scale
Millon Adolescent Clinical Inven-
tory (MACI)
Millon Adolescent Personality
Inventory
Millon Behavioral Health Inven-
tory (MBHI)
Millon Clinical Multiaxial Inven-
tory-II (MCMI-II)

test *(cont.)*

Milwaukee Academic Interest
Inventory (MAII)
Mini Inventory of Right Brain
Injury (MIRBI)
Mini-Mental State Examination
Minimum Auditory Capabilities
(MAC) Test
Minimum Essentials Test (MET)
Minnesota Child Developmental
Inventory (MCDI)
Minnesota Clerical Assessment
Battery
Minnesota Engineering Analogies
Test (MEAT)
Minnesota-Hartford Personality
Assay (MHPA)
Minnesota Importance Question-
naire
Minnesota Infant Development
Inventory
Minnesota Job Description Ques-
tionnaire (MJDQ)
Minnesota Manual Dexterity Test
Minnesota Multiphasic Personality
Inventory (MMPI)
Minnesota Multiphasic Personality
Inventory, Adolescent
(MMPI-A)
Minnesota Multiphasic Personality
Inventory, Second Edition
(MMPI-2)
Minnesota Percepto-Diagnostic
Test (MPDT)
Minnesota Preschool Scales
Minnesota Rate of Manipulation
Tests
Minnesota Satisfaction Question-
naire (MSQ)
Minnesota Satisfaction Scales
(MSS)

test *(cont.)*

Minnesota Scholastic Aptitude Test (MSAT)

Minnesota Spatial Relations Test (MSRT)

Minnesota Teacher Attitude Inventory (MTAI)

Minnesota Test for Differential Diagnosis of Aphasia

Minnesota Test of Aphasia

Minnesota Vocational Interest Inventory (MVII)

Miskimins Self-Goal-Other Discrepancy Scale

misplaced objects test

Missouri Children's Picture Series (MCPS)

Missouri Kindergarten Inventory of Developmental Skills

Modern Language Aptitude Test

Modern Occupational Skills Test (MOST)

Modified Health Assessment Questionnaire (MHAQ)

Modified Vygotsky Concept Formation Test

Modified Word Learning Test (MWLT)

Monaural Loudness Balance (MLB) Test

Monitoring Basic Skills Progress (MBSP)

Monotic Word Memory Test (MWMT)

Montgomery and Asberg Depression Rating Scale (MADRS)

month of year test

Mooney Problem Check List (MPCL)

Morbid Anxiety Inventory (MAI)

Mother-Child Relationship Evaluation (MCRE)

test *(cont.)*

Mother/Infant Communication Screening (MICS)

Motivational Patterns Inventory

Motivation Analysis Test (MAT)

Motor-Free Visual Perception Test (MVPT)

Motor Impersistence Test (MIT)

Motor Steadiness Battery

Movement Disorder Questionnaire

Mullen Scales of Early Learning

Multidimensional Aptitude Battery

Multidimensional Assessment of Gains in School (MAGS)

Multidimensional Assessment of Philosophy of Education (MAPE)

multidimensional scale for rating psychiatric patients (MSRPP)

Multidimensional Self Concept Scale (MSCS)

Multifactor Leadership Questionnaire (MLQ)

multi-item test

Multilevel Informal Language Inventory

Multilingual Aphasia Examination (MAE)

Multiphasic Environmental Assessment Procedure (MEAP)

Multiphasic Personality Inventory (MPI)

Multiple Sleep Latency Test (MSLT)

multiplication table test

Multiscore Depression Inventory (MDI)

Murphy-Meisgeier Type Indicator for Children (MMTIC)

Music Achievement Tests 1, 2, 3, and 4 (MAT)

Musical Aptitude Profile (MAP)

Myers-Briggs Type Indicator (MBTI)

Nalline test

test *(cont.)*

Names Learning Test (NLT)
name the date test
naming common objects test
National Adult Reading Test,
    Second Edition (NART)
National Business Competency
    Tests
National Educational Development
    Tests
National Occupation Competency
    Testing (NOCTI)
National Police Officer Selection
    Test (POST)
Natural Process Analysis
Naylor-Harwood Adult Intelligence
    Scale (NHAIS)
need a sentence test
Need for Cognition Scale
NEO Five Factor Inventory
Neonatal Behavioral Assessment
    Scale (NBAS)
Neonatal Behavioral Assessment
    Scale with Kansas Supplements
    (NBAS-K)
NEO Personality Inventory, Re-
    vised (NEO-PI-R)
Neurobehavioral Cognitive Status
    Examination
Neurobehavioral Rating Scale
neuropsychological battery of tests
Neuropsychological Screening
    Exam
Neuropsychological Status Exami-
    nation
neuropsychometric test
Neuroticism Scale Questionnaire
    (NSQ)
Neurotic Personality Factor Test
    (NPFT)
New Jersey Test of Reasoning
    Skills

test *(cont.)*

New Mexico Attitude Toward
    Work Test (NMATWT)
New Mexico Career Planning
    Testing (NMCPT)
New Mexico Job Application
    Procedures Test (NMJAPT)
New Mexico Knowledge of Occu-
    pations Test (NMKOT)
New York University Parkinson
    Disease Scale
NIH Stroke Scale
NOCTI Teacher Occupational
    Competency Test: Child Care
    and Guidance
NOCTI Teacher Occupational
    Competency Test: Mechanical
    Technology
Non-Language Learning Test
Non-Language Multi-Mental Test
Nonreading Aptitude Test Battery
    (NATB)
Non-Reading Intelligence Tests,
    Levels 1-3 (NRIT)
Non-Verbal Ability Tests (NAT)
Normative Adaptive Behavior
    Checklist
norm-referenced test
Norris Educational Achievement
    Test (NEAT)
North American Depression Inven-
    tories for Children and Adults
Northwestern Syntax Screening
    Test (NSST)
Northwestern University Children's
    Perception of Speech Test
Northwick Park Index of Indepen-
    dence in ADL
Nottingham Extended ADL Index
Nottingham Health Profile
Nottingham Ten-Point ADL Scale
NU Auditory Test Lists 4 and 6

test *(cont.)*

number 3 traced on patient's palm
test

Numerical Attention Test (NAT)

Nurse Aide Practice Test

Nurses' Observation Scale for
Inpatient Evaluation (NOSIE)

OARS Multidimensional Functional Assessment Questionnaire
(OMFAQ)

Object Classification Test (OCT)

Objective-Analytic Batteries

objective test (OT)

Object Relations Technique

Object Sorting Scales (OSS)

object sorting test (OST)

objects test

O'Brien Vocabulary Placement
Test

Obsessive-Compulsive Personality
Disorder Subscale from Millon
Clinical Multiaxial Inventory II

Obsessive Compulsive Subscale of
the Comprehensive Psycho-
pathological Rating Scale

Occupational Ability Patterns
(OAPs)

Occupational Aptitude Survey and
Interest Schedule, Second
Edition–Aptitude Survey
(OASIS-2 AS)

Occupational Aptitude Survey and
Interest Schedule, Second
Edition–Interest Survey
(OASIS-2 IS)

Occupational Check List (OCL)

Occupational Environment Scales,
Form E-2

Occupational Interests Explorer
(OIE)

Occupational Interests Surveyor
(OIS)

test *(cont.)*

Occupational Roles Questionnaire
(ORQ)

Occupational Stress Indicator
(Research Version) (OSI)

Occupational Test Series–Basic
Skills Tests

Offer Parent-Adolescent Questionnaire, The

Offer Self-Image Questionnaire for
Adolescents (OSIQA)

Offer Self-Image Questionnaire,
Revised (OSIQ-R)

Office Skills Test

Ohio Tests of Articulation and
Perception of Sounds (OTAPS)

Ohio Vocational Interest Survey
(OVIS), Second Edition

Ohio Work Values Inventory
(OWVI)

OISE Picture Reasoning Test
(PRT)

Oliphant Auditory Discrimination
Memory Test (OADMT)

Oliphant Auditory Synthesizing
Test (OAST)

Omnibus Personality Inventory
(OPI)

Opinions Toward Adolescents
(OTA)

Oral Language Evaluation, Second
Edition

Oral Language Sentence Imitation
Diagnostic Inventory (OLSIDI)

Oral Language Sentence Imitation
Screening Test (OLSIST)

Oral-Motor/Feeding Rating Scale

Oral Verbal Intelligence Test
(OVIT)

Ordinal Scales of Psychological
Development

Organic Integrity Test (OIT)

test *(cont.)*

Organizational Climate Index
Organizational Culture Inventory
(OCI)
Organizational Test for Professional Accounting
Organizational Value Dimensions Questionnaire (OVDQ)
Organization Health Survey
Orleans-Hanna Algebra Prognosis Test
Otis-Lennon Mental Ability Test (OLMAT)
Otis Quick Scoring Mental Abilities Tests
Ottawa School Behavior Check List (OSBCL)
Overcontrolled Hostility Scale (OHS)
Oxford STA Scale
Paced Auditory Serial Addition Test (PASAT)
PACG Inventory
Pain and Distress score (PAD)
Pain Apperception Test (PAT)
Pair Attraction Inventory (PAI)
Pantomime Recognition Test (PRT)
paragraph recall test
Parallel Spelling Tests
Paranoia "6" Scale
Paranoid Sensitivity Profile
Parent-Adolescent Communication Scale
Parental Acceptance-Rejection Questionnaire
Parent as a Teacher Inventory (PAAT)
Parent Attachment Structured Interview
Parent Attitude Scale (PAS)

test *(cont.)*

Parent Awareness Skills Survey (PASS)
Parent Effectiveness Training (PET)
Parenting Stress Index
Parent Interview for Child Syndrome (PICS)
Parent Opinion Inventory
Parent Perception of Child Profile (PPCP)
Parent Rating of Student Behavior
Parent-Teacher Questionnaire (PTQ)
Partner Relationship Inventory (PRI)
Patient Rated Anxiety Scale (PRAS)
Patient Rated Disability Scale
Patient Rated Impairment Scale
Patient Rated Overall Life Impairment
Patterned Elicitation Syntax Screening Test (PESST)
Patterned Elicitation Syntax Test
Paykel Life Events Scale
PDI Employment Inventory
Peabody Developmental Motor Scales and Activity Cards
Peabody Individual Achievement Test (PIAT)
Peabody Mathematics Readiness Test
Peabody Picture Vocabulary Test (PPVT)
Pediatric Early Elementary Examination
Pediatric Examination of Educational Readiness at Middle Childhood
Pediatric Extended Examination at Three (PEET)

test *(cont.)*
  Pediatric Speech Intelligibility Test
  Peer Nomination Inventory of
    Depression
  Peer Profile
  Perception of Ability Scale for
    Students (PASS)
  Perception of Illness Scale
  Perception-of-Relationships-Test
    (PORT)
  Perceptual Maze Test
  Perceptual-Motor Assessment for
    Children & Emotional/Behavior
    Screening Program (P-perfor-
    mance test
  Perceptual Organization Deviation
    Quotient (PODQ)
  Performance Assessment of Syntax
    Elicited and Spontaneous
    (PASES)
  Performance Efficiency Test
  Performance Intelligence Quotient
    (PIQ)
  Performance I.Q. Score
  Performance Levels of a School
    Program Survey
  Performance Scale Scores
  Perley-Guze Hysteria Checklist
  Personal and Role Skills (PARS)
  Personal Assessment of Intimacy
    in Relationships (PAIR)
  Personal Attributes Questionnaire
    (PAQ)
  Personal Experience and Attitude
    Questionnaire (PEAQ)
  Personal Experience Screening
    Questionnaire (PESQ)
  Personal Inventory of Needs
  Personality Adjective Check List
    (PACL)
  Personality Assessment Inventory
    (PAI)

test *(cont.)*
  personality assessment system
    (PAS)
  Personality Diagnostic Question-
    naire-Revised (PDQ-R)
  Personality Factor Questionnaire
    (PFQ)
  Personality Inventory for Children
    (PIC), Revised
  Personality Rating Scale (PRS)
  Personality Research Form (PRF)
  personality test
  Personal Locus of Control (PLC)
  Personal Orientation Inventory
    (POI)
  Personal Preference Scale (PPS)
  Personal Problems Checklist for
    Adolescents (PPC)
  Personal Relationship Inventory
    (PRI)
  Personal Resource Questionnaire
    (PRQ)
  Personal Strain Questionnaire
    (PSQ)
  Personal Values Abstract (PVA)
  personal values inventory (PVI)
  Personnel Reaction Blank
  Personnel Security Preview (PSP)
  Personnel Selection Inventory
  Personnel Tests for Industry (PTI)
  Phelps Kindergarten Readiness
    Scale (PKRS)
  Philadelphia Head Injury Question-
    naire (PHIQ)
  Phoneme Discrimination Test
    (PDT)
  Phonological Process Analysis
    (PPA)
  Photo Articulation Test (PAT)
  Physical and Architectural Features
    Checklist
  Physical Tolerance Profile (PTP)

test *(cont.)*

Physiognomic Cue Test (PCT)
Picha-Seron Career Analysis
(PSCA; PSCA-CP; PSCA-OP;
PSCA-PP)
Pickford Projectives Pictures (PPP)
Pictorial Test of Intelligence (PTI)
picture arrangement (PA) subtest
Picture Articulation and Language
Screening Test (PALST)
picture completion (PC) subtest
Picture Identification for Children-
Standardized Index (PICSI)
Picture Identification Test (PIT)
Picture Interest Exploration Survey
(PIES)
Picture Sound Discrimination Test
Picture Speech Discrimination Test
Picture Spondee Threshold Test
Picture Story Language Test
(PSLT)
Piers-Harris Children's Self-
Concept Scale
Pimsleur Language Aptitude
Battery
Pin Test, The
Planning Career Goals (PCG)
Politte Sentence Completion Test
Pollack-Branden Inventory: For
Identification of Learning
Disabilities, Dyslexia and
Classroom Dysfunction
Porch Index of Communicative
Ability (PICA)
Porch Index of Communicative
Ability in Children (PICAC)
Porteus Maze Test (PMT)
Portland Digit Recognition Test
(PDRT)
Portland Problem Behavior
Checklist–Revised
Portuguese Speaking Test (PST)

test *(cont.)*

Position Analysis Questionnaire
(PAQ)
Positive and Negative Syndrome
Scale (PANSS)
Posttraumatic Stress Disorder Scale
Potential for Addiction Index
Practical Maths Assessments
Pragmatics Profile of Early Com-
munication Skills
Pragmatics Screening Test
Predictive Ability Test (PAT)
Predictive Screening Test of
Articulation
Preliminary Diagnostic Question-
naire
Premarital Communication Inven-
tory (PCI)
Pre-Professional Skills Test
Preschool and Kindergarten
Interest Descriptor
Preschool Behavior Questionnaire
(PBQ)
Preschool Development Inventory
Preschool Language Assessment
Instrument (PLAI)
Preschool Language Scale (PLS)
Preschool Language Screening
Test
Preschool Screening Test
Preschool Speech and Language
Screening Test
Prescriptive Reading Inventory
(PRI)
Present State Examination (PSE)
presidents test
Prevocational Assessment and
Curriculum Guide (PACG)
Prevocational Assessment Screen
(PAS)
Primary Language Screen, The
(TPLS)

test *(cont.)*

Primary Measures of Music Audiation

Primary Self-Concept Inventory (PSCI)

Primary Test of Cognitive Skills (PTCS)

Primary Visual Motor Test (PVMT)

Printing Performance School Readiness Test (PPSRT)

Priority Counseling Survey (PCS)

Problem Experiences Checklist

Problem of Immediate Gratification

Procedures for the Phonological Analysis of Children's Language

Process Diagnostic (PD)

Process for the Assessment of Effective Student Functioning

Process Skills Rating Scales (PSRS)

Processing Word Classes

Professional and Administrative Career Examination (PACE)

Professional and Managerial Position Questionnaire (PMPQ)

Professional Employment Test (PET)

Professional Sexual Role Inventory (PSRI)

Profile of Adaptation to Life

Profile of Mood States (POMS)

Profile of Nonverbal Sensitivity (PONS)

Profile of Out-of-Body Experiences (POBE)

Prognostic Value of Imitative and Auditory Discrimination Tests

Progress Assessment Chart of Social and Personal Development (PAC)

test *(cont.)*

Progressive Achievement Tests of Listening Comprehension (PATLC)

Progressive Achievement Test of Mathematics [Revised] (PATM)

Progressive Achievement Tests of Reading [Revised]

Projective Assessment of Aging Method

projective test

Prosody-Voice Screening Profile (PVSP)

proverb interpretation test

proverbs test

Psychasthenia "7" Scale

Psychiatric Diagnostic Interview

Psychiatric Evaluation Form (PEF)

Psychiatric Evaluation Profile (PEP)

Psychiatric Knowledge and Skills Self-Assessment Program (PKSAP)

Psychiatric Status Rating Scale

Psychiatric Status Schedule (PSS)

psychoacoustic testing (PAT)

Psycho-Educational Evaluation

Psychoeducational Profile Revised (PEP-R)

Psycho-Epistemological Profile (PEP)

Psycholinguistic Rating Scale

Psychological Distress Inventory

psychological examination

Psychological Screening Inventory (PSI)

psychological test (testing)

Psychopathic Deviance "4" Scale

psychophysiological test

Psychosocial Adjustment to Illness Scale (PAIS)

test *(cont.)*

Psychosocial History Screening Questionnaire (PHSQ)
Psychotherapy Competence Assessment Schedule (PCAS)
Psychotherapy Supervisory Inventory
Psychotic Inpatient Profile (PIP)
Psychotic Reaction Profile (PRP)
Pupil Rating Scale: Screening for Learning Disabilities (PRS)
Pupil Record of Education Behavior (PREB)
Purdue Pegboard Dexterity Test
Purdue Perceptual-Motor Survey (PPMS)
Purdue Student-Teacher Opinionaire (PSTO)
Purdue Teacher Opinionaire (PTO)
Purpose in Life Test (PIL)
Pyramid Scales
Quality of Life Questionnaire (QLQ)
Quality of Well-Being Scale
Questionnaire of Basic Personality Supports
Questionnaire on Resources and Stress for Families with Chronically Ill or Handicapped Members
Quick Neurological Screening Test
Quick Phonics Survey (QPS)
Quick Picture Vocabulary Test (QPVT)
Quickscreen
Quick Screening of Mental Development
Quick Screen of Phonology (QSP)
Quick-Score Achievement Test
Quick Test (QT)
Quick Word Test

test *(cont.)*

Rand Functional Limitations Battery
RAND Patient Satisfaction Questionnaire
Rand Physical Capacities Battery
Rapidly Alternating Speech Perception Test (RASP)
Rathus Assertiveness Scale
Rating Inventory for Screening Kindergartners (RISK)
Rating Scale of Communication in Cognitive Decline (RSCCD)
Readiness Scale–Self Rating and Manager Rating Forms
Reading Comprehension Battery for Aphasia
Reading Comprehension Inventory
Reading Expectancy Screening Scales (RESS)
Reality Check Survey (RCS)
reality testing
Reasons for Living Inventory (RLI)
recall 5 items after 5 minutes test
recall of information test
recent memory test
Receptive-Expressive Emergent Language Test, Second Edition (REEL-2)
Receptive-Expressive Observation Scale (REO)
Receptive One Word Picture Vocabulary Test (ROWPVT)
Recognition Memory Test
Recognition vs. Recall
Rehabilitation Indicators (RIs)
Reitan Evaluation of Hemispheric Abilities and Brain Improvement Training
Reitan-Indiana Neuropsychological Test Battery for Adults

test *(cont.)*

Reitan-Indiana Neuropsychological Test Battery for Children

remote memory test

Repeated Test of Sustained Wakefulness (RTSW)

Resident and Staff Information Form

Responsibility and Independence Scale for Adolescents (RISA)

Retirement Descriptive Index (RDI)

reverse digit span recall test

Reynell-Zinkin Scales: Developmental Scales for Young Handicapped Children, Part 1 Mental Development

Reynolds Adolescent Depression Scale (RADS)–Revised

Reynolds Child Depression Scale (RCDS)

Rey-Ostereith Complex Figure Test

Right-Left Orientation Test (RLO)

Riley Articulation and Language Test (RALT)

Riley Inventory of Basic Learning Skills (RIBLS)

Riley Motor Problems Inventory

Riley Preschool Developmental Screening Inventory (RPDSI)

Ring and Peg Tests of Behavior Development

Rinne Hearing Conduction Test

Rivermead ADL Test

Rivermead Behavioral Memory Test (RBMT)

Rivermead Mobility Index

Rivermead Motor Assessment

Rivermead Perceptual Assessment Battery

Robbins Speech Sound Discrimination and Verbal Imagery Type Tests

test *(cont.)*

Robert's Apperception Test for Children (RATC): Supplementary Test Pictures for Black Children

Roeder Manipulative Aptitude Test

Rogers Criminal Responsibility Scale

Rogers Personal Adjustment Inventory, UK Revision

Rokeach Value Survey (RVS)

Romberg Test

Rorschach cards

Rorschach Content Test (RCT)

Rorschach Inkblot Test

Rorschach Projective Technique

Rorschach test (Exner Scoring System)

Rosenberg Self-esteem Scale (RSES)

Rosenzweig Picture-Frustration Study (RPFS)

Ross Information Processing Assessment

Ross Test of Higher Cognitive Processes

Roswell-Chall Auditory Blending Test

Roswell-Chall Diagnostic Reading Test of Word Analysis Skills: Revised and Extended

rotation test

Rothwell-Miller Interest Blank

Rotter Incomplete Sentences Blank (RISB), Second Edition

Rotter Sentence Completion Test (RSCT)

Rucker-Gable Educational Programming Scale (RGEPS)

Rule Eleven Psych Evaluation

Russell Version Wechsler Memory Scale

test *(cont.)*

Rust Inventory of Schizotypal Cognitions

Rutler-Graham Psychiatric Interview

Rutter-B questionnaire

Safran Student's Interest Inventory (SSII), Third Edition

Salamon-Conte Life Satisfaction in the Elderly Scale (LSES)

Sales Attitude Check List (SACL)

Sales Personality Questionnaire (SPQ)

Sales Style Diagnostic Test

Salience Inventory (SI) (Research Edition)

SCALE (Scales of Creativity and Learning Environment)

Scaled Curriculum Achievement Levels Test (SCALE)

Scale for Assessment of Negative Symptoms (SANS)

Scale for Assessment of Positive Symptoms (SAPS)

Scale for Assessment of Thought, Language, and Communication

Scale for Emotional Blunting (SEB)

Scale of Social Development

Scales for Early Communication Skills for Hearing-Impaired Children (SECS)

Scales of Independent Behavior

Schaie-Thurstone Adult Mental Abilities Test

SCAN-TRON Reading Test

Schedule for Affective Disorders and Schizophrenia (SADS)

Schedule for Affective Disorders and Schizophrenia–Change (SADS-C)

test *(cont.)*

Schedule for Affective Disorders and Schizophrenia–Lifetime (SADS-L), Third Edition

Schedule for Affective Disorders and Schizophrenia for School Age Children (K-SADS-P)

Schedule of Growing Skills

Schedule of Recent Experience

Schizophrenia "8" Scale

schizotypy scale

Scholastic Abilities Test for Adults (SATA)

Scholastic Aptitude Test (SAT)

School Administrator Assessment Survey

School-Age Depression Listed Inventory

School and College Ability Test (SCAT)

School and College Ability Tests II & III

School Apperception Method

School Assessment Survey (SAS)

School Atmosphere Questionnaire (SAQ)

School Attitude Survey (SAS)

School Attitude Test (SAT)

School Climate Inventory

School Environment Preference Survey

School Handicap Condition Scale (SEH)

School Interest Inventory

School Library/Media Skills Test

School Motivation Analysis Test (SMAT)

School Problem Screening Inventory (SPSI)

School Readiness Screening Test

School Readiness Survey

test *(cont.)*

School Situation Survey (SSS)
School Social Skills Rating Scale
(S3 Rating Scale)
Schubert General Ability Battery
Schutz Measures
Schwabach Test
Science Research Associates
Mechanical Aptitudes
Scott Mental Alertness Test
screening articulation test
Screening Assessment for Gifted
Elementary Students–Primary
(SAGES-P)
Screening Children for Related
Early Educational Needs
(SCREEN)
Screening Deep Test of Articulation
Screening Instrument for Targeting
Educational Risk (SIFTER)
Screening Kit of Language Devel-
opment (SKOLD)
Screening Procedure for Emotional
Disturbance (Draw A Person)
(DAP:SPED)
Screening Speech Articulation Test
Screening Test for Assignment of
Remedial Treatments (START)
Screening Test for Auditory
Comprehension of Language
(STACL)
Screening Test for Auditory
Perception
Screening Test for Auditory
Processing Disorders
Screening Test for Developmental
Apraxia of Speech
Screening Test for Educational
Prerequisite Skills (STEPS)
Screening Test for Identifying Cen-
tral Auditory Disorders (SCAN)

test *(cont.)*

Screening Tests for Young Chil-
dren and Retardates (STYCAR)
Screening Test of Academic Readi-
ness
Screening Test of Adolescent Lan-
guage
S-D Proneness Checklist
SEARCH: A Scanning Instrument
for the Identification of Potential
Learning Disability
Seashore Rhythm Test
Seasonal Pattern Assessment Ques-
tionnaire (SPAQ)
SEED Developmental Profiles
Seeking of Noetic Goals Test
Selective Reminding Test
Self-Administered Dependency
Questionnaire (SADQ)
Self-Assessment Depression (scale)
(SAD)
Self-Assessment in Writing Skills
Self-Concept and Motivation Inven-
tory (SCAMIN)
Self-Concept as a Learner (scale)
(SCAL)
Self-Concept Scale
Self-Consciousness Scale
Self-Control Inventory
self-criticism scale
Self-Description Questionnaire II
(SDQII)
Self-Esteem Index (SEI)
Self-Esteem Questionnaire
Self-Perception Inventory (SPI)
Self-Perception Profile for Children
self-rating test
self-report personality inventories
Senf Comrey Ratings of Extra
Educational Needs
Senior Apperception Technique

test *(cont.)*

Senior Apperception Test (SAT)
Sensation-Seeking Scale (SSS)
Sense of Coherence Questionnaire
Sensory Integration and Praxis
Tests (SIPT)
Sentence Closure Test
sentence completion test
Sentence Repetition Test
Sequenced Inventory of Language
Development (SILD)
Sequential Assessment of Mathematics Inventories: Standardized
Inventory
sequential multiple analysis (SMA)
Sequential Tests of Educational
Progress, Series III (STEP-III)
Serial Digit Learning Test (SDL)
serial sevens (7's) test
serial threes (3's) test
Sex Knowledge and Attitude Test
(SKAT)
Sexual Compatibility Test (SCT)
Sexual Functioning Index (SFI)
Sexuality Preference Profile (SPP)
Shapes Analysis Test (SAT)
Sheltered Care Environment Scale
Shipley Institute of Living Scale
(SILS)
Shipley Personal Inventory (SPI)
Shipman Anxiety Depression Scale
(SADS)
Short Employment Tests
Shortened Edinburgh Reading
Tests
Short Imaginal Processes Inventory
(SIPI)
Short Increment Sensitivity Index
(SISI)
Short Michigan Alcoholism
Screening Test (SMAST)

test *(cont.)*

short orientation-memory-concentration (OMC) test
Short Portable Mental Status Questionnaire (SPMSQ)
Short-Term Auditory Retrieval and
Storage Test (STARS)
Short Test for Use with Cerebral
Palsy Children
Sickness Impact Profile (SIP) Test
similarities mental status test
Similes Test
Singer-Loomis Inventory of Personality (SLIP)
Single and Double Simultaneous
Stimulation Test
Sixteen Personality Factor Questionnaire, Fifth Edition (16PF)
Skill Indicators (SKIs)
Skill Scan for Management Development
SKILLSCOPE for Managers
Sklar Aphasia Scale: Revised
Slingerland College-Level Screening
for the Identification of Language Learning Strengths and
Weaknesses
Slingerland Screening Tests (SST)
for Identifying Children with
Specific Language Disability
Slosson Articulation Language Test
with Phonology (SALT-P)
Slosson Children's Version Family
Environment Scale
Slosson Drawing Coordination Test
Slosson Intelligence Test for Children and Adults
Slosson Intelligence Test–Revised
(SIT-R)
Slosson Oral Reading Test–Revised
(SORT-R)

test *(cont.)*

Slosson Test of Reading Readiness (STRR)

Smith-Johnson Nonverbal Performance Scale

Smoking Behavior Questionnaire (SBQ)

Smoking-Habit Related Activities Questionnaire

Social Adaptation Status (SAS)

Social Adequacy Index (SAI)

Social Adjustment Scale II

Social Adjustment Self-Report Scale (SAS-RS)

Social and Occupational Functioning Assessment Scale (SOFAS)

Social and Prevocational Information Battery (SPIB)

Social Behavior Assessment Inventory (SBAI)

Social Behavior Assessment Schedule

Social Climate Scales (SCS)

Social-Emotional Dimension Scale

Social Intelligence Test

Social Interaction Scale

Social Introversion "0" Scale

Social Readjustment Rating Scale (SRRS)

social relations (SRT) test

Social Reticence Scale

Social Skills Rating System (SSRS)

social stress and functionability inventory (SSFI)

SOI Learning Abilities Test: Screening Form for Gifted

Somatic Inkblot Series

Somatic "3" Scale

Sorting of Figures Test (SOFT)

Southern California Motor Accuracy Test, Revised

test *(cont.)*

Southern California Postrotary Nystagmus Test

Southern California Sensory Integration Tests

Spadafore Diagnostic Reading Test

Spanish Computerized Adaptive Placement Exam (S-CAPE)

span recall test

SPAR Spelling and Reading Tests, Second Edition

Spatial Orientation Memory Test (SOMT)

Special Aptitude Test Battery (SATB)

SPECTRUM-I: A Test of Adult Work Motivation

Speech and Language Evaluation Scale (SLES)

Speech and Language Screening Questionnaire (SLSQ)

Speech Discrimination in Noise

Speech Improvement Cards

Speech-Language Pathology Evaluation Assessment

Speech Questionnaire

Speech Sound Memory Test

Speech-Sounds Perception Test

Speech with Alternating Masking Index (SWAMI)

spell-a-word-backwards test

Spelling Grade Rating

Spelling Scale (British Ability Scales)

Spielberger Anxiety Inventory

Spielberger State-Trait Anger Expression Inventory

Spiritual Well-Being Scale (SWBS)

SRA Achievement Series, Forms 1-2

SRA Arithmetic Test

test *(cont.)*
SRA Nonverbal Form
SRA Pictorial Reasoning Test
SRA Reading Test
SRA Verbal Form
Staff Burnout Scale for Health
Professionals
STAI-Y
Standardized Assessment of De-
pressive Disorders (SADD)
standardized test (ST)
Standardized Test of Computer
Literacy (STCL)
Standard Progressive Matrices
Stanford Achievement Test (SAT)–
Abbreviated Version–8th
Edition
Stanford-Binet Intelligence Scale
(SBIS): Form L-M
Stanford Diagnostic Mathematics
Test
Stanford Early School Achieve-
ment Test, Second Edition
Stanford Hypnotic Clinical Scale
for Children
Stanford Hypnotic Susceptibility
Scale (SHSS)
Stanford Profile Scales of Hypnotic
Susceptibility, Revised
Stanton Survey
State–Trait Anger Expression
Inventory (STAXI)
State–Trait Anger Scale (STAS)
State–Trait Anxiety Inventory
(STAI)
State–Trait Anxiety Inventory for
Children (STAIC)
State–Trait Personality Inventory
(STPI)
status examination
Status Indicators (SIs)
Stein Sentence Completion (SSC)
test

test *(cont.)*
Stenger Test
Stenographic Skill-Dictation Test
Stephens Oral Language Screening
Test (SOLST)
Steps Up Developmental Screening
Program
stimulant challenge test
Stimulus Recognition Test
Stone and Neale Daily Coping
Assessment
Story Articulation Test
Street Survival Skills Questionnaire
Strength of Grip Test
Stress Audit
Stress Evaluation Inventory
Stress from Life Experience (SFLE)
Stress Impact Scale (SIS)
Stress Response Scale
Strong-Campbell Interest Inventory
(SCII)
Stroop Color and Word Test
Structural Analysis of Social
Behavior
Structured and Scaled Interview to
Assess Maladjustment (SSIAM)
Structured Clinical Interview for
DSM-IV Axis I Disorders:
Clinician Version (SCID-CV)
Structured Clinical Interview for
DSM-IV Axis II: Personality
Disorders (SCID-II)
Structured Clinical Interview for
DSM-IV: Dissociative Disorders
(SCID-D), Revised
Structured Interview of Reported
Symptoms (SIRS)
Structured Photographic Articulation
Test Featuring Dudsberry
(SPAT-D)
Structured Photographic Expressive
Language Test-II (SPELT-P)

test *(cont.)*

Structure of Intellect Learning
Abilities Test–Form P (Primary)
Student Opinion Inventory (SOI)
Student Orientations Survey (SOS)
Student Talent and Risk Profile
(STAR Profile)
Study Attitudes and Methods
Survey (SAMS)
Study of Values (SV)
STYCAR Hearing Test (SHT)
STYCAR Language Test (SLT)
STYCAR Vision Tests (SVT)
Style of Leadership Survey
Style of Management Inventory
Style of Mind Inventory (SMI)
Subjective Treatment Emergent
Side Effects Scale
Substance Abuse Problem Checklist
Substance Abuse Questionnaire
(SAQ)
Substance Abuse Subtle Screening
Inventory (SASSI)
Suicide-Depression Proneness
Checklist (SDPC)
Suicide Intervention Response
Inventory
Suicide Opinion Questionnaire
(SOQ)
Suicide Probability Scale
Suinn Test Anxiety Behavior Scale
(STABS)
Supervisory Behavior Description
(SBD)
Supervisory Practices Inventory
Supervisory Practices Test (SPT)
Suprathreshold Adaptation Test
(STAT)
Survey of Employee Access (SEA)
Survey of Interpersonal Values
(SIV)
Survey of Organizations

test *(cont.)*

Survey of Personal Values
Survey of School Attitudes
Survey of Study Habits and
Attitudes (SSHA)
Survey of Work Values, Revised,
Form U
sweep-check test
Swinging Story Test
Symbol Digit Modalities Test
(SDMT)
Symbolic Play Test (SPT), Second
Edition
Symptom Checklist-90-Revised
(SCL-90-R)
Symptom Rating Scale (SRS)
Synthetic Sentence Identification
Test
Szondi Test
Tactile Finger Recognition Test
(TFRT)
Tactile Form Recognition Test
(TFRT)
Tactual Performance Test (TPT)
TARC Assessment System
Task Assessment Scales
Task-Oriented Assessment
Taylor-Johnson Temperament
Analysis
Taylor Manifest Anxiety Scale
(TMAS)
Teacher Attitude Inventory (TAI)
Teacher Evaluation Scale (TES)
Teacher Feedback Questionnaire
Teacher Occupational Competency
Test: Child Care and Guidance,
NOCTI
Teacher Occupational Competency
Test: Mechanical Technology,
NOCTI
Teacher Opinion Inventory

test *(cont.)*
Teacher's School Readiness
Inventory (TSRI)
Teacher Stress Inventory
Teaching Style Inventory
Team Effectiveness Survey (TES)
Tell-Me-A-Story (TEMAS)
Temperament and Values Inventory
Temperament Assessment Battery
for Children
Temple University Short Syntax
Inventory (Revised) (TUSSI)
Tennessee Self-Concept Scale
(TSCS)
Test Anxiety Inventory (TAI)
Test Anxiety Profile
Test Anxiety Scale
Testing-Teaching Module of Auditory Discrimination (TTMAD)
Thackray Reading Readiness Profile (TRRP)
theatrical test
thematic picture test
Thematic Apperception Test (TAT,
T.A.T.)
Thematic Aptitude Test (TAT)
Thinking Creatively in Action and
Motion
Thinking Creatively with Sounds
and Words (TCSW)
Thinking Disturbance Factor
(TDF)
"Thinking Good" Profile
This I Believe (TIB) test
Three-Dimensional Block Construction Test (3DBCT)
Three Minute Reasoning Test
3-R's Test
three-stage command test
Thurstone Temperament Schedule
Time Compressed Speech Test

test *(cont.)*
Timed Behavioral Rating Sheet
(TBRS)
Timed Stereotypes Rating Scale
Time Perception Inventory
Time Problems Inventory
Time-Sample Behavioral Checklist
(TSBC)
Time Use Analyzer
Tinker Toy Test
TMJ Scale
T.M.R. Performance Profile for
the Severely and Moderately
Retarded
TOEFL Test of Written English
Token Test for Aphasia
Token Test for Children
Token Test for Receptive
Disturbances in Aphasia
tolerance test
Tone Decay Test
Tone in Noise (TIN)
Toronto Alexithymia Scale
Toronto Functional Capacity Questionnaire (TFCQ)
Torrance Tests of Creative Thinking (TTCT)
Trailmaking Tests (Forms A & B)
Trainer's Assessment of Proficiency (TAP)
Trait Evaluation Index
Transactional Analysis Life Position Survey (TALPS)
Transition Behavior Scale (TBS)
Trauma Symptom Checklist for
Children Ages 8-15
Trites Neuropsychological Test
Battery
Twenty Statements Test (TST)
tyramine challenge test
understanding of similarities test

test *(cont.)*

United States Employment Service Interest Inventory (USES-II)

University Residence Environment Scale (URES)

Utah Test of Language Development (UTLD)

Valpar Work Sample Battery

Values Inventory for Children (VIC)

Vancouver Family Survey (VSF)

Verbal and Oral Language Ability

Verbal Auditory Screen for Children test (VASC)

Verbal Comprehension Deviation Quotient (VCDQ)

Verbal Intelligence Quotient (VIQ)

Verbal I.Q. Score

Verbalizer-Visualization Questionnaire (VVQ)

Verbal Language Development Scale

Verbal Perceptual Speed

Verbal Scale Scores

Verdun Depression Rating Scale (VDRS)

vestibular function test

Vineland Adaptive Behavior Scales

Vineland Social Maturity Scale (VSMS)

Visual-Auditory Screening test for Children (VASC)

Visual Aural Digit Span (VADS) Test

visual choice reaction time test

visual evoked response test

visual field test

Visual Form Discrimination Test (VFDT)

Visual Memory Score (VMS)

Visual-Motor Gestalt Test (VMGT)

test *(cont.)*

Visual-Motor Integration Test (VMIT)

Visual-Motor Sequencing Test (VMST)

Visual Neglect Test

Visual Pattern Completion Test

Visual Perceptual Speed

Visual Reinforcement Audiometry

Visual Search and Attention Test (VSAT)

visual threat test

Vocabulary Comprehension Scale

Vocational Apperception Test (VAT)

Vocational Evaluation and Work Adjustment (VEWA)

Vocational Interest and Sophistication Assessment (VISA)

Vocational Interest Blank (VIB)

Vocational Interest Inventory and Exploration Survey

Vocational Interest Questionnaire (VIQ)

vocational interest schedule (VIS)

Vocational Opinion Index (VOI)

Vocational Planning Inventory (VPI)

Vocational Preference Inventory (VPI)

Voc-Tech Quick Screener (VTQS)

Vulpé Assessment Battery

Vygotsky Concept Formation Test, Modified

Wachs Analysis of Cognitive Structures

Wahler Physical Symptoms Inventory

Wahler Self-Description Inventory (WSDI)

Wakefield Self-Assessment Depression Inventory

test *(cont.)*

Walker-McConnell Scale of Social Competence and School Adjustment

wall chart vision test

WAQ (Work Attitudes Questionnaire)

Ward Atmosphere Scale (WAS)

Ward Behavior Rating Scale (WBRS)

Waring Intimacy Questionnaire (WIQ)

Washington Speech Sound Discrimination Test (WSSDT)

Wasserman test

Watson-Glaser Critical Thinking Appraisal (WGCTA)

Ways of Coping Scale

Weak Opiate Withdrawal Scale (WOWS)

Weber Advanced Spatial Perception (WASP)

Weber Test

Wechsler Adult Intelligence Scale, Revised (WAIS–R)

Wechsler-Bellevue Scale (WBS)

Wechsler Intelligence Scale for Children, Third Edition (WISC-III)

Wechsler Memory Scale, Revised

Wechsler Memory Scale, Russell Version

Wechsler Preschool and Primary Scale of Intelligence (WPPSI)

Wechsler Scales

Weiss Comprehensive Articulation Test

Weiss Intelligibility Test

Weller-Strawser Scales of Adaptive Behavior for the Learning Disabled

Welsh Figure Preference Test

test *(cont.)*

Wepman Auditory Discrimination Test

Wesman Personnel Classification Test

Western Aphasia Battery (WAB)

Western Personality Inventory

Western Personnel Tests

What I Like to Do: An Inventory of Students' Interests (WILD)

Whitaker Index of Schizophrenic Thinking (WIST)

WHO Handicap Scales

Wide Range Achievement Test 3 (WRAT3)

Wide Range Assessment of Memory and Learning

Wide Range Employment Sample Test (WREST)

Wide Range Intelligence and Personality Test (WRIPT)

Wide Range Interest–Opinion Test (WRIOT)

Wiggins Content Scale (WCS)

Wilson-Patterson Attitude Inventory (WPAI)

Wisconsin Card-Sorting Test (WCST)

WISC-R Split-Half Short Form, Second Edition

Wittenborn Psychiatric Rating Scale (WITT, WPRS)

Wolfe Microcomputer User Aptitude Test

Wonderlic Personnel Test

W-1/W-2 Auditory Tests

Woodcock-Johnson Achievement Tests (WJAT)

Woodcock-Johnson Psycho-Educational Battery–Revised (WJ-R)

Woodcock Language Proficiency Battery–English Form

test *(cont.)*

Woodcock Language Proficiency Battery–Revised (WLPB-R)

Woodcock Reading Mastery Tests–Revised (WRMT-R)

Word Association Test

Word Intelligibility by Picture Identification (WIPI)

Word Processing Test

Word Processor Assessment Battery

Word Recognition Test

word retrieval test

Word Search

Work Attitudes Questionnaire (WAQ)

Work Environment Preference Schedule (WEPS)

Work Environment Scale, Second Edition (WES)

Work Information Inventory (WII)

Work Interest Index

Work Motivation Inventory (WMI)

Work Skills Series Production (WSS)

Work Values Inventory (WVI)

World of Work Inventory (WWI)

Worse Premorbid Adjustment Scale

write a sentence test

Written Language Assessment

W-22 Auditory Test

Yale-Brown Obsessive-Compulsive Scale (YBOCS)

Yerkes-Bridges test (YBT)

Zung Self-Rating Depression Scale

testamentary capacity

Test Anxiety Inventory (TAI)

Test Anxiety Profile

Test Anxiety Scale

testicle, undescended

testicular hypofunction

testing, functional gain

Testing-Teaching Module of Auditory Discrimination (TTMAD)

testis pain, psychogenic

Test Orientation Procedure (TOP)

testosterone

test protocol

test-retest reliability coefficient

tetanic convulsion

tetanic stimulation

tetany

tetrahydrocannabinol (THC) dependence

tetrahydrol-soquinoline (THIQ)

Teutonomania

Teutonophobia

Teutophobia

"Texas pot" (cannabis)

"Texas tea" (cannabis)

"Tex-mex" (cannabis)

text

nonobtrusive

obtrusive

pragmatic

textual operant

texture responses

TF (transvestic fetishism)

TFCQ (Toronto Functional Capacity Questionnaire)

TFRT (Tactile Finger Recognition Test)

TFRT (Tactile Form Recognition Test)

TGA (transient global amnesia)

T-group (sensitivity-training group)

thaasophobia

Thackray Reading Readiness Profile (TRRP)

Thai marijuana

"Thai sticks" (cannabis)

thalamic epilepsy

thalassomania

thalassophobia
thanatomania
thanatophobia
thanatos (death instinct)
THC (tetrahydrocannabinol) elevation
  screen
Theater of Spontaneity (Stegreiftheater)
theatrical test
theatricality
theatromania
theatrophobia
theft
Thematic Apperception Test (TAT)
Thematic Aptitude Test (TAT)
Thematic Content Modification
  Program (TCMP)
thematic paralogia
thematic paraphasia
thematic picture test
thematic role
theme
  common
  grandiose
  self-derogatory
theomania
theophobia
the oral-nasal acoustic ratio (TONAR)
theory (pl. theories)
  Adler
  adlerian
  aggressive behavior
  allenian
  Allport group relations
  anxiety sensitivity
  attachment
  biolinguistic language
  cognitive
  constitutional bisexuality
  continuum
  cybernetic
  decision

theory *(cont.)*
  double blind
  empiricist
  etiology of
  field
  focal conflict
  frequency hearing
  Freud
  freudian
  game
  gestalt
  hearing
  information
  innateness
  item response (IRT)
  libido
  Jung; jungian
  Klein suffocation alarm
  language innateness
  language learning
  learning
  mixture
  motor learning
  nativist
  object relations
  personal construct
  personality
  phonation
  place
  place hearing
  psychoanalytic
  psycholinguistic
  psychological
  rankian
  resonance-volley
  rogerian
  social dominance
  speech innateness
  stuttering
  taftian
  telephone (volley)
  telephone hearing

theory *(cont.)*
  traveling wave hearing
  violence
  volley
  volley hearing
  X-bar
therapeutic agent
therapeutic alliance
therapeutic approaches for deceitfulness
therapeutic botulinum neurotoxin
therapeutic atmosphere
therapeutic community
therapeutic crisis
therapeutic drug holiday
therapeutic effect
therapeutic error signal (TES)
therapeutic group
therapeutic impasse
therapeutic milieu
therapeutic modality
therapeutic processes
therapeutic program
therapeutic recreation (TR)
therapeutic role
therapeutic trial
therapeutic window
therapist
  active
  auxiliary
  language
  occupational
  passive
  recreation
  speech
  voice
therapy (pl. therapies)
  activity group (AGT)
  adjunctive
  adjuvant
  adolescent group
  adult group

therapy *(cont.)*
  agonist
  allenian
  anaclitic
  art
  aversion
  behavioral
  behavior marital (BMT)
  bioenergetic
  biological
  branching steps in
  brief stimulus (BST)
  carbon dioxide
  child group
  client-centered
  cognitive
  cognitive-behavioral (CBT)
  color
  combined
  conditioning
  conjoint
  contextual
  convulsive
  corrective
  couples
  dance
  deliberate
  diagnostic (Dx)
  dialectical behavior
  drug
  dual-sex
  ego-state
  electroconvulsive (ECT)
  electroconvulsive shock
  existential
  experimental
  exploratory
  exposure-based
  expressive
  extended family (EFT)
  family (FT)
  fluency shaping

therapy *(cont.)*
  focused expressive
  gestalt
  group
  group adjustment (GAT)
  implosive
  individual (IT)
  Indoklon
  insight
  insulin coma (ICT)
  light
  lithium
  long-term
  major role (MRT)
  marital
  marriage
  megavitamin
  Metrazol shock
  milieu
  Morita
  multiple
  music (MT)
  myofunctional
  narrative
  neuro-
  nonconfrontive
  nondirective
  occupational (OT)
  operant
  orthomolecular
  passive
  pharmaco-
  pharmacological
  play
  play group (PGT)
  positive reinforcement
  precision
  primal
  programmed
  psychedelic
  psychiatric somatic
  psychoanalytic

therapy *(cont.)*
  psychological
  psychopharmacological
  psychovisual
  quadrangular
  rankian
  rapid-eye
  rational (RT)
  rational emotive (RET)
  reality
  reality-oriented
  relationship
  relaxation
  rogerian
  SET (support, empathy, truth)
  sex
  shock (ST)
  sleep
  social
  social network
  socioenvironmental
  somatic
  speech
  suggestion
  symptomatic
  systematized assertive (SAT)
  systemic assertive (SAT)
  talk
  theta-criterion
  thought field
  tongue thrust
  total push
  vitamin
  will
there-and-then
thermal noise
thermal stimulus
thermophobia
theta activity, EEG
theta criterion
theta index
theta rhythm

theta wave
thiamine deficiency encephalopathy
    (TDE)
thickened speech
"thing" (cocaine; heroin; drug of
    choice)
thinking
    abstract
    alogical
    archaic-paralogical
    autistic
    avoid
    black-and-white
    circular
    clear
    combinative
    conceptual
    concrete
    creative
    delusional
    dereistic
    difficulty
    disordered
    disorganized
    distorted
    distortion of inferential
    eccentric
    erratic
    futuristic
    idiosyncratic
    illogical
    impoverishment in
    inferential
    magical
    marginal
    odd
    prelogical
    primary process
    ritualistic
    suicidal
    symbolic
    tangential

thinking *(cont.)*
    vague
    wishful
thinking ability, impaired
Thinking About My School
thinking compulsion
Thinking Creatively in Action and
    Motion
Thinking Creatively with Sounds and
    Words (TCSW)
Thinking Disturbance Factor (TDF)
"Thinking Good" Profile
thinness, drive for
thioxanthene
thioxanthene derivatives
THIQ (tetrahydrol-soquinoline)
third nervous system
third octave filter
third position
thirst drive
"thirst monsters" (re: crack users)
"thirteen" (cannabis)
This I Believe (TIB) test
thixophobia
thoracic respiration
"thoroughbred" (re: drug dealer)
thoroughness, reliability, efficiency,
    analytic (ability) (TREA)
thought (pl. thoughts)
    alien
    blasphemous
    categorical
    coherent stream of
    compulsive
    considered
    constriction of
    delusional
    diminution of
    disconnected
    distressing
    disturbing
    errant

thought *(cont.)*
  fluency of
  focus of
  impoverished
  inappropriate
  incomprehensible
  interruption of
  intrusive
  lost in
  obsessional
  painful
  persistent
  poverty of
  poverty of content of
  preoccupation of
  pressing
  productivity of
  racing
  recurrent
  repeated
  self-deprecating
  speed of
  stream of (SOT)
  suicidal
  syncretic
  syntaxic
  train of
  trend of
  unacceptable
  uncontrollable
  unrelated
  wandering
  wide circles of
thought blockade
thought broadcasting
thought content
thought control
thought deletion
thought deprivation
thought disorder
thought disturbance
thought form

thought insertion
thoughtless
thoughtlessness
thought patterns
thought period
thought process disorder
thought processes
  bizarre
  concrete
  egocentric
  linear
thought reading
thought reform
thoughts and beliefs
thoughts of death
thought stopping
thought transference
thought withdrawal
threat of death
threat, suicide
threat test, visual
threatening behavior
threatening comment
threatening hallucination
threatening voices
Three-Dimensional Block Construction Test (3DBCT)
3-factor dimensional model of schizophrenia
Three Minute Reasoning Test
3-R's Test
three-stage command test
three-step task
three times daily (t.i.d.; 3/d)
threshold
  absolute
  acoustic reflex
  audibility
  auditory
  detectability
  detection
  differential

threshold *(cont.)*
  discomfort
  equivalent speech reception
  false
  feeling
  intelligibility
  intelligible
  noise detection (NDT)
  pain
  pure tone air-conduction
  pure tone bone-conduction
  reflex
  sensory
  speech awareness (SAT)
  speech detectability (SDT)
  speech detection (SDT)
  speech reception (SRT)
  stimulus
  taste
  tickle
  vibrotactile
threshold for speech
threshold level, hearing (HTL)
threshold shift
  permanent (PTS)
  temporary
threshold shift masking technique
threshold shift method
throat clearing
"thrust" (isobutyl nitrite)
thrust, tongue
"thrusters" (amphetamine)
thrusting, pelvic
"thumb" (cannabis)
thumb
  cerebral
  rule of
thumb position, cortical
thumb-sucking
Thurstone Temperament Schedule
thyroarytenoid muscle
thyroepiglottic muscle

thyrohyoid muscle
thyroid cartilage
thyroid cartilage shaving
thyroid delirium
thyrotoxicosis
TIB (This I Believe) test
"tic" (phencyclidine in powder form)
tic (pl. tics)
  articulatory
  body
  breathing
  child problem
  chronic motor
  complex motor
  complex vocal
  compulsive
  convulsive
  current
  facial
  habit
  lid
  motor
  motor-verbal
  occupational
  past
  primary
  psychogenic
  simple motor
  simple vocal
  spasm
  tardive
  Tourette
  transient
  vocal
tic de pensée
tick-borne viral encephalitis
"ticket" (lysergic acid diethylamide)
tickle threshold
tic-like behavior
tic-like facial grimace
tic orbicularis
"tic tac" (phencyclidine)

t.i.d. (three times daily)
tidal air
tidal volume
"tie" (re: drug injection)
TIES (The Instructional Environment
   Scale)
ties with reality
timbre
timbromania
time
   losing
   quality
   reaction
   reflex
   response
   reverberation
   sense of
   voice onset (VOT)
   voice termination (VTT)
time and motion studies
Time Compressed Speech Test
Timed Behavioral Rating Sheet
   (TBRS)
time deixis
Timed Stereotypes Rating Scale
time management
time of evaluation
time-out (TO)
time patterning of speech
time patterns
Time Perception Inventory
time, place and person (TP & P)
time preceding evaluation
time pressure
Time Problems Inventory
times (x)
times a day (x day)
Time-Sample Behavioral Checklist
   (TSBC)
time sense
Time Use Analyzer
time zone

time-zone-change syndrome
timidity
timing mechanisms, endogenous abnormalities in sleep-wake
timing of sleep
"tin" (re: cannabis container)
TIN (Tone in Noise)
tin ear
tingling sensation
Tinker Toy Test
tinnitus (cocaine-related)
tip-of-the-tongue phenomenon
"tish" (phencyclidine)
"tissue" (crack)
tissue, connective
tissue damage
"titch" (phencyclidine)
TL (team leader)
TLA (RBH Test of Learning Ability)
TLAC (Test of Learning Accuracy in
   Children)
TLC (Test of Language Competence)
TLC (total lung capacity)
TLC-C (Test of Language Competence
   for Children)
TLC-Learning Preference Inventory
TM (team member)
TMA (analog of amphetamine/
   methamphetamine)
TMAS (Taylor Manifest Anxiety
   Scale)
TMH (trainable mentally handicapped)
TMJ (temporomandibular joint)
TMJ Scale
T.M.R. Performance Profile for the
   Severely and Moderately Retarded
"T.N.T." (fentanyl; heroin)
TO (time out)
TOA (Bay Area Functional Perfor-
   mance Evaluation, Second Edition)
TOAL (Test of Adolescent Language)
to-and-fro tremor

tobacco addiction
tobacco dependence
tobacco use disorder
tocophobia
TOEFL Test of Written English
toilet training
  delayed
  lax
"toilet water" (inhalant)
"toke" (re: cannabis use; cocaine use)
token economy
token economy reward
token reward
Token Test for Aphasia
Token Test for Children
Token Test for Receptive
  Disturbances in Aphasia
"toke, to" (re: smoking cannabis)
"toke up" (re: cannabis use)
TOLD (Test of Language Development)
TOLD-I:2 (Tests of Language Development—Intermediate, Second
  Edition)
TOLD-P:2 (Tests of Language Development—Primary, Second Edition)
TOLD-2 (Tests of Language Development, Second Edition)
tolerance level
tolerance of drug
tolerance potential
  high
  low
tolerance range
tolerance, sound
tolerance test
tolerance threshold for speech
tomboy behavior
tomboyishness
tomomania
tomophobia
tonal spectrum

TONAR (the oral-nasal acoustic ratio)
"toncho" (octane booster which is
  inhaled)
tone (pl. tones)
  biofeedback
  complex
  contour
  difference
  emotional
  glottal
  inhibitory
  level
  modal
  partial
  pure
  register
  simple
  warble
tone air-conduction
tone air-conduction threshold
tone audiometer
  pure
  brief (BTA)
tone average
tone bone-conduction threshold
tone control
tone deafness
tone decay
Tone Decay Test
Tone in Noise (TIN)
tone of feelings
tone of voice
tongue
  bifid
  dorsum of
  fissured
  forked
  grooved
  hypertonic
tongue clucking
tongue dysfunction stuttering
tongue habits

tongue height
tongue press
tongue protrusion
tongue thrust
tongue-thrust therapy
tongue-tie
tongue tremor
TONI (Test of Nonverbal Intelligence)
tonic block (in stuttering)
tonic-clonic convulsion
tonic-clonic movement
tonic-clonic seizure
tonic foot reflex
tonic seizure
tonitrophobia
tonometer
tonsil
  palatine
  pharyngeal
tonsillectomy and adenoidectomy
  (T&A)
"tooies" (amobarbital/ secobarbital)
"tooles" (barbiturate)
"tools" (re: equipment for injecting
  drugs)
"toot" (cocaine)
"tooties" (barbiturate)
"Tootsie Roll" (heroin)
TOP (Test Orientation Procedure)
topectomy
"top gun" (crack)
"topi" (mescaline)
topic shift
  abrupt
  gradual
topics, emotionally laden
TOPL (Test of Pragmatic Language)
topographic mapping
topographical agnosia
topography
topophobia

TOPOSS (Tests of Perception of
  Scientists and Self)
"tops" (cannabis; mescaline)
"torch" (cannabis)
"torch cooking" (re: cocaine use)
"torch up" (re: cannabis use)
Toronto Alexithymia Scale
Toronto Functional Capacity
  Questionnaire (TFCQ)
"torpedo" (crack and cannabis)
torpid idiocy/idiot
torque
Torrance Tests of Creative Thinking
  (TTCT)
torsional wave
torsiversion
torsiversion of teeth
torticollis, psychogenic
torture
TOSF (Test of Oral Structures and
  Functions)
"toss up" (re: crack prostitute)
total communication
total laryngectomy
total lung capacity
totally disabled
"totally spent" (methylenedioxymethamphetamine hangover)
total push therapy
total response index (TRI)
totem and taboo
"toucher" (re: crack user)
touch perception
touch sensation
  light
  loss of
touching (communication pattern)
tough love
tough-minded tendency
tough poise
Tourette disorder

Tourette syndrome, tardive
Tourette tic
"tout" (opium)
TOWER (Testing, Orientation and
    Work Evaluation for
    Rehabilitation)
TOWL (Test of Written Language)
toxic action
toxic amblyopia
toxic-confusional state
toxic deafness
toxic delirium
toxic dementia
toxic effect of drug
toxic effects
    acute
    chronic
toxic encephalopathy
toxic hepatitis
toxic hypoxia
toxic injury
toxic insanity
toxicity, drug
toxic levels
toxic lithium tremor
toxic nystagmus
toxic psychosis
toxic reaction
toxic retinoneuropathy
toxic substances
toxicological analysis
toxicophobia
toxin-provoked amnesia
toxins, exposure to
toxiphobia
toxophobia
"toxy" (opium)
TPLS (The Primary Language
    Screen)
TP & P (time, place and person)
TPS (Test of Pragmatic Skills—
    Revised)

TPT (Tactual Performance Test)
TR (therapeutic recreation)
traces, memory
trachea (pl. tracheae)
tracheobronchial tree
tracheoesophageal fistula, Blom-Singer
tracheosophageal puncture
tracheosophageal speech
tracheotomy
tracing
    abnormal EEG
    I (interrupted tracing)
"track" (re: drug injection)
"tracks" (re: drug injection)
tract
    extrapyramidal
    nasal
    needle
    pyramidal
    respiratory
    vocal
trading sex
traditional belief; value
traditional grammar
traditional phonetic analysis
traditional society
"tragic magic" (crack dipped in phen-
    cyclidine)
tragus (pl. tragi)
trailing images
Trailmaking Tests (Forms A & B)
"trails" (re: lysergic acid diethylamide
    use)
Trainer's Assessment of Proficiency
    (TAP)
training
    Anxiety Control (ACT)
    Anxiety Management (AMT)
    assertiveness
    auditory
    autogenic
    clinical

training *(cont.)*
  cognitive self-hypnosis
  cultural
  ear
  general relaxation
  hypnotic relaxation technique
  neurofeedback
  occupational skill
  Parent Effectiveness (PET)
  improvement
  sensitivity
  social skill
  toilet
  trait factors
  visual
  vocational
training discrimination
training group (T-group), sensitivity
training units
  auditory
  speech
train of thought
trait (pl. traits)
  cognitive personality
  dominant
  ego-syntonic
  interpersonal personality
  intrapsychic personality
  paranoid
  personality
  temperament
Trait Evaluation Index
trait factors
trance
  dissociative
  hysterical
  involuntary state of
  possession
trance disorder, dissociative
trance identification, deep
trancelike behavior
trance logic

trance state, possession
trance symptom, possession
"trank" (phencyclidine; barbiturate)
tranquil
tranquility
tranquilizer
  butyrophenone-based
  major
  minor
  phenothiazine-based
tranquilizer abuse
tranquilizer drug dependence
transaction
transactional analysis (TA)
Transactional Analysis Life Position
  Survey (TALPS)
transactional psychotherapy
transcortical aphasia
transcortical apraxia
transcortical mixed aphasia
transcortical motor aphasia
transcortical sensory aphasia
transcription
  broad
  close
  narrow
  phonemic
  phonetic
transcultural psychiatry
transderivational search
transducer
transducing
transfer
  correctional (C.T.)
  intersensory
transference
  analysis of
  extrasensory thought
  negative
  positive
  thought
  traumatic

transference behavior
transference feelings
transference love
transference neurosis
transference paradigms
transference relationship
transferred meaning
transformation (T)
transformational grammar, generative
Transformational Leadership Development Program
transformationally related
transformational rule
transformer
transgendered
transgenerational role of giving
transgress
transgressions, behavioral
transient amnesic
transient auditory hallucinations
transient auditory illusions
transient distortion
transient depressive reaction
transient global amnesia (TGA)
transient hallucinatory experience
transient hypersomnia
transient ideas of reference
transient ideation
transient image
transient insomnia
transient ischemic attack (TIA)
transient mental states
transient organic psychosis
   delirious
   delusional
   depressive
   epileptic
   hallucinatory
   paranoid
transient psychosis
transient tactile hallucinations
transient tactile illusions

transient tic disorder of childhood
transient vibration
transient visual hallucinations
transient visual illusions
transillumination
transistor
transition
   life-cycle
   normal
   sleep-wake
   vowel-consonant
transitional change
transitional objects
transitional sleep
transitional stuttering
Transition Behavior Scale (TBS)
transition process
transitive verb
transitory mania
translating
translocation mongolism
transmethylation
transmissible agent
transmission of ideas by language
transmission of schizophrenia, familial
transmitted disease, sexually (STD)
transsexual (TS)
transsexual voice
transsexualism
transverse arytenoid muscle
transverse hermaphroditism
transverse muscle of tongue
transverse orientation
transverse temporal gyri
transverse wave
transversion of teeth
transvestic fetishism (TF)
transvestic phenomena
transvestic subculture
transvestism
transvestite
"trap" (re: drug concealment)

T ratio
trauma
  acoustic
  birth
  brain
  cerebral
  childhood
  closed head
  CNS (central nervous system)
  craniocerebral
  extreme
  head
  laryngeal
  occult head
  physical
  psychic
trauma and PTSD, early-age
trauma-induced delirium
trauma-specific reenactment
Trauma Symptom Checklist for
  Children Ages 8-15
traumatic amnesia
traumatic anesthesia
traumatic brain injury (TBI)
traumatic cataracts
traumatic delirium
traumatic dementia
traumatic encephalopathy, progressive
traumatic epilepsy
  early
  late
traumatic event, reexperienced
traumatic experience, unconscious
  processing of
traumatic headache
traumatic idiocy
traumatic injury
traumatic memories
traumatic neurosis
traumatic psychosis
traumatic seizure
traumatic separation

traumatic stress, serious
traumatic stressor
traumatic themes through repetitive
  play, expression of
traumatic transference
traumatophobia
"travel agent" (lysergic acid diethylamide supplier)
traveling wave hearing theory
"trays" (re: drug containers)
TREA (thoroughness, reliability,
  efficiency, analytic [ability])
treatment
  active
  adequate
  antidepressant
  appropriate
  cognitive-behavioral
  communication/cognition
  daily
  diet
  drug
  educational
  electroshock (EST)
  exercise
  family
  light (for winter depression)
  medical
  methadone maintenance
  Metrazol shock
  moral
  neuroleptic
  nutrition
  ongoing
  orthomolecular
  pharmacological
  pharmacotherapeutic
  prescribed
  prolonged sleep
  prophylactic
  proposed
  psychiatric

treatment *(cont.)*
  psychodynamic
  psychopharmacological
  psychosocial
  psychotherapeutic
  refusal to provide
  regressive electroshock (REST)
  rehabilitation
  residential
  shock
  somatic
  specific
  subcoma insulin
  symptomatic
  ultrasound
treatment frequency
treatment modality
  focused expressive therapy
  gestalt therapy
  psychodrama
Treatment of Depression Collaborative Research Program
treatment plan (TrPl)
treatment-refractory schizophrenia
treatment refusal
treatment response
treatment selection
treat, refusal to
tredecaphobia
tree, tracheobronchial
trees, decision
trembling voice
tremens, delirium (DT, DTs, Dt's, dt's)
tremophobia
tremor
  action
  benign essential
  cerebellar
  cerebral outflow
  coarse
  counting-money

tremor *(cont.)*
  cps (cycle per second)
  dystonic
  end point
  essential
  essential cerebellar
  essential cerebral
  facial
  familial
  fine
  fine postural
  flapping
  hand
  head and neck
  hepatic encephalopathy
  heredofamilial
  hysterical
  intentional
  kinetic
  lip
  metabolic
  no-no
  nonparkinsonian
  nonpharmacologically induced
  nontoxic lithium
  oscillating
  parkinsonian
  perioral
  physiologic
  physiological
  pill-rolling
  positional
  postural
  preexisting
  progressive cerebellar
  rest
  resting
  rhythmic
  rubral
  senile
  shaking
  small-amplitude rapid

tremor *(cont.)*
  static
  striatocerebral
  substance withdrawal
  sustention/intention
  terminal
  to-and-fro
  tongue
  toxic lithium
  vocal
  voice
  volitional
  writing
  yes-yes
tremulous cerebral palsy (CP)
tremulous movement
tremulousness
tremulous speech
trend of thought
trends
  anxiety
  paranoid
  phobic
TRI (total response index)
triad
trial (pl. trials)
  dosage reduction
  field
  medication
  placebo medication
  standing
  therapeutic
trial and error, vicarious (VTE)
trial home visit
triangles of conflict
triangular wave
trichinophobia
trichomania
trichopathophobia
trichophagia
trichophobia
trichorrhexomania

trichotillomania-induced alopecia
tricyclic antidepressant (TCA, TCAD)
tricyclic antipsychotic (TCA)
tricyclic drug
tridecaphobia
trigeminal nerve (cranial nerve V)
trigeminal neuralgia
trigger an obsession
triggering mechanism
triggering stimulus
trigger reaction
trill consonant formation
trim of adenoid
"trip" (alpha-ethyltryptamine; lysergic
  acid diethylamide)
trip, drug
triphthong
"trippier" (more intoxicating)
triskaidekaphobia
trismus
trisomy
tristimania
Trites Neuropsychological Test
  Battery
TROCA (tangible reinforcement of
  operant conditioning audiometry)
trochaic stress
trochlear nerve (cranial nerve IV)
tromomania
"troop" (crack)
trophobolene (injectable steroid)
troubled marriage
troubled relationship
troublesome
troubling experience
trough levels, peak and
troughs of waves
TrPl (treatment plan)
TRRP (Thackray Reading Readiness
  Profile)
"TR-6's" (amphetamine)

truancy
  school
  socialized childhood
  unsocialized childhood
truant
"truck drivers" (amphetamine)
truculence
truculent
true amnesia
true aphasia
true apnea
true belief
true folds, polypoid degeneration of
  the
true hermaphroditism
true language
true perception
true vertigo
true vocal folds
truncate
truncation, predicate
trusting relationship
truth disclosure
"truth serum" (scopolamine)
trypanophobia
TS (Tourette syndrome)
TS (transsexual)
TSBC (Time-Sample Behavioral
  Checklist)
TSCS (Tennessee Self-Concept Scale)
T-score range
TSI (Test of Social Inferences)
TSRI (Teacher's School Readiness
  Inventory)
TST (Twenty Statements Test)
"TT1," "TT2", "TT3" (phencycli-
  dine)
TTCT (Torrance Tests of Creative
  Thinking)
TTMAD (Testing-Teaching Module of
  Auditory Discrimination)
TTO (Test of Temporal Orientation)

tube
  auditory
  eustachian
  tympanotomy
  ventilation
tube microphone, probe
tubercle, acoustic
tuberculophobia
tuberous sclerosis
tubular vision
"tuie" (barbiturate)
Tuke, William (1732-1819)
tumescence
  nocturnal penile (NPT)
  penile
tumor
  brain
  brain stem
  eighth nerve
tumultuous
tunnel vision
turbinate bone
  inferior
  interior
  medial
  supreme
  sphenoidal
  superior
"turbo" (crack and cannabis)
turbulence
  family
  nasal
turbulent
"turf" (re: drug-buying place)
"turkey" (amphetamine; cocaine)
"Turkish green" (cannabis)
Turkomania
turmoil, emotional
"turnabout" (amphetamine)
"turned on" (introduced to drugs)
Turner syndrome
turning against self (TAS)

TUSSI (Temple University Short
 Syntax Inventory), Revised
"tutti-frutti" (flavored cocaine)
twang, nasal
TWCS (Test of Work Competency
 and Stability)
"tweak" (methamphetamine-like
 substance)
"tweaker" (re: crack user; methcathinone)
"tweaking" (drug-induced paranoia;
 re: amphetamine use)
"tweak mission" (re: crack acquisition)
Twelve Step Program
"twenty" ($20 rock of crack)
"twenty-five" (lysergic acid diethylamide)
Twenty Statements Test (TST)
2,5-DMA (analog of amphetamine/
 methamphetamine)
TWF (Test of Word Finding)
TWFD (Test of Word Finding in
 Discourse)
twice a day (2/d, b.i.d.)
twilight epilepsy
twilight state
 confusional
 epileptic
 psychogenic
twin (pl. twins)
 conjoined
 dizygotic
 fraternal
 identical
 monozygotic
 Siamese
twin language
twirling of objects
"twist" (cannabis cigarette)
twist, octave
"twistum" (cannabis cigarette)

twitch, twitching
 facial
 focal
 involuntary
 muscle
 rhythmical
"two for nine" (two $5 vials of crack
 for $9)
two-person interview team
two-tone voice
two-word stage
Tx (treatment)
tympanogram classification
 Feldman model
 Jerger model
tympanophonia
tympanoplasty
tympanostomy
tympanotomy tube
type A personality
type B personality
type I alcoholic (late onset)
type I error
type 1 trauma
type II alcoholic (early onset)
type II error
type 2 trauma
type of symptom
 mixed
 motor
 seizure
 sensory
types of sexual encounters
typical absence seizure
typical age
typical seizure
typomania
tyramine challenge test
tyrannical decision making
tyrannophobia
tyranny of silence

U, u

u (unit)
UA (urinalysis)
UC (unit clerk)
UCI (usual childhood illnesses)
UCL (uncomfortable loudness level)
"ugly" body parts
UL (unauthorized leave)
ulcer
    contact
    psychogenic duodenal
    psychogenic gastric
    psychogenic peptic
"ultimate" (crack)
ultradian rhythms
ultrasonic frequency
ultrasound treatment
ululation
UM (unmarried)
umbo
unaggressive conduct disorder
unaggressive undersocialized reaction
unaided augmentative communication
unanalyzable
unaspirated sounds
unauthorized leave (UL)
unawareness of environment
unbearable

unbecoming
unbiased information
unbound pronoun
uncertain, uncertainty
uncharacteristically
uncinate convulsion
uncinate seizure
"uncle" (Federal agents)
"Uncle Milty" (barbiturate)
uncomfortable loudness level (UCL)
unconditioned reflex
unconditioned response
unconditioned stimulus
unconscious, collective
unconscious concern
unconscious conflict
unconscious homosexuality
unconsciousness conversion
unconscious processing
unconscious rage
uncontrollable action
uncontrollable sleep attacks
uncontrollable thoughts
uncontrolled
uncoordinated gait
uncooperative
uncoupling, nasal

uncued behavior
underachievement disorder, academic
underachiever
underbite malposition of teeth
undercontrol
  behavioral
  emotional
underdose
underextension
underlip
underlying emotional issues
underlying structure
underproductive speech
undersocialized conduct disorder
  aggressive type
  unaggressive type
undersocialized reaction
  aggressive
  unaggressive
undersocialized runaway reaction
undersocialized socialized disturbance
  aggressive type
  unaggressive type
understanding
  shared
  speech
  word (WU)
Understanding and Managing Stress
understanding of similarities test
understatement (figure of speech)
understimulating environment,
  academically
understimulation, environmental
undetermined origin (UO)
undifferentiated schizophrenia
undifferentiated-type conduct disorder
undisciplined self-conflict
undisturbed nocturnal sleep
undoing (defense mechanism)
undue social anxiety
unemployable
unethical behavior

unexpected behavior
unexpected death
unexpected (uncued) panic attacks
unexpected response
unexplained absence from work
unexplained pain
unfamiliar place
unfilled pauses in speech
unformed visual hallucination
ungiving, emotionally
ungiving parent
ungrammatical sequence
unhappiness, patterns of pervasive
uniformly progressive deterioration
unilateral abductor paralysis
unilateral adductor paralysis
unilateral brief pulse ECT
unilateral cleft lip
unilateral cleft palate
unilateral focus
unilateral headache
unilateral hermaphroditism
unilateral migraine headache
unilateral neglect
unilateral organic neglect
unilateral paralysis
unilateral seizure
unilateral sine wave ECT
unilateral spatial neglect
unilateral visual neglect
unimodal
unimproved
unintelligible speech
unintended effect
unintended sleep
unintentional daytime sleep episodes
unintentionally produced symptoms
uninterrupted period of illness
unipolar depression
unipolar disorder
unipolar psychosis
unisensory

unit (pl. units)
  addictive disease (ADU)
  auditory training
  family
  intensive care (ICU)
  intensive treatment (ITU)
  life change (LCU)
  loudness
  maximum security
  psychiatric intensive care (PICU)
  relational
  sensation (SU)
  speech training
unit clerk (UC)
unit restriction (UR)
unit secretary (US)
United States Employment Service
  Interest Inventory (USES-II)
United States Pharmacopeia (USP)
United States Public Health Service
  (USPHS)
universal grammar
universal quantifier
universality
universals
  formal
  language
  substantive
universals theory, linguistic
University Residence Environment
  Scale (URES)
unjustified
unjustified doubts of loyalty
unjustified doubts of trustworthiness
unkempt appearance
unkempt manner
"unkie" (morphine)
unknown language
unknown substance-induced mood
  disorder
unlawful behavior
unmarried (UM)

unmet dependency needs
unmet needs
unmitigated echolalia
unnatural cheerfulness
unobtrusive
unplanned pregnancy
unpleasant hallucination
unpredictability
unpredictable
unproductive mania
unprotected sex
unpublished data sets
unpurposeful behavior
unquiet
unreactive pupils
unreal
unrealistic
unreality, feeling of
unreasonable belief
unreasonable fear
unreasonable idea
unreasonable demand
unreasoning
unrefreshing sleep
unrelated thoughts
unreliability
unreliable
unrelieved agitation
unresolved conflict
unresolved grief
unresolved loss
unresponsive patient
unresponsive state
unrest
unrounded vowel
unruffled
unsanctioned response
unshakable belief
unshakable preoccupation
unsocialized aggressive disorder
unsocialized aggressive reaction
unsocialized childhood truancy

unspecified bipolar I disorder
unspecified psychological factors
unspecified-type delusions
unspecified-type dyssomnia
unspecified-type personality disorder
unstable affect
unstable attachments
unstable personality disorder
unstable relationship
unstable self-image
unsteady gait
unstressed syllable deletion
unstressed vowel
unsystematized delusion
untimely death
untreated episode
untriggered agitation
unusual rare detail response (dr)
unvoiced speech
unwanted child
unwanted pregnancy
unwarranted idea
unwillingness to speak
UO (undetermined origin)
"up against the stem" (re: cannabis
   addiction)
"up in the clouds"
upbringing
upper bound
upper limit of age at onset
upper partial
upper respiratory infection (URI)
"uppers" (amphetamine)
"uppies" (amphetamine)
"ups" (amphetamine)
"ups and downs" (barbiturate)
upset
   emotionally
   excessively
   mental
upward masking
upwardly mobile

UR (unit restriction)
UR (Utilization Review)
uranophobia
uranoplasty
uranoschisis
urban psychiatry
uremic convulsion
URES (University Residence
   Environment Scale)
urges
   intense sexual
   masochistic sexual
   persistent inappropriate
   persistent intrusive
   sexual
URI (upper respiratory infection)
urinalysis (UA)
urinary incontinence
urinary MHPG
urination
   pain during
   public
urine drug screen
urophobia
urticaria, psychogenic
US (unit secretary)
U.S. (see *United States*)
usage doctrine
use
   drug
   language
use disorder
   alcohol
   amphetamine
   anxiolytic
   cannabis
   cocaine
   hallucinogen
   hypnotic
   inhalant
   nicotine
   opioid

use disorder *(cont.)*
  PCP
  psychoactive substance
  sedative
  substance
use of aliases
USES (United States Employment
  Service)
USES-II (United States Employment
  Service Interest Inventory)
Usher's syndrome
"using" people
USP (United States Pharmacopeia)
USPHS (United States Public Health
  Service)
usual activities
usual childhood illnesses (UCI)
Utah Test of Language Development
  (UTLD)

uteromania
uterus pain, psychogenic
utility
  clinical
  expected (EU)
utilization review (UR)
UTLD (Utah Test of Language
  Development)
"utopiates" (hallucinogens)
utricle
utterance
  holophrastic
  mean length of (MLU)
  mean relational (MRU)
  polymorphemic
  telegraphic
uvula (pl. uvulae)
uvular muscle
"uzi" (crack)

V, v

"V" (Valium)
V (verbal)
VA (Veterans Administration) domicil-
    iary
vaccinophobia
vacuous affect
V Adj (vocational adjustment)
V Adm (Veterans Administration)
vaginismus
    acquired type
    functional
    generalized type
    lifelong type
    situational type
vagrancy
vagrant
vague communication
vague speech
vagus nerve (cranial nerve X)
validating variables
validation (communication pattern),
    consensual
validity
    concurrent
    construct
    content
    criterion-related

validity *(cont.)*
    descriptive
    discriminant
    ecological
    external
    face
    factorial
    intervening
    predictive
Valpar Work Sample Battery
value (pl. values)
    educational
    foreign
    high
    idealized
    monetary
    moral
    nontrivial
    personal
    prognostic
    sentimental
    sharing of
    social
    status
    symbolic
    traditional
value judgment

Values Inventory for Children (VIC)
valve, velopharyngeal
variability, intra-subject
variable
   criterion
   dependent
   independent
   intervening
   predictor
   preexisting cognitive
   quantitative
   validating
variable behavior
variance, analysis of (ANOV, ANOVA)
variant seizure, petit mal
variation
   conative negative (CNV)
   free
   linguistic
   physiological functional
   phonetic
VASC (Verbal-Auditory Screen for Children) test
vascular dementia
vascular headache
vascular-type headache
vasculogenic loss of erectile functioning
vasectomy
vasocongestion of pelvis
vasomotor headache
VAT (Vocational Apperception Test)
VC (vital capacity)
VC (vowel-consonant)
VCDQ (Verbal Comprehension Deviation Quotient)
VD (venereal disease)
VDRS (Verdun Depression Rating Scale)
VE (vocational evaluation)
vegetative life
vegetative neurosis
vegetative state

vegetative symptoms
vehicle for communication
vela (pl. of velum)
velar area consonant placement
velar insufficiency
velar tail
velarized consonant
velars, backing to
velocity, particle
velopharyngeal closure
velopharyngeal competence
velopharyngeal incompetence
velopharyngeal insufficiency
velopharyngeal port
velopharyngeal valve
velum
venereal disease (VD)
venereophobia
vented earmold
ventilate concerns
ventilation during sleep
ventilation, impaired
ventilation tube
ventilatory control
ventral cochlear nucleus
ventricular dysphonia
ventricular fold
ventricular function
ventricular phonation
ventriculus laryngis
VEP (visual evoked potential) brain test
VER (visual evoked response) brain test
veracity
verb (parts of speech)
   auxiliary
   helping
   intransitive
   linking
   main
   modal

verb *(cont.)*
  modal auxiliary
  performative
  secondary
  transitive
verbal (V) (parts of speech)
verbal ability
verbal abuse
verbal agnosia
verbal agraphia
verbal amnesia
Verbal and Oral Language Ability
verbal aphasia
verbal apraxia
verbal auditory agnosia
Verbal Auditory Screen for Children
  test (VASC)
verbal behavior
verbal communication
Verbal Comprehension Deviation
  Quotient (VCDQ)
verbal comprehension factor (V factor)
verbal expression
verbal fluency
Verbal Intelligence Quotient (VIQ)
Verbal I.Q. Score
verbalization of feelings
verbalizations
  paucity of
  sparsity of
Verbalizer-Visualization Questionnaire
  (VVQ)
Verbal Language Development Scale
verbal language quotient
verbal learning
verbally mediated function
verbally mediated skills
verbal mediation
verbal memory
verbal, numerical, and reasoning
  (V, N, R)

verbal operant
verbal paraphasia
Verbal Perceptual Speed
verbal play
verbal reinforcement
verbal scale (VS)
Verbal Scale Scores
verbal technique
verbal visual agnosia
verbatim
verbigeration
verbomania
verborum, delirium
verbous
verb phrase
Verdun Depression Rating Scale
  (VDRS)
veridical dream
vermiform movement of tongue
vermillion border
vermiphobia
vernacular
Vernet syndrome
vertebrobasilar insufficiency
vertical canal
  anterior
  posterior
vertical-gaze palsy
vertical muscle of tongue
vertical nystagmus
vertiginous seizure
vertigo
  labyrinthine
  true
vestibular canal
vestibular folds
vestibular function
vestibular hallucination
vestibular hydrops
vestibular membrane
vestibular migraine headache
vestibular movement

vestibular window
vestibule
vestibuli
  fenestra
  scala
vestibulocochlear nerve
Veterans Administration (VA, V Adm)
Veterans Hospital (VH)
veterinary steroid
  abolic
  dianabol
  equipose
  finajet/finaject
  parabolin
  winstrol V
VEWA (Vocational Evaluation and
  Work Adjustment)
V factor (verbal comprehension factor)
VFDT (Visual Form Discrimination
  Test)
VH (Veterans Hospital)
VI (Visual Imagery)
viable alternative
VIB (Vocational Interest Blank)
vibrant consonant
vibration
  forced
  free
  glottal
  sympathetic
  symptomatic
  transient
  vocal fold
vibration meter
vibration sensation
vibrator, bone-conduction
vibratory cycle
vibrometer
vibrotactile aids
vibrotactile hearing aid
vibrotactile response
vibrotactile threshold

VIBS (vocabulary, information, block
  design, similarities)
VIC (Values Inventory for Children)
vicarious trial and error (VTE)
vice-like pain
vicious cycle
vicissitudes of life
victim
  abuse
  child neglect
  condition of
  crime
  intended
  rape
victimization
victimize
victim role
victim syndrome
Vienna Psychoanalytic Society
VIESA (Vocational Interest, Experience and Skill Assessment), Second
  Edition
view
  intropunitive
  Pollyanna-like
  psychobiological
vigilance
vigil, coma
vigorous
Vineland Adaptive Behavior Scales
Vineland Social Maturity Scale
  (VSMS)
violate, violation
violation of age-appropriate societal
  norms
violation of rules, serious
violation of the rights of others,
  pattern of
violations
  nonsexual boundary
  sexual boundary

violence
    alcohol-related
    alleviating
    domestic (D-V)
    drug-related
    family
    workplace
violent acts
violent agitation
violent behavior
violent death
violent outburst
violent personal assault
"viper's weed" (cannabis)
VIQ (Verbal Intelligence Quotient)
VIQ (Vocational Interest Question-
    naire)
viral encephalopathy
Virgin Mary visions
virgule
VIS (vocational interest schedule)
VISA (Vocational Interest and
    Sophistication Assessment)
visage, scanning
viscera (sing. viscus)
visceral disorder
visceral nervous system
visceral swallowing
vision
    altered
    blurred
    darkening
    double
    entopic
    foveal
    hemifield of
    impaired
    tubular
    tunnel
    Virgin Mary
vision disparity
vision test, wall chart

visit
    trial home
    weekend
visitation rights
vista responses
visual acuity
visual agnosia
    apperceptive
    associative
    verbal
visual alexia
visual amnesia
visual aphasia
visual area
Visual-Auditory Screening test for
    Children (VASC)
visual aura
Visual Aural Digit Span (VADS) Test
visual center
visual closure
visual cue
visual discrimination
visual disorders
visual disturbance
visual epilepsy
visual evoked potential (VEP) test
visual evoked response (VER) test
visual field construction
visual field cut
visual field defect
visual field disturbance
visual field exam
visual field test
Visual Form Discrimination Test
    (VFDT)
visual form of Wernicke aphasia
visual hallucination
    formed
    transient
    unformed
visual hearing
visual illusions

visual image
Visual Imagery (VI)
visual impairment
visualization, speech
visualized
visual letter dysgnosia
visual listening
visual literacy
visual loss
   complete
   hysterical
   partial
visual memory
Visual Memory Score (VMS)
visual memory span (VMS)
visual method
visual-motor coordination
Visual-Motor Gestalt Test (VMGT)
visual-motor impairment
visual-motor integration
Visual-Motor Integration Test (VMIT)
Visual-Motor Sequencing Test (VMST)
visual-motor tasks
visual motor test (see *test*)
visual neglect
Visual Neglect Test
visual number dysgnosia
visual obstruction
Visual Pattern Completion Test
visual pattern recognition
visual perception
visual perceptual skills
Visual Perceptual Speed
visual prodrome
visual pursuit movement
visual radiation
Visual Reinforcement Audiometry
visual reproduction
visual retention test (see *test*)
Visual Search and Attention Test
   (VSAT)
visual seizure

visual sensations
visual sensory modality
visual-spatial acalculia
visual-spatial distortion
visual-spatial memory
visual stimulation
visual stimulus
visual symptoms
Visual-Tactile System of Phonetic
   Symbolization
visual threat test
visual training
visuospatial disorders
visuospatial disorientation
visuospatial problem solving
visuospatial processing
visuospatial stimuli
vital capacity (VT)
vital energy
vital signs (VS)
vitamin deficiency
vitamin therapy
vivid dream image
vivid dream recall
vivid hallucination
VMGT (Visual-Motor Gestalt Test)
VMI (Visual-Motor Integration)
VMIT (Visual-Motor Integration Test)
VMS (Visual Memory Score)
VMS (visual memory span)
VMST (Visual-Motor Sequencing
   Test)
V, N, R (verbal, numerical, reasoning)
vocabulary
   core
   limited
Vocabulary Comprehension Scale
vocabulary language quotient
vocabulary test (see *test*)
vocal abuse
vocal attack

vocal bands
vocal behavior
vocal constriction
vocal cord dysfunction
vocal cord paralysis
vocal cords
vocal efficiency
vocal effort
vocal fatigue
vocal focus
vocal fold approximation
vocal fold paralysis
vocal folds
  bowed
  false
  true
vocal fold vibration
vocal fry
vocalic alliteration
vocalic glide
vocalization
vocal mode
vocal muscle
vocal nodules
  polypoid
  sessile
vocal organs
vocal phonics
vocal pitch abnormality
vocal play
vocal production
vocal range
vocal register
vocal rehabilitation
vocal resonance
vocal tic
vocal tract
vocal tremor
vocational achievement
vocational adjustment (V Adj)
Vocational Apperception Test (VAT)
vocational environment

vocational evaluation (VE)
Vocational Evaluation and Work
  Adjustment (VEWA)
vocational functioning
vocational goal-setting
vocational guidance
Vocational Interest and Sophistication
  Assessment (VISA)
Vocational Interest Blank (VIB)
Vocational Interest Inventory and
  Exploration Survey
Vocational Interest Questionnaire
  (VIQ)
vocational interest schedule (VIS)
Vocational Opinion Index (VOI)
Vocational Planning Inventory (VPI)
Vocational Preference Inventory (VPI)
vocational rehabilitation (VR)
vocational rehabilitation and education
  (VR&E)
Vocational Rehabilitation Services
  (VRS)
vocational strain
vocational training
Voc-Tech Quick Screener (VTQS)
"vodka acid" (lysergic acid diethylamide)
Vogt-Spielmeyer idiocy
VOI (Vocational Opinion Index)
voice (pl. voices)
  active
  adolescent
  altered
  chest
  esophageal
  eunuchoid
  falsetto
  gravel
  guttural
  hearing
  hearing God's
  inspiratory

voice *(cont.)*
  light
  muffled
  mutation
  negative
  passive
  pejorative
  pulsated
  shaking
  shaky
  threatening
  tone of
  transsexual
  trembling
  two-tone
voice audiometry
  live
  monitored live
voice clinician
voiced consonant
voiced feature English phoneme
voice disorder
  cul de sac
  denasality
  hyperrhinolalia
  hyperrhinophonia
  mixed nasality
  rhinolalia aperta
  rhinolalia clause
voice disorder of assimilated nasality
voice disorder of phonation
voice disorder of resonance
voice fatigue
voice hostility
voice instructions
voiceless consonant
voice murmuring
voice onset time (VOT)
voice pathologist
voice prints
voice register
voice shift

voice termination time (VTT)
voice therapist
voice tone focus
voice tremor
voices inside head
voices outside head
voicing of consonants
Vol Adm (voluntary admission)
volatile
volitional drinking
volitional movement
volitional oral movement
volitional tremor
volition, hedonic
volley hearing theory
volley theory
volt
volubility, excessive
voluble
volume
  air
  expiratory reserve (ERV)
  inspiratory reserve (IRV)
  lung
  residual (RV)
  respiratory
volume control
  automatic (AVC)
  manual
volume depletion
volume unit meter (VU meter)
voluntary admission (Vol Adm)
voluntary hospitalization
voluntary hysterical overbreathing
voluntary motion
voluntary motor functioning
voluntary movement peculiarities
voluntary muscle movement
voluntary mutism
voluntary napping phenomenon
voluntary retention
voluntary sensory functioning

volunteer bias
vomer skull bone
vomiting
    psychogenic
    self-induced
    "voodoo death"
VOT (voice onset time)
vowel
    accented
    back
    cardinal
    central
    close
    front
    high
    indefinite
    interconsonantal
    lax
    light
    lip rounded
    long
    low
    mid
    narrow
    nasalized
    neutral
    obscure
    open
    postconsonantal
    preconsonantal
    pure
    retroflex
    rounded
    short
    stressed
    syllabic
    tense
    unrounded
    unstressed
vowel assimilation

vowel-consonant (VC)
vowel-consonant syllable
vowel-consonant transitions
vowelize
vowel neutralization
vowel quadrilateral
vowel shift
voyeur
voyeurism
voyeuristic activity
voyeuristic behavior
voyeuristic sexual behavior
voyeuristic sexually arousing fantasy
VPI (Vocational Planning Inventory)
VPI (Vocational Preference Inventory)
VR (vocational rehabilitation)
VR&E (vocational rehabilitation and
    education)
VRS (Vocational Rehabilitation
    Services)
VS (verbal scale)
VS (vital signs)
VSAT (Visual Search and Attention
    Test)
VSMS (Vineland Social Maturity
    Scale)
V_T (tidal volume)
VTE (vicarious trial and error)
VTQS (Voc-Tech Quick Screener)
VTT (vocal termination time)
vulgar language
vulnerability
    genetic
    narcissistic
Vulpé Assessment Battery
VU meter (volume unit meter)
VVQ (Verbalizer-Visualization Ques-
    tionnaire)
Vygotsky Concept Formation Test,
    Modified

W, w

W (word fluency)
WAB (Western Aphasia Battery)
"wac" (phencyclidine on cannabis)
Wachs Analysis of Cognitive Structures
"wack" (phencyclidine)
"wacky weed" (cannabis)
waddling gait
wage earner
Wahler Physical Symptoms Inventory
Wahler Self-Description Inventory
    (WSDI)
WAIS (Wechsler Adult Intelligence
    Scale)
WAIS-R (Wechsler Adult Intelligence
    Scale–Revised)
WAIS-R Block Design Test
Wakefield Self-Assessment Depression
    Inventory
wakefulness
    intermittent
    state of full
    subjective sensation of
wakefulness epochs
wakefulness quiet
wakefulness resting
wakeful state
"wakeups" (dextroamphetamine sulfate)

waking EEG
waking frequency
Walker-McConnell Scale of Social
    Competence and School Adjust-
    ment
wall, alveolar
wall chart vision test
wandering, aimless
wandering thoughts
wane, wax and
waning, waxing and
WAQ (Work Attitudes Questionnaire)
war
    not prisoner of (NPOW)
    Persian Gulf
    prisoner of (POW)
    Vietnam
warble tone
ward
    disturbed
    psychiatric
Ward Atmosphere Scale (WAS)
Ward Behavior Rating Scale (WBRS)
ward clerk (WC)
warfare, psychological (PW)
Waring Intimacy Questionnaire (WIQ)
warm-wire anemometer

war neurosis
war-related stress
Wartenberg reflex
WAS (Ward Atmosphere Scale)
Washington School of Psychiatry
Washington Speech Sound Discrimination Test (WSSDT)
WASP (Weber Advanced Spatial
Perception)
wastage, air
"wasted" (murdered)
"wasted" (re: drug influence)
"water" (methamphetamine; phencyclidine)
water balance in schizophrenia
water, body
water deprivation
water drinking, compulsive
water intoxication
watershed area
Watson-Glaser Critical Thinking
Appraisal (WGCTA)
Watson, John B. (1878-1958)
watt
"wave" (crack)
wave (pl. waves)
    alpha
    aperiodic
    beta
    brain
    complex
    cosine
    damped
    delta (on EEG)
    diffracted
    diphasic
    electromagnetic
    excitation
    Hertz positive spike
    incident
    in-phase
    Jewett

wave *(cont.)*
    longitudinal
    negative spike
    nonperiodic
    notched
    periodic
    polyphasic
    pure
    reflected
    refracted
    simple
    sine
    sinusoidal
    slow
    sound
    sound pressure
    spike-like
    standing
    theta
    torsional
    transverse
    triangular
    troughs of
wave filter
waveform distortion
wavelength
wave on EEG
wave strains
wax and wane
waxing and waning
wax weak stress
waxy flexibility
Ways of Coping Scale
Wb (well-being)
WBRS (Ward Behavior Rating Scale)
WBS (Wechsler-Bellevue Scale)
WC (ward clerk)
WCS (Wiggins Content Scale)
WCST (Wisconsin Card-Sorting Test)
W/D (withdrawal)
weak ego control
weakness of extremity

Weak Opiate Withdrawal Scale
  (WOWS)
weak parent
weak stress
weak syllable deletion
weak-willed
weapon
wearing-off effect of drugs
webbing
Weber Advanced Spatial Perception
  (WASP)
Weber Test
web, laryngeal
Wechsler Adult Intelligence Scale
  (WAIS)
Wechsler Adult Intelligence Scale–
  Revised (WAIS-R)
Wechsler-Bellevue Scale (WBS)
Wechsler Intelligence Scale for Children, Third Edition (WISC-III)
Wechsler Memory Scale, Revised
Wechsler Memory Scale, Russell
  Version
Wechsler para Adultos, Escala de
  Inteligencia (EIWA)
Wechsler Preschool and Primary
  Scale of Intelligence (WPPSI)
"wedding bells" (lysergic acid diethyl-
  amide)
"wedge" (lysergic acid diethylamide)
Wednesday Evening Society
"weed" (cannabis; phencyclidine)
"weed tea" (cannabis)
weekend drinking
weekend headache
weekend hospital
weekend pass
weekend visit
weight-control program
weight fluctuations
weight gain
"weightless" (re: crack influence)

weight loss
weight loss aids
weight perception
Weiss Comprehensive Articulation
  Test
Weiss Intelligibility Test
Welch Allyn AudioScope
well-articulated speech
well-being (Wb)
  exaggerated feeling of
  feeling of
  sense of (Wb)
  sensation of
well-being scale
Weller-Strawser Scales of Adaptive
  Behavior for the Learning Disabled
well-formed outcome
well-formed delusion
well-motivated
well-systematized delusional system
Welsh Figure Preference Test
Wepman Auditory Discrimination
  Test
WEPS (Work Environment Prefer-
  ence Schedule)
Wernicke aphasia, visual form of
Wernicke area 22, 39, 40
Wernicke dementia
Wernicke encephalopathy
Wernicke-Korsakoff encephalopathy
Wernicke-Korsakoff syndrome
WES (Work Environment Scale,
  Second Edition)
Wesman Personnel Classification Test
Western Aphasia Battery (WAB)
western equine viral encephalitis
Western Personality Inventory
Western Personnel Tests
wet brain syndrome, alcoholic
wet dream
wet hoarseness
Wever-Bray phenomenon

Weyer, Johann (1515-1588)
WGCTA (Watson-Glaser Critical
  Thinking Appraisal)
"whack" (phencyclidine and heroin)
What I Like to Do: An Inventory of
  Students' Interests (WILD)
"wheat" (cannabis)
"when-shee" (opium)
"whippets" (nitrous oxide)
whipping
whisper
  buccal
  forced
  soft
  stage
whispering, involuntary
whistle feedback
Whitaker Index of Schizophrenic
  Thinking (WIST)
"white" (amphetamine)
"white" (cocaine)
"white ball" (crack)
"white boy" (heroin)
"white cloud" (crack smoke)
"white cross" (amphetamine; methamphetamine)
"white dust" (lysergic acid diethylamide)
"white ghost" (crack)
"white girl" (cocaine; heroin)
"white-haired lady" (cannabis)
"white horizon" (phencyclidine)
"white horse" (cocaine)
"white junk" (heroin)
"white knuckling" sobriety
"white lady" (cocaine; heroin)
"white lightning" (lysergic acid
  diethylamide)
white matter
  long spinal
  periventricular
  subcortical

white matter diseases
white matter hyperintensity
"white mosquito" (cocaine)
white noise
"white nurse" (heroin)
"whiteout" (isobutyl nitrite)
"white Owsley's" (lysergic acid
  diethylamide)
"white powder" (cocaine; phencyclidine)
"white stuff" (morphine)
"white sugar" (crack)
"white tornado" (crack)
White, William Alanson (1870-1937)
"whiz bang" (cocaine and heroin)
WHO (World Health Organization)
WHO Handicap Scales
whole word repetition
wide-band noise
wide-based gait
wide circles of thoughts
Wide Range Achievement Test 3
  (WRAT3)
Wide Range Assessment of Memory
  and Learning
wide range audiometer
Wide Range Employment Sample
  Test (WREST)
Wide Range Intelligence and
  Personality Test (WRIPT)
Wide Range Interest–Opinion Test
  (WRIOT)
wide-set eyes
widowhood
wife-to-husband aggression
Wiggins Content Scale (WCS)
WII (Work Information Inventory)
WILD (What I Like to Do: An Inventory of Students' Interests)
wild behavior
"wild cat" (methcathinone and
  cocaine)

Willis paracusis
willpower
will therapy
Wilson disease
Wilson-Patterson Attitude Inventory
(WPAI)
windigo (culture-specific syndrome)
windigo psychosis
window
    cochlear
    oval
    round
    therapeutic
    vestibular
"window glass" (lysergic acid diethyl-
    amide)
"window panes" (lysergic acid diethyl-
    amide)
windpipe
wing-beating tremor
"wings" (cocaine; heroin)
Wing symbol
winking syndrome, spasmodic
winter depression
WIPI (Word Intelligibility by Picture
    Identification)
WIQ (Waring Intimacy Questionnaire)
wired on cocaine
WISC (Wechsler Intelligence Scale for
    Children)
Wisconsin Card-Sorting Test (WCST)
WISC-R (Wechsler Intelligence Scale
    for Children-Revised)
WISC-R Split-Half Short Form,
    Second Edition
WISC-III (Wechsler Intelligence Scale
    for Children–Third Edition)
wish (pl. wishes)
    cross-gender
    disturbing
    intense

WIST (Whitaker Index of Schizo-
    phrenic Thinking)
"witch" (cocaine; heroin)
"witch hazel" (heroin)
withdrawal
    alcohol
    amphetamine
    anchor signs of
    anxiolytic-type
    apathetic
    caffeine
    cocaine
    drug
    hypnotic-type
    interpersonal
    narcotic
    nicotine
    opioid
    physiological signs of
    prevention of
    sedative-type
    signs of
    social
    substance
    thought
withdrawal adjustment reaction
withdrawal criteria
withdrawal delirium
    alcohol
    anxiolytic
    hypnotic
    sedative
    substance
withdrawal disorder
withdrawal from social affairs
withdrawal hallucinosis
withdrawal insomnia
withdrawal movement
withdrawal reaction of adolescence
withdrawal reaction of childhood
withdrawal seizure

withdrawal signs and symptoms
withdrawal state
withdrawal syndrome
  alcohol
  characteristic
  drug
withdrawal tremor
withdrawn catatonic schizophrenia
within normal limits (WNL)
witness, expert
WITT (Wittenborn Psychiatric Rating
  Scale)
Wittels, Fritz (1880-1950)
Wittenborn Psychiatric Rating Scale
  (WITT, WPRS)
WJAT (Woodcock-Johnson Achieve-
  ment Tests)
WJPTB (Woodcock-Johnson Psycho-
  educational Test Battery)
WJ-R (Woodcock-Johnson Psycho-
  Educational Battery, Revised)
WLPB-R (Woodcock Language
  Proficiency Battery, Revised)
WMI (Work Motivation Inventory)
WMS (Wechsler Memory Scale)
WNL (within normal limits)
"wobble weed" (phencyclidine)
"wolf" (phencyclidine)
Wolfe Microcomputer User Aptitude
  Test
"wollie" (crack and cannabis)
Wonderlic Personnel Test
W-1/W-2 Auditory Tests
Woodcock-Johnson Achievement Tests
  (WJAT)
Woodcock-Johnson Psycho-Educational
  Battery, Revised (WJ-R)
Woodcock Language Proficiency
  Battery, English Form
Woodcock Language Proficiency
  Battery, Revised (WLPB-R)

Woodcock Reading Mastery Tests,
  Revised (WRMT-R)
word (pl. words)
  ambiguous
  back-formation
  base
  broken
  class
  clipped
  closed-class
  coin new
  complex
  compound
  content
  feared
  filler
  form
  function
  glossal
  heterogeneous
  homogenous
  inappropriate
  interstitial
  Jonah
  lexical
  loan
  monosyllabic
  multi-syllable
  nonsense
  nonsensical
  onomatopoetic
  open-class
  paradigmatic
  PB (phonetically balanced)
  pivot
  polysyllabic
  portmanteau
  process
  relational
  root
  sign

word *(cont.)*
  simple
  split
  spondee
  standard
  structure
  syntagmatic
  telescoped
word accent
word approximation
word association
Word Association Test
word attack
word-attack skills
word blindness
word calling
word classes
word coinage
word configuration
word count
word deafness
  developmental
  pure
word discrimination score
word finding
word-finding ability
word-finding difficulty
word-finding problem
word-finding skills
word identification speed
Word Intelligibility by Picture
  Identification (WIPI)
word paradigm
Word Processing Test
Word Processor Assessment Battery
word production, stressful
Word Recognition Test
word repetition, senseless imitative
word retrieval problem
word retrieval task
word salad
Word Search

word sequence
word sets
word substitution
word test (see *test*)
word understanding (WU)
word writing
workaholic
Work Attitudes Questionnaire (WAQ)
work disability
work dysfunction
Work Environment Preference
  Schedule (WEPS)
Work Environment Scale, Second
  Edition (WES)
work group
Work Information Inventory (WII)
"working" (re: crack dealing)
working alliance
"working half" (re: crack weights)
working out
working relationship
working through
work inhibition
Work Interest Index
Work Motivation Inventory (WMI)
workplace violence
work-related hearing loss
work-related problem
"works" (re: equipment for injecting
  drugs)
workshop, sheltered
Work Skills Series Production (WSS)
Work Values Inventory (WVI)
World Health Organization (WHO)
world of reality
World of Work Inventory (WWI)
World Psychiatric Association (WPA)
"worm" (phencyclidine)
worry, worrying
  constant
  excessive
  focus of

worry *(cont.)*
  hyperresponsible
  uncontrolled
Worse Premorbid Adjustment Scale
worse sleep continuity
worth, inflated
worthlessness, feelings of
wound
  gunshot (GSW)
  self-inflicted (SIW)
wounded-victim syndrome
WOWS (Weak Opiate Withdrawal Scale)
WPA (World Psychiatric Association)
WPAI (Wilson-Patterson Attitude Inventory)
WPPSI (Wechsler Preschool and Primary Scale of Intelligence)
WPRS (Wittenborn Psychiatric Rating Scale)
WRAT3 (Wide Range Achievement Test 3)
"wrecking crew" (crack)
WREST (Wide Range Employment Sample Test)
WRIOT (Wide Range Interest-Opinion Test)
WRIPT (Wide Range Intelligence and Personality Test)
wrist cutting

write-a-sentence test
writer's cramp
writing
  consonantal
  sound
  syllabic
  word
writing ability
writing disorder
writing tremor
written English
written expression
Written Language Assessment
written language quotient
WRMT-R (Woodcock Reading Mastery Tests, Revised)
"wrong" sex
wryneck
WSDI (Wahler Self-Description Inventory)
WSS (Work Skills Series Production)
WSSDT (Washington Speech Sound Discrimination Test)
W-22 Auditory Test
WU (Word Understanding)
WUSCT (Washington University Sentence Completion Test)
WVI (Work Values Inventory)
WWI (World of Work Inventory)

X, x

x (times)

"X" (amphetamine; cannabis; methylenedioxymethamphetamine)

X-bar theory

xenomania

xenophobia

xerophobia

"X-ing" (methylenedioxymethamphet-amine)

X-linkage

X-linked dominance

X syndrome, fragile

"XTC" (ecstasy) (methylenedioxy-methamphetamine)

Y, y

"yahoo/yeaho" (crack)
"Yale" (crack)
Yale-Brown Obsessive-Compulsive
  Scale (YBOCS)
Yale Global Tic Severity Scale
yawning, psychogenic
yawn-sign approach
YBOCS (Yale-Brown Obsessive-
  Compulsive Scale)
YBR (Yellow Brick Road)
YBT (Yerkes-Bridges test)
Y-cord hearing aid
year of birth (YOB)
year old *or* years old (y.o.)
"yeh" (cannabis)
"yellow" (lysergic acid diethylamide;
  barbiturate)
"yellow bam" (methamphetamine)
Yellow Brick Road (YBR)
"yellow bullets" (pentobarbital)
"yellow dimples" (lysergic acid
  diethylamide)
"yellow dolls" (pentobarbital)
"yellow fever" (phencyclidine)
"yellow jacket" (barbiturate)

"yellows" (barbiturate)
"yellow submarine" (cannabis)
"yellow sunshine" (lysergic acid
  diethylamide)
"yen pop" (cannabis)
"Yen Shee Suey" (opium wine)
"yen sleep" (re: lysergic acid diethylamide use)
"yerba" (cannabis)
"yerba mala" (phencyclidine and
  cannabis)
Yerkes-Bridges test (YBT)
YES (Youth Enjoying Sobriety)
"yesca" (cannabis)
"yesco" (cannabis)
yes-no question
yes-yes tremor
"yeyo" (cocaine)
"yimyom" (crack)
y.o. (years old)
YOB (year of birth)
yoke, alveolar
youth counselor
Youth Enjoying Sobriety (YES)

Z, z

0 (zero morpheme)
"Z" (1 ounce of heroin)
z (dram)
"Zacatecas purple" (cannabis)
"zambi" (cannabis)
ZDS (Zung Depression Scale)
zealot
zelophobia
"zen" (lysergic acid diethylamide)
"zero" (opium)
zero amplitude
zero, audiometric
zero cerebral
zero hearing level
zero level
zero morpheme (0)
zest, loss of
"zig zag man" (lysergic acid diethyl-
    amide; cannabis)
"zip" (cocaine)

"zol" (cannabis cigarette)
"zombie" (phencyclidine)
"zombie dust" (phencyclidine)
"zombie weed" (phencyclidine)
zone
    erogenous
    time
"zooie" (re: cannabis equipment)
"zoom" (phencyclidine; cannabis and
    phencyclidine)
zoomania
"zoomers" (re: dealers in fake crack)
zoophil psychosis
zoophilia (bestiality)
zoophobia
zoster meningitis, herpes
Zung Self-Rating Depression Scale
zygomatic bones
zygomatic skull bones
zygosity (dizygotic and monozygotic)

Appendix I

Sample Reports

The following sample reports have been constructed from information gleaned from many transcribed sources and the DSM-IV criteria. The emphasis is on the different formats of the reports and on wording of diagnoses in the DSM-IV classification system. The content of the reports does not depict the actual circumstances of specific individuals. In the sample reports in this appendix, the DSM-IV codes with an asterisk (*) represent coding changes to the DSM-IV classification system, which became effective October 1, 1996, and January 1, 1997. The multiaxial evaluation criteria for each Axis are as follows:

AXIS I: Clinical disorders and other conditions which may be a focus of clinical attention. These include disorders usually first diagnosed in infancy, childhood, or adolescence; delirium, dementia, amnestic and other cognitive disorders; mental disorders due to a general medical condition; substance-related disorders ("E Codes" optionally may be coded here for medications prescribed at therapeutic dose levels that cause substance-induced disorders); schizophrenia and other psychotic disorders; mood disorders; anxiety disorders; somatoform disorders; factitious disorders; dissociative disorders; sexual and gender identity disorders; eating disorders; sleep disorders; impulse-control disorders NOS (not otherwise specified); and adjustment disorders.

AXIS II: Personality disorders, including mental retardation and learning disabilities. The personality disorders include paranoid, schizoid, schizotypal, antisocial, borderline, histrionic, narcissistic, avoidant, dependent, obsessive-compulsive, and personality disorder NOS (not otherwise specified).

AXIS III: General medical conditions. This Axis should always contain (1) the general medical condition with the appropriate ICD-9-CM or ICD-10 code, with optional "E Code" for medications prescribed at therapeutic dose levels that cause substance-induced disorders, or (2) "None" when no general medical condition exists, or (3) "Deferred" when additional medical information is pending.

AXIS IV: Psychological and environmental problems. These include problems with the primary support group, social environment, education, occupation, housing, economics, access to health care services, interaction with the legal system and crime, and other psychosocial and environmental problems.

AXIS V: Global Assessment of Functioning Scale (GAF Score)

INITIAL PSYCHIATRIC EVALUATION   SAMPLE REPORT I

PATIENT #123459   PAGE 1
DATE OF ADMISSION: 01-02-97
DATE OF EVALUATION: 01-03-97
ATTENDING PHYSICIAN: A. Smith, M.D.

CHIEF COMPLAINT: "My drug dependency is costing me my job."

HISTORY OF PRESENT ILLNESS: This 29-year-old white female
comes in with a history of migraine headaches, cerebral infarct with
seizure, and opioid and anxiolytic substance dependence. Current daily
prescription drug use includes 6 morphine sulfate tablets, 18 tablets of
diphenhydramine, and 16 alprazolam tablets. She takes 3 tablets of
triazolam nightly. Her drug dependency dates to 1994. She notes
increased tolerance to drugs. Prescriptions have been obtained from
multiple physicians. On withdrawal, she variously experiences symptoms such as mania or hypomania, an "achy feeling" in the back and
legs, irritability, craving, headaches, insomnia, cold sweats, and
decreased energy. Suicidal ideas occur while on medication, but she
has not acted on them. She feels depressed when on medication.
Delusions and hallucinations are denied. She complains of cervical
radicular pain, often awakening at night with hand numbness and
tingling. She also complains of lumbosacral spine pain radiating into
the legs during waking hours.

PAST MEDICAL HISTORY: Allergies: None. Surgeries: T&A in
1977. Medical Illnesses: Head injury as a teenager due to a gymnastic
accident; migraine headaches with scintillating scotoma beginning at
that time. She had a cerebral infarct in 1993 with subsequent seizure
disorder for several months. Her cerebral infarct, attributable to her
migraines, resulted in left-sided loss of mobility, dysphagia, and
expressive aphasia resolving over time. In early 1994, she suffered
severe neck and back strain/sprain in a car accident.

PSYCHIATRIC HISTORY: This is her first psychiatric admission.
Her outpatient treatment intermittently dates from late 1994 to mid-
1996. Currently, she has been taking paroxetine 20 mg p.o. each day
and the above abused drugs, as well as using diazepam.

INITIAL PSYCHIATRIC EVALUATION   SAMPLE REPORT 1

PATIENT #123459   PAGE 2

PHARMACOLOGICAL HISTORY: Amitriptyline HCl, propranolol HCl, and verapamil provided no migraine headache relief. Ergot alkaloids helped some, as have oxycodone and other opiates. Prior biofeedback and relaxation techniques were unsuccessful.

SOCIAL HISTORY: Patient is separated and feels socially isolated. She reports being abused emotionally and physically by her husband. Divorce proceedings are ongoing. She works as a telemarketer. Her manic/hypomanic state is impacting on her job performance.

REVIEW OF SYSTEMS: Significant for migraine headaches, back pain radiating into the lower extremities, as well as neck pain with hand numbness and tingling.

MENTAL STATUS EXAMINATION TODAY: Patient is alert and oriented. No hallucinations or delusions. No formal thought disorder. No homicidal or suicidal ideas but has feelings of alienation. Mood is hypomanic. Her affect is somewhat blunted though labile. Her fund of knowledge is within normal limits. She uses language and syntax appropriately. She interprets proverbs correctly. Memory is intact. She can do serial 7's and 4-digit number reversal. Insight into her problems is fair. Judgment is good. Eye contact is good.

DSM-IV MULTIAXIAL ADMISSION DIAGNOSES:

AXIS I	304.00	Opioid dependence
	304.10	Anxiolytic (benzodiazepine) dependence
	292.84	Opioid-induced mood disorder, with mania or hypomania, onset during withdrawal
	293.84*	Anxiety disorder due to continuous neck pain, back pain and migraine headaches; fears recurrent cerebral infarct.
	V61.12*	Physical abuse by spouse
AXIS II	V71.09	No diagnosis, avoidant personality features
AXIS III	346.00	Migraine headaches
	723.4	Cervical radiculopathy
	724.4	Lumbosacral radiculopathy
	292.0	Opioid and anxiolytic drug withdrawal

INITIAL PSYCHIATRIC EVALUATION   SAMPLE REPORT 1

PATIENT #123459   PAGE 3

AXIS IV   Spousal abuse, pending divorce, and job loss
AXIS V   GAF=50 (current)

PLAN/RECOMMENDATIONS: Patient is admitted for inpatient
detoxification and treatment of mood and anxiety disorders with
associated symptoms. Counseling will continue for her spousal abuse
issues. A neurology consult is ordered for her radicular pains and
migraines. Paroxetine medication will be monitored; opiates are
discontinued. Laboratory work has been ordered.

A. Smith, M.D. (Date)
DD: 01/03/97 DT: 01/03/97:md

DISCHARGE SUMMARY   SAMPLE REPORT 2

PATIENT #123456   PAGE 1
DATE OF ADMISSION: 12-27-96
DATE OF DISCHARGE: 01/01/97 Against Medical Advice
ATTENDING PHYSICIAN: J. Jones, M.D.

DSM-IV MULTIAXIAL ADMISSION DIAGNOSES:

AXIS I	296.62	Bipolar I disorder, most recent episode mixed, moderate severity
	304.60*	Phencyclidine dependence
	304.0	Heroin dependence
	V62.83*	Physical abuse by adult other than partner
AXIS II	V71.09	No diagnosis, borderline personality features
AXIS III	401.1	Hypertension, essential
	786.59	Chest pain
	414.00*	Atherosclerotic heart disease
	250.00	Diabetes mellitus, adult-onset, non-insulin dependent
	042.1*	HIV infection, with candidiasis, by history
AXIS IV	Homeless; unemployed; physically abused	
AXIS V	GAF=25 (on admission)	

IDENTIFYING INFORMATION: This 51-year-old single Caucasian male is homeless and unemployed. He receives Social Security Disability income and Medicare.

HISTORY OF PRESENT ILLNESS: This man was initially seen seven months ago for a manic episode. Currently he presents with manic and depressed episodes ongoing for one week. He details several grandiose, delusional concerns about aliens trying to kill him and complaints of chest pain resulting from the aliens "shooting" him. He reports living on the streets and being physically abused on a regular basis by a fellow drug user. He admits to sharing needles, using PCP and heroin, and having tested HIV positive. His affect is labile. The patient's past medical history includes diabetes, hypertension, possible angina, and ASHD.

MENTAL STATUS EXAMINATION ON ADMISSION: The patient was poorly groomed and malodorous. He was excited and uncooperative. He

DISCHARGE SUMMARY   SAMPLE REPORT 2

PATIENT #123459   PAGE 2

presented with pressured speech, flight of ideas, loosening of associations, and tangentiality. Mood was sweeping. Affect was extremely
labile. There was no suicidal or homicidal ideation. He exhibited
grandiose and delusional thought content with paranoia.

PHYSICAL EXAMINATION: Internal medicine consult was obtained
for his poorly controlled high blood pressure, diabetes, and skin infection. His heart disease was stable. His chest discomfort had diminished.

LABORATORY DATA: Fasting glucose of 160. Chest x-ray normal.
EKG revealed right bundle branch block.

HOSPITAL COURSE: Patient was admitted voluntarily. Initially, the
patient was compliant with his lithium medication and adjustments in
medications recommended by the internist. The patient showed rapid
improvement; however, he shortly became medication noncompliant
and refused all additional blood work, including a lithium level. His
manic and depressive episodes continued, as did his grandiose and
delusional states. He was uncooperative and became verbally abusive
to staff. He signed a 24-hour notice to be discharged. He subsequently
agreed to see his primary care physician and restart his medications
after discharge. He was not a danger to self or others.

MENTAL STATUS EXAMINATION ON DISCHARGE: Patient was
alert and agitated. Grooming and hygiene were poor. Eye contact was
75%. Mood was dysphoric. Affect was labile. He denied suicidal or
homicidal ideation. Thought content continued grandiose and delusional without hallucinations. Judgment and insight were poor. Cognitive
testing was not done due to lack of cooperation.

DSM-IV MULTIAXIAL DISCHARGE DIAGNOSES:
AXIS I   296.62   Bipolar I disorder, most recent episode mixed,
                         moderate severity
              304.60*   Phencyclidine dependence
              304.0   Heroin dependence
              V62.83*   Physical abuse by adult other than partner

DISCHARGE SUMMARY   SAMPLE REPORT 2

PATIENT #123459   PAGE 3

AXIS II	V71.09	No diagnosis, borderline personality features
AXIS III	401.1	Hypertension, essential
	414.00*	Atherosclerotic heart disease
	250.00	Diabetes mellitus, adult-onset, non-insulin dependent
	042.1*	HIV infection, with candidiasis, by history
AXIS IV	Homeless; unemployed	
AXIS V	GAF=25	(at discharge)

DISCHARGE PLAN: Patient had all his current medications with him upon admission. These were returned to him. He is currently medication noncompliant. No additional medications were prescribed on discharge, as arrangements for him to see his primary care physician the next day were already in place. Additional blood work was to be done including lithium level. Any adjustment in his lithium dosage would be made once the results of his lithium level were known. A referral for follow-up outpatient psychiatric care was given. The staff assisted patient with post-discharge lodging.

J. Jones, M.D.   (Date)
DD: 01/01/97 DT: 01/02/97:md

Appendix II

Muscles of the Larynx, Palate, Pharynx, Respiration, and Tongue

Note: The Latin singular form *musculus,* with its modifiers, is used when a single muscle or a single pair of muscles is described. In a few instances, multiple pairs of muscles are described. In these instances the plural form *musculi* with its modifiers is used.

Muscles of the Larynx

Extrinsic Muscles (suprahyoid)

digastric muscle, anterior (musculus digastricus anterior)
digastric muscle, posterior (musculus digastricus posterior)
geniohyoid muscle (musculus geniohyoideus)
mylohyoid muscle (musculus mylohyoideus)
stylohyoid muscle (musculus stylohyoideus)

Extrinsic Muscles (infrahyoid)

omohyoid muscle, anterior (musculus omohyoideus anterior)
omohyoid muscle, posterior (musculus omohyoideus posterior)
sternohyoid muscle (musculus sternohyoideus)
sternothyroid muscle (musculus sternothyroideus)
thyrohyoid muscle (musculus thyrohyoideus)

Muscles of the Larynx *(continued)*

Intrinsic Muscles

aryepiglottic muscle (musculus aryepiglotticus)
arytenoid muscle, oblique (musculus arytenoideus obliquus)
arytenoid muscle, transverse (musculus arytenoideus transversus)
cricoarytenoid muscle, lateral (musculus cricoarytenoideus
    lateralis)
cricoarytenoid muscle, posterior (musculus cricoarytenoideus
    posterior)
cricothyroid muscle (musculus cricothyroideus)
thyroarytenoid muscle (musculus thyroarytenoideus)
thyroepiglottic muscle (musculus thyroepiglotticus)
vocal muscle (musculus vocalis)

Muscles of the Palate

glossopalatine muscle (musculus palatoglossus)
elevator muscle of soft palate (musculus levator veli palatini)
pharyngopalatine muscle (musculus palatopharyngeus)
tensor muscle of the soft palate (musculus tensor palati *or*
    musculus tensor veli palatini)
uvular muscle or muscle of the uvula (musculus uvulae)

Muscles of the Pharynx

constrictor muscle of pharynx, inferior (musculus constrictor
    pharyngis inferior)
constrictor muscle of pharynx, middle (musculus constrictor
    pharyngis medius)
constrictor muscle of pharynx, superior (musculus constrictor
    pharyngis superior)
salpingopharyngeal *or* salpingopharyngeus muscle (musculus
    salpingopharyngeus)
stylopharyngeal *or* stylopharyngeus muscle (musculus
    stylopharyngeus)

Muscles of Respiration

Inhalation (Quiet) Muscles

external intercostal muscles (musculi intercostales externi)
scalene muscle, anterior (musculus scalenus anterior)
scalene muscle, middle (musculus scalenus medius)
scalene muscle, posterior (musculus scalenus posterior)
elevator muscles of rib (musculi levatores costarum)

Inhalation (Forced) Muscles

serratus anterior muscle (musculus serratus anterior)
serratus posterior inferior muscle (musculus serratus posterior inferior)
serratus posterior superior muscle (musculus serratus posterior superior)
pectoral muscle, greater (musculus pectoralis major)
pectoral muscle, smaller (musculus pectoralis minor)
latissimus dorsi muscle (musculus latissimus dorsi)
subclavian muscle (musculus subclavius)
sternoclavicular muscle (musculus sternoclavicularis)
sternocleidomastoid muscle (musculus sternocleidomastoideus)

Exhalation Muscles

oblique muscle of abdomen, external (musculus obliquus externus abdominis)
oblique muscle of abdomen, internal (musculus obliquus internus abdominis)
internal intercostal muscles (musculi intercostales interni)
iliocostal muscle of thorax (musculus iliocostalis thoracis *or* musculus iliocostalis dorsi)
lumbar iliocostal muscle (musculus iliocostalis lumborum)

Muscles of the Tongue

Extrinsic Muscles

genioglossal muscle (musculus genioglossus)
hyoglossal (hyoglossus) muscle (musculus hyoglossus)
palatoglossus muscle (musculus palatoglossus)
styloglossus muscle (musculus styloglossus)

Intrinsic Muscles

longitudinal muscle of tongue, inferior (musculus longitudinalis
    inferior linguae)
longitudinal muscle of tongue, superior (musculus longitudinalis
    superior linguae)
transverse muscle of tongue (musculus transversus linguae)
vertical muscle of tongue (musculus verticalis linguae)

The Authors

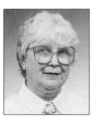

Mary Ann D'Onofrio earned credentials as a certified medical transcriptionist (CMT) and accredited record technician (ART) in 1980. She continues to be certified as a CMT. She maintained her ART credential for 12 years while active in the health information field. Her experience as a medical transcriptionist and coder/analyst of medical records dates from 1972. In addition to her hospital-based medical transcription and medical record technician activities, she has specialized in transcription for physician clients in the fields of cardiology, rehabilitative medicine, ophthalmology, neurology, and psychiatry/psychology. She holds a master's degree in information/library science (AMLS) from the University of Michigan.

An active member of AAMT since 1980, she received the Distinguished Member Award in 1984. Her regular columns for the *Journal of AAMT*, including "What's Your MT Quotient" and "Scope," appeared for six years. She has been a contributing author to Health Professions Institute's *Perspectives* magazine. Her first joint venture with her daughter Elizabeth was as editor of the AAMT *Annotated Bibliography* (1981). She has been listed in Marquis' *Who's Who in the West* and *Who's Who of American Women*.

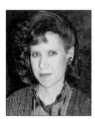

Elizabeth D'Onofrio joined the field of medical transcription in 1988, with a specialty in psychiatry/psychology. A graduate of the University of Arizona, she is co-owner with Mary Ann of MED-COMM Associates, L.L.P., which operates their medical transcription business. Elizabeth is a former member of the Health Professions Institute staff and has also been a contributing author to *Perspectives* magazine.

Mary Ann's hobbies are photography and desert gardening. She has four children and four grandchildren. Elizabeth writes fiction and nonfiction. She has an avid interest in the theater, cinema, and television production. In 1993 they established a division of MCA, called Ema of Tucson, a fine jewelry and apparel design firm. They both enjoy attending the world renowned Gem and Mineral Show in Tucson each February.